Prospective Longitudinal Research

An Empirical Basis for the Primary Prevention of Psychosocial Disorders

Edited by

SARNOFF A. MEDNICK, Ph.D., Dr. Med.
Professor, University of Southern California
Director, Psykologisk Institut, Kommunehospitalet, Copenhagen
Consultant in Mental Health to the WHO Regional Office for Europe

and

ANDRÉ E. BAERT, M.D.
Regional Officer for Mental Health, WHO Regional Office for Europe

Assistant Editor
BARBARA PHILLIPS BACHMANN, M.A.
Social Science Research Institute, University of Southern California

Published on behalf of the
World Health Organization Regional Office for Europe

Oxford New York Toronto Melbourne
OXFORD UNIVERSITY PRESS
1981

Oxford University Press, Walton Street, Oxford OX2 6DP

OXFORD LONDON GLASGOW
NEW YORK TORONTO MELBOURNE WELLINGTON
KUALA LUMPUR SINGAPORE JAKARTA HONG KONG TOKYO
DELHI BOMBAY CALCUTTA MADRAS KARACHI
NAIROBI DAR ES SALAAM CAPE TOWN

© *English language edition Oxford University Press 1981*

British Library Cataloguing in Publication Data
Prospective longitudinal research. – (Oxford medical publications).
  1. Psychiatry – Longitudinal studies
  I. Mednick, Sarnoff Andrei
  II. Baert, André E III. World Health
Organization. Regional Office for Europe
IV. Series
  616.8'9'00722   RC437.5   79-41242

ISBN 0-19-261184-4

Phototyeset in V.I.P. Times by Western Printing Services Ltd, Bristol
Printed in Great Britain at the University Press, Oxford
by Eric Buckley, Printer to the University

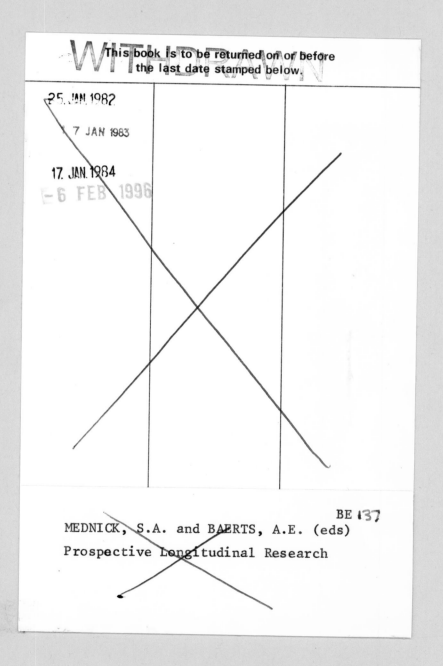

BE 137

MEDNICK, S.A. and BAERTS, A.E. (eds)

Prospective Longitudinal Research

OXFORD MEDICAL PUBLICATIONS

Prospective Longitudinal Research

Foreword

Leo A. Kaprio,
WHO Regional Director for Europe

Europe is facing a critical problem: the tremendous burgeoning of the number of chronically ill who are being maintained and treated by our health care systems. The suffering of these individuals and the cost of their care is a huge burden which will not decrease in the foreseeable future. Rather than attempt to attack the roots of this nearly overwhelming problem, our national efforts currently are aimed almost exclusively at improving treatment and maintenance. These efforts, while highly praiseworthy, paradoxically enough serve to increase the number of chronically ill and the total amount of suffering. This increase in need further taxes our treatment–technology research inventiveness. In this manner, advances in treatment–maintenance technology and increases in the number of chronically ill reciprocally augment each other in an inexorable manner. The consequences of allowing this spiralling to continue have some potentially unpleasant moral, social, and economic implications.

To attack the roots of this problem we must devote some increasing proportion of our research resources to work on the primary prevention of these chronic ailments. An important tool in our understanding of the bases of these conditions and the possibilities of their prevention is longitudinal, prospective research.

Prospective, longitudinal research projects are delicate, long-term enterprises which have special scientific, administrative, and financial needs. The potential value and limitations of these projects and the conditions under which they prosper and best serve humanity have not been sufficiently considered. This volume may serve to generate a more focused interest in prospective research and aid in the establishment of intra- and international co-ordination and communication in this area.

Contents

List of Contributors

GUSTAV AMNELL, Ph.D., M.D., Department of Public Health, University of Helsinki, SF 00200 Helsinki 29, Finland.

C. AGUÉ, Ph.D., Psychiatric Clinic, University Cery, 1008 Prilly-Lausanne, Switzerland.

JULES ANGST, Prof., M.D., Psychiatric University Clinic Zurich, Research Department, PO Box 68, Lenggstrasse 31, CH-8029 Zurich, Switzerland.

TERTTU ARAJÄRVI, M.D., Department of Child Psychiatry, University of Helsinki, Lastenlinnantie, SF 00250 Helsinki 25, Finland.

ELENA ARBORE, M.D., Child and Youth Hygiene Department, Institute of Hygiene and Public Health, Str. Dr. Leonte 1–3, Bucharest, Romania.

CHRISTIAN ASTRUP, M.D., Gaustad Sykehus, Boks 22, Gaustad, Oslo 3, Norway.

E. ATKINS, M.Sc., MRC Unit on Environmental Factors in Mental and Physical Illness, London School of Economics, 20 Hanway Place, London W1P 0AJ, United Kingdom.

ANDREÉ E. BAERT, M.D., Regional Officer for Mental Health, World Health Organization Regional Office for Europe, 8, Scherfigsvej, DK-2100 Copenhagen ø, Denmark.

JOHANN BINDER, Psychiatric University Clinic Zurich, Research Department, PO Box 68, Lenggstrasse 31, CH-8029 Zurich, Switzerland.

TOR BJERKEDAL, M.D., M.P.H., Institute of Hygiene, University of Oslo, Gydas Vei 8, Oslo 3, Norway.

SIGURJON BJORNSSON, Ph.D., Department of Psychology, University of Iceland, Reykjavík, Iceland.

GILLIAN BROWN, B.A., Research Social Worker, Department of Child and Adolescent Psychiatry, Institute of Psychiatry, University of London, London SE5 8AF, United Kingdom.

ROGER BYRING, M.D., II Department of Pediatrics, University of Helsinki, Helsinki 29, Finland.

OLIVER CHADWICK, Ph.D., Research Psychologist, Department of Child and Adolescent Psychiatry, Institute of Psychiatry, University of London, London SE5 8AF, United Kingdom.

NORA CHARITOS-FORSTER, Ph.D., 75 Cos Cob Avenue, Cos Cob, Connecticut 06807, USA.

N. CHERRY, M.Phil., M.I.S., MRC Unit on Environmental Factors in Mental and Physical Illness, London School of Economics, 20 Hanway Place, London W1P 0AJ, United Kingdom.

IRINA CHIRIAC, M.D., Child and Youth Hygiene Department, Institute of Hygiene and Public Health, Str. Dr. Leonte 1–3, Bucharest, Romania.

Ms. ANGELA CHITU, Child and Youth Hygiene Department, Institute of Hygiene and Public Health, Str. Dr. Leonte 1–3, Bucharest, Romania.

V. ČIPEROVÁ, M.D., ILF, subkatedra dětské neurologie, 14629 Prague, Czechoslovakia.

GILBERT CLINCKE, Ph.D., Department of Developmental Psychology, Blandijnberg 2, 9000 Ghent, Belgium.

L. CIOMPI, Ph.D., Psychiatric Clinic, University Cery, 1008 Prilly-Lausanne, Switzerland.

HANS CURMAN, M.D., Karolinska Institutet, Barn- och ungdomspsykiatriska kliniken, S:t Görans sjukhus, 112 81 Stockholm, Sweden.

J. P. DAUWALDER, Psychiatric Clinic, University Cery, 1008 Prilly-Lausanne, Switzerland.

WILLIAM DE COSTER, Ph.D., Department of Developmental Psychology, Blandijnberg 2, 9000 Ghent, Belgium.

ROBERT DEROM, Ph.D., Department of Obstetrics, Akademisch Zienkenhuis, De Pintelaan 135, 9000 Ghent, Belgium.

MIEKE DE ZUTTER, Ph.D., Department of Developmental Psychology, Blandijnberg 2, 9000 Ghent, Belgium.

J. DITTRICHOVÁ Ph. D., Ústav pro péči o matku a dítě, 14710 Prague, Czechoslovakia.

MARTA DONNER, M.D., Department of Paediatrics, Stenbackstreet 11, University of Helsinki, Finland.

J. W. B. DOUGLAS, B.M., B.Sc., MRC Unit on Environmental Factors in Mental and Physical Illness, London School of Economics, 20 Hanway Place, London W1P 0AJ, United Kingdom.

ANDERS DUNÉR, Ph.D., University of Stockholm, Department of Psychology, Box 6706, 113 85 Stockholm, Sweden.

STURE ENBERG, Ph.D., Swedish School of Social Work, Topeliuksenkatu 16, Helsinki 25, Finland.

INGEMAR FÄGERLIND, Ph.D., Institute for the Study of International Problems in Education, University of Stockholm, Fack, S-10405 Stockholm 50, Sweden.

D. P. FARRINGTON, Ph.D., Institute of Criminology, 7 West Road, University of Cambridge, Cambridge CB3 9DT, United Kingdom.

W. FELDER, M.D., Psychiatric University Clinic Zurich, Research Department, PO Box 68, Lenggstrasse 31, CH-8029 Zurich, Switzerland.

KEN FOGELMAN, B.A., Principal Research Officer, National Children's Bureau, 8 Wakley Street, Islington, London EC IV 7QE, United Kingdom.

R. FREY, M.D., Psychiatric University Clinic Zurich, Research Department, PO Box 68, Lenggstrasse 31, CH-8029 Zurich, Switzerland.

ANITA GOETHALS, Ph.D., Department of Developmental Psychology, Blandijnberg 2, 9000 Ghent, Belgium.

IRVING I. GOTTESMAN, Ph.D., Professor and Director, Behavioural Genetics Centre, Department of Psychology, University of Minnesota, Minneapolis, Minnesota 55455, USA.

ERNEST M. GRUENBERG, M.D., Dr. P.H., Professor and Chairman, Department of Mental Hygiene, Johns Hopkins School of Hygiene and Public Health, 615 North Wolfe Street, Baltimore, Maryland 21205, USA.

OLLE HAGNELL, M.D., Professor of Psychiatry, Department of Social and Forensic Psychiatry, University of Lund, S:t Lars sjukhus, 220 06 Lund, Sweden.

TORE HÄLLSTRÖM, M.D., Assistant Professor of Psychiatry, Department of Psychiatry I, University of Gothenburg, Sahlgrenska sjukhuset, S-413 45 Gothenburg, Sweden.

MOGENS HAUGE, M.D., Professor of Clinical Genetics, University of Odense, Arvepatologisk Institut, J.B. Winsløwsvej 17, DK - 5000 Odense C, Denmark.

MILUŠE HAVLINOVA, Ph.D., Institute of Hygiene and Epidemiology, Prague 10, Šrobarova 48, Czechoslovakia.

LÁRUS HELGASON, M.D., Kleppsspítalin, P.B. 1429, Reykjavík, Iceland.

TÓMAS HELGASON, M.D., Kleppsspítalin, P.B. 1429, Reykjavík, Iceland.

ERIK HØGH, Dr. Scient. Soc., Associate Professor of Sociology,

Sociological Institute, University of Copenhagen, Linnésgade 22, DK 1361 Copenhagen K., Denmark.

MATTI O. HUTTUNEN, M.D., Department of Psychiatry, University of Helsinki, Lapinlahdentie, SF 00180 Helsinki 18, Finland.

RAYMOND ILLSLEY, Ph.D., MRC Medical Sociology Unit, Institute of Medical Sociology, Westburn Road, Aberdeen AB9 2ZE, United Kingdom.

JACK INGHAM, Ph.D., MRC Unit for Epidemiological Studies in Psychiatry, University Department of Psychiatry, Royal Edinburgh Hospital, Morningside Park, Edinburgh EH10 5HF, United Kingdom.

BJORN JACOBSEN, M.D., Psykologisk Institut, Psychiatric Dept., Kommunehospitalet, 1399 Copenhagen, Denmark.

FRANTIŠEK JANDA, M.D., Dr. Sc., Institute of Hygiene and Epidemiology, Prague 10, Šrobarova 48, Czechoslovakia.

CARL-GUNNAR JANSON, Ph.D., Department of Sociology, University of Stockholm, 106 91 Stockholm, Sweden.

V. KAPALIN, Ph.D., Institute of Hygiene and Epidemiology, Šrobarova 48, Vinehrady, Prague 10, Czechoslovakia.

JAAKKO KAPRIO, M.D., Department of Public Health Science, University of Helsinki, Haartmaninkatu 3, SF-00290 Helsinki 29, Finland.

HEINZ KATSCHNIG, Ph.D., Psychiatrische Universitatsklinik, Lazarettgasse 14, 1097 Vienna, Austria.

H. C. G. KEMPER, Ph.D., University of Amsterdam, Jan Swammerdam Instituut, Eerste C. Huygensstraat 20, Amsterdam, The Netherlands.

K. E. KIERNAN, M.Sc., MRC Unit on Environmental Factors in Mental and Physical Illness, London School of Economics, 20 Hanway Place, London W1P 0AJ, United Kingdom.

JOE KIFF, B.A., MRC Unit for Epidemiological Studies in Psychiatry, University Department of Psychiatry, Royal Edinburgh Hospital, Morningside Park, Edinburgh EH10 5HF, United Kingdom.

GUNNAR KLACKENBERG, M.D., Associate Professor, Head of Department of Child Psychiatry, Karolinska sjukhuset, 104 01 Stockholm, Sweden.

MARKKU KOSKENVUO, M.D., Department of Public Health Science, University of Helsinki, Haartmaninkatu 3, SF-00290 Helsinki 29, Finland.

LINDA LERESCHE, Sc.D., Research Scientist, Johns Hopkins School of Hygiene and Public Health, 615 North Wolfe Street, Baltimore, Maryland 21205, USA.

B. LOHMEYER, M.D., Psychiatric University Clinic Zurich, Research Department, PO Box 68, Lenggstrasse 31, CH-8029 Zurich, Switzerland.

R. LÜTHI, Ph.D., Institute for Social and Preventive Medicine, University of Berne, Switzerland.

HÓLMFRÍDUR MAGNÚSDÓTTIR, M.D., Kleppsspítalin, P.B. 1429, Reykjavík, Iceland.

DAVID MAGNUSSON, Ph.D., University of Stockholm, Department of Psychology, Box 6706, S-113 85 Stockholm, Sweden.

DAVID MAY, Ph.D., Department of Psychiatry, University of Dundee, Ninewells Hospital, Dundee, DD2 1UD, United Kingdom.

BILL McGARVEY, Ph.D., Social Science Research Institute, University of Southern California, 950 W. Jefferson Blvd., Los Angeles, California 90007, USA.

BIRGITTE R. MEDNICK, Ph.D., Assistant Professor, Department of Education, University of Southern California, Los Angeles, California 90007, USA, and Psykologisk Institut, Kommunehospitalet, 1399 Copenhagen, Denmark.

SARNOFF A. MEDNICK, Ph.D., Dr. Med., Center for Longitudinal Research, Social Science Research Institute, University of Southern California, Los Angeles, California 90007, USA, and Director, Psykologisk Institut, Kommunehospitalet, 1399, Copenhagen, Denmark.

MARIE MEIERHOFER, Dr. Med., Dr. Phil., Institut für Psychohygiene im Kindesalter, Albisstrasse 117, 8038 Zürich, Switzerland.

NIELS MICHELSEN, M.D., University of Copenhagen, Institute of Social Medicine, Juliane Mariesvej 32, 2100 Copenhagen, Denmark.

KATARINA MICHELSSON, M.D., Department of Paediatrics, Stenbackstreet 11, University of Helsinki, Finland.

PATRICK MILLER, Ph.D., MRC Unit for Epidemiological Studies in Psychiatry, University Department of Psychiatry, Royal Edinburgh Hospital, Morningside Park, Edinburgh EH10 5HF, United Kingdom.

ROGER MISES, M.D., Professeur à l'Université Paris-Sud, Chef du département de psychologie et de psychiatrie de l'enfant, Fondation Vallée, 7, rue Benserade, 94250 Gentilly, France.

CARL GUSTAF NILSSON, M.D., Department of Medical Chemistry, University of Helsinki, Siltav. penger 10, Helsinki 17, Finland.

MARIE NOVOTNA, M.D., Institute of Hygiene and Epidemiology, Prague 10, Šrobarova 48, Czechoslovakia.

INGVAR NYLANDER, M.D., Karolinska Institutet, Department of Child and Youth Psychiatry, S:t Görans sjukhus, 112 81 Stockholm, Sweden.

AILEEN O'HARE, M. Soc. Sc., Medico-Social Research Board, 73 Lower Baggot Street, Dublin 2, Ireland.

ROGER PERRON, Dr. es Lettres et Sc. Hum., Maître de Recherches au CNRS, Laboratoire d'Etude Génétique de la Personnalité, Fondation Vallée, 7, rue Benserade, 94250 Gentilly, France.

MARTIN A. PLANT, Ph.D., Alcohol Research Group, University Department of Psychiatry, Royal Edinburgh Hospital, Morningside Park, Edinburgh EH10 5HF, United Kingdom.

BIRTE PRAHL-ANDERSEN, Ph.D., Professor of Orthodontics. Vrije Universiteit, De Boelelaan 1115, PO Box 7161, 1007 MC Amsterdam, The Netherlands.

MIROSLAV PROKOPEC, Ph.D., Dr. Sc., Institute of Hygiene and Epidemiology, Prague 10, Šrobarova 48, Czechslovakia.

DAVID QUINTON, M.A., Department of Child and Adolescent Psychiatry, Institute of Psychiatry, University of London, London SE5 8AF, United Kingdom.

ILARI RANTASALO, M.D., Department of Public Health Science, University of Helsinki, Haartmaninkatu 3, SF-00290 Helsinki 29, Finland.

STEPHEN A. RICHARDSON, Ph.D., Department of Pediatrics and Community Health, Albert Einstein College of Medicine, 1300 Morris Park Avenue, Bronx, New York 10461, USA.

DAVID H. ROSEN, M.D., Shetland Health Study, Langley Porter Institute, University of California Medical Center, San Francisco, California 94143, USA.

MICHAEL RUTTER, M.D., F.R.C.P., F.R.C. Psych., D.P.M., Professor of Child Psychiatry, Department of Child and Adolescent Psychiatry, Institute of Psychiatry, University of London, London SE5 8AF, United Kingdom.

PER-ANDERS RYDELIUS, M.D., Department of Child and Youth Psychiatry, S:t Görans Sjukhus S-112 81 Stockholm, Sweden.

M. L. SAMPHIER, MRC Medical Sociology Unit, Institute of Medical Sociology, Westburn Road, Aberdeen AB9 2ZE, United Kingdom.

SVERKER SAMUELSSON, M.D., Department of Psychiatry I, University of Gothenburg, Sahlgrenska sjukhuset, S-413 45 Gothenburg, Sweden.

E. ALFRED SAND, M.D., Professeur de Médecine sociale et de Prophylaxie criminelle, Ecole de Santé publique, Université libre de Bruxelles, 808 Route de Lennik, 1070 Bruxelles, Belgium.

SEPPO SARNA, Ph.D., Department of Public Health Science, University of Helsinki, Haartmaninkatu 3, SF-00290 Helsinki 29, Finland.

C. SCHARFETTER, Prof., M.D., Psychiatric University Clinic Zurich, Research Department, PO Box 68, Lenggstrasse 31, CH-8029 Zurich, Switzerland.

LYDIA SCHEIER, Dr. Phil., Marie Meierhofer Institut für daskind, Rieterstrasse 7, 8002 Zurich, Switzerland.

DAVID SHAFFER, M.B., M.R.C.P., M.R.C. Psych., D.P.M., Director, Division of Child Psychiatry, Department of Mental Hygiene, Psychiatric Institute, 722 West 168th Street, New York, N.Y. 10032, USA.

MARTIN SIEBER, Ph.D., Psychiatric University Clinic Zurich, Research Department, PO Box 68, Lenggstrasse 31, CH-8029 Zurich, Switzerland.

DAG SÖRBOM, Ph.D., University of Uppsala, Department of Statistics, PO Box 513, S-751 20 Uppsala, Sweden.

ELENA STANCIULESCU, Ph.D., Child and Youth Hygiene Department, Institute of Hygiene and Public Health, Str. Dr. Leonte 1–3, Bucharest, Romania.

JÓN G. STEFÁNSSON, M.D., Kleppsspítalin, P.B. 1429, Reykjavík, Iceland.

Z. ŠTEMBERA, M.D., Dr. Sc., Ústav pro péči o matku a dítě, 14710 Prague, Czechoslovakia.

G. TANASESCU, Ph.D., Child and Youth Hygiene Department, Institute of Hygiene and Public Health, Str. Dr. Leonte 1–3, Bucharest, Romania.

MICHEL THIERY, M.D., Department of Obstetrics, Akademisch Zienkenhuis, De Pintelaan 135, B-9000 Ghent, Belgium.

HANS THOMAE, Ph.D., Psychologisches Institut, Universitat Bonn An der Schlosskirchel, 53 Bonn, Federal Republic of Germany.

BARBARA THOMPSON, Ph.D., MRC Medical Sociology Unit, Institute of Medical Sociology, Westburn Road, Aberdeen AB9 2ZE, United Kingdom.

ALMA THORARINSON, M.D., Kleppsspítalin, P.B. 1429, Reykjavík, Iceland.

PEKKA TIENARI, M.D., Psychiatric Clinic, University of Oulu, Oulu, Finland.

J. TOMANOVÁ, Ústav pro péči o matku a dítě, 14710 Prague, Czechoslovakia.

ANDRE VANDIERENDONCK, Ph.D., Department of Developmental Psychology, Blandijnberg 2, 9000 Ghent, Belgium.

ÅGE VILLUMSEN, M.D., Surgical Department, The Deaconess Hospital, Copenhagen, Denmark.

V. VLACH, M.D., ILF, subkatedra dětské neurologie, 14629 Prague, Czechoslovakia.

DEBORAH J. VOORHEES-ROSEN, R.N., Shetland Health Study, Langley Porter Institute, University of California Medical Center, San Francisco, California 94143, USA.

J.-C. VUILLE, M.D., Institute for Social and Preventive Medicine, University of Berne, Switzerland.

M. E. J. WADSWORTH, Ph.D., MRC Unit on Environmental Factors in Mental and Physical Illness, London School of Economics, 20 Hanway Place, London W1P 0AJ, United Kingdom.

DERMOT WALSH, M.B., F.R.C. Psych., F.F.C.M., F.F.C.M.I., D.P.M., Medico-Social Research Board, 73 Lower Baggot Street, Dublin 2, Ireland.

PETER WEDGE, M.A., Deputy Director, National Children's Bureau, 8 Wakley Street, Islington, London EC1V 7QE, United Kingdom.

D. J. WEST, M.D., Ph.D., Institute of Criminology, 7 West Road, University of Cambridge, Cambridge CB3 9DT, United Kingdom.

FIONA WILSON, Ph.D., MRC Medical Sociology Unit, Institute of Medical Sociology, Westburn Road, Aberdeen AB9 2ZE, United Kingdom.

PREBEN WOLF LL.M., Associate Professor of Sociology, Sociological Institute. University of Copenhagen, Linnésgade 22. DK 1361 Copenhagen K, Denmark.

GUNNEL WREDE, Ph.D., Forskningsintitutet, Svenska handelshögskolan, Arkadiagatan 22, SF-00100 Helsingfors 10, Finland.

ANNELI YLINEN, M.D., Department of Paediatrics, Stenbackstreet 11, University of Helsinki, Finland.

BENGT ZACHAU-CHRISTIANSEN, M.D., Professor, Department of Paediatrics, State University Hospital (Rigshospitalet), Copenhagen, Denmark.

J. ZEZULÁKOVÁ, M.D., Ústav pro péči o matku a dítě, 14710 Prague, Czechoslovakia.

R. J. VAN ZONNEVELD, M.D., Ph.D., Director Bureau Raad voor Gezondheidsresearch TNO, Reader in Social Geriatrics at the University of Leiden and the Agricultural University of Wageningen, Juliana van Stolberglaan 148, Postbus 297, The Hague 2076, The Netherlands.

Part I

Introduction

1. Place of longitudinal research in the WHO European Region long-term programme on mental health

ANDRÉ E. BAERT

The World Health Organization European Region comprises 32 countries with a total population of about 850 million people. The geographical, social, economic, political, and historical diversity explain the wide variety of mental health problems found in the Region and the wide range of approaches needed to tackle them.

Major overall mental health problems in the WHO European region

The care of the mentally ill has traditionally been the responsibility of the public authorities, mainly because in the past these patients were considered dangerous. As a consequence there are still more than one million people in mental hospitals in the WHO European Region. A quarter of the establishments have more than 1000 beds, and the large size of these mental hospitals leads to impersonal custodial regimes, lack of privacy, and absence of social and intellectual stimulation. Although the trend in most WHO member states in the European Region towards community-oriented delivery of mental health care continues, the pace of this development varies and the process is nowhere complete. Figure 1.1 gives an overview of the wide variations in the provision of psychiatric

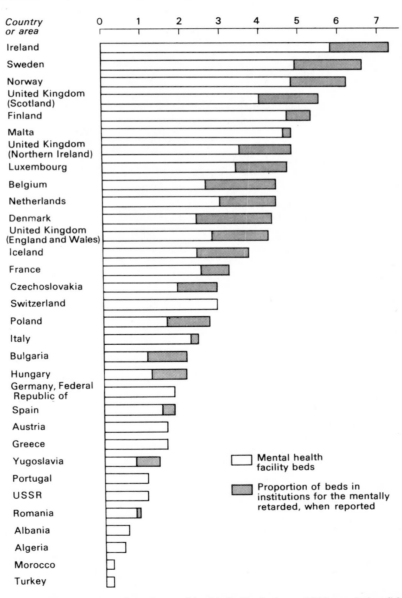

Fig. 1.1 Reported number of mental health facility beds per 1000 population (May 1976).

beds per 1000 population. There was a 35-fold difference in 1972 among the 31 countries responding to a WHO questionnaire (May 1976).

As the European Region faces the demographic phenomenon of an absolute and relative increase in its older population, there is a growing demand for various types of medical and social care for chronic patients. Information collected in pilot studies in some European countries indicates that about 20 per cent of the population may have recourse to mental health services in the course of a lifetime and that every third hospital bed is used for a patient suffering from a mental disorder.

Mental health legislation has not kept up with changes in mental health care and is sometimes in dissonance with other social legislation. Many countries still do not adequately formulate the mental health component in their national health policies while the monitoring and management of mental health care are frequently unsatisfactory.

A second major group of mental health problems is linked to certain behaviour patterns and life styles. Effects of excessive alcohol consumption appear at an earlier age while the aggregate level of alcohol consumption is increasing together with multiple drug misuse. The annual alcohol consumption in the European Region varies from an equivalent of about 0·5 litre of pure alcohol *per capita* to 16 litres (see Fig. 1.2). The number of deaths by suicide is of the same magnitude as those from road traffic accidents, each estimated at about 100 000 in 1974.

The concept of mental health stresses its public health and social aspects rather than linking it only to mental diseases and to psychiatry as a separate specialty that can be applied only in special institutions. There is steadily increasing evidence that behaviour patterns such as smoking, over-eating, excessive use of alcohol and drugs, extended exposure to psychosocial stresses, loneliness, and even sedentariness are common factors in certain noncommunicable diseases such as arteriosclerosis, hypertension lung cancer, various other forms of physical illness, and increased dependence on mental health care (Commission of the European Communities 1978). In spite of the enthusiasm of some investigators, technologies for primary prevention have failed, and huge public health campaigns are insufficiently assessed or evaluated.

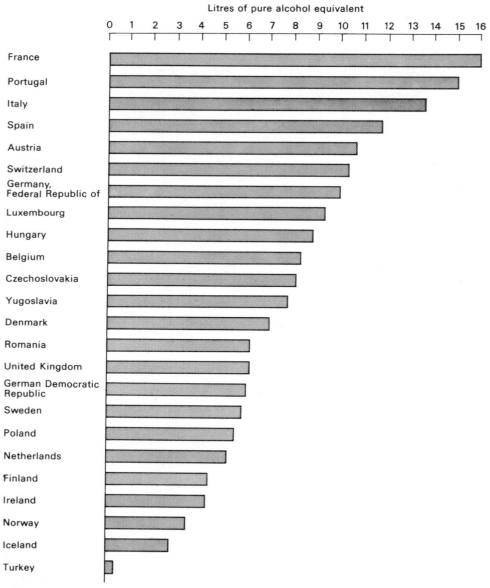

FIG. 1.2 Annual *per capita* consumption of alcohol in 24 European countries (1968–70) (from Bruun *et al.* 1977).

The long-term programme in mental health of the WHO Regional Office for Europe

At its twentieth session in 1970 and at its twenty-third session in 1973, the WHO Regional Committee for Europe approved proposals for a long-term programme in mental health covering the years 1970–80, with projections up to 1983.

The six detailed objectives selected are:

(1) The strengthening of the *mental health component* within national health policies;
(2) The promotion of *community mental health* care and its integration with other community services;
(3) The promotion of mental health in specific *high-risk groups and situations*;
(4) The prevention of *alcohol and drug dependence*;
(5) An improvement in the *training* of mental health workers and administrators;
(6) The development of *primary prevention* programmes.

Accordingly, a number of subprogrammes were developed as a coherent series of studies, working groups, symposia, publications, training courses, and conferences together with direct assistance to countries in the form of courses, consultantships, fellowships, and expert advice, where appropriate, and with a network of pilot study areas in selected member states. Publications and documents relating to the different projects of the long-term programme of the WHO Regional Office for Europe are given at the end of this volume.

The need for primary prevention and for mental health programme evaluation

The energetic development of medical technology has actually increased the prevalence of a variety of chronic illnesses and handicaps because it allows us to prolong life. This in turn has created a greater need and demand for medical services, giving rise to an ever-increasing spiral of demands, needs, and services. There is increasing awareness among decision-makers that the cost spiral must be stopped and that society could be better served by devoting more effort to research on methods of primary prevention. The change in emphasis from medication to mental health promotion has increased the demand for further knowledge about psychosocial factors, the influence of the environment on health, and the effects of changes in life style on the use of the medical services and on drug consumption.

One important line of research on prevention is concerned with early detection of populations at risk and the development of intervention techniques to reduce the probability of morbidity in these populations. The prospective longitudinal approach is most suitable for the elaboration of methods of early detection. A large representative sample of a population is studied intensively early in life and then followed until some members of the population sample develop the morbid condition under study. By going back to the original assessment it is possible to identify the individual and environmental characteristics that distinguish those who later succumb to the illness or deviation in question from those who do not. Such research has a contribution to make in understanding the aetiology of mental illness and in planning research on promotion of mental health.

Apart from being a basic research tool in psychiatry, education, and somatic development, the prospective longitudinal approach is vital for monitoring, assessing, and evaluating the impact of all health, including mental health, programmes. It may be suggested that no major national mental health programme should be launched without providing for, within the allocated budget, an evaluation employing the prospective longitudinal method. However, it is for their administrative as well as for their scientific value that such studies are essential. As Douglas (1976) pointed out, the question is whether we wish to know to what extent the new medical, social, educational or other services and programmes fulfil their stated objectives and intentions.

As many longitudinal cohort studies exist in Europe, it was felt that a co-ordinated description of them would advance the goal of establishing common methodology, terminology, and criteria, and stimulate further studies.

This survey of prospective longitudinal research may serve as an introduction to the subject for those responsible for evaluating health and social action, as well as those engaged in research on primary prevention.

2. Methods of ascertainment of longitudinal projects in this survey

S. A. MEDNICK and A. E. BAERT

The procedure employed in the development of this volume comprised three stages: tracing and locating as many prospective longitudinal studies as possible in the European Region, approaching selected individual project leaders inviting them to contribute a description, and screening, editing, and commenting upon these contributions.

Tracing and locating

In order to locate as many longitudinal studies as possible we engaged in the following activities:

Literature survey. A MEDLARS search was instituted yielding a total of 927 titles. Titles of potential interest were selected and copies requested together with copies of articles mentioned in papers. This provided a list of key persons carrying out or directing longitudinal cohort studies.

Letter to ministries of health. The Regional Office for Europe sent a circular letter to the ministries of health of all 32 member countries of the European Region giving some background information and requesting details about longitudinal projects 'which have involved the identification and assessment of relatively large populations, which have been or could be subject to follow-up study'. Ministries were also asked to indicate the names of project directors so that we could correspond directly with them to obtain detailed information.

Letter to medical research councils of the member countries of the European Region. A letter circular similar to that sent to ministries of health, together with attached list of investigators already traced, was also sent to national medical research councils and to the European Co-ordinating Centre for Research and Documentation in Social Sciences asking for additional names of project directors.

The overall response to the letters of enquiry varied. Researchers in several countries had made extensive use of the longitudinal research method while other countries had few or no researchers performing such studies. Largely owing to language difficulties, contacts with countries in Eastern Europe and with some in southern Europe were rather few but some contributors were eventually enlisted. It became obvious that in many member countries the health authorities, and even the national research council were not aware of longitudinal projects conducted within the countries. This indicates one of the difficulties involved in intracountry, and thus intercountry, co-ordination and collaboration.

Direct contacts with project directors and selection

For each project ascertained by the methods mentioned above a letter was sent to the principal investigator requesting copies of published articles or other descriptions of the project. The project material was reviewed and some critical research sites with ongoing relevant cohort studies were visited in order to make certain that the projects fulfilled the preset criteria. To be included in the survey a project had to meet the following conditions.

(1) To be prospective and longitudinal;
(2) To involve registration of information on individuals of a cohort at at least two points in their lives (also included were some ongoing projects that had definite follow-up plans);
(3) To allow some flexibility in methodological considerations. This was especially true in the case of studies in certain substantive areas;
(4) To take some account of the geographical location of projects so as to make the survey as representative as possible of the whole European Region.

When deemed appropriate investigators were invited to submit project descriptions for inclusion in the final report. Investigators were given considerable freedom in the length and form of their articles. However, the authors were asked to use a questionnaire (see Table 2.1) as a checklist for the history and rationale of the project, population sample, methodology, results related to theory

TABLE 2.1
Questionnaire sent to contributors to this study

Title of project: Date:

Who answered this questionnaire:

I   *Scientific personnel*
        1. Who began the project? when did the project begin?
        2. With what objective?
        3. Who are now the directors of the project and what are their special interests?
II   *Questions relative to national settings*
        1. Is there a central register for: criminality? mental health? suicide? death?
        2. If so, how far back does it go? How accurate is it? (What empirical tests have been made of its accuracy?)
        3. How available are these registers? What procedures are necessary to gain access to them? Does the project have access to these registers?
        4. What is done in these registers about dead individuals (i.e., are the records discarded or transferred?).
III   *Information on the index sample*
        1. How is it defined?
           (a) Year of birth of index subjects; geographical delimitation;
           (b) At what age were they identified by the project?
           (c) In what ways is the cohort not complete?
        2. How is the problem of drop-outs (e.g. non-co-operation, death) handled?
IV   *Contact of sample*
        1. What governmental or institutional approval was obtained?
        2. Was the sample personally contacted? How was sample contacted? How was the purpose of the project explained? Were the mass media utilized to inform the sample?
        3. Was there an offer of information feedback or services or reward made to the sample?
V   *Ethical considerations*
        1. Protection of subjects' anonymity;
        2. Responsibility regarding public use of findings.
VI   *Background information*
        1. Information regarding the parents and grandparents of the subject:
           (a) Are they registered? How complete is the registration?
           (b) Is there information recorded as to: social deviance? major physical illnesses? stability of the family? social class?
        2. Other information.

VII   *Assessment of the cohort* (if there has been a personal assessment)
        1. How often have index subjects been assessed? List of years.
        2. List of assessment devices at each assessment. Details of non-standard assessment devices. Details of special follow-up procedures.
        3. How co-operative were subjects? Per cent subject loss at each assessment. Representativeness of remainder.
VIII   *Status of the data*
        1. Are the data: in raw form? coded? punched? on tape?
        2. Could the subject be identified now for purposes of follow-up?
IX   *Data analysis and reports*
        1. What data analyses have been completed?
        2. Are there publications? a publication list?
X   *Special problems encountered*
        1. In funding; how is project funded?
        2. In following subjects;
        3. In staffing;
        4. In data analysis (resulting from size of data array);
        5. In subject co-operation;
        6. In co-operation with national or local administrative units.
XI   *Special advantages of project*
        It is hoped that the answers to this question will be useful in the preparation of a statement of the advantage of longitudinal research in contributing to the early detection and prevention of mental health problems and social deviance.
XII   Would the current investigators be interested in contacts with other European longitudinal projects for purposes of establishing cross-national reliability of findings and maximum exploitation of available data?
XIII   *Administrative considerations*:
        1. What administrative unit is responsible for the project?
        2. Utilization of the project
           (a) Training
           (b) Other
        3. Long-term guarantees of funding? Is there a fixed termination date?
XIV   *Impact of project*
        If the project is old enough, has there been an impact on public health, education, welfare, legal system etc.?

and results with social applications, the problems, advantages, limitations, and current status of each project and to write a narrative description that would be suitable for publication in a scientific journal. A tentative outline of the final report was also attached to indicate to the different authors where their articles would be placed.

Screening, editing, and commentary

The projects vary widely in complexity and scope. Some have been undertaken by experienced researchers assisted by larger research teams; others were undertaken by individual investigators. All groups maintained contact with their study cohorts despite financial and professional difficulties and, sometimes, lack of interest, by administrators and research councils. In reviewing project descriptions we could occasionally glimpse the qualities of steadfast heroism which this work has required.

Three experts in different disciplines were invited to write a commentary chapter on the 70 accepted project descriptions from the viewpoint of their particular discipline—namely, as epidemiologist, child psychiatrist, and (ontogenetic) psychologist; these commentaries are found in Part IV of this volume.

Comments on the procedure

The terminology used in the letter of enquiry to ministries of health and national research councils was for many not clear or was not considered within their jurisdiction. In these cases a negative reply was received.

With regard to contacts with ministries and national research councils, it became obvious that most were insufficiently aware of the ongoing prospective longitudinal research in their country and were pleased to receive the list of investigators. These official contacts have thus proven most useful in informing the WHO member states of existing longitudinal research and the interest of the Regional Office for Europe in promoting longitudinal research.

In many cases there was difficulty in locating studies because in many countries it is not the ministry of health, nor even the national medical research council, that is responsible for prospective longitudinal research but another ministry, agency, or foundation—a ministry of education, justice, or social affairs, or a national centre for infancy, for example. The need for communication, co-ordination, and co-operation within the national administration was again made apparent. Furthermore, without such co-ordination there is a risk of overlapping or repetitive research.

Most useful for tracing and locating prospective longitudinal projects were the individual contacts with researchers and participation in international conferences by which participants were made aware of similar ongoing research not only in their own countries but even in their own university. This again points to the lack of co-ordination on the local level and among researchers themselves.

As evidenced by the bulk of this volume, we succeeded in locating many projects—many more than anticipated. Investigators generally showed great enthusiasm for a volume describing longitudinal research in order to promote communication and co-operation on an international level, and to close the gap between researchers and public health administrators.

Part II

Longitudinal research methods

3. Methods of prospective, longitudinal research

SARNOFF A. MEDNICK

Between 1959 and 1962, the 9125 children born at a University Hospital in Copenhagen formed the subject population for a longitudinal perinatal project (Zachau-Christiansen and Ross 1975). Of the 7407 mature births (birthweight over 2500 g), 305 (4·12 per cent) of the neonates evidenced neurological symptoms (convulsions, respiratory distress, limpness, etc.). In 215 of these cases the symptoms were mild and disappeared after the fifth day of life. These 215 children and their mothers were discharged with no further treatment or special comment. This is apparently a common clinical practice. It assumes that the neonates had 'grown out of it'; it also avoids labelling the infant as brain damaged.

When these 215 children reached 10–12 years of age, 11 per cent ($N=24$) of them (and matched controls) were brought in for an intensive assessment. The investigators wished to determine if any adolescent behavioural or neurological difficulties were associated with the fleeting, mild, neonatal neurological symptoms. Compared to controls the neonatally-deviant children were in trouble; 71 per cent evidenced moderate neurological disturbance; only 8 per cent of the controls were so afflicted (Mednick and Michelsen 1977). The neonatally-deviant children also had serious cognitive and social difficulties (Mednick 1977). It seems likely that the children's preadolescent problems were, at least in part, related to their neonatal symptoms. If these children had been selected by a researcher as 'school problems' and compared to controls (without school problems) their social isolation might have been noted as a correlate and possible cause of their difficulties. The longitudinal study suggests an earlier factor which could conceivably be a partial cause of both the social isolation and the school difficulties.

This study illustrates an important potential public health application of the longitudinal, prospective design. Adequately replicated, these findings suggest one possible source of some of the school and MBD problems we observe in childhood. It suggests a simple, reliable method of early detection of some of these future problem children. Early detection offers the opportunity to select such risk children for attempts at prevention of future social, intellectual and educational difficulties. In public health terms, even partially successful early intervention in 4 per cent of live mature births could represent a huge economy in human suffering and societal resources. It seems possible that unless we intervene, these neonatally-deviant infants will not be underrepresented among our future delinquents, mentally disturbed, and social losers.

The study also illustrates a major problem with long-term research. It took 10–12 years to develop these findings. This is a long time to wait, a long time for research councils to feed and maintain the longitudinal study, a long time for the professional researcher to postpone publication-gratification. The cross-sectional study is quicker; we could have noted and published the social correlates of these school and social problems in a quick assessment completed in just a few weeks. But it is like the old story of the man who loses his keys in the dark alley. It may seem more tempting and more convenient to search under the street light 50 metres away. But not if you really want to find the keys.

This study of neonates represents the type of longitudinal research which identifies deviants early in life and determines their outcome by follow-up procedures. Longitudinal research takes other forms.

Types of longitudinal research and their advantages

Organizations and classifications of types of research are almost never extremely useful or productive. But a certain abhorrence of a Table of Contents totally innocent of traces of organization has prompted a search for meaningful clusters or types among the longitudinal research described in this volume. Happily, several methods of classification have been suggested in the literature, including grouping by type of design and nature of subject population (Wall and Williams 1970). A clustering first by type of design and then by method of selection of subjects resulted in an organization which was least unsatisfactory. This organization is summarized in Table 3.1.

TABLE 3.1

Summary table of European longitudinal studies[1]

Investigators	Country	Year of birth of cohort	Number of subjects
A. Correlative Longitudinal Research			
1. Normal, representative populations			
a. Prospective birth cohort studies			
Atkins, Cherry, Douglas, Kiernan, Wadsworth	Britain	1946	5362
Fogelman, Wedge	Britain	1958	16 000
Aräjarvi, Huttunen	Finland	1975–6	5500
Amnell	Finland	1955	6789
Bjerkedal	Norway	1967–76	630 000
Illsley, Wilson, May[2]	Scotland	1950–5	15 000
Illsley, Thompson, Samphier[2]	Scotland	1949 and ongoing	120 000
Chiriac, Arbore, Chitu	Romania	1969	123
Tanasescu, Chiriac, Stanciulescu	Romania	1932–71	325 000

Investigators	Country	Year of birth of cohort	Number of subjects
De Coster, Clincke	Belgium	1974–6	560
B. Mednick, Michelsen, Zachau-Christiansen, Villumsen	Denmark	1959–61	215
T. Helgason	Iceland	1895–7	5395
b. Prospective school-age cohort studies			
Janson	Sweden	1953	15 117
Høgh, Wolf	Denmark	1953	12 270[3]
Prahl-Andersen	The Netherlands	1961, 1963–4, 1966–7	486
Kemper	The Netherlands	1963, 1964	665
Magnusson, Dunér	Sweden	1950, 1952, 1955	3315

Table 3.1—*contd*

Investigators	Country	Year of birth of cohort	Number of subjects
Rutter, Graham, W. Yule, Tizard, Whitmore, Rigley[4]	England	1953–5	2200
Rutter, Maughan, Mortimore, Ouston, Gray, B. Yule[5]	England	1960	1000
Björnsson	Iceland	1950–61	1100
Farrington, West	England	1951–4	411[6]
Fägerlind	Sweden	1928	1544
Thomae	Federal Republic of Germany	1945–6	2800

c. Prospective adult cohort studies

Hallström, Samuelsson	Sweden	1914, 1918, 1922, 1930	1622[7]
Binder, Angst	Switzerland	1958, 1959	600
van Zonneveld	The Netherlands	1856–90	3149
Thomae	Federal Republic of Germany	1890–1905	222
Sieber, Angst	Switzerland	1952	841
Plant	Scotland	1919–59	300

d. Prospective community cohort studies

Voorhees-Rosen, Rosen	Scotland	1916–60	533
Astrup	Norway		3125
Hagnell	Sweden	1854–1957	3563

2. Non-representative populations

a. Normal birth cohort studies

Sand	Belgium	1955–8	265
Prokopec, Havlínová, Novotná	Czechoslovakia	1956–60	287
Klackenberg	Sweden	1955–8	212

b. Specialized cohort studies

i. Twin cohorts[8]

Kaprio, Koskenvuo, Sarna, Rantasalo	Finland	before 1958	32 000
Hauge	Denmark	1870–1930	75 000
De Coster, Vandierendonck, De Zutter, Thiery, Derom	Belgium	1965–72	411

ii. Adoptee cohort

Jacobsen, Schulsinger	Denmark	1922–47	14 500

iii. First-cousin study

T. Helgason, Manúsdóttir	Iceland	1879–1966	1951

iv. Birth difficulty, neonatal brain damage studies

Donner, Ylinen, Michelsson	Finland	1971–4	300/year

Investigators	Country	Year of birth of cohort	Number of subjects
Štembera, Zezuláková, Dittrichová, Tománová	Czechoslovakia	1970–2	1163
De Coster, Goethals, Vandierendonck, Thiery, Derom	Belgium	1972–3	80

v. Follow-up studies of deviants

a. Epidemiological studies

L. Helgason	Iceland	1901–53	2388
O'Hare, Walsh	Ireland		120

b. Patient studies

Curman, Nylander	Sweden	1933–53	2268
Ingham, Miller, Kiff	England		800
Ciompi, Agué, Dauwalder	Switzerland	1976	81
Stefánsson	Iceland		501
Angst, Scharfetter	Switzerland	before 1960	273
Angst, Frey, Felder, Lohmeyer	Switzerland	1880–1945	404
Richardson	Scotland	1951–5	589
Rutter	England	1941–55	126
Chadwick, Brown, Shaffer, Rutter	England	1960–71	90
Rutter, Yule, Berger, Hersov, Hemsley, Howlin, Holbrook, Sussenwein[9]	England	1961–70	32
Mises, Perron	France	1958–62	20
Rydelius	Sweden	1951–62	149
Rydelius	Sweden	1947–50	52
Thorarinsson, T. Helgason	Iceland	1908–62	3000

vi. Children at risk

Wrede, Byring, Enberg, Huttunen, Mednick, Nilsson	Finland	1960–4	212
Tienari	Finland		210
Mednick, Schulsinger, Venables	Denmark	1942–52	311
Rydelius	Sweden	1945–54	392
Rutter, Quinton	England	1951–67	556
Charitos-Forster	Switzerland	1956–61	122
Quinton, Rutter, Dowdney, Liddle, Mrazek[10]	England	1952–7	300
Dixon[11]	England	1968–71	78

B. Experimental–manipulative research

Vuille, Lüthi	Switzerland	1975	600
Scheier, Meierhofer	Switzerland	1961–5	20
Mednick, Schulsinger, Venables	Mauritius	1969	1800

---

[1] Table 3.1 is arranged in the same order as the contents of the book.
[2] These studies are reported in Chapter 11.
[3] Males only.
[4] Isle of Wight studies reported in Chapter 21.
[5] Inner London studies reported in Chapter 21.
[6] Males only.
[7] Females only.
[8] Number of subjects represents individuals, not twin pairs.
[9] Home-based treatment project, reported in Chapter 55.
[10] A follow-up study reported in Chapter 65.
[11] The institution-reared and fostered children study reported in Chapter 65.

Correlative vs. experimental–manipulative design. Perhaps the broadest differentiation classifies longitudinal studies as being *correlative and non-interventive* as opposed to being *experimental–manipulative* research. Most projects are correlative; that is, early characteristics or experiences are noted and correlated with outcomes at later stages of development. Among the correlative projects one can differentiate between those based on normal, unselected, representative populations and those which are non-representative and based on special or deviant groups. Also included in this latter category are those projects using normal birth cohorts which are rather small, but very intensively studied.

Some projects attempt a more or less systematic intervention aimed at preventing later illness or deviance. They, of course, include a follow-up assessment of differential outcome. Regrettably, such systematic intervention projects are relatively few in number.

Correlative longitudinal research

The basic definition of a longitudinal project requires some assessment of the subjects at a minimum of two points in their lives. The points of measurement should be relatively widely spaced (months or years, rather than minutes or hours). The designs in this section are correlative; this is mentioned to de-emphasize the occasional imputing of causality to relationships discovered in longitudinal research.

Normal representative populations.
The normal representative populations mentioned in Table 3.1 tend to be large (in the thousands). The *national birth populations* are defined by all births in a nation within a given time period. The 1946 and 1958 British cohorts (Chapters 6 and 7) defined their populations as all births in Britain in a given week in March. This is also true for the 1970 cohort which is unfortunately not included in this volume. The Norwegian Birth Register (Chapter 10) includes all births in the Kingdom of Norway. But a birth cohort may also be established on the basis of all the births in a metropolitan area within a given time period (typically a year) Chapters 8, 9, 11, and 12). *Perinatal projects* often include all births at large obstetrical departments for a period of some years (Chapter 14). *Community cohorts* will take all individuals of all ages living in a given moderate size community (Chapters 32, 33, and 34).

This large cohort project design is the ideal method for most research purposes. It is ideal for a number of reasons:

1. *Representativeness.* A profound advantage of the large, normal, representative-population cohort studies is the generalizability of the obtained results. For example, investigators have established a relationship between certain autonomic nervous system factors and antisocial behaviour (Siddle 1977). These findings have been noted in a variety of highly selected abnormal populations. Their applicability to a general population could justifiably be questioned. In Chapter 6 Wadsworth presents a demonstration of the existence of a similar relationship in the 1946 British birth cohort. This one statement from a representative population supports the generalizability of the previously published work.

2. *Multipurpose.* The large population cohorts have a great advantage in that they can be multipurpose. The oldest of these studies, the 1946 British cohort has been quite successful in developing a multipurpose stance over the years. As the other projects in this volume mature they will also be suitable for this type of exploitation. Since the populations are large, they can be used to determine early signs of later deviance for almost any social or medical condition which has a prevalence of more than 1 per cent in the population. This suggests that in the planning stages of a new project, a cross-disciplinary group of scientists (and funding agencies?) should be involved. It is important that research councils keep in mind and encourage this possible multidisciplinary utilization of

birth cohorts. It can result in great economies (which will please the funding agencies) and in important opportunities to study the interaction of disparate variables (which will please the scientists).

A corollary of a project's being multipurpose is the possibility of utilizing it for studies totally unforeseen at its inception. For example, the study by B. Mednick (based on the Danish Perinatal Project) cited in the introduction to this chapter demonstrates the usefulness of neonatal neurological signs in prediction of preadolescent behavioural and neurological difficulties. This utilization was unforeseen at the inception of this project. Douglas is now working with the 1946 British birth cohort to find childhood distinguishing characteristics of individuals who are now suffering psychiatric difficulties (personal communication). The Aberdeen Delinquency Study (Chapter 11D) by May, takes advantage of that cohort to elaborate the early characteristics of delinquents. A birth cohort can also yield information on the ultimate outcome of a variety of early anomalies (e.g., low birth weight, small for dates, neonatal neurological difficulties, developmental retardation) or early social circumstances (e.g., parental separation).

3. Complete sampling. A great advantage of longitudinal projects, especially the large birth cohorts, is the fact that they have identified a total population. Those individuals who later become institutionalized or who die have already been identified in the original population. It is possible to be aware of their absence in any subsequent assessment of the population. In comparison, in a typical cross-sectional study these individuals would simply be overlooked. This could lead to some disabling biases in the results and conclusions of such studies.

4. *Loss of subjects.* A related problem in longitudinal research is the inevitable loss of subjects through emigration, residential mobility, or lack of willingness to co-operate. A strength of the *birth cohort* method is that there is some knowledge regarding who it is one has lost in the course of the study. It is frequently possible to find out the reasons for the loss. In most projects these missing cases have been shown to be individuals with some form of psychiatric or social deviance.

5. *Incidence and prevalence.* The representative cohorts are clearly ideal for the development of incidence and prevalence rates for almost all of the attainments and afflictions of humans. This type of application is clear in the Iceland project by Helgason (Chapter 15) and the Helsinki project by Amnell (Chapter 9). The community cohort studies (Chapters 32–34) also present information useful in determination of incidence and prevalence rates.

6. *Social changes.* The study by Rosen and Rosen (Chapter 32) illustrates the use of community longitudinal projects in evaluating the effects of social change. The Shetland Islands, a relatively sheltered area of Scotland, are being changed by the introduction of a large oil industry. The effects on the mental health of the population can be evaluated by this project. An ongoing longitudinal project can evaluate the effect of changes in educational systems, and the effects of the introduction of health or social welfare plans.

Non-representative populations

Smaller normal birth cohorts. The smaller birth cohorts (Chapters 35, 36, and 37) typically consist of one to three hundred subjects who are described in great detail in terms of their development of physical growth, cognitive functioning, and personality behaviour. Because of the size of the smaller cohorts it is possible for them to undertake extremely intensive and repeated assessments. They are specially well adapted for disclosing discontinuities and plateaus in growth curves of physical and mental processes. Unfortunately, the size of the samples studied in these smaller birth cohorts restricts the yield of psychiatric or social deviants. Because of the intensity of assessments, however, such studies might be very useful for generating hypotheses regarding factors predisposing to adult outcome.

Specialized cohorts. The *specialized cohorts* tend to be aimed very specifically at answering certain questions. The primary purpose of establishing *twin cohorts* (Chapters 38, 39, and 40) is, of course, the estimation of the heritability of traits or conditions. The longitudinal following of twins can yield a variety of special comparisons not otherwise available. If monozygotic twins are discordant for an abnormality, the data on their life circumstances can yield information on predispositional environmental factors. The findings of such a study would be completely unbiased by genetic factors. Much the same may be said for the adoptee cohorts (Chapter 41). They are also mainly developed to explore genetic hypotheses. The following of *adoptees* can reveal relationships between deviant behaviour and early separation from the biological parents and foundling home experience relatively independent of (or in interaction with) genetic background. Cross-fostering designs can compare the influence of genetic and certain environmental conditions on later deviance.

Perinatal damage cohorts (Chapters 43, 44, and 45) may be of special interest since they frequently demonstrate long-term consequences of neonatal anomalies. They can lead to work on the primary prevention of the perinatal damage and/or intervention to reduce the probability of negative long-term consequences.

Long-term study of groups of *identified patients or antisocial individuals* (Chapters 48–60) can provide information on outcomes, changes in diagnosis and recidivism. If the patients or clients have been assigned to a variety of treatments, the follow-up might hint at the long-term differential effects of these treatments (taking into consideration the problems of differential assignment to treatments). If the patients are intensively examined early, then the relationship between these early symptoms and signs and follow-up status can suggest methods of prognosis.

Longitudinal, prospective studies of *children at risk* have certain advantages. Such children may be at risk because of parental deviance (Chapters 61–5) or because of some deviant early experience (Chapters 65 and 66). They are typically studied in childhood or early adolescence before they themselves evidence deviance. These early assessments are only minimally contaminated by the consequences of the abnormality. Children of schizophrenic parents (Chapters 61, 62, and 63) have a 10–15 per cent risk of themselves becoming schizophrenic; but they have not yet experienced the drugs, hospitalization, misery, and failure often associated with being schizophrenic. Consequently, their assessments and reports by observers are not influenced by these factors or knowledge that the individuals have been diagnosed. Young children of alcoholics (Chapter 64), some of whom later will themselves become alcoholic, do not have the physiological damage which will very likely accompany their future heavy drinking. When some of these high-risk individuals succumb to alcoholism childhood characteristics which distinguish them from their more fortunate fellow high-risk individuals cannot be attributed to the *effects* of heavy drinking. These characteristics may be useful in early detection of future alcoholics. These 'predisposing' characteristics may suggest hypotheses relating to aetiology. The only advantage of the risk design over the study of normal, representative populations is the higher yield of deviant individuals in the study. This means that in order to eventually obtain a sample of alcoholics or schizophrenics of a given size, one can begin with a smaller total cohort. This can be of great importance if time-consuming assessments are envisioned.

Experimental–manipulative research

A great source of difficulty for the researcher interested in studying the causes of mental illness or social deviance is the unavailability of the experimental–manipulative approach. For example, we cannot and will not, for research (or any other) purposes, inflict conditions on children which we suspect might cause mental illness. But research on primary prevention affords us the opportunity to utilize the experimental–manipulative method. Systematic research in this area has hardly begun. In view of the somewhat limited success of the treatment of mental illness and in view of the human suffering and societal cost involved, primary prevention research seems a viable and as yet relatively unexplored possible solution. Chapters 67–9 give some taste of the possibilities.

Longitudinal research and causal statements

If longitudinal research takes on an interventive nature then it becomes experimental–manipulative. Assuming proper controls and research design, certain types of causal statements may be made concerning the conclusions of such research. However, most longitudinal research is correlative. In such research there can be no attempt to *prove* causal relationships. Because of the time frame involved in longitudinal research, however, certain factors can sometimes be discredited as possible causes. If, for example, jailed adult criminals evidence serious EEG disturbances but these EEG disturbances were not present before these individuals began their criminal careers, then we might better attribute the EEG disturbances to correlates of criminal behaviour (e.g., head injuries). (By specifying adults we mean to minimize the influence of maturational factors.) If on the other hand, the EEG disturbances were a distinguishing characteristic of the criminals in their premorbid state, then the EEG factors can be considered among the possible causal variables.

Longitudinal research: problems and recommendations

Problems

1. *Financial and administrative.* Perhaps the most common criticism of longitudinal studies has been the high cost and the difficult long-term financial commitment which must be made by a granting agency. In addition, the administrative continuity of the projects very often is difficult to maintain. Typically these two problems are not independent. Despite the fact that the allegation regarding high costs for longitudinal projects has been very freely and frequently made, no one has actually cost-accounted this factor to support his statement. While some longitudinal projects have been exceptionally expensive (United States Collaborative Project) the classic English studies (Chapters 6 and 7), the Finnish studies (Chapters 8 and 9), the Aberdeen study (Chapters 11 A, B, C, D) and the Danish study (Chapter 14) have been conducted at surprisingly low cost.

The largest cost in a longitudinal project is the initial assessment of the subjects. If apparatus is to be used it will be purchased at this initial stage; the initial assessment will typically encompass the largest number of individuals in the cohort. It will also require the longest and most expensive training period for the staff. In the simplest form of longitudinal projects, the assessment of final outcome (mental illness, criminality, school performance, socio-economic level, personality characteristics, etc.) is the only required additional step. If only the initial and outcome assessments are made, costs per year can be very modest. More frequently, however, assessments of the population can be profitably undertaken at intermediate stages of the research.

If, in planning of the project, the work is multidisciplinary such that information relating to a large number of social and medical deviances can be obtained, then the basic cost for each of these subareas can be very substantially reduced. In any case, when one compares the cost of gathering this information and its potential use in prevention, with the suffering involved and the cost of the care, feeding, and treatment of deviant populations, it is likely that such research costs are a very good investment.

2. *Obsolescence.* One serious problem to which all longitudinal research is subject is that measures and theories which seem important at the inception of the project may seem terribly dated and misdirected twenty years later. It is good advice for the individual intending to begin longitudinal research to keep his theory fairly general and his choice of measures fairly eclectic and not allow himself to be totally dominated by any specific theoretical orientation. The researcher is wise if he records raw data from his subjects. That is to say, he should record actual verbalizations rather than just the coding of attitudes and opinions; he should record raw physiological data on magnetic tape rather than only complex derivatives. The basic raw data is more likely to be meaningful or rescorable 20 years hence.

3. *Problems in non-age-specific interpretations.* In the 1946 British cohort, Douglas reports that the experience of the child (age 0–2 years) in breathing polluted air did not result in significantly more coughing or bronchitis in later adolescence. At age 25, however, those who had been subjected to highly polluted air in childhood did evidence significantly more coughing and bronchitis (personal communication). This is an instance of a sleeper effect; the effect of an antecedent factor does not show itself until a later period of life. Conclusions regarding the influence of a childhood factor in a longitudinal study should not be made in an absolute manner. The Douglas study shows us that such conclusions should be restricted to their age-specific period. As another example, there is reason to suspect that delinquency may not have the same origins as adult criminality. It is possible, therefore, that factors which relate to delinquency may be different from those which relate to adult criminality. Thus, if an antecedent factor is not associated with an increase in the probability of delinquency, this does not mean that it will be unrelated to adult criminal behaviour in the same population.

4. *Population flux.* After some years of population shifts it is possible that a large birth or school cohort could grow less than representative of a current population. For example, in northern Europe the recent and large scale influx of guest workers from the south could render a birth cohort which began in the early 1940s unrepresentative of the current population. Of course the cohort would still be representative of the 1940 native birth population. The cohort could also be supplemented by judicious sampling of the new immigrants.

In the case of large amounts of emigration and in the absence of population registers, the investigator could find it difficult to locate his population after some years. Sending birthday and Christmas cards will help in learning when the subject changes residence. The addresses and telephone numbers of a number of relatives and friends of the subject will aid in locating him in the case of residence changes.

5. *Publication.* One frequently mentioned problem of longitudinal research projects has been the difficulty of achieving publication of their findings. Some reasons are fairly clear; the exciting pay-off for most of these projects only comes when the subjects reach adult age, have attained or failed to attain certain life goals, or have manifested or not manifested certain deviance. However, the longitudinal researcher can explore the possibility of exploiting certain short-term goals. For example, if the longitudinal researcher is interested in criminality he might take delinquency as a short-term goal. If he is interested in mental illness, he might take adjustment in school as a short-term goal.

6. *Repeated measures.* In some longitudinal projects the same measures are administered repeatedly to the subjects. This of course entails a danger of the measurement itself changing the subject. Typically however this danger is a minimal one. When we observe the difficulty of noting a significant effect of years of psychotherapy with schizophrenics, it seems unlikely that our one, two, three, or four interviews in a lifetime will significantly alter our subject populations. Of course, under certain circumstances and under some special testing conditions it is conceivable that the repeated measurement effect could be important. It is also possible to assess the effect with controls who have less frequent assessments.

Specific recommendations

1. *Behaviour genetics* has taught us that we can frequently better understand the workings of environmental variables when we have controlled or reduced genetic variance (see Chapter 72). Where possible and conceivably appropriate, investigators should obtain information on family background for mental illness, and social deviance. Where possible, variance attributable to these sources should be taken into consideration.

2. *Registers.* Whenever possible, public registers for criminality, mental illness, obstetrical records, hospitalizations records, etc. should be utilized. In many cases it is more reliable to ascertain and describe these events via public records than via interview techniques.

3. *Statistics.* Human lives are complex and multidetermined. Our methods of analysis of the influences on these lives should be of the same order of complexity as our hypothesized determinants. After the mandatory careful examination of distributions and univariate relationships, multivariate analysis should be a natural next step. We are fortunate in that Jöreskog has designed structural equation models which are especially appropriate for analysis of longitudinal data (see Chapters 4 and 5). His latest edition of LISREL (IV) is especially easy to apply and interpret.

4. *Biological measures.* With the exception of the perinatal projects, most longitudinal projects in the behavioural sciences have not been especially oriented toward biological variables. In contrast to an interview, a paper and pencil test, or a questionnaire, biological measures tend to be relatively intrusive and messy. One must often make a hole in the subject to draw some body fluids; the processing of biochemical analyses has been expensive and time-consuming.

At this point, however, technical advances in biochemical analysis techniques have reduced the amount of fluids necessary and increased the yield of substances which can be assayed. 'Neurometrics' (John *et al.* 1977) has developed to a point where computer processing of neurophysiological data makes relatively large-scale assessments of central nervous system functioning feasible. The same can be said for assessment of autonomic nervous system functioning.

The longitudinal researcher should consider these measures where appropriate.

General recommendations

1. *Advisory board.* In Chapter 70 Gruenberg and LeResche recommend that at the inception of every longitudinal project an advisory board of outside distinguished scientists be appointed to help the investigators. They suggest that the advisory board be independent of the grant-giving agency so that the exchanges between the scientists and the advisory board can be uninhibited by financial considerations. It would probably be of some use if the advisory board were cross-disciplinary. Any large longitudinal study should be considered multipurpose. It is best if it were planned this way. The cross-disciplinary advisory board could provide the professional contacts necessary to properly exploit multidisciplinary opportunities.

2. *Sharing of data*. The longitudinal projects are almost all funded by public sources. The investigators should consider these data as a type of public property (in a limited sense). Of course, the investigators' aims and interests must first be taken into account, but whenever possible the investigator should be open to the exploitation of 'his' data or 'his' population by outside, responsible scientists. Perhaps this volume will catalyse such productive interactions.

3. *Public information*. In the Örebro Project (Chapter 20) Magnusson and Dunér made great efforts to enlist the co-operation of the public in their longitudinal research project. Their cohort was school-based and required repeated testing. They gained the co-operation of the newspapers, political and school officials, as well as the families of the children involved. Their effort was highly successful in this regard. It is not clear that such publicity is useful or wise in all longitudinal projects; but in general, an open stance, such as these investigators took, will repay itself in co-operation on the part of the prospective subjects. It is also possible, however, that in some studies such wide publicity might produce problems which otherwise would not arise. It is, in any case, an important matter for each investigator to consider with respect to his project.

4. *Flexibility*. From the planning stages of a longitudinal project, it is useful for the investigator to be as flexible as possible. It is important to remember that some of the outcomes which will be related to the antecedent factors in the project may not evidence themselves for twenty years. The investigator will be wise to formulate hypotheses in a very general form and admit, among his antecedent measures, variables which are not necessarily directly and specifically suggested by his theoretical orientation. During the course of the study it is important to make use of opportunities which present themselves for gathering of additional information on the subjects.

Summary

Within the framework of a classification of prospective, longitudinal research the various types of studies have been described. Some of the advantages of these types of research have been briefly outlined. The chapter closes with some recommendations for researchers.

4. A statistical model for analysis of longitudinal data: LISREL

DAG SÖRBOM

Introduction

A longitudinal study is characterized by the fact that the same individuals or observational units are measured on two or more occasions. This research design undoubtedly leads to several difficulties which concern the collection of data. In recent years there has been growing agreement among researchers that these difficulties can be disregarded when related to the gain in information that is available from a longitudinal study. To assimilate this gain there is a need for careful analysis of the data, but methodological problems in the statistical analysis of the data are also inherent in the longitudinal design. In this chapter a statistical model called LISREL (see e.g. Jöreskog and Sörbom 1976a, 1977) and a computer program (see Jöreskog and Sörbom 1976b) are described, which have been developed as tools for the analysis of data of the kind that arises from longitudinal studies.

Latent variables

The term latent is used to indicate that the variable referred to is in some way not directly measurable, in the sense that variables like height and weight of a person are measurable. Latent variables are inherent in most analyses of data in the social sciences because the concepts used are often unmeasurable. There are two principal reasons for this: (i) we have no instrument that can measure the variable exactly, and (ii) the concept we are interested in is in fact non-existent. As examples of the latter we can consider concepts such as socio-economic status, intelligence, verbal ability, spatial ability, and permanent income. All these concepts have in common that they are more or less defined by the very process we claim is measuring them. Thus, the variables which are measured and used in an analysis can broadly be considered to contain two sources of variability, one from the concept we are studying and one from error. This error is in turn a composite of two different kinds of

error, namely a measurement error and an operational error. The distinction between these two categories of error is not always clear-cut. However, the former is usually associated with reliability; that is, if the same or very similar measurement procedure is used twice, we are not guaranteed that exactly the same value will be observed both times. The latter kind of error is associated with validity; that is, our measurements are not measuring exactly what we intended them to measure. In both cases we need more information than is contained in a single measure. A common way to handle this is to collect information from several similar measures and to consider the common parts of the measures or variables to be a better measure of what we are interested in. These common parts can be interpreted as a new set of variables, unobserved or latent variables, and the main focus is on the relations among these rather than among the observed variables.

In Fig. 4.1 a typical simple situation is depicted. To be explicit: Suppose we want to study the interrelationship between intelligence and socio-economic status. These two variables are typically unobservable, they exist in reality only as constructs defined by the variables we believe are measuring them. In Fig. 4.1 the observed variables are denoted by squares and the latent variables by circles. The arrows indicate the direction of influence. For example, we assume that the latent variable ξ influences the two observed variables x_1 and x_2. The observed values of x_1 and x_2 are also influenced by the errors ε_1 and ε_2, respectively. These errors are to be con-

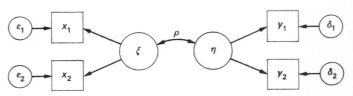

FIG. 4.1. The model for the measurement of two latent variables by four observable variables.

sidered as all that remains in the observed variables after the influence of the latent variable has been accounted for. Thus, they consist of pure measurement errors as well as of other influences on the observed variables that are not directly associated with the latent variables. For example, if ξ is intelligence and x_1 and x_2 are two intelligence tests, the measurement error parts can be regarded as those influences on x_1 and x_2 which are due to the conditions that were present on the occasion when the tests were administered, and which were not intended when the tests were constructed. The operational error part could be interpreted as that part of the two tests that is not common to both of them, that is x_1 might be a test which is aimed more at measuring verbal ability, whereas x_2 might be more like a test for numerical ability. In this case ε_1 would be supposed to contain some part of the verbal ability of the testee and ε_2 some numerical ability. The use of the two intelligence tests x_1 and x_2 should be clear: We have constructed a variable, ξ, which should be more adequate as a measure of intelligence than any of the tests x_1 and x_2 used separately.

Analogously, the two variables y_1 and y_2, being measures like occupational status, income, home background, can be used to construct the variable η, socio-economic status. The main focus is on the interrelationship; e.g. the correlation $\rho_{\xi\eta}$ between ξ and η, denoted in the figure by a curved two-headed arrow, indicating that there is no interpretation of the direction of cause. It should be clear from the discussion above that this correlation is more truthful as a description of the relationship between intelligence and socio-economic status than any of the observable correlations between x- and y-variables.

The above description of latent variables is concerned with the situation when we have quite good information about our measurable variables, that is, when we have rather specific knowledge as to which observed variable is measuring which latent variable. In this case we are saying that we are conducting a *confirmatory* study. However, latent variables have also been used in situations when we have only vague ideas of the structure of the relationships among the observed variables. We are speaking of *exploratory* studies when we assume that the interrelations among a number of observed variables could in some sense be explained by a number of latent variables, the number of which is assumed to be smaller than the number of observed variables. The introduction of the latent variables is then aimed at getting a more parsimonious description of data than is possible by a study of the observed interrelationships among the observed variables.

The model concept

Figure 4.1 can also be used as an illustration of a model for observable variables. A model is simply a description of the relationships among the variables; this means that we are assuming certain restrictions for the relations among the entities involved. In Fig. 4.1 for example it is stated that there is no direct influence of x_1 on y_1; any such influence is assumed to be mediated by ξ and η, and it is assumed that there are no relations between the errors and so on.

The model in Fig. 4.1 can be conceived as being composed of two kinds of models, a *measurement model* describing the relationships among the latent variables and the variables measuring them, and a *structural equation model* describing the relations among the latent variables. It is this latter model that it is often our main objective to study.

The LISREL model

LISREL is an abbreviation of LInear Structural RELationships. The LISREL model is particularly designed to handle models for latent variables. In LISREL we are working with two sets of latent variables, namely a set of dependent variables denoted by η and a set of independent variables, denoted by ξ. These variables are assumed to be measured by two sets of observable variables, y measuring η and x measuring ξ. The simplest possible situation is depicted in Fig. 4.1. Here two variables, y_1 and y_2, are measuring η, and two variables, x_1 and x_2, are measuring ξ. The structural equation model is

$$\eta = \gamma\xi + \zeta. \tag{1}$$

The dependent latent variable η is assumed to be explained by the independent latent variable ξ except for an error ζ. The measurement model for the η-variable is

$$y_1 = \eta + \varepsilon_1 \tag{2a}$$
$$y_2 = \eta + \varepsilon_2$$

and, for the ξ-variable,

$$x_1 = \xi + \delta_1 \tag{2b}$$
$$x_2 = \xi + \delta_2.$$

That is, the observable variables x and y are assumed to be composed of two parts, one 'true' part, η or ξ, and one error part, ε or δ.

The model described in eqns (1) and (2) is the simplest meaningful model that can be handled by LISREL and is discussed here to give an indication of the kind of problems the model is intended to be used with. In the general case, when there are m η-variables and n ξ-variables, and there are more than two x- and y-variables, the interpretation of the different parts of the model is similar to the one above. Thus, we are mainly studying relations among the η- and ξ-variables of the following general form:

$$\beta_{11}\eta_1 + \beta_{12}\eta_2 + \ldots + \beta_{1m}\eta_m = \gamma_{11}\xi_1 + \gamma_{12}\xi_2 + \ldots + \gamma_{1n}\xi_n + \zeta_1 \tag{3a}$$
$$\beta_{21}\eta_1 + \beta_{22}\eta_2 + \ldots + \beta_{2m}\eta_m = \gamma_{21}\xi_2 + \gamma_{22}\xi_2 + \ldots + \gamma_{2n}\xi_n + \zeta_2$$

$$\beta_{m1}\eta_1 + \beta_{m2}\eta_2 + \ldots + \beta_{mm}\eta_m = \gamma_{m1}\xi_1 + \gamma_{m2}\xi_2 + \ldots + \gamma_{mn}\xi_n + \zeta_m$$

which with use of the notation of matrix algebra can be written

$$\beta\eta = \Gamma\xi + \zeta. \tag{3b}$$

In eqn (3) we can see that in the general case we have added a possibility for relations among the η-variables as expressed by the β-coefficients.

The measurement model for p y-variables can be written

$$y_1 = \lambda_{11}\eta_1 + \lambda_{12}\eta_2 + \ldots + \lambda_{1m}\eta_m + \varepsilon_1 \tag{4a}$$
$$y_2 = \lambda_{21}\eta_1 + \lambda_{22}\eta_2 + \ldots + \lambda_{2m}\eta_m + \varepsilon_2$$

$$y_p = \lambda_{p1}\eta_1 + \lambda_{p2}\eta_2 + \ldots + \lambda_{pm}\eta_m + \varepsilon_p$$

or in matrix notation

$$y = \Lambda_y\eta + \varepsilon. \tag{4b}$$

The measurement model for the x-variables is similar to eqn (4).

Equations (3) and (4) give the structure of the model in its most general form for m dependent latent variables, n independent latent variables, p observed y-variables and q observed x-variables. There are no restrictions imposed on the relations within each set of errors in the model. Thus, there may be correlations among the ζ-variables, as well as among the ε- and δ-variables. A specific model to be analysed is set up by specifying which of the parameters are to be fixed and which are to be estimated. For the model in Fig.

4.1 we have $m = n = 1$ and $p = q = 2$, and thus, the general model in this case is

$$\beta_{11}\eta_1 = \gamma_{11}\xi_1 + \zeta$$
$$y_1 = \lambda_{y_{11}}\eta_1 + \varepsilon_1$$
$$y_2 = \lambda_{y_{21}}\eta_1 + \varepsilon_2$$
$$x_1 = \lambda_{x_{11}}\xi_1 + \delta_1$$
$$x_2 = \lambda_{x_{21}}\xi_1 + \delta_2,$$

(5)

and the model in Fig. 4.1 is specified by stating

$$\beta_{11} = 1$$
$$\lambda_{y_{11}} = \lambda_{y_{21}} = \lambda_{x_{11}} = \lambda_{x_{21}} = 1.$$

By adding the restrictions that ε_1 and ε_2 are uncorrelated and that δ_1 and δ_2 are uncorrelated we have explicitly specified the model depicted in Fig. 4.1.

Within the LISREL model we have one further possibility to specify models, namely, by restricting some parameters to be equal to each other. For example, if the two x-variables in Fig. 4.1 have the same proportion of contribution from the 'true' variable ξ, we might specify that the variances of δ_1 and δ_2 are equal. That is to say that the two x-variables have the same reliability.

The LISREL program

The aim of an analysis of data is usually to get a more comprehensive description of what has been measured by the data, and to test whether the data show indications that some specific hypotheses about the analysed model are tenable or not.

By the use of the LISREL computer program (see Jöreskog and Sörbom 1976b) we can get estimates of the parameters of the model and their standard errors, which can be seen as indicators of how precisely we have been able to estimate our parameters. These standard errors can also be used to ascertain whether or not a parameter makes a significant contribution to the model by testing if the parameter is significantly different from zero or not. In addition a run with the LISREL program supplies us with a measure of the overall fit of the model to the data. This measure, being approximately distributed as a χ^2-variable, allows us to judge whether an estimated model as a whole can be regarded as describing our data satisfactorily or not. By studying differences in this measure for different models it is possible to choose among the models. For example, the model in Fig. 4.1 can be estimated with unequal variances for δ_1 and δ_2. Then we can estimate the model once more with the restriction that these variances be equal. This latter model will have a higher χ^2-value, but if it is not significantly different from the χ^2 for the previous model we can not reject the hypothesis of equal variances, and hence the possibility that the two variables x_1 and x_2 have equal reliabilities.

Often it happens that the model used for the first analysis of a set of data does not fit very well in the sense that it results in a significant χ^2. There are several conceivable reasons for this. An obvious one is that in the specification of the model we have overlooked some significant relations, that is that there are parameters that we have specified to be equal to zero which in fact are different from zero, or we have specified parameters to be equal which in fact are unequal. With the program it is possible to obtain indicators which show which of the specified zeros are most likely not to be equal to zero and which equalities are most likely not to hold. These indicators are the first-order derivatives, and a high value of a derivative for a specified zero indicates that it should be incorporated in the set of parameters to be estimated.

Thus, the program gives two ways of improving a model: (1) by deleting relations that are not significant in order to get a more parsimonious description of the data; and (2) by adding relations in order to get a better fit to the data. The model we start with should

include, as far as is possible, all the information we have about our data. However, the analysis often shows that we have to reformulate our model in order to improve it with respect to different aims as exemplified above. In many instances it has been apparent that the final model is quite different from the initial one. This means that the analysis is more or less an exploratory one, which in turn implies that, if we want our results to be generally applicable, we must test the model with a new, independent set of data.

The LISREL model for longitudinal data

The structure of the variables inherent in a longitudinal study can be described schematically as in Fig. 4.2. We are mainly interested in the change over time in the set of variables called criterion

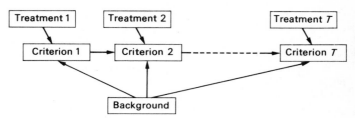

FIG. 4.2. A typical structure for a longitudinal study.

variables in Fig. 4.2. Between each of the T occasions the observational units have been exposed to some kind of treatment, and we want to study the influence of this treatment on the criterion variables. However, we also often have information from a set of variables X which we know affect the criterion variables, although we are not interested in this effect. These variables, referred to as background variables, are incorporated in the analysis mainly to make the analysis more precise. The background variables are also used to eliminate pre-existing differences among observational units. For example, in studies in the social sciences it is often impossible to get data from groups of individuals that are equivalent before a treatment. In this case the background variables are used to single out the group differences so they will not be confused with the effects of treatment.

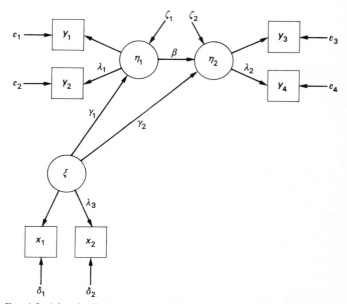

FIG. 4.3. A longitudinal study with a criterion measured on two occasions and with one background variable. All latent variables are measured by two variables each.

Most commonly the LISREL model treats the criterion variables as η-variables and the treatment and background variables as ξ-variables. However, in many instances there is no quantifiable treatment variable; e.g. a treatment is given to one group of individuals and a second group, the control group, is given no treatment at all. In this case we may treat the data from each group separately.

As discussed above, the variables in Fig. 4.2 are often not directly observable and we only have observed variables which are indicators of some latent variables. A simple example of the longitudinal design for two occasions, with no treatment variable and with two indicators for each latent variable is shown in Fig. 4.3. Our criterion variables are denoted by η_1 and η_2 and the background variable by ξ. We are mainly concerned with the relation between η at occasion 2 and η at occasion 1, that is with the parameter β in the structural equation

$$\eta_1 = \gamma_1\xi + \zeta_1$$
$$\eta_2 = \beta\eta_1 + \gamma_2\xi + \zeta_2.$$

For more complex examples of the use of the LISREL model and the LISREL computer program, see Chapter 69. An example of the application of the LISREL programme follows in Chapter 5.

5. School desegregation and peer acceptance: an application of LISREL to longitudinal data

BILL McGARVEY

Introduction

As Sörbom has suggested in Chapter 4, the LISREL model is a very general hypothesis-testing framework which is highly appropriate for longitudinal researchers. The present chapter provides two fairly simple examples which should help demonstrate the model's utility in a practical context.

The data for these examples are drawn from the author's dissertation, and represent an application of the LISREL model to the study of longitudinal factors in school desegregation. While the data provide an interesting substantive and applied base from which to operate, the inferences about desegregation which flow from these models should be treated as tentative. Originally, these data were collected by Gerard and Miller (1975) as part of a massive, comprehensive study of the effects of school desegregation—the Riverside School Study (RSS). One of the areas of importance to these researchers concerned the antecedents of classroom acceptance, as it was assumed by earlier researchers (e.g., Coleman *et al.* 1966) that such peer acceptance was conducive to, and/or necessary for the 'lateral transmission of achievement values'—a process presumed to be of benefit to the minority child.

Subjects for the present data were 241 white and 117 minority children attending the Riverside, California school district in the academic years 1965–6 (Year 1 herein) and 1966–7 (Year 2 herein). Their initial grades ranged from kindergarten through fifth grade. The children were measured on several dimensions, of which only a few are analysed here. Minority students in the present analyses were selected as subjects here because they were attending segregated schools in Year 1 and desegregated schools in Year 2. The question of essential interest in the present analyses revolves around the effects of pre-desegregation academic ability on the acceptance of minority children in the desegregated classroom. To examine this question, ten measures have been selected. They are listed in Table 5.1, along with the relevant second-order partial

TABLE 5.1

Second-order partial correlations, means, and standards deviations†

Measure	Acronym	SPOP66	WPOP66	PPOP66	SPOP67	WPOP67	PPOP67	VACH66	PEAIQ66	RAVIQ66
Seating choices 1966	SPOP66		0·608	0·485	0·306	0·279	0·129	0·074	0·106	0·340
Work choices 1966	WPOP66	0·540		0·401	0·280	0·281	0·041	0·078	0·108	0·179
Play choices 1966	PPOP66	0·562	0·526		0·146	0·171	0·173	0·146	0·066	0·085
Seating choices 1967	SPOP67	0·459	0·320	0·313		0·534	0·261	−0·035	−0·021	−0·020
Work choices 1967	WPOP67	0·412	0·469	0·313	0·641		0.280	0·145	0.095	0·121
Play choices 1967	PPOP67	0·368	0·337	0·369	0·601	0·480		0·181	−0·075	−0·123
Verbal achievement	VACH66	0·255	0·278	0·155	0·199	0·281	0·204		0·336	0·197
Peabody vocabulary	PEAIQ66	0·126	0·119	0·104	0·125	0·130	0·119	0·392		0·161
Raven matrices	RAVIQ66	0·005	0·096	−0·026	0·099	0·199	0·082	0·404	0·408	
White mean		4·120	3·979	3·892	3·963	4·129	3·900	108·112	110·876	107·423
Minority mean		3·701	3·718	3·932	3·026	2·786	3·667	94·513	92·376	93·880
White S.D.		2·583	2·626	3·224	2·465	2·567	3·284	14·339	12·419	14·332
Minority S.D.		2·102	2·038	2·518	1·684	1·665	2·663	9·563	9·554	12·859

† Initial grade and sex are partialled out; minority intercorrelations are above the main diagonal, while white intercorrelations are below the main diagonal.

correlations (controlling for initial grade and sex), means and standard deviations for whites and minorities. A short description of each follows.

Constructs and measures

Peer acceptance. According to Moreno (1934) and others, perhaps one of the best ways to assess acceptance or popularity is through tallied peer nominations—the essence of sociometry. In each classroom where a subject could be found, all children were asked three questions:

(1) If you could sit next to anybody in this class, who would it be (i.e., seating choice, or SPOP)?;

(2) If you could pick anybody in this class to do school work with, who would it be (i.e., work choice, or WPOP)?;

(3) If you could pick anybody in this class to be on your ball team at recess, who would it be (i.e., play choice, or PPOP)?

Each child in the class made three choices for each question. Each Riverside school study subject's sum of choices received from classmates was then computed for each school year. For further discussion, see Gerard *et al.* (1975).

Academic ability. Two standard measures of academic ability on which the RSS sample were tested included: (1) the Raven Progressive Matrices (RAVIQ); and (2) the Peabody Picture Vocabulary Test (PEAIQ). State-mandated achievement tests were also administered to the children each school year. Sundry in label and protean in composition, these tests are more fully described elsewhere (see for example, Singer *et al.* 1975). Present analyses utilized the standardized verbal achievement test scores (VACH).

An inspection of means suggests that white and minority students received about the same number of choices pre-desegregation; post-desegregation, however, whites received a greater number of choices than minorities. Measured white academic ability was greater than that of minorities on all three variables of interest.

But the question of further interest here is whether being a brighter student aided in classroom acceptance in Year 2—for both whites and minorities. To address this question in more detail, we turn to one of the plausible structural models which could underlie this data.

A LISREL model

It is often convenient to depict hypothesized structural models through path diagrams. In Fig 5.1, note that the three unmeasured constructs 'academic ability' (ACDABIL), 'peer acceptance 1' (PRACCP1), and 'peer acceptance 2' (PRACCP2) are depicted in circles, while the measured variates are depicted in rectangles.† The arrows from the circles to the squares denote the factor loadings (or alternatively, path coefficients) of the measured variables. The additional paths from the δs and εs denote the combined measure-specific and random error components of each variate. The algebra of LISREL, discussed in Chapter 4 by Sörbom as well as in Jöreskog and Sörbom (1977), treats the data in terms of *measurement equations* and *structural equations*. The measurement equations relate the observed variates to the constructs, while the

---

† It should be apparent to the reader that this is not the only plausible model here. The assumption of causal precedence which argues for the academic ability-to-peer-acceptance-1 linkage is certainly not like the temporal sequence linking popularity at time 1 with popularity at time 2. An alternative model, of course, would label *both* academic ability and peer acceptance 1 as exogenous (independent) variables, due to their synchronicity of measurement. For purposes of example, and given the theoretical position that whatever academic ability the child possesses is determined prior to acceptance, the models have been constructed as depicted here.

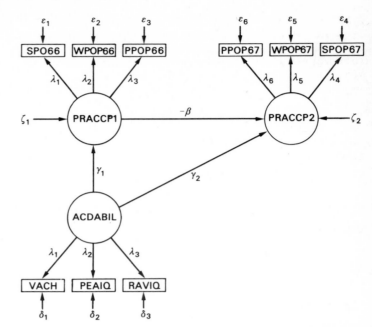

FIG. 5.1. A general model for testing the effects of academic ability on peer acceptance.

structural equations depict the relationships between the constructs. It should be noted, however, the LISREL makes all parameter estimates (in both the measurement and structural equations) simultaneously. The present data may be depicted in LISREL algebra as follows:

1. The measurement equation for the set of dependent variables (y).

$$\begin{bmatrix} \text{SPOP66} \\ \text{WPOP66} \\ \text{PPOP66} \\ \text{SPOP67} \\ \text{WPOP67} \\ \text{PPOP67} \end{bmatrix} = \begin{bmatrix} \lambda_1 & 0 \\ \lambda_2 & 0 \\ \lambda_3 & 0 \\ 0 & \lambda_4 \\ 0 & \lambda_5 \\ 0 & \lambda_6 \end{bmatrix} \cdot \begin{bmatrix} \text{PRACCP1} \\ \text{PRACCP2} \end{bmatrix} + \begin{bmatrix} \varepsilon_1 \\ \varepsilon_2 \\ \varepsilon_3 \\ \varepsilon_4 \\ \varepsilon_5 \\ \varepsilon_6 \end{bmatrix} \quad (1)$$

$$\underset{\sim}{y} = \underset{\sim}{\Lambda_y} \cdot \underset{\sim}{\eta} + \underset{\sim}{\varepsilon}$$

while for the independent variables (x), the measurement equation looks like

$$\begin{bmatrix} \text{VACH} \\ \text{PEAIQ} \\ \text{RAVIQ} \end{bmatrix} = \begin{bmatrix} \lambda_1 \\ \lambda_2 \\ \lambda_3 \end{bmatrix} \cdot \begin{bmatrix} \text{ACDABIL} \end{bmatrix} + \begin{bmatrix} \delta_1 \\ \delta_2 \\ \delta_3 \end{bmatrix} \quad (2)$$

$$\underset{\sim}{x} = \underset{\sim}{\Lambda_x} \cdot \underset{\sim}{\xi} + \underset{\sim}{\delta}$$

2. The structural equation for this data looks like

$$\begin{bmatrix} 1 & 0 \\ \beta & 1 \end{bmatrix} \cdot \begin{bmatrix} \text{PRACCP1} \\ \text{PRACCP2} \end{bmatrix} = \begin{bmatrix} \gamma_1 \\ \gamma_2 \end{bmatrix} \cdot \begin{bmatrix} \text{ACDABIL} \end{bmatrix} + \begin{bmatrix} \zeta_1 \\ \zeta_2 \end{bmatrix} \quad (3)$$

$$\underset{\sim}{B} \cdot \underset{\sim}{\eta} = \underset{\sim}{\Gamma} \cdot \underset{\sim}{\xi} + \underset{\sim}{\zeta}$$

By structuring the analyses around this general model, some very interesting tests and inferences can be made.

Within the LISREL-IV program there are actually eight matrices which are employed in the simultaneous theoretical decomposition of the observed variance–covariance or correlation matrix. Involved with the measurement equations are the $\underset{\sim}{\Lambda_y}, \underset{\sim}{\Lambda_x}, \underset{\sim}{\theta_\varepsilon}$, and

θ_δ matrices. The parameter estimates within these matrices reflect the communalities ($\underset{\sim}{\Lambda}_y$ and $\underset{\sim}{\Lambda}_x$) and errors ($\underset{\sim}{\theta}_\varepsilon$ and $\underset{\sim}{\theta}_\delta$) associated with each of the observed measures. The four matrices β, Γ, $\underset{\sim}{\Phi}$, and $\underset{\sim}{\Psi}$, reflect:

(1) The relationships among the dependent latent variables ($\underset{\sim}{\beta}$);
(2) The partial regression coefficients between the independent and dependent latent variables ($\underset{\sim}{\Gamma}$);
(3) The variances and covariances of the independent latent variables ($\underset{\sim}{\Phi}$);
(4) The variances and covariances among the unmeasured residuals ($\underset{\sim}{\Psi}$).

There is a great deal of versatility and a wide variety of options in the nature of these matrices which the LISREL-IV user can select. To illustrate, consider the following results from the minority and white data. The matrix set-ups are given in Table 5.2.

TABLE 5.2
Pattern matrices for LISREL

Variable	Matrix		
	$\underset{\sim}{\Lambda}_y$		
SPOP66	1·0†	0	
WPOP66	λ_1	0	
PPOP66	λ_2	0	
SPOP67	0	1·0†	
WPOP67	0	λ_3	
PPOP67	0	λ_4	
	$\underset{\sim}{\Lambda}_x$		
VACH66	λ_5		
PEAIQ66	λ_6		
RAVIQ66	λ_7		
	$\underset{\sim}{\beta}$		
PRACCP1	1·0	0·0	
PRACCP2	β	1·0	
	$\underset{\sim}{\Gamma}$		
PRACCP1	γ_1		
PRACCP2	γ_2		
	$\underset{\sim}{\Phi}$		
ACDABIL1	1·0		
	$\underset{\sim}{\Psi}$		
PRACCP1	ψ_{11}		
PRACCP2	0·0	ψ_{22}	
	$\underset{\sim}{\theta}_\varepsilon$		
SPOP66	ε_1		
WPOP66	0	ε_2	
PPOP66	0	0	ε_3
SPOP67	0	0	0 ε_4
WPOP67	0	0	0 0 ε_5
PPOP67	0	0	0 0 0 ε_6
	$\underset{\sim}{\theta}_\delta$		
VACH66	δ_1		
PEAIQ66	0	δ_2	
RAVIQ66	0	0	δ_3

† To fix the scale of the unmeasured variable, the assumption here is that it is measured in the same metric as SPOP. For further discussion, see Jöreskog and Sörbom (1977).

Minority data

In Fig. 5.2 the relevant coefficients as computed by LISREL-IV are depicted. (This data represents the standardized solution, wherein the variances of the endogenous, or dependent, variables are fixed to be 1·0). The X^2 test of fit suggests that for the minority data, the hypothesized overall model is doing an acceptable job of fitting the data ($X^2 = 34.85$, $df = 24$, $p = 0.0707$)†. The LISREL-IV pro-

† The reader should note that the usual logic of hypothesis-testing is reversed here. Instead of seeking statistical significance, the desired outcome in certain maximum-likelihood structural covariance analyses is non-significance. While this reversal may seem difficult to accept, there are further complications in terms of Type 1 – Type 2 error reversals and a unique loss function.

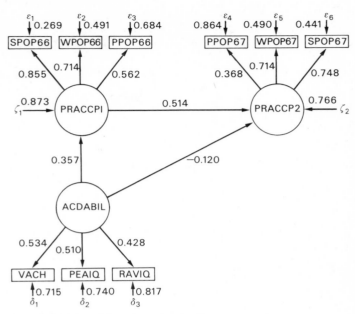

FIG. 5.2. Initial model results, minority data.

gram also calculates the standard error of each estimated parameter, so that separate significance tests and/or confidence-intervals around the parameters can be constructed. The only non-significant parameter computed here involves the direct path from academic ability to peer acceptance at Time 2 (unstandardized $\gamma = -0.090$, S.E. $= 0.124$, standardized $\gamma = -0.120$). Otherwise, the parameter estimates suggest the observed measures share a good deal of common variance (hence, the significant factor loadings) and the constructs are related. Substantively, these results suggest that the academic ability of minority children may aid in their becoming popular in the segregated classroom (in more familiar R^2 terms, academic ability appears to account for 12·7 per cent of the variance in initial popularity). This initial popularity in a segregated school certainly aids in peer acceptance in the desegregated school ($\beta = 0.514$)‡, but simply being bright may actually be little or no help whatsoever.

White data

While it does not offer a strictly appropriate control group for adequate inferences about the effects of desegregation, the white data for this model will serve both interesting substantive and heuristic purposes. The results from an initial test of the model in Fig. 5.1 with the white data are depicted in Fig. 5.3. (This is again, a standardized solution.) The overall fit of the model, however, is not very good ($X^2 = 61.82$, $df = 24$, $p = 0.0000$). But this event allows us to explore both the data and some LISREL-IV features further.

In an effort to aid exploratory research, the user can request the LISREL-IV program to print residuals and first-order derivatives. The object of LISREL, of course, is to determine some population variance–covariance matrix, $\underset{\sim}{\Sigma}$, based on the observed sample matrix, $\underset{\sim}{S}$, and the theoretical/methodological constraints placed on the solution. These printed residuals reflect the differences ($\underset{\sim}{\Sigma}$ - $\underset{\sim}{S}$), and offer some more exact indication where the model is not fitting. But an inspection of residuals is insufficient; hence the first-order derivatives must be considered conjointly with the residuals. Such an inspection here indicated that some measure-specific autocorrelation of the work-popularity variable was being underestimated. To examine the plausibility of this

‡ One of the peculiarities of the LISREL algebra is that the components within the θ matrix are reversed in sign from the 'true' nature.

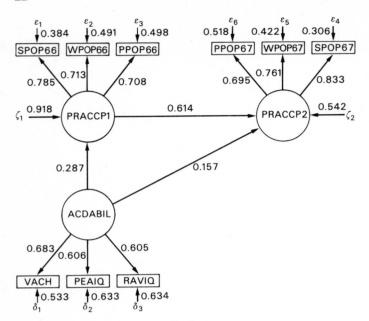

FIG. 5.3. Initial model results, white data.

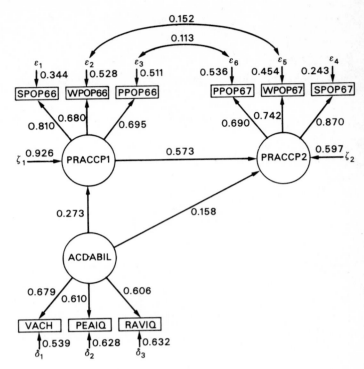

FIG. 5.4. Final model results, white data.

proposition, the appropriate off-diagonal parameter in the $\underset{\sim}{\theta}_\varepsilon$ (theta epsilon) matrix was freely estimated (i.e., not pre-set to zero).

This correlated residual term did appear to be contributing significantly to an improved fit. The second X^2 goodness-of-fit statistic dropped sharply from 61·82 to 46·14 ($df=23$, $p=0.0029$). As the difference in X^2 figures (15·68) is a X^2 test with one degree of freedom (and an associated $p<0.001$), and because the newly estimated parameter exceeded twice its standard error, it was deemed worth retaining.

But, while improved, the model still does not appear to be adequately fitting the data. In another attempt to improve the fit, the first-order derivatives and residuals were inspected. This examination suggested that the measure-specific components of the play popularity variable (PPOP66–PPOP67) were correlated. To take this very likely possibility into account, the relevant $\underset{\sim}{\theta}_\varepsilon$ parameter was freely estimated.

The results of these two additional model assumptions are displayed in Fig. 5.4. All estimated parameters here differ significantly from zero, and the model's fit is improved over the two earlier versions ($X^2=38.44$, $df=22$, $p=0.0164$). But it is still not doing a totally adequate job. Inspection of the minimization function F, and the size of the residuals suggested, however, that the white model was doing as good—or better—than the minority model. But the size of the white sample ($N=243$) is more than twice the size of the minority sample ($N=117$). It is this difference in sample sizes which has generated the impression of a 'poor' fit.

This case demonstrates exactly the sensitivity of the X^2 test to larger sample sizes. As I have argued elsewhere (McGarvey 1977), this means the X^2 test is important but should not be treated as the sole criterion of fit. In short, the final white model is doing acceptably well. A great deal more exploration might be made here, including the assumption of equal factor loadings and error terms.

There are a great many similarities between the white and minority models. The most glaring departure, however, concerns the direct path from academic ability to peer acceptance 2. For the minorities, it was negative (albeit non-significant), while for whites it was significantly positive. Hence, for whites, the data support the notion that academic ability is conducive to popularity in Year 2 not just by increasing peer acceptance in Year 1, but also by making an 'independent' contribution. Again, this does not appear to be the case for minority students. Their academic ability alone does not appear to be making them any friends in the desegregated schools. On the contrary, it may well work *against* their acceptance.

Summary

In this chapter, some minor explication and application of the LISREL model to longitudinal research has been presented. We have seen both the confirmatory and exploratory natures of the model (and the LISREL-IV computer program), in an analysis of the effects of academic ability upon peer acceptance in both segregated and desegregated schools. The sensitivity of the X^2 test to sample size has also been demonstrated, as well as the relative validity of the tested models. As long as longitudinal researchers are forced to rely on essentially correlational data which is contaminated by measurement error, the variety and generality of the LISREL model make it a preferred data-analytic tool. While the nature of each researcher's design and data may dictate a variety of models to be tested, the LISREL model may have something to offer to all.

Part III

Descriptions of longitudinal projects

A. Correlative longitudinal research
1. Normal, representative populations
a. Prospective birth cohort studies

6. The 1946 British birth cohort: an account of the origins, progress, and results of the National Survey of Health and Development

E. ATKINS, N. CHERRY, J. W. B. DOUGLAS, K. E. KIERNAN, and M. E. J. WADSWORTH

This chapter describes a national birth cohort study (The National Survey of Health and Development) and gives an account of the contributions it has made and is making to our understanding of abnormal behaviour. As the assessment of the value of this study must be reached through an understanding of the type of data collected and the methods used we have spent some pages describing this study. More detailed information will be found elsewhere (Douglas 1976).

Development of the study

The 5362 members of this birth cohort were born in England, Wales, and Scotland between the 3rd and 9th of March 1946, two years before the introduction of the National Health Service. The Royal Commission on Population needed answers to certain questions about the maternity services and the cost of having children, and it was decided to carry out a study by asking health visitors (community nurses) to interview mothers and complete questionnaires about all births occurring in one week. Health visitors were thought particularly appropriate since they worked in every part of the country, visited in the course of their normal duties more than 90 per cent of homes in which new births occurred, and had first-hand knowledge of the maternity and child welfare services as well as access to records. The interviews were completed between May and September 1946 and the results published in 1948 (Population Investigation Committee).

A short-term follow-up of this group was planned to examine the many social differences in infant and child morbidity and mortality. As funds were limited a sample was drawn. In order not to be restricted in making comparisons between children born of parents with different occupational levels a sample was taken which included all the non-manual workers' families, all the families of agricultural workers, and a randomly selected one-in-four sample of the remaining families, giving a sample of 5362 children. About half of these children had parents who were non-manual workers. Illegitimate children and twins were excluded. While the initial intention was to study this group for five years, the value of the information obtained was such that the term has been successively extended, the last contact (with 88 per cent of survivors still living in Great Britain) being made in 1977.

Two follow-up studies were carried out during the pre-school years, when children were aged two years and four years. On both occasions health visitors interviewed mothers at home using a structured and largely pre-coded questionnaire. The main aims of these studies were to obtain factual information about the development of the children, the accidents and illnesses they had, the circumstances of their families, and their use of welfare services and nurseries. Information was also gathered on the mother's employment, her hours of work, and the arrangements she made for looking after children.

The first follow-up study set a pattern that was repeated in following years. As the children grew older, school doctors, school teachers, youth employment officers, and the children themselves reported back to us. The aim was to make contact every two years or more frequently, and to continue to collect information that was largely factual. With school entry the focus of interest moved to educational progress. For four years the primary school teachers kept running records of school absences which were checked with the mothers. The first testing of ability and attainment was carried out when the children were eight. They completed, under their teacher's supervision, tests of mechanical reading, sentence completion, vocabulary, and picture intelligence. The National Foundation for Educational Research chose the tests and was responsible for checking and standardizing the results. Similar testing programmes were repeated when the children were aged eleven and fifteen, and at the ages of thirteen and fifteen their teachers were asked to rate a large number of items of behaviour in and out of the classroom. The heads of both primary and secondary schools described the school facilities available and the occupational group from which their pupils were drawn. During this time the medical interest of the survey was maintained. Complete records were kept of accidents, hospital admissions, and attendance at clinics, and four special medical examinations were undertaken by the school doctors when the children were aged six, seven, eleven, and fifteen years. All hospital admissions were checked with the institutions concerned.

The statutory school-leaving age for this sample was fifteen years, and by the end of the summer term 1961, half were in employment. These early leavers were seen by youth employment officers who carried out detailed interviews for the National Survey. Children who stayed on at school were contacted through their teachers. Thereafter, yearly contact was maintained by mail questionnaire followed up if necessary by calls from health visitors.

When the survey members were twenty-six years of age, trained and adequately briefed professional interviewers visited the homes and asked about the family and household structure, religious beliefs, training for work, type of employment (including levels of skill and responsibility), and earnings. Questions were also asked about the social origins, education, and employment history of the husband or wife, the survey member's views of society, and his membership of clubs and other organizations. Two tests were also given for a second time—the Watts–Vernon reading test first given at 15, and the short version of the Maudsley Personality Inventory first given at 16. A summary of all contacts with the survey members from birth to age 26 is given in Table 6.1.

Table 6.1

Overview of data collected since 1946

Age of child	Interview with mother	Medical examination	School information	Tests	Questionnaires, inventories by child
4–6 weeks	Antenatal care, mother's education and work, baby care, confinement, post-natal care, father's occupation.				
2 years	Child's development and health, mother's health.				
4 years	Accidents and health, hospital stay, use of welfare services.				
6 years	Accidents, health, toilet training habits, sleep and play, parents, education, school absence, and sickness record.	General examination and history; laterality.	School absence record.		
7 years	School absence through sickness and holidays.	General examination and history.	Sex and size of class, parents' interest, school absence record.		
8 years	Accidents, health, hospital and clinic attendances, school absence, attitudes to secondary schools, households and family.		School absence record.	Ability and attainment.	
9 years	Similar to 8 years.		School absence record.		
10 years			Streaming, class size, achievement and behaviour, parents' interest and home environment.		
11 years	Similar to 8 years.	General examination and history, sexual development, medical examination of 'controls'.	School facilities buildings, environment, record of transfer to secondary school.	Ability and attainment.	
13 years			Child's achievement, ratings of attitudes to work, behaviour, habits, personality.		Job ideas, hobbies, and interests. Personality inventory.
15 years	As in previous interviews, plus attitudes of parents to work and further education of child.	General examination and history, sexual development.	Ratings as at 13 years, school-leaving and guidance on careers, school facilities.	Ability and attainment.	Occupational interest inventory, attitudes to jobs and further education.
16 years			School-leaving and examinations, school-leaving of 'controls'.		

Table 6.1—*contd*

Survey members who had left full-time education			Survey members who were still in full-time education		
Age	Other Information	Questionnaires, interviews by youngster	Age	School, college information	Questionnaires
17 years	YEO rating of training, vocational guidance received. Technical college: course facilities.	Job choice, job history, training, apprenticeship, technical education, ambitions, pay, hobbies, health, M.P.I.	16 years	School-leaving, examinations, attendances.	Course, future career, part-time jobs, hobbies, health, M.P.I.
18 years	Technical college: course and achievement.	Job history and technical education. Job history of controls.	17 years	School-leaving, examinations, attendances.	
			18 years	School-leaving, examinations, attendances.	
19 years	Technical college: course and achievement.	Health visitor interview; health, marriage, babies, use of medical services, job history, technical education.	19 years	School-leaving examinations, attendances.	Health visitor interview; same as for those not in full-time education.
			19 years or more	Examination record, plans for further studies. Undergraduate group discussions.	Degree course details, vacation jobs, health, M.P.I.

All survey members		
Age	Other information	Questionnaires, interviews by members
20 years	Universities and colleges: course and achievement.	Postal questionnaire: similar to 19 years plus chest trouble and smoking, heights, and weights.
21 years	Parents' and sibs' eyesight.	Correspondence college information.
22 years	Universities and colleges: course and achievement.	Postal questionnaire: similar to 19 years, plus income and housing.
23 years		Postal questionnaire: similar to 19 years.
24 years	Universities and colleges: course and achievement.	
25 years		Postal questionnaire: similar to 20 years, plus income.
26 years	Checking of all recent hospital admissions. Clarification of education queries.	Marriage, children, housing, heights and weights, home and work stress, nervous troubles, religion, training, employment of spouse, father, father-in-law, spouse's education, perceptions of society, voting, membership of unions, and other organizations.

All survey members with a child of 4 years or more. Since 1969 an intensive interview has been carried out with each survey member (or, if a man, his wife) within six months of her first child reaching 4 years. A further interview and reading test is being carried out as these children reach 8 years.

In parallel with the main survey, a second-generation study was begun in 1969. This involves the families of all survey members when their first-born singleton children reach the ages of 4 and 8. This study makes use of the unique opportunity presented by the National Survey to record the behaviour of its respondents as parents, and to relate this information to the existing collection of life history data. Our findings on experience in the early years of life in the first generation consistently show their importance in educational achievement and in later illness and behaviour. It is, therefore, important to ask, as the second-generation study does, whether members of the original cohort whose early experiences have been shown to affect their later life also differ in the way they bring up their children and conduct their family life. This study is carried out in homes by professional interviewers, and in addition to questions put to mothers about family life, child-rearing, health

and sickness, preparation for school, and school experience, the children take three tests of attainment at age 8 years, and these are the same tests as those taken by the survey member parent at this age.

Losses and possible sources of bias

In a longitudinal study it is important to consider the extent of loss through refusals or failure to trace and the extent to which the characteristics of the sample may have been altered by the very fact that they were being kept under observation.

Losses. In the National Survey of Health and Development losses have been low—after 26 years they amount to 12 per cent. This is partly because in a national sample internal migration is not a source of loss, and partly because contact has been maintained at intervals of less than two years up to age 26, so that even after they left the educational system it has been possible to maintain contact with the survey members. Those lost to the survey through refusal or failure to trace are not substantially different from those we have kept in touch with. There is a slight excess loss of manual workers, particularly those in semi-skilled and unskilled occupations, but the resulting bias is not large enough to be a source of concern. More likely to be serious are hidden biases which may never be detected; for example parents who withdrew their child because they considered him or her stupid, or parents afraid that home visits would show dissension in the family.

Possible distortion through repeated study. There are dangers that members of a longitudinal study will be influenced by the fact of their inclusion. Questions relating, for example, to standards of care and health, use of the services, or educational or occupational aspirations may change parental attitudes and behaviour. Frequent medical examinations may lead to the treatment of conditions which otherwise would remain undetected. Repeated tests of ability and attainment may leave children with a test sophistication that others do not have. It is essential that any longitudinal study should be able to check these kinds of bias. The National Survey provided for a partial check by taking a quarter of the manual working class children, that is to say one-third of those rejected from the final sample, as a control group. Only two minor differences have so far been found—those in the control group being less likely than those in the main sample to have been prescribed glasses or to have had speech therapy.

Possible distortion in sampling method. It could also be argued that a sample of a complete week's births is in many ways not representative of a whole year's births. Respiratory infections in early infancy, for example, are likely to be fewer among those born in the spring than in the autumn, and so are accidental burns which are particularly likely to occur when a child is learning to walk. The season of the year is also important in relation to the age of entering school since those born between April and August may have up to a year more primary education than those born between September and December, and the results of this may show in reading and attainment. As it is possible and not unusual to leave school at the statutory leaving age, the date of birth also affects job opportunities for early leavers. While any season of the year has both advantages and disadvantages, the advantages predominate for those born in the spring.

Results

This chapter's aim is to discuss the contributions that a birth cohort study is making to psychiatric and related research. A more general discussion of results is however advisable to illustrate methods which could well be applied to psychiatric problems, though they have not as yet been so applied. A list of all publications can be obtained from the authors. The following comments on results refer to only a few of them. These comments are in two sections; the first describes a few studies of general interest and the second focuses on work that has some direct relevance to the study of abnormal behaviour.

Results of general interest

Local inequalities. The first study of this sample gave striking evidence of the variation in services provided by different maternity and child welfare authorities, and the lack of information about the effect of these differences on local maternal and child morbidity. The diversity of local provision in Britain has been defended as

providing natural experiments which can be used to see the effectiveness of different types of service. But if there is no assessment of the outcome this is a frivolous defence. Local variations were also evident in the provision of selective secondary school places, and the then Ministry of Education attributed them to differences in the local availability of independent schools and the unequal geographical distribution of ability. Both these explanations were found to be false in this study. Indeed, geographical variation in the provision of selective school places accounted for approximately half the social inequalities in secondary school selection, after taking account of ability. It was also argued that when selective schools were in short supply alternative courses would be provided in secondary modern schools and technical colleges. This, however did not hold and the adverse effects of local education deficiencies on achievement have been cumulative as these young people grew older. There is no reason to believe that the introduction of comprehensive education has fundamentally altered local differences in the quality of teaching or the overall level of educational provision, but it has made such differences more difficult to detect. Yet, unless these geographical inequalities are removed, the social inequalities will remain whatever type of secondary education we have, because those who value education for their children will move, if they can afford to do so, to areas where the services are known to be good. Where people live in Britain still influences their survival, health, education, and employment.

Selective education. The children in this sample were among the last to go through a wholly selective system of secondary education, and in order to understand the subsequent changes it is important to be able to look closely at the extent of support that a selective system gave or failed to give. Cherry (1974) has shown that Survey members' levels of ambition, as shown by preferences for jobs of high or low status, were influenced by the social classes from which the schools drew their pupils, as well as by the types of family individual pupils came from. For the same type of child the level of ambition is lower in schools which draw their pupils predominantly from the manual working class than in schools which have a more mixed or middle class catchment. This, however, only applied to secondary modern schools and in grammar schools the level of ambition was independent of the social composition of the school. In this sense the grammar schools in predominantly working class catchment areas were giving support to their pupils from whatever type of family they came.

The link between early events and illness and later health and behaviour. Chest illnesses in childhood were found to be linked with the current level of smoke pollution in the air and also with overcrowding in the home. Those with a history of early chest illness were more likely than others to complain of coughs at twenty years, and this association increased in strength as they grew older. At twenty-five years not only was the association of cough with early chest illness stronger than at twenty, but other circumstances in childhood such as smoke pollution and poor home conditions, which were not associated with the prevalence of symptoms at twenty, began to appear as pre-disposing factors in adult respiratory illness. It seems as if the aetiology of chronic bronchitis may extend back to lung damage in early childhood which has been silent in the intervening years (Kiernan *et al.* 1976).

The possibility that early illnesses or early traumatic events may have a postponed rather than an immediate effect emphasizes the need for longitudinal studies. Without them serious misconceptions may arise.

Topics of psychiatric interest

In the National Survey, 2 per cent of the sample had been treated, by the age of 26 years, as psychiatric in-patients—a further 18 per cent of young men and women had consulted a doctor about a nervous or psychiatric problem during the previous 12 years. Amongst those without such psychiatric difficulties, 20 per cent felt that, at 26 years, they were under some or severe nervous strain in their job or in their home or personal lives. This high toll of psychiatric distress is not the full picture; other survey members had a history of prolonged bed-wetting, of poor adjustment at school, of persistent job-changing, or of brushes with the law. The longitudinal data collected in the National Survey provide the opportunity to examine this wide range of related assessments, all having direct implications for mental health.

Early separation and adjustment problems. Some of the first, and clearest, reports of the effects of early separation in this sample arose from studies of enuresis. Rowntree (1955) showed that broken homes were associated with bed-wetting. This finding was extended in later studies of the same group (Douglas 1970, 1973). Children whose fathers had died were at no greater risk of bed-wetting at any age (4–15 years), and the frequent absence of a father had no apparent effect on the rate of enuresis. However, when the break was caused by divorce or separation, or by the death of the mother, a highly significant increase in rate was found. In this group, the highest proportions of bed-wetters were amongst those living in foster homes or institutions, or whose mothers remarried. Much lower rates (although still higher than in unbroken families) were found for those living with their mother alone. A more detailed analysis of the findings on delinquency and broken homes has been completed by Wadsworth (1979a). In relation to delinquency and broken homes it was found that a break before 4 years and 3 months was significantly associated with later delinquency in boys. Experience of parental divorce or separation or maternal death by this age was associated with an increased likelihood of committing officially reported sexual or violent offences, and to a lesser extent serious acquisitive crimes, by age 21 years. Other studies of enuresis in this cohort have shown no clear relationship between the birth of a younger child and the prevalence, at $4\frac{1}{4}$ years, of regular bed-wetting (Blomfield and Douglas 1956). Wadsworth (1979b) found a marked increase in delinquency amongst those boys whose relationship with their mother was disturbed, by age 4 years, by a subsequent birth. The arrival of a new baby also appeared to affect the response of a child to hospital admissions before the age of 5 years (Douglas 1975, see below). Wadsworth found that the effect of an early break (by divorce or separation) on delinquency is maintained after statistical adjustment for all available changes in material circumstances. Most interestingly, he also finds (Wadsworth 1976) a lower pulse rate, in a mildly stressful situation, amongst boys from homes with early breaks, whether or not they become delinquent. Low pulse rates are also found amongst delinquents from unbroken homes who commit crimes of violence or sexual offences. The death of the father appears to have little or no effect on enuresis or delinquency. However, current work suggests that the marriage and fertility patterns of girls without fathers are markedly different from those from unbroken homes. A study of ill and disabled parents (Douglas *et al.* 1968) also suggests untoward effects of the death of the father. Boys and girls whose fathers died following a protracted illness, had markedly depressed scores on tests of ability and attainment at 15 years even after allowance for family circumstances such as housing (shown by Rowntree 1955, to deteriorate following a break in the family).

Fortunately only a small proportion of children in the survey (5 per cent) experienced a break in their parents' marriage before they reached the age of 5 but many more (20 per cent) entered hospitals before this age. The effects of such admissions have been extensively studied by Douglas (1975). He found that both single admissions of more than a week's duration and repeated admissions between the age of 6 months and $3\frac{1}{2}$ years were related at 13 and 15 years to troublesome (but not nervous) behaviour in school, accord-

ing to teachers' ratings, and to low reading scores at 15 years. Long or repeated admissions to hospitals were also related to delinquency and to frequent job-changing amongst early school leavers, but only when a hospital admission had also occurred after the 5th birthday. First admissions after the age of 5 did not lead to an increase in any of the measures of poor adjustment in adolescence. This study also shows that poor adjustment was more likely to result from early hospital admissions if a new baby had been born in the previous 6 months. In addition, it appears that only children (possibly over-protected), those competing with older sibs, and those whose mothers started to work outside the home about the time of hospital admission, were particularly vulnerable to later effects. Children whose mothers had started work some time before the admission (and who, it might be thought, had become used to alternative care) were somewhat protected from the effect of hospital admissions.

Other factors associated with poor adjustment. Although early hospitalization does relate to poor adjustment, a number of other medical factors—persisting disability (Douglas 1975), low birth weight (Douglas and Gear 1976), and measles (Douglas 1964b)—do not appear to increase the likelihood of a child being rated as poorly adjusted by his teachers. Birth spacing and social class also had little effect on teachers' ratings at age 15 (Douglas *et al.* 1968b), although they have been shown by Wadsworth (1978) to relate to delinquency. Working class girls are more likely than girls from middle class homes to be bed-wetters up to the age of 11 years (Blomfield and Douglas 1956). Working class girls are also more likely to have pre-marital conceptions. Features of the school are statistically related to measures of adjustment; delinquency was less amongst those who had attended primary schools with a good academic record, and pupils at secondary modern schools were rated as more aggressive than selective school pupils. It is also of interest that children up to 11 years of age who have been in many accidents are more likely to be rated by secondary school teachers as being aggressive (Douglas *et al.* 1968). Backward children who later entered ESN schools were frequently seen by teachers as experiencing particular difficulties in getting along with other children at the primary schools.

The effects of poor adjustment. Several of the studies already mentioned have used poor school adjustment to explain other forms of behaviour. Thus the poor reading scores of those with early hospital admissions were largely accounted for by reports of a poor attitude to school work, and delinquents were reported to have significantly worse adjustment at school than other boys. In a further study (Cherry 1976b) boys and girls with low school attendance and poor tractability in the last year at school, were shown to be less likely than other early school leavers to settle at work. Douglas *et al.* (1968b) found that 15 year olds rated by their teachers as being either nervous or aggressive, who were reported as having certain symptoms (stammering, nail biting, thumb sucking, and so on), or who chose many neurotic responses on a self-report inventory, all had lower scores on the ability and attainment tests completed at 8, 11, and 15 years. The only group, however, who showed a progressive deterioration in test performance during their years at school were those unfavourably identified on all 3 assessments (teachers' ratings, symptoms, and neuroticism scores).

The study of hospitalization showed that the outcome of early separation could be manifested in a number of ways, any one child being likely to show only one 'symptom' of maladjustment. This variety of response was also found in studies of delinquency and of persistent job-changing. Those who had had many jobs by age 18 were found, in the following 7 years, to be more likely than other young workers to have an illegitimate child, to enter upon a marriage that had broken by age 26, to spend much time unemployed, or to report psychiatric problems. Similarly those boys incorrectly predicted as delinquent, by a discriminant analysis using data on early disruption, had a higher prevalence of admission to psychiatric hospitals, and of stomach, peptic and duodenal ulcers, and colitis by age 26 years (Wadsworth 1978). Finally, men who obtained high neuroticism scores at age 16, who had recorded psychiatric problems between 15 and 26 years of age, and who lived under stress in their personal lives, were more likely than other men in full time work to report occupational stress. Neuroticism (and extroversion) also increases the probability of cigarette smoking, neurotic introverts being least likely to give up the habit (Cherry and Kiernan 1976). Other analyses being carried out suggest a slight social class gradient amongst survey members consulting a doctor with nervous problems. Middle class survey members are more likely than manual workers to report such visits to the doctor. An even stronger social class gradient in the same direction was found to reflect reports of nervous strain.

Future studies

The information on psychiatric illness, checked with hospital records, has only recently become available, and work has now started on the relationship between overt psychiatric stress to the age of 26 years, early separation, and social and employment factors. The National Survey sample is to be followed up for at least a further ten years, and one of its main concerns will be the changing incidence of psychiatric illness in the years leading to middle-age. For studies of psychiatric adjustment, the next years of the cohort's life will also be of great importance, and will provide information on the latent effects of early experience that could be obtained by no other method.

Conclusions on the potential contribution of the 1946 cohort to the study of psychiatric illness

The 1946 cohort should provide an exceptional opportunity to test hypotheses about the relation between disturbing or traumatic events and manifestations of psychiatric illness. Not only are major events and the general circumstances of life recorded concurrently or nearly so, but those who show psychiatric disturbance can be compared with a complete population. Our information on psychiatric hospital inpatient admissions is satisfactory as we have been able to check the information provided by the sample members with the Department of Health's Psychiatric Register and with the hospitals concerned. It is less satisfactory for those who went no further than their family doctor or those who did not seek any

treatment. No doubt our information on these persons can be improved. It might also be possible to use a screening inventory and follow it up with a psychiatric interview, although this would be expensive and difficult to organize.

All life events that have appeared to us as major have been recorded, but we do not know whether the survey members themselves also perceived these as major events or whether they would have seen other and apparently more trivial events as outstanding. Our information on home circumstances is detailed, ranging from health visitors' assessments of care to the extent of help given by husbands and others, sleeping arrangements, and household amenities. We have not attempted to assess the quality of the marriages though much can be inferred from the part played by the husband in the day-to-day running of the home or in contacts with his child. While our data lack subtlety they are sufficient to test some of the hypotheses that relate life events to the onset of psychiatric illness. Moreover our wide range of information at all ages allows us to look at associations that could only come from a longitudinal study, e.g. the sharing of a parent's bedroom or bed after a bereavement, followed by ejection on remarriage. We can also observe the extent to which events that for some people are associated with nervous illness are in others associated with different types of disturbance (for example educational failure, delinquency, job instability, or unusual patterns of marriage and fertility), some of which may themselves be mediating factors in the later development of psychiatric illness.

Lastly there are two later birth cohorts in Britain, started in 1958 and 1970. In time these studies will enable us to see changes in the prevalence of different types of psychiatric illness in the country as a whole as well as in different sections of the population. We will also be able to assess the impact of new services and policies, and gauge how far they are meeting the needs of those they were intended to help. It could be maintained that these answers will be long, perhaps too long, in coming, but this is the nature of the situation and quick answers are not worth having. While the expenditure involved may appear large when measured against the cost of many short-term research projects, these expenses are small when measured against the cost of the services that are being assessed.

Because of their unique value in assessing the effectiveness of new policies it would be worthwhile to establish a series of national longitudinal cohort studies spaced apart by ten or fifteen years. Comparisons between the studies would then show relationships between the establishment of new services and later changes in health, growth, and behaviour. With careful planning this method will continue to advance scientific knowledge in psychiatry and other branches of medicine and the human sciences.

7. The National Child Development Study (1958 British cohort)

KEN FOGELMAN and PETER WEDGE

Introduction

Many people have been involved in this study over the years and we have tried to reflect their contribution in this chapter. In particular we should like to thank those many past and present colleagues on whose work we have drawn liberally.

The 16 000 subjects of this interdisciplinary project are now aged nineteen; information was obtained at the time of their birth and on three further occasions, the last at the age of sixteen. In a number of respects this study followed a pattern not dissimilar to that of a longitudinal study of children born in one week twelve years earlier

(Douglas, 1964a) except that in the case of the project described in this chapter the total sample of births has been followed up throughout, enabling special studies of particular groups to be carried out, and in our study we did not maintain regular contact with the subjects but retraced them at each follow-up.

Historical origins

In 1958, a study was mounted by the National Birthday Trust Fund of all births in England, Scotland, and Wales in the week 3–9

March, 1958. At that time the British perinatal mortality rate, that is the proportion of babies who were either stillborn or died within seven days of birth, was 35 per 1000 births, and the main purpose of the study was to examine social and obstetric factors associated with such deaths. To this end, the study successfully obtained information on some 98 per cent of the total births (about 17 000) registered as occurring during that week.

By investigating the factors related to mortality risk and the well-being of the new-born baby, this research demonstrated many facts which are now commonplace and was able to give numerical precision to often observed relationships. It showed, for example, that the risk of a perinatal death was 50 per cent higher than average if the mother was having her fifth or subsequent baby, and was 30 per cent higher in mothers who smoked heavily during pregnancy compared to non-smokers. The major findings of the perinatal study are summarized in two books. (Butler and Alberman 1969; Butler and Bonham 1963).

Twelve years previously, in 1946, a team led by J. W. B. Douglas had also studied children born in Britain during the same week, and subsequently has followed up about a third of the sample at regular intervals. The success of this study prompted considerable interest in the possibility of following up the 1958 cohort of births.

Strong representations from Dr Pringle, Director of the National Children's Bureau, Professor Butler, an eminent paediatrician, and Professor Wall, then Director of the National Foundation for Educational Research, were made to a Government committee set up to look into primary school education (the Plowden Committee). Following this, in 1964, the Department for Education and Science agreed to commission the National Children's Bureau to collect information on all these children when they were seven. This follow-up study of all the surviving children became known as the National Child Development Study (NCDS), and the first major publication also appeared as an Appendix to the Plowden Committee report (Pringle *et al.* 1966). At the time the study was instituted the aims were summarized as follows:

Short-term

(a) To study the educational, behavioural, emotional, social, and physical development of a large and representative group of British children in order to gather normative data; to investigate the complex interrelationships between the many facets, both normal and deviant, of children's development; and to report the incidence of handicaps with the provision currently being made.

(b) To utilize the uniquely comprehensive perinatal data, already available, in an evaluation of the relationships between conditions during pregnancy and at birth, both medical and social, and the development of children in all its aspects at the age of 7 years.

Long-term

(a) To explore the constancy and change in the pattern of children's development longitudinally, and to investigate the associated educational, environmental, and physical factors.

(b) To follow the progress—over a long period—of those children who at birth might be considered at risk in order to evaluate possible latent effects; and also to examine any post-natal factors, environmental, educational, or medical, which may minimize a handicap.

(c) To identify and follow the progress of children who at 7 years of age are already handicapped or showing signs of difficulty: those who because of adverse social or other circumstances might be considered at risk of becoming educationally backward or socially deviant; and those who display exceptional talent or aptitude.

(d) To evaluate the efficiency of medical and educational provisions for handicapped, deviant, and exceptional children.

(e) To identify groups of children of special interest, including many of of those identified under (c) and (d) above, so that intensive studies may be mounted by expert teams. This would permit much more detailed and comprehensive investigation of the factors involved against a backcloth of the necessarily cruder data gathered in the follow-up of the whole cohort.

The longitudinal structure of the study

Explicit in the above aims is the intention that in addition to the general study of the entire cohort there would be special studies of appropriate subgroups. We shall return to this question in a later section (Related Studies), concentrating first on the mainstream work.

To date there have been three full follow-ups of the entire cohort. As already mentioned the first took place in 1965, when the children were aged seven. To a certain extent this date was dictated by circumstances in that it coincided with the interest of the Plowden Committee and thus with the availability of finance. However it also coincides with an important stage in the progress of British school children. For most children in Britain primary schooling covers the ages from five to eleven (twelve in Scotland). This is further subdivided into the infant period (usually from five to seven) and the junior period (from eight to eleven). These periods of education generally take place in distinct schools or in separate departments within one primary school. Thus at the time of the first follow-up, the majority of the NCDS children would be in their final year of infants' schooling and about to transfer to a new department or new school.

The second follow-up was planned to coincide with the next major change in most British children's schooling. The age of eleven, for most English and Welsh children (but not Scottish), marks the end of primary schooling and transfer to secondary schools, and it was in the final year of their junior schooling (1969) that the second follow-up took place.

The third and most recent follow-up took place in 1974, the year in which the members of the cohort reached their sixteenth birthday, and their final year of compulsory schooling (the minimum leaving age having just been raised from fifteen and the NCDS cohort being part of the year-group first affected by this decision).

All three follow-ups have explored medical, educational, and social aspects (described in detail in a later section), and have been mounted by the National Children's Bureau, a London-based independent, interdisciplinary organization which is engaged in a wide range of research and other work.

Resources, staffing and co-operation

The siting of the study in a single institution responsible for its execution is undoubtedly one reason why it has been able to continue. Another reason can be found in the relatively high degree of centralization of education, health, and welfare services in Britain, which has helped to make it possible to maintain contact with almost all of the children in the study. Although much of the responsibility for the provision of these services has lain with Local Authorities at town, city and county levels, there is considerable co-ordination by central government; and local staff are used to providing information to central agencies.

Funds for each of the major follow-ups have come mainly from public sources such as the Department of Education and Science, the Department of Health and Social Security, and the Social

Science Research Council. Additional grants for specific analyses or for the study of special groups have come from a variety of sources—other government departments, several private trusts, and, recently, the U.S. National Institute of Education in Washington, D.C. While the study has managed to obtain the money for specific projects which enables it to continue, it has not so far proved possible to secure long-term financial support, and hence to carry out the kind of forward planning which would most benefit the study.

In general the funding has been adequate to enable the study to progress satisfactorily, although for the second follow-up it proved possible to obtain only enough money to mount the follow-up, collect the data, and carry out preliminary analysis. Fortunately, it subsequently became possible to remedy this, as the funds for the third follow-up allowed for a sufficiently large research team to continue to analyse the data already collected at the same time as preparing for the next stage, and additionally various related studies were mounted (see below).

Inevitably in a study of this size and duration there has been considerable staff turnover, although stability and continuity have been provided by the siting of the study in the National Children's Bureau. In particular Dr Mia Pringle, the Bureau's Director, has been closely involved with the study since its inception. Further continuity has been provided by the involvement of Professor Neville Butler who directed the original perinatal study and co-directed the first and second follow-ups, Professor Ronald Davie, who was Senior Research Officer at the time of the first follow-up and then co-director as well as Deputy Director of the Bureau at the time of the second, Professor Harvey Goldstein who was part-time Statistician during the first follow-up, and then became and remained until recently the Bureau's Principal Statistician, and Peter Wedge who was Senior Research Officer at the time of the second follow-up and is now Deputy Director of the Bureau. In addition, Professors Butler and Davie have been and continue as Honorary Consultants to the study, together with Professors Wall, Healey, and Tanner.

Changes in the research team responsible for the day-to-day work in the study have tended to coincide with the transition from work on one follow-up to preparation for the next. For example, there has been only one change among the present eight members of the research team since the beginning of the third follow-up, but on the other hand, only one of the eight was working on the study when the second follow-up was being carried out.

As well as changes in actual personnel there has been substantial variation in the size of the research team. For example at the time of its inception in 1965 there were three researchers with the support of one part-time statistician, and now in 1977 there are eight researchers and two statisticians.

From the point of view of those working on the study perhaps one of its most stimulating attributes has been the multi-disciplinary composition of the research team, resulting from both the general aims of the study set out above, and the philosophy of the National Children's Bureau. The academic disciplines of the present research team encompass education, medicine, psychology, biology, sociology, social work, and statistics.

Like many projects this study depends on the support and involvement of a wide range of professionals and professional organizations representing those concerned with child development and children's services. At appropriate stages throughout the study we have discussed our intentions with relevant bodies and invited the support of them and their members for our work.

Maintaining and tracing the sample

Other longitudinal studies have put major efforts, often very sucessfully, into maintaining permanent, ongoing contact with their subjects. For three main reasons such an approach would not have been the most efficient one for the NCDS. First, there is the sheer size of the sample (over 16 000), which would make the exercise extremely expensive. Second, the period between follow-ups has never been less than four years, so that the effort would not be justified by the frequency with which information has been collected. Third, the sample for each follow-up consists of all those now in the country who were born in the week 3–9 March, 1958 (that is, not only the original birth cohort, but all those born in the same week who have entered the country subsequently). Those new to the study would therefore have to be identified and traced at each stage in any case.

In Britain it is not permitted to utilize census and other similar information obtained by central and local government. Data linkage such as practised in some countries is not possible and thus our strategy has been to trace the children afresh for each stage of the study. The basic procedure has been to circulate all schools to ask them to inform us of the name and home address of all children on their registers with a relevant date of birth. In the case of state schools, this was carried out on our behalf by local education authorities, while the Bureau contacted independent schools directly. Once these school lists were returned to the Bureau they had then to be matched with the records from previous follow-ups so that the serial number identifying each child for all stages of the study could be allocated.

This brief summary gives no indication of the detailed work often necessary—the misspelt names, the uncertainties about dates of birth, the difficulties of identifying with certainty which of the children with identical names and birth-dates is the correct one to match with earlier information when both have changed their addresses and schools frequently, and the inevitable, countless reminder letters.

At each follow-up, approximately 90 per cent of the NCDS children were traced by this basic procedure. Further steps were then taken to trace the remainder. Local Health Authorities supplied the names of children outside the school system for whose care they were responsible, last known addresses were written to and newspapers carried requests for parents to contact us. Finally the names of those few remaining who had been in the study previously, but with whom no contact had been made this time, were submitted to the National Health Service Central Register who were able to inform us of any death or emigrations of which we had not previously known.

We have throughout the study considered it essential that no information be obtained about the children or their families without the knowledge and consent of the parents. Therefore, at each follow-up, as soon as a child was traced, a letter was sent to parents informing them that a further follow-up was to take place, indicating its general nature and asking them to let us know if they did not wish to take part. It was possible, as some did, to opt out of only part of the follow-up, or out of only the current follow-up, or to request to take no further part at all in the study. The replies are discussed further below (see Response section).

Methods of data collection

At each of the three follow-ups, information has been obtained from four main sources: the children themselves, the parents, Local Authority Medical Officers, and schools.

A more detailed account of the data collected is given below, but in summary:

At age seven, the child's direct contribution to the study was limited to the completion of tests administered in school, but at age eleven and sixteen each child also completed a questionnaire.

At each age the parents (in fact most commonly the mother alone) were interviewed in the home by a Local Authority Health Visitor, who completed a pre-coded form in the course of the interview.

At each age, each child received a full medical examination from a Local Authority Medical Officer, who again completed a pre-coded form, additionally using some information available from medical records to help in compiling a medical history.

At each age, the schools (usually the headteacher and class-teacher(s)) completed a questionnaire providing information on the school and on the study child.

The lists below give an indication of the contents of these instruments. However, they are not exhaustive, and it is clearly not possible here to go into considerable detail on each variable.

Tests

At seven

Southgate reading test (Southgate 1962)—a test of word recognition and comprehension particularly suited to identifying backward readers.
Copying designs test—to obtain some assessment of the child's perceptuo-motor ability.
Drawing a man test (Goodenough 1926)—as an indication of the child's general mental and perceptual ability.
Problem arithmetic test (Pringle *et al.* 1966).

At eleven

General ability test (Douglas 1964b)—containing verbal and non-verbal items.
Reading comprehension test—constructed by the National Foundation for Educational Research in England and Wales (NFER) specifically for use in this study.

At sixteen

Reading comprehension test—same test as at eleven.
Mathematics test—constructed by the NFER for use with this age group.

The unreferenced tests are unpublished, but copies and technical details are available from the National Children's Bureau.

Study child's questionnaire

At eleven, this was relatively brief, and contained questions on leisure activities and attitudes to school. Each child was also asked to write a short composition on the life he imagined he would be leading at the age of 25.

At age sixteen a more substantial questionnaire included questions on: attitudes to school and to methods of punishment in school, future educational and occupational expectations and aspirations, reasons for leaving school and choosing a job, school absences, self-ratings in school subjects, spare-time work, income and pocket money, intentions about marriage and having children, sex education and preparation for parenthood, leisure activities, family relationships, smoking and drinking, and handedness.

Parental interview

There have been variations from age to age, but in general the following areas have been covered: family composition, father's and mother's occupation, length of parents' education, smoking habits, aspirations and expectations for child's future education and occupation, family relationships, parent–school contacts, sources of income and indices of poverty (including at age sixteen only, details of household income), housing circumstances, child's general health and information on accidents, hospital admissions and visits to doctor, and details of medical history relating to vision, hearing,

speech therapy, convulsions, asthma, migraine, enuresis, psychiatric problems, dental care, and pubertal development.

At ages eleven and sixteen parents also answered questions which combine to give an index of behaviour in the home (Rutter *et al.* 1970b). Individual items of this scale also provide useful information, for example concerning truancy.

Medical examination

The medical officer obtained information on aspects of medical history, similar to that obtained from parents. He or she recorded the results of tests of near and distant vision, hearing, speech, and motor co-ordination and measured the child's height and weight. In the course of a systematic examination, results were recorded of any findings relating to skin conditions, hernias, respiratory tract infections and any defects in the cardiovascular system, the alimentary tract, the urogenital system, bones and joints, and the neuromuscular system.

At eleven and sixteen, the medical officers assessed the child's pubertal development.

School questionnaire

For obvious reasons, there has been considerable variation in detail according to the age of the child, but, in general, the areas covered include type and size of school, social composition and academic record of school, provision for sex education and career advice, parent–school contacts, disciplinary methods used, size and nature of child's class, ability ratings, likely examination entries, details of any special provisions for the child, attendance records, prediction of future educational and occupational progress, and ratings of parental interest.

At each age teachers completed a standardized instrument to provide a description of the child's behaviour in school. At seven and eleven, this was the Bristol Social Adjustment Guide (Stott 1963), and at sixteen the school version of the home behaviour scale referred to above was used.

Response

All involved in longitudinal studies are very aware of the importance of maintaining a good response rate. Where analyses incorporate information collected on several occasions, poor response rates can have a dramatic effect on the numbers available with sufficiently complete data to be included in an analysis. Further, as one of the aims of the NCDS is to provide normative data at each age, it is important also to be able to demonstrate that the responding sample retains the national representativeness of the original cohort.

The response rates obtained by the NCDS are summarized in Table 7.1. Since the target population for each follow-up or sweep consists essentially of those known to be alive and in the country at the time of the previous follow-up (although not precisely, since children born in the same week but newly in the country are also included), the main figures to note in Table 7.1 are the 91·2 per cent on whom information was obtained at seven, 90·9 per cent at eleven and 87·3 per cent at sixteen. The probable reasons for this slight decline are interesting and demonstrate some of the practical problems met by studies of this kind.

Of course, those who refused to take part were not required to give any reason for this, but in fact two reasons were mentioned fairly frequently at the 16-year follow-up. The first reason given stems from the fact that the school year in which our work was taking place was the one in which many children were preparing for the public examinations taken by the majority of British school children at this time. Some parents clearly felt that our requests would place extra stress on their children which they preferred to

TABLE 7.1

Basic distributions (percentages)

	Age	Total	N	Some data	Refusal	No data†	Untraced†	Emigrant at sweep‡	Deaths since and including previous sweep
(a)	Birth All children	100·0	17 733	98·2		1·8		—	—
(b)	7 years All children	100·0	18 118	85·0	0·5	7·7		2·3	4·5
	(Excluding deaths and emigrants)	100·0	16 883	91·3	0·5	8·3		—	—
(c)	11 years All children	100·0	18 365	83·3	4·5	3·9		3·8	4·5
	(Excluding deaths and emigrants)	100·0	16 835	90·0	4·9	4·1		—	—
(d)	16 years All children	100·0	18 578	79·5	6·2	2·3	3·1	4·3	4·7
	(Excluding deaths and emigrants)	100·0	16 915	87·3	6·7	2·5	3·4	—	—

† At the ages of 7 and 11 years, for technical reasons, the separate figures for 'no data' and 'untraced' are unavailable.
‡ Some of the emigrants at earlier ages returned later and are included in the above figures. In all 1013 had ever emigrated by the age of 16 (5·5 per cent of the sixteen-year-old total).

avoid. Many such refusers did not appear antipathetic to the study in general and often expressed their willingness to take part again in any later stage.

Second, the carrying out of a National Census in 1971—three years before our follow-up—had created considerable public discussion and some adverse publicity concerning privacy and confidentiality. It was clear that for a small minority this was the cause of animosity to surveys in general—including the National Child Development Study.

The increase in those who were traced, but for whom no further data were obtained, was probably in part due to a more passive kind of refusal—people who did not actually write, but were not co-operative when approached for information—but undoubtedly this was exacerbated to some extent by the reorganization of local government in this country on 1 April 1974. This meant that staff who were responsible for forwarding our material to schools, medical officers, and health visitors could often find themselves working for a new authority and with totally different responsibilities, and this exactly at the time when the circulation of our material was at its height. Of course, we had taken some steps to cope with this, and local authority staff dealt with the situation splendidly, but a few children were missed as a result.

Although the overall response rate compares well with other surveys, the proportion without data is quite large enough to introduce the possibility of bias in the responding sample. It is in this area that longitudinal studies have an advantage which is too rarely stressed. By their nature they can establish the characteristics of the non-responding group by using data from an earlier stage on subjects missed from the current stage.

Extremely detailed analyses of this kind have been carried out in relation to the latest follow-up (Fogelman 1976). There has been found to be no bias in the responding sample at sixteen in relation to parent's education, occupation, attitudes, and aspirations for the child, or indices of physical development. There is a slight relationship with physical circumstances of the home, and the largest biases are found in relation to minority groups of disadvantaged children. For example, children who had been receiving special education because of handicap and children born illegitimately are slightly underrepresented at sixteen. Although such biases indicate the need for caution, they are not very large. For example 3·4 per cent of the total cohort are known to have been born illegitimate, whereas the figure for those with information at sixteen is 3·2 per cent.

In addition to such checks on representativeness it is possible to repeat longitudinal analyses using data collected up to the age of eleven, but omitting those for whom data were not obtained at sixteen. This has been done for several such analyses, and in no case has led to any significant change in the results obtained.

Thus the general picture is satisfactory. Of course this is not quite the whole story, since it has been in terms of those with some information compared to those with none. There may yet be particular questions or instruments for which the response pattern differs from that found overall, and hence the need for continuous monitoring in the context of specific analyses.

Related studies

The description of the study given so far has been restricted to the major follow-ups of the entire cohort. As well as charting general patterns of development, the aims included the intention to mount more intensive studies of groups of special interest. Indeed, one reason for following-up the entire cohort has been to increase the possibility of sufficient numbers in such groups. There have been several related studies, ranging from those which have carried out special analyses of the data already collected to those where it has been possible to go back to the subjects and collect further information relevant to the specific circumstances of the group concerned. In general such studies have been separately funded and staffed, although recently it has been possible to do some such work within the resources of the main study team (see Current Work section).

Related studies which have taken place to date include:

Adopted and illegitimate children
    Studies of the progress to age seven of these two groups (which of course overlap) have been reported (Crellin *et al.* 1971; Seglow *et al.* 1972). An extension of this work is currently in progress (see Current Related Studies section).
Gifted children
    The progress to age eleven of children identified as exceptional by a variety of criteria (Hitchfield 1974) is summarized under Findings from Related Studies. Further work to the age of sixteen is described under Current Related Studies.
Children in one-parent families
    The findings to the age of eleven have been reported in two books

(Ferri 1976; Ferri and Robinson 1976; see also Some Findings below) and the study is now being extended to age sixteen by the main study team (see Current Work section).

Physically and mentally handicapped children

A number of projects described below under Some Findings from Related Studies.

Children in care

Following the collection of further information on these children at seven, the main study team has recently published findings on their progress to the age of eleven (Essen *et al*. 1976; Richardson 1977a; see also Findings section).

Socially disadvantaged children

A study of children experiencing the extremes of adverse home circumstances at the age of eleven (Wedge and Prosser 1973), and summarized below under Findings.

Regional differences in children's development

Carried out at the age of eleven and investigating the relationship between children's development and demographic, environmental and expenditure patterns of the areas in which they live; this work is described in Donnison and Soto (in press).

Feasibility study of the educational progress of children in selective and non-selective secondary schools

A study which is just beginning and is described below under Current Related Studies.

Prediction of educational failure

Described below under Current Related Studies.

Statistical methods of analysing change

A methodological study being done in conjunction with the above.

Early work experiences of handicapped school leavers

A study which has involved a further follow-up of a sub-group since the third major follow-up, and which is described below under Current Related Studies.

Some findings from the main study

Clearly it is possible here to give only a brief selection of the findings which the study has produced to date. A more comprehensive impression of the areas within which work has been done can be gained from the titles in the list of publications at the end of this chapter.

The reader will notice that not all the findings described capitalize on the longitudinal aspect of the study. The major part of the first topic, and all of the second depend on data collected at one point in time only. Nevertheless these are analyses to which the study was thought to be particularly suited, because of the size and representativeness of the sample.

Smoking during pregnancy

It has been known since the 1950s that mothers who smoke during pregnancy tend to have lighter babies than those who do not, the average birthweight difference being somewhat less than 200 g. Since lower birthweight is known to be associated with increased perinatal mortality, investigators have been looking for mortality differences associated with smoking. Two problems soon became apparent. First, the sample of births would have to be very large—of the order of several thousands—to detect the small differences anticipated. Secondly, there appeared to be conflicting evidence even among the studies using a large sample. Some studies, usually of the babies of relatively well-off groups of women, showed very small mortality differences, whereas others, generally among poorer groups, showed much larger differences, with up to 50 per cent higher mortality among the children of smokers.

The original survey of births also studied the perinatal deaths occurring in Britain in the months of March, April, and May 1958, a total of about 7000. For the purpose of comparing the mortality rates of babies of smokers and non-smokers, the combined data provide estimates and significance tests as accurate and sensitive as those derived from a simple sample of births numbering about 150 000. In this sense, therefore, it is well placed to resolve some of the apparently contradictory results.

Among mothers who were married to men in the upper social classes the perinatal mortality rate was only 10 per cent higher for children of smokers than for those of non-smokers, whereas for all babies it was 28 per cent higher. In addition, the more privileged groups have a smaller proportion of low-birthweight babies (under 2000 g), among whom a further average decrease of about 200 g brings a much greater increase in mortality risk than among those with a modal birthweight of about 3400 g. Thus for less privileged groups of women where a relatively large proportion of low-birthweight babies is expected, we should also expect a greater increase in perinatal mortality associated with smoking. Since approximately the same average decrease in birthweight is noted in all studies irrespective of social class, this seems a plausible explanation for the discrepant findings.

There remains the question of whether this association of smoking during pregnancy with birthweight and mortality is causal, or the result of a link with another factor, such as the constitution of the mother. It is ultimately impossible to resolve the question using only epidemiological evidence, but it was possible to rule out some of the other factors. After making allowance for social class, maternal age, maternal height, number of previous births, and length of gestation, the birthweight and mortality differences between babies of smokers and non-smokers remained virtually unchanged.

A further finding is also consistent with a causal link: of the women who were smoking at the beginning of pregnancy, about 20 per cent had given up smoking by the fourth month. In terms of both birthweight and mortality, their babies fared as well as the babies of mothers who had never smoked at all. If we reject a causal explanation for this finding then we are led to postulate a further factor or factors which predispose some women towards smoking and then giving it up during pregnancy and also towards decreased risk of mortality in their babies, with those mothers who continue to smoke (Goldstein 1975).

In a follow-up analysis the characteristics of children of smokers and non-smokers at the ages of seven and eleven were examined. At both ages it was found that the children of mothers who smoked heavily during pregnancy (10 or more cigarettes a day) were on the average about 1·5 cm shorter than the children of non-smokers. This difference was almost halved, however, when allowance was made for the associated factors mentioned above.

Class size

Davie *et al*. (1972) provide a detailed account of the analysis of differences associated with size of class among the children in the cohort who were seven years old in 1965. It is a well known fact among researchers that despite a considerable number of studies over the past few years or so—mostly in the United States—there is very little evidence which demonstrates that small classes produce better attainments. In this country, two earlier studies (Morris 1966; Wiseman 1967) had found that in the primary schools they studied there was, perversely, an association between small classes and lower attainment. Because these results appeared somewhat anomalous, it was decided to use the large sample within the NCDS to carry out an analysis which could take fuller acount of many of the factors which might otherwise have contaminated the analysis. First a number of groups of children were excluded: children in independent schools, children in 'streamed' classes (or in special schools, or in classes for the handicapped), and those who had had nursery schooling. In addition, children in Scottish schools were excluded because preliminary results suggested that rather more were in large classes; the Scottish children were also markedly better readers at seven than the English or Welsh. Second, the analysis was designed to take account of school size and type, length of schooling, social class, and interest of parents. All the children were allocated to groups according to their class size: small classes (30 or less), medium-sized classes (31–40), or large classes (41 or more). Three measures were selected for the analyses: the South-gate Group Reading Test score; a problem arithmetic test score; and a measure of the children's behaviour and adjustment in school—the Bristol Social Adjustment Guide. Describing the researchers' expectations Davie (1971) writes:

> Having taken all the steps outlined, there was a quiet confidence that the results would show previous research to have been oversimplified and misleading. The analyses would confirm, it was felt, what every practising teacher knows to be the case. However, this confidence was misplaced.
>
> For the children in infant departments of junior-with-infant schools there were no differences between the class size groups on any of the measures used. More surprisingly, of the children in infants schools, those in 'large' classes had the highest reading and arithmetic attainments and those in 'small' classes had the lowest. This, it will be remembered, was after allowance had been made for all the other factors. There were no differences in behaviour and adjustment for the groups.

Although demonstrating associations rather than a causal relationship, there was a considerable controversy raised among professional educators when these findings were first published. Like many other pieces of research they prompt more questions than they answer. However, it is clear that whatever may be desirable in terms of teachers' working conditions or conditions appropriate to particular methods of teaching, a general reduction in class size cannot automatically or necessarily be assumed to be followed by any rise in standards of attainment in reading or arithmetic.

Nocturnal enuresis

In the course of the parental interview at the seven-year-old follow-up the parents were asked whether the study child had 'wet at night after five years of age', and at the eleven-year-old follow-up they were asked whether the child had 'wet at night in the past month'. From the responses to these questions it was found that 10·7 per cent of the cohort were enuretic between the ages of five and seven years, but only a third of these (3·5 per cent) were still enuretic at eleven. A further 1·3 per cent reported dry when they were seven, were enuretics at eleven, making a total of 4·8 per cent enuretics at eleven years. More boys than girls were wet at eleven although there was no difference between the sexes at seven.

The association between enuresis and environmental factors, factors indicating delayed development and the children's attainment and behaviour, were examined, and comparisons were also made according to the age at which the child was enuretic.

Both seven-year-old enuretics who cleared up (early bed-wetters) and eleven-year-old enuretics were more likely to have larger families and be later-born, to be from the working classes, and to live in over-crowded homes, but only early bed-wetters were more likely to share a bed. Early bed-wetters tended to have been slow at learning to walk and to talk although there were no such differences among the eleven-year-old enuretics. Proportionately more eleven-year-old enuretics than non-enuretics were in one-parent families or had been in the care of the local authority, but this did not apply to such an extent to early bed-wetters.

Analyses of behaviour and attainment in school were carried out in which allowance was made for the environmental characteristics shown above to be related to enuresis. Both groups of enuretics were more likely to be reported by both their parents and their teachers as showing more difficult behaviour when they were eleven than non-enuretics, and this was especially marked for the eleven-year-old enuretics. There were also slight differences in

their attainment test scores at age eleven, again with the children who were enuretic at the time having the lowest average scores, and non-enuretics the highest average scores.

The conclusions of this study were that social, developmental, and psychiatric factors are each associated with enuresis but the extent of this association varies with different groups of children, in particular with the age at which the children are enuretic (Essen and Peckham 1976).

Age of starting school

In an earlier report on the National Child Development Study (Pringle *et al.* 1966) the authors commented on differences in children's attainment at seven years associated with the age at which school was started. All the children in the cohort attained the age of five in March 1963 and for the purposes of analysis they were divided into early starters (age 4 years 6 months to 4 years 11 months) and later starters (age 5 years 0 months to 5 years 6 months). It is perhaps not surprising that differences in test scores were found between the two groups of children who, while of precisely the same age, had been exposed to differing amounts of educational experience. More interesting, however, is the question of long-term effects. Specifically, are differences in age of starting school found to be associated with the attainment of children at the age of eleven? The short answer is that they are.

Fogelman and Gorbach (1978) conclude that 'at the age of eleven children who started school before their fifth birthday will be some two or three months ahead of those who started school after their fifth birthday in terms of general ability, reading comprehension, and mathematics attainment'. Their analyses took account of social class, family size, region, parents' education, interest in child's education, housing conditions, school and class size, sex, and attendance rate at age seven.

The differences between these two groups of children amount to only about a quarter of the differences between children of professional/ managerial fathers, and those with fathers in unskilled manual occupations; on the other hand, in comparison with other school variables which might be amenable to legislation or policy the differences associated with age of starting school are not dissimilar to those associated with size of class.

Seemingly, one group of children gain an educational advantage over another simply because of parental pressure, local administrative convenience, or chance. Further, the findings suggest that these same children tend to be from groups whose social backgrounds give them educational benefits anyway. One starting date for all children might be more equitable (as in Scotland), or alternatively a policy of positive discrimination is not difficult to devise. In any event, it is interesting that these variations in starting date are still detectable at age eleven, and it remains to be seen whether analysis of attainment at sixteen will still reveal similar differences associated with age of starting school eleven years earlier.

Longitudinal analysis of social factors associated with changes in educational attainment

An earlier cohort study, the National Survey of Health and Development, which followed up a sample of children born in one week of 1946, demonstrated differences associated with different family sizes and father's occupation on tests of reading vocabulary and intelligence at the age of eight, and additionally in arithmetic at age eleven (Douglas 1964b). Furthermore, these differences were found by Douglas to persist through secondary school to the age of fifteen (Douglas *et al.* 1968b). Similar findings emerged from the NCDS in that social class and family size were associated with large differences in school attainment at the age of seven (Davie *et al.* 1972) and eleven (Fogelman 1975).

Fogelman and Goldstein (1976) addressed themselves to the question of whether the differences between these groups change as the children progress through school. They sought to establish whether children of low social class and large families show a once and for all difference, which is stable throughout their education, or whether the gap between them and their peers became wider or narrower. In fact, Douglas concluded that the average test scores made by children in four social classes differed more widely at eleven than they did at eight, but that with regard to family size there was 'no evidence that children from large families deteriorated in their test performance . . . (showing that the influence of family size on the level of the test score has exerted its full effect by eight years)' (Douglas 1964b). Fogelman and Goldstein used social class, family size, and attainment measures at seven and eleven years of age and their analysis was able to take account of changes in these social factors. Their data confirmed Douglas's findings on social class and additionally showed that family size exhibits a continuing association with attainment test scores between the ages of seven and eleven. Further, they demonstrated that social mobility and increase in family size are also associated with test scores in the expected directions. In a comment on social class the authors point out that in addition to the well known differences between the children of manual and non-manual groups, those from upwardly mobile families improve their attainment scores relative to those in static families, who in turn improve relative to those from downwardly mobile families.

Clearly, these findings are important for educational planners and theorists although, like other findings based on the NCDS data, these results represent average differences which actually exist among children and do not necessarily imply a cause-effect relationship. Furthermore, they are dependent on assumptions about the comparability of tests designed for use at different ages.

Linguistic maturity

Strictly speaking, the analyses carried out under this heading require neither a longitudinal study (although there is considerable scope for extension in this way) nor a large, nationally representative sample, since they are concerned with data from a single follow-up, and have involved a detailed analysis of a sample of just 500 of the children's essays. However they have proved to identify a rich vein of research, of considerable interest to the academic community. This demonstrates the importance of a flexibility of approach, a willingness to devote some resources to an unanticipated area, difficult as this is in an organization such as the National Children's Bureau where each project needs to be specifically funded.

At the eleven-year follow-up children were asked to 'Imagine that you are now 25 years old. Write about the life you are leading, your interests, your home life and your work at the age of 25'. One use made of these compositions was to analyse a sample for writing productivity and syntactic maturity (Mean T-Unit Length, in Hunt 1970). These two measures were further examined for associations with other variables which commonly preoccupy child development and educational researchers. Writing productivity was strikingly associated with most of these variables, including social class, sex, reading comprehension and general ability test scores, teachers' subjective impressions of oral work, use of books, number work and general knowledge, family size, and spare-time reading. Syntactic maturity was associated only with reading books for leisure, reading comics, newspapers and magazines, number work, and (weakly) with both verbal and non-verbal components of the general ability test. Thus there were no significant associations between syntactic maturity and social class, reading comprehension, family size, and teachers' impressions other than number work. These results have been interpreted in the context of recent theories of syntactic development and syntactic divergence (Richardson *et al.* 1976; Richardson 1977a, b).

Some findings from related studies

The related studies selected for brief description demonstrate the range of such work, from those analysing only data collected, to those where further field-work has been carried out to collect more specifically relevant information.

Children in one-parent families

Ferri (1976) provides a wealth of detail about the circumstances of the group of children who have grown up in a one-parent family and about the relative educational attainment of a group commonly accepted to be deprived. She found that a straightforward comparison between one and two parent children in terms of their attainment and adjustment showed that, in each area, the one-parent group were doing significantly less well. However, she demonstrated that there were marked differences in the background and environment of children from one or two parent families, and many of the background factors which were particularly characteristic of one-parent children (for example, low social class, poor housing, having been in care) had been shown to be related to lower attainment in school, and to poorer social adjustment. She therefore analysed her data to take account of such differences between the two groups of children and as a result the differences between the two groups in school attainment and social adjustment were greatly narrowed.

Children living with widowed mothers and fatherless illegitimate children no longer differed significantly from their peers in two-parent families. In both these fatherless groups, but especially among the illegitimate children, those whose mothers were in full-time employment showed better attainment and adjustment than children whose mothers were not working or were employed only part time. This trend did not appear among children in two-parent families, suggesting that perhaps in the case of these lone mothers, the material and social/psychological benefits of employment were related, directly or indirectly to comparatively favourable development in their children.

Motherless children on the other hand, and those who were fatherless as a result of marital breakdown, still showed a rather poorer level of development than two-parent children even after disadvantaging background factors had been taken into account. In both these cases, however, differences in development which were associated with family situation *in itself* were small by comparison with differences due to social and environmental factors. One particularly striking finding to emerge from this part of her study was the importance of economic hardship, measured by whether or not a child received free school meals, as a factor associated with the relatively poor performance of children from fatherless homes. Hence the relatively poor school attainment and social adjustment of one-parent children seemed to owe much more to the disadvantaging circumstances *associated with* one-parent family status than to the fact of being brought up by a lone mother or father. Again, this is an important finding which has implications not just for the support services needed to enable lone parents to care adequately for their children, but also for the expectations which the wider community, and particularly the professional educator, has for the one-parent child in the educational system. To supplement this heavily data-based aspect of the study, interviews were carried out with a sample of the lone fathers and lone mothers, to obtain their comments on their situation (Ferri and Robinson 1976).

Mentally and physically handicapped children

There have been related studies of a number of groups of physically and mentally handicapped children from within the cohort. Some have been relatively simple and descriptive (Pearson and Peckham 1972), using the comprehensiveness and representativeness of the NCDS data to establish prevalence rates for particular conditions.

Others have looked in greater depth at the circumstances and progress of particular groups, for example those with hearing difficulties (Sheridan 1972; Peckham *et al.* 1972), or speech defects (Butler *et al.* 1973; Sheridan 1973; Peckham 1973), the mentally retarded (Frew 1972; Frew and Peckham 1972) and children who had experienced convulsions (Ross 1973).

At the age of seven, children with moderate bilateral hearing impairment or marked deafness in one ear only were found to be disadvantaged in school compared with their normally hearing classmates. However the problems which they experienced were considerably fewer than those of children with speech difficulties but normal hearing. The latter not only obtained lower scores on tests of school attainment, but also showed a significantly higher prevalence of visual defects, general motor inco-ordination, and emotional instability. According to their mothers' reports they had shown considerable delay in walking and talking.

When the incidence of speech defects was related to the provision of speech therapy there proved to be considerable regional and social variation in the extent to which these needs were being met. For example, approximately four times as many children of un-skilled manual workers as children of professional workers were reported as having speech problems, whereas the amount of speech therapy provided to the two groups was virtually the same.

Further examination of the same children at the age of eleven showed that whereas those children with moderate hearing difficulties showed improvement, children with speech defects continued to have considerable problems, not only with verbal communication, but also with school attainment (Sheridan and Peckham 1975). The authors of that work concluded:

There can be no doubt that more effective identification of children with speech and language difficulties at or before school entry is necessary and that this must be associated with comprehensive pediatric, audiological, visual and educational assessment, practical parent guidance, vigorous speech therapy and one-to-one remedial teaching in favourable surroundings.

Socially disadvantaged children

For the purposes of this project a functional view of social disadvantage was employed; thus, using in particular the data gathered at seven and at eleven years, the concern of this study was with children in families where there had been a low income, poor housing, five or more children, or only one parent figure. Information about the importance of each of these family circumstances was already available from previous research, including some at the Bureau. This project, however, aggregated such circumstances and examined the overlap between them. What was known to be a considerable problem could now be seen as a much more serious one; for example, by the age of eleven, 23 per cent of the children were known to have been living in poor housing, and at the same time 14 per cent were living in low income families. But, putting these together, it was shown that poverty of income or of housing affected some 30 per cent of all the children. The study also found that 23 per cent of the children had, by the age of eleven, grown up in a family with five or more children or with only one parent figure.

The socially disadvantaged included those who had experienced this atypical family situation, had lived in a low income family, and had experienced bad housing. It comprised 6 per cent of the nationally representative sample and this group was compared with the much larger group of children who fell into none of the three categories mentioned.

The dimensions of disadvantage were then shown to extend from before birth through health factors, accommodations, family circumstances, and school experience, as well as physical development and educational attainment. The report of this study (Wedge and Prosser 1973) was designed to make a popular impact in itemizing the massive accumulation of additional hardships that were found to confront the group of socially disadvantaged children in almost every aspect of their daily lives; the report avoided statistical sophistication and contained a large number of photographs and diagrams in a very slim volume. At the time of publication it was featured widely in media reports, and subsequently has been the subject of press articles and reports on radio and television.

Gifted children

In this study, the term gifted was widely interpreted to include not only children of high general ability but also those outstanding in any one of a range of specific abilities, such as mathematics, art, music, or sports. A substantial proportion of children with fathers in semi-skilled or unskilled manual occupations was included to counteract the usual under-representation of these groups. Information collected when the children were seven provided the basis from which the gifted and able children were identified although some of the 238 children included were selected following parents' letters after a public invitation through the press.

Each of the children was interviewed by an educational psychologist with the aim of assessing each child in general and specific areas of knowledge or behaviour. Parents were interviewed about their child's schooling, interests, hobbies, friends, personal qualities and general behaviour, their child's future, education, employment, and their own education.

Gifted children were found not to be losing out through being in ordinary schools—although the study recommended ways in which schools and teaching skills might be improved for the benefit of all the children, including the gifted. Criticisms that gifted and able children were often unidentified and unprovided for were said to be largely unfounded, but parents' and children's views were felt to be important if reasonable and accurate assessments were to be made. Parents of gifted children tended to have positive attitudes to early education, and middle class children who were gifted were shown to have a distinct advantage over working class children in their facility with verbal tests (Hitchfield 1974). This work is now being extended to age sixteen (see Current Related Studies section).

Children in care

Although conceptually a related study in which the collection of further data at seven was separately funded and staffed, the eleven-year work was carried out within the main study team.

At age seven the special study was set up to look at those children who had been received into the care of either a local authority or a voluntary society because their parents were unable to care for them at home. A question to parents at the seven-year-old follow-up identified these children, and additional information was then collected in respect of them (2·1 per cent of the cohort). This included details of their experiences of being in care, such as the age at which they were first received into care, and their placements in foster homes or children's homes (Mapstone 1969).

By the time the children were eleven a further 1·3 per cent of the cohort were known to have been in care, but of those in care at an earlier age not necessarily all were still living away from their parents at the time of the eleven-year-old follow-up—by then over 80 per cent of them were no longer in care.

The children who had been in care by eleven years were compared with those who had not, in terms of their home and family characteristics, their school attainment, and their behaviour both at home and at school. Comparisons were also made according to the age at which the child was first received into care. Children who had been in care at any age tended to be living in a materially and economically disadvantaged situation when they were eleven. They were likely to be in large families, often with only one parent, in families with a low income, in poor housing, and a large proportion had fathers in semi- or unskilled manual jobs. Children in these

difficult home circumstances have been shown previously to perform poorly at school and to show difficult behaviour even if they
have not been in care (Wedge and Petzing 1970). Therefore these
factors were allowed for in the analyses of attainment and
behaviour.

Children who had been in care, in particular if this was before
they were seven, had lower average scores in tests of reading and
mathematics taken when they were eleven than those never in care.
In the tests of reading and mathematics taken at age seven the
children who were not received into care until after this age already
had lower than average scores. Their scores did not then deteriorate
relatively between the ages of seven and eleven even though this
was the period during which they spent some time in care. However
during this period the attainment of the group who had been in care
before they were seven did drop further behind that of the children
never in care. These findings together suggest that the low attainment was associated with factors other than the experience of care
itself (Essen *et al.* 1976). In many respects the results on adjustment to school showed a similar pattern to those on attainment.
Children in care had higher scores (indicating less conforming
behaviour) than those not in care, both at the seven-year and the
eleven-year follow-ups. This was so both for the group who had
already been in care by the age of seven and for those who were not
in care until later. However the pattern differed from that for
attainment: the gap between the school adjustment scores of both
the in care groups and of the children who had not been in care
widened between the ages of seven and eleven. This suggests that
the less conforming behaviour of children in care is related to
factors both outside and within the experience of care itself. The
analyses of behaviour at home showed inconclusive results
(Lambert *et al.* 1977).

Current work of the main study team

During preparations for the follow-up at sixteen years, discussions
took place between the researchers and an Advisory Group, containing representatives of the sponsors and other Government
departments concerned with children and young people, in order to
determine the priorities for analyses of the data. Given the extent
and variety of NCDS data, decisions had to be taken about what
specific topics should be investigated within the current grant. By
this exercise, sixteen such topics were identified and can be divided
into three groups. The first four, which are also generally less
extensive than the remainder, are cross-sectional in that they predominantly use data collected at the age of sixteen only. It could be
said that they do not capitalize on the strengths of the study, but
they are concerned with information which is of immediate importance and interest to the sponsors and other policy-makers. Furthermore all four are undoubtedly topics which will inform and
contribute to any future development of the study and could therefore develop into longitudinal analyses in conjunction with data
which we hope will be collected at a later stage.

The next eight are concerned with longitudinal patterns of
development of the entire cohort, as indeed are the final four, but
the latter are distinct as being studies of special subgroups. Of
course they do use the data for the remainder of the cohort for
comparison purposes.

The transition from school to work and further education
The sixteen-year-olds provided information on four broad variables relevant to these analyses: the job aspired to; the job they
thought likely; their reasons for choosing a job; their plans for
continuing their education. Each of these is being related to a
number of personal, social, and school variables (e.g. sex, social
class, region, type of school, career advice in the school) as well as to

parents' and teachers' aspirations and expectations for the child.
From this should develop a joint analysis in an attempt to identify
the most important influences on the dependent variables.

Family relationships and attitudes to the family
The young people and their parents answered questions on relationships within the family and on the amount of disagreement over
specific issues. The simple and joint distributions of the replies will
be examined in order to provide a picture of the pattern of relationships and the degree of harmony within the family. Their association with such background factors as sex, social class, and family
size will then be examined, as well as their relationship with the
sixteen-year-olds' own plans for future family life.

Smoking and drinking among sixteen-year-olds
We have information on cigarettes smoked per week and on type,
quantity, and place of recent alcoholic drink. Analyses are examining: distributions, sex, regional, and social class differences; the
relationship between parents' and children's smoking; the relationship between smoking and drinking and income from spare-time
work and pocket money; the relationships between smoking and
drinking and type of school, attainment, emotional symptoms, and
respiratory infections.

Self-rated knowledge of birth, contraception, and venereal disease
Information was provided by the school and the sixteen-year-olds
on the extent of lessons in school on such topics. The latter also
answered questions on other sources of such information and their
satisfaction with the information which they had received. These
data are being used: to identify groups of children according to
whether they have received teaching in school on these topics and
whether they feel they have sufficient knowledge, and then to
examine their background characteristics and the characteristics of
their schools; to identify other sources of knowledge which complement, or substitute, lessons to give a feeling of sufficient knowledge;
to examine the relationship between knowledge on these topics and
attitudes to future family life.

Longitudinal patterns of school attainment
This work falls into two complementary but distinct parts. The first
is an extension of the work by Fogelman and Goldstein described
above (Some findings from the main study) and is addressed to
the question of whether the widening gaps in attainment which
were found between ages seven and eleven among children from
different social backgrounds continue in the same pattern to the age
of sixteen. Are differences which develop between the ages of
eleven and sixteen greater than those which developed between
ages seven and eleven? Such questions are being investigated in
relation to sex, social class, region, and family size.

The second part is concerned with the prediction of relative
attainment and the latter's stability over time. How common is it for
children who are doing relatively poorly at age seven or eleven to be
successful at age sixteen, and vice versa? What are the characteristics of such children and how do they compare with those who
perform consistently well or poorly?

Longitudinal patterns of behaviour
This work also can be considered in two parts, the first of which is
analogous to the second group of attainment analyses described
above. Considering ratings of behaviour at home and at school
separately, changes in reported behaviour over time are being
examined, and the major background factors associated with
change identified. Further, at each age, the relationship between
home and school ratings is being examined, and the background
factors associated with discrepancies identified.

The second part is investigating the relationship of behaviour ratings and other possible predictors with such outcomes at age sixteen as psychiatric referral and getting into trouble with the police.

Growth in height and weight

This consists of two sets of parallel analyses: one with height and the other with weight for height as the dependent variable. For brevity the following refers to height only. The first set examines the relationship between height at age sixteen and height at ages seven and eleven, and the background factors related to rate of growth between these ages. This includes investigation of the relationship between puberty and growth from ages eleven to sixteen. The second set examines how changes in background factors during the child's life influence growth between the three age levels.

School characteristics and attainment and adjustment

A range of characteristics of secondary schools are being related, singly and jointly, and allowing for children's ability before entry to the school, to reading and mathematics scores, attitude to school, and parental satisfaction with the school. The characteristics being studied include: type of school; teacher/pupil ratio; size of class (for English and Math lessons); whether co-educational; age range of school; size of school; teacher turnover; use of corporal punishment; opportunities for parental contact.

Housing and home amenities

The following housing variables are available from the study: crowding, amenities (bathroom, indoor lavatory, hot water supply), tenure and type of accommodation. The following questions are being explored: What proportions of children are in each type of housing situation at age sixteen and what are their background characteristics? How do these compare with the corresponding figures at ages seven and eleven and with other available figures? What are the characteristics of children whose housing improves, deteriorates, remains good or remains poor over the period from ages seven to sixteen? What are the differences in attainment, adjustment, and growth among children with different housing patterns over that period? Which housing variables appear to be most important in influencing attainment etc. by the age of sixteen?

Vision screening and vision defects

This work entails:

(a) A descriptive analysis of visual acuity at age sixteen—to include an analysis of distant and near visual acuity, with and without glasses, within sex and social class;
(b) An examination of changes in visual acuity from age seven to sixteen;
(c) A more detailed scrutiny of the records of children who have a visual acuity of 6/24 or worse in their better eye, to investigate, for example, their educational progress and the prevalence of other physical handicaps.

School attendance and truancy

We have five indices of attendance and truancy at age sixteen: parents', teachers' and pupils' reports and actual attendance rates in the past two autumn terms. Using these we are:

(a) Looking at the interrelationships among them and with reported medical causes of absence;
(b) Examining the relationship between absenteeism and background factors such as sex, social class, region, etc;
(c) Comparing the poor attenders and truants with others in terms of such variables as desired school-leaving age, attitudes to school, aspirations for the future, leisure activities, and spare-time work;

(d) Examining the relationship between absenteeism and the characteristics of schools;
(e) Investigating the association of absenteeism at age sixteen with absenteeism at earlier ages;
(f) Investigating the association between absenteeism at all ages and attainment and behaviour at age sixteen.

Ability-grouping in the school

The school supplied information on its philosophy concerning the formation of classes, i.e. whether children were taught in mixed-ability groups, or were grouped according to their ability in particular subjects, or streamed so that a child took all lessons in one class formed according to ability. The school's method of ability-grouping is being related to: other characteristics of the school; the academic progress made by children between ages eleven and sixteen and their aspirations and expectations for the future; the characteristics of children according to the ability range of the classes in which they are studying English and mathematics at age sixteen; the range of measured ability at age sixteen.

Children with asthma

The main purpose of these analyses is to identify the prevalance of asthma at different ages and to study the use made by the parents of children with asthma of medical services for investigation and treatment of this condition. It is hoped that time will also allow the investigation of the impact of asthma on educational progress, etc., and the relationship of asthma to other medical conditions.

Speech and language problems

These analyses are investigating the association with speech defect, at age sixteen, of a range of social and physical variables; the persistence of speech defect from ages seven to sixteen; factors associated with improvement between these ages; the relationship between speech defect and hearing attainment.

Immigrant children

Two groups can be defined and compared with children born in Great Britain to parents born in this country:

(a) Children born overseas with at least one parent born overseas, further subdivided according to country of origin and length of time in this country;
(b) Children born in this country to parents born overseas.

Analyses encompass the following areas: housing and financial situation; parental and children's attitudes and aspirations about education and work; height and weight and puberty ratings; health problems such as vision, hearing and respiratory problems; school attainment at age sixteen; and changes in attainment between ages eleven and sixteen, after allowing for background factors including whether English is spoken in the home; discrepancies between teachers' ratings and attainment test results. For those who came to Britain before age eleven, we shall also explore whether differences from non-immigrants in housing and attainment changed between ages eleven and sixteen.

Children in one-parent families

These analyses extend and build upon those recently reported for these children up to the age of eleven and described earlier. Specifically they:

(a) Identify the proportions in anomalous parental situations at age sixteen and examine patterns over the period from birth to age sixteen;
(b) Compare these findings with those from the study of children born in 1946;
(c) Examine differences between one- and two-parent families

in their financial and work situation (including the sixteen-year-olds' pocket money and spare-time income);

(d) Compare children in one- and two-parent families in terms of their plans for future employment and education and attitudes to future family life;

(e) Investigate the relationship between parental situation and children's attainment, behaviour, and adjustment.

Current related studies

The descriptions below are of studies which are using the NCDS cohort and data, but which are funded and staffed separately from the main study work described above.

Study of illegitimately born and of adopted children and their families

This study is concerned with the development of eleven-year-olds who were born illegitimate, some of whom were subsequently adopted, and includes comparison with children who were legitimately born. Two previous studies explored the development of these two groups of children up to the age of seven, comparing them with their peers (Pringle 1967). This new study is making similar cross-sectional comparisons between illegitimate children who were adopted and those who remained with their mothers, and is also examining longitudinally any changes in development between the ages of seven and eleven to discover whether the differences found at seven years have increased or diminished four years later.

Developmental differences between the groups of children are expected to persist but variations within and between the illegitimate and adopted groups are expected to relate to the environmental circumstances in which the children are growing up. Of particular interest is the family situation of the children, not only at age eleven but at birth and at age seven, and the relationship of social class, income, and housing to different family structures. The previous study found that by the age of seven both groups of children had been socially mobile, but in opposite directions. In the current study the various test scores of the children will be examined according to stability and change in social class position from birth, through seven to eleven years.

Study of gifted children

The earlier study (described above) is now being followed up with work to assess the progress of the gifted children over the period from seven to sixteen years. Their performance will be compared with their peers, and an assessment made as to whether they have progressed as might have been predicted from their performance at seven and eleven or whether there has been marked improvement or deterioration in their achievements up to age sixteen. Further, the study will explore the existence of any special developmental, personality, or scholastic problems arising from or linked with the special talents of these children, as well as their specific interests, attitudes, and vocational intentions.

Prediction of educational failure

This study is examining the effect of educational, social, and environmental factors on the changes in educational attainment between the ages of seven, eleven, and sixteen; and how educational failure at age sixteen can be predicted by using both educational and socio-environmental factors. It has already been shown that at any given age there are differences in attainment between children from different social backgrounds and that changes in attainment between the ages of seven and eleven are also associated with social class and family size, with children in the more disadvantaged groups falling further behind as they get older.

The present study is extending these analyses by studying measures of poverty (determined largely by eligibility for welfare assistance grants) and measures of different educational provision. The latter will include characteristics of the school such as size, average class-size, type of school, and provision of special help for children with particular needs. It is hoped that this research will provide reliable and useful predictors of particular relevance to compensatory education programmes.

Employment experiences of handicapped school leavers

The main aim of this project is to explore the reasons for success as well as failure to get or keep a satisfying job among a sample of some 450 handicapped and 100 non-handicapped young people, aged eighteen. The study was commissioned by the Warnock Committee, set up by the Government in 1974 to study the educational needs of handicapped children. It is hoped that the report will be included in the evidence on which the Warnock Committee will base its recommendations for the future use of resources in educating handicapped young people and preparing them for employment.

The group of school-leavers in this study was drawn from the NCDS and includes those ascertained as physically and mentally handicapped who were receiving special education at sixteen years, and also a small number of those young people who, while not having received special education would have benefited from it, in the opinion of their teachers. The group of 100 non-handicapped young people were included for comparative purposes.

The lengthy interview schedules contain a wealth of information about the education and work history of the young people as well as the views of their parents and themselves about the usefulness or otherwise of career services and advice received on further education or training. In addition the research team has carried out small-scale inquiries among employers, industrial training boards, and a sample of staff in different types of schools. These will make it possible to give a picture of the difficulties which handicapped young people present to employers and schools, and of any special facilities provided.

Feasibility study of educational progress of children in selective and non-selective secondary schools

At the time of writing, this study is just on the point of starting, and will examine the adequacy of the numbers of children within the NCDS sample in different types of secondary schools.

In Britain, about 60 per cent of secondary school pupils are educated in schools which, nominally, cater for the entire ability range (comprehensive schools), while the remainder are in schools for which pupils are selected according to ability. The last two decades have been a period of transition from an almost exclusively selective system to a predominantly comprehensive one, with the result that local authorities differ in the kind of secondary education offered. In many areas the two systems still co-exist. Attempts to compare the attainment of pupils in comprehensive and selective schools have usually been confounded by the inability to control or make proper allowance for factors such as the initial attainment and social background of pupils entering the two systems and for the effects on comprehensive schools of 'creaming'. Some, at least, of these factors can be taken into account in a longitudinal study which includes information about pupils' attainment *before* entering secondary school as well as on relevant social factors and attainment at the age of sixteen.

It is envisaged that in a subsequent study comparisons will be made in terms of such variables as: attainment test scores; teachers' ratings of attainment and behaviour; career aspirations; educational aspirations; attendance record; and attitudes to school. Possible control variables include the pupil's sex, social class, region, measures of attainment at the age of eleven, the year in which the school became comprehensive, and a number of other school characteristics such as size, age-range, social mix, and teacher/pupil ratio.

Publication and dissemination

A complete list of the ten books and 124 chapters and papers which have arisen from the study to date may be obtained by writing to the authors. In addition to the usual channels of publication through books and journal articles, which are given first priority, the contents of the list demonstrate the importance the National Children's Bureau has always placed on additionally presenting summaries of findings in more popular outlets, so that they are available to policy-makers, field professionals, and the general public who would not normally turn to academic sources.

Apart from such conventional methods of dissemination there are three particular aspects of the study worthy of mention.

(1) We are very aware of our dependence on local authority staff, teachers, doctors, and health visitors for local administration of the study, the carrying out of interviews and examinations, and the completion of questionnaires. We therefore feel it important that special efforts are made to acquaint them with the fruits of their labour. To this end, it has been possible for the funding of the study to include a small amount to enable the purchase of sufficient reprints and their distribution to local authorities. Because of costs, this has generally had to be limited to articles, but we were able to distribute free copies of our most recent book, *Britain's sixteen-year-olds*, in this way.

(2) We are of course at least equally dependent on the co-operation of the subjects themselves and their parents and it is perhaps even more important that they should know what we are writing about them, both for ethical reasons and for the more pragmatic purpose of maintaining their interest in the study. Of course whenever we are writing to the entire cohort for any reason we take the opportunity to inform them of recent developments and publications. However on two occasions so far it has proved possible to go beyond this. At the time of the publication of the major, general report on seven-year findings—*From birth to seven*—and again for the preliminary report of sixteen-year findings—*Britain's sixteen-year-olds*—a national Sunday newspaper carried a lengthy illustrated summary of the findings in its colour supplement. In place of the usual fee the Bureau accepted copies of the supplement and the cost of posting one to each of the young people in the study.

(3) This aspect is concerned not with dissemination of findings, but with dissemination of the actual data. In the hope that a wider exploitation of the material may occur without breaching the confidentiality of the information, a magnetic tape with a copy of the data from the perinatal survey and from the first and second follow-ups has been provided by the National Children's Bureau for the Social Science Research Council Survey Archive at Essex University. It is intended to add the third follow-up data in due course. Bona fide researchers can gain access to the data in this way, with background assistance supplied where practicable by the study researchers themselves. The SSRC Survey Archive has a reciprocal arrangement with archives in other countries, so these data can be made available to researchers outside the United Kingdom.

The future

From the inception of the study it has been the intention to follow-up the group of young people in this study into adulthood, and the determination to do so remains as strong as ever. However, there is no detailed research design and no assured funding to enable this intention to be implemented. Those of us involved in the study are convinced that with this, as with other major longitudinal studies, the benefits in terms of increased knowledge multiply with successive follow-ups. Further, development itself does not end at some arbitrary point in childhood or adolescence but continues through life; it is important therefore to have some purchase on answers to questions such as: what kind of children become what kind of citizens, workers, or parents? How do adults themselves develop over time and is this related to aspects of childhood? In what ways does one birth cohort of adults differ in these respects from cohorts born earlier?

However, as mentioned above, the funding of the National Child Development Study has in the past never been assured for more than four years at one time. In the absence of any firm commitment of future funding, the danger is that the research design is perceived only in immediate and pragmatic terms, and that because of a lack of security the research team itself periodically changes and loses a stability and continuity which would be advantageous for the research itself. Therefore, the researchers have had to make assumptions about what might be possible if events should prove favourable for future work on the study. This planning, in turn, has had to be founded, not on any idealistic notion upon what the future could bring, but on a more realistic appraisal of what could be possible.

Before turning to the matter of research that might now be carried out using the National Child Development Study, it is perhaps important to mention one factor which complicates the raising of funds which would enable this study to continue; namely, the fact that it is interdisciplinary in nature. This interdisciplinary character seems to inhibit a specific disciplinary interest, such as a single Government Department, from promoting further work; the task of obtaining support from two or more sponsoring Government Departments or trust funds is much more complex and lengthy, as well as being less likely to prove fruitful. This is in no sense an argument for failing to carry out interdisciplinary studies in an interdisciplinary institution, such as the National Children's Bureau. On the contrary, it is an argument for providing a policy towards such longitudinal studies which recognizes that the best return from any national comprehensive study is that it be planned as a long-term, even life-time, venture and that support should be provided for a core of research staff whose task would include the continual development of the study and the preparation of follow-ups at various points in time; these follow-ups might well require additional staff who would concentrate on a particular phase of the study only.

Given that this is not the situation which obtains for the National Child Development Study, what would be a viable scheme for future work? This would seem to us to fall into two distinct parts, the first being concerned with the exploitation of data already gathered, and the second with the collection of further data on the cohort as they get older.

Exploitation of data already available

Longitudinal studies seem to have been singled out for special criticism because of a tendency to gather data which is then not analysed. In the case of the National Child Development Study it has been decided, on principle, at times to collect information which it was expected might not be analysed immediately but which would prove valuable should future funding become available.

At the time of preparation of this account the follow-up carried out at sixteen years is almost complete and it is clear that much valuable data will be unexploited, particularly with respect to special groups of children with particular needs. Thus one object which remains is to obtain funding to enable further analysis to be carried out on, for example, children who are handicapped, who have been adopted, or have grown up in public care, who have a known criminal record, or have been mentally ill; in each case the opportunity arises to explore the backgrounds of these different groups of children to shed more light on the problems which they have and how such problems have come about. The aetiology and epidemiology of such conditions comprise gaps in our knowledge which, if filled, could lead to the development of policies to improve the circumstances of such groups of children, young people, and adults in the future. Further studies could explore the ways in which medical, educational, and social services have been used by different groups in different parts of Britain to illuminate both the nature of the group utilizing services and the territorial injustices involved in the services as delivered.

Gathering new data

The difficulties of developing a comprehensive plan for the long-term future of the study are discussed above. What follows is a suggestion for work which could be carried out within the next decade, when the cohort is moving into and through their twenties.

This stage of life is one when most young adults are marrying, having children, and hence forming households and becoming established in their job and career. It is a period of high geographic mobility as well as occupational and social mobility. Any study should therefore focus on these characteristics and the attitudes, intentions, aspirations, and experiences of the cohort in relation to the range of data already collected on their social, environmental, educational, and health attributes from birth onwards. Data could be obtained on family structure, household formation, housing aspirations, geographic mobility, employment patterns, health, aspects of educational choice and mobility, post-sixteen schooling, further and higher education; such data could be analysed both cross-sectionally and longitudinally in order to inform future demographic, housing, and employment projections in the light of interdisciplinary background factors.

Such a study could address itself to the ways in which fertility is associated with housing, employment, or social, educational, and medical background. It could examine the relationship between expressed housing preferences, tenure options, and past housing experiences. It could consider the view that socially deprived children are likely to continue to be housing disadvantaged in early adulthood. Further, if appropriate, special studies could be carried out amongst minority groups (rather than concentrating on the essentially normal population) such as those exposed to particular housing stress, or people in single person households, or single parents. The study might explore ways in which job choice, school attainments, further and higher education and training, and basic education and earlier experiences are inter-related. Topics that could be examined might include the ways in which housing availability is itself related to job choice, the readiness of individuals to move to seek work, the aspirations of young women in the employment market, the relationship of job aspiration and the present occupation to aspects of physical and educational development in childhood.

Turning to education, it could be important to explore the further

and higher education of the young adults, and to relate this and their job experiences, etc., to aspects of education and home background in childhood. Analyses could explore day-release, apprenticeship, adult education, public examination results, late development, aspirations, and earlier educational attainments.

Given the considerable volume of information about the health and physical development of the cohort in childhood it would also be important to attempt to measure adult health, and to relate both earlier health and physical development to, for example, use of health and personal social services, attitudes to smoking and family planning, the take-up of social welfare benefits, and fertility rates, etc.

While it is clear that such a study could add significantly to knowledge of the circumstances, aspirations, and experiences of young adults in relation to their own earlier backgrounds, such a study would present a host of technical problems both of a methodological nature and of a practical kind for the team involved in it. The technical difficulties of analysis and interpretation are well known, and alternative solutions to them are continually being tried out. On the other hand, the practical difficulties are more problematic. For example, the study has succeeded well to date in enlisting the co-operation of the subjects, in part because they have been in schools and hence have been relatively easy to contact; now that this is no longer the case, there must be uncertainty concerning the success with which a tracing exercise could be carried out, and the response that could be obtained.[†]

Certainly, whatever the problems, the National Children's Bureau would welcome the opportunity to attempt their solution in continuing to study this nationally representative group.

Additional references

Essen and Ghodsian (1977); Fogelman (1978*a*); Peckham and Pearson (1977); Lambert (1977*a*); Richardson *et al.* (1977); Pearson and Lambert (1977); Lambert and Pearson (1977); Lambert (1977*b*); Essen and Lambert (1977); Walker and Lewis (1977); Pearson and Richardson (1978); Essen *et al.* (1978*a*); Tibbenham *et al.* (1978*a*); Fogelman *et al.* (1978); Essen *et al.* (1978*b*); Lambert (1978*a*); Ghodsian and Lambert (1978); Sherridan and Peckham (1978); Fogelman (1978*b*); Peckham and Butler (1978); Fogelman (1978*c*); Fogelman *et al.* (1978); Lambert (1978*b*); Essen (1978); Calnan *et al.* (1978); Tibbenham *et al.* (1978*b*); Essen *et al.* (1978); Fogelman (1979); Essen *et al.* (1979); Hutchison *et al.* (1979); Essen and Fogelman (1979)

† In fact, since this account was first written, a feasibility study has been mounted which entailed attempting to trace and interview a 5 per cent sub-sample of the cohort at the age of twenty. As a result we are now confident that it is possible to carry out a successful interview with at least 75 per cent of the subjects, and that any bias in the responding sample will be small. The National Children's Bureau is currently negotiating funds for a further full follow-up.

---

8. Pregnancy and birth complications in the aetiology of psychiatric disorders with a special reference to the temperament of the children: a description of the Finnish prospective epidemiological study

TERTTU ARAJÄRVI and MATTI O. HUTTUNEN

Introduction

There is substantial evidence that pregnancy and birth complications (PBC) may play some role in the aetiology of a number of child and adult psychiatric disorders (Lilienfield *et al.* 1955; Pollack

and Woerner 1966; Woerner *et al.* 1973; Pollin and Stabenau 1968; Mednick *et al.* 1971; Cohler *et al.* 1975). The research has, however, not yet been able to give answers concerning the aetiological specificity of these complications of a very different nature. Neither has it been possible to rule out that the increased frequency of PBC of the mothers and the psychiatric disorders of the children would stem from a common genetic or social factor rather than that these phenomena would have a direct cause–effect relation. The analysis of the role of the various genetic and environmental factors has been made even more difficult by the fact that most of the relevant research has been done with a relatively small group of subjects with a high genetic risk for the psychiatric disorders. It has been suggested that future research should be directed more towards the identification of factors such as the nature and extent of maternal life-event stress or anxiety that are likely to affect the course of the pregnancy and childbirth (Garmezy 1974; Cohler et al. 1975).

Children have been shown to have different inborn modes of behaviour and temperaments (Thomas et al. 1968; Chess et al. 1973; Buss and Plomin 1975). These temperament characteristics of the children have been demonstrated to be relatively stable and to affect the interaction of the child with his parents and peers. It has been postulated that some of these temperament characteristics increase the risk of the child developing behaviour disorders, especially if his mode of behaviour is not understood to reflect his inborn temperament (Thomas et al. 1968). The inborn temperament of children is probably mostly of genetic origin (Buss and Plomin 1975), but the influence of various environmental events during the foetal and neonatal time on the temperament has not been studied. Still, research with animals has eminently shown the importance of prenatal factors in the development of the mode of animal behaviour (Joffe 1969). One of the present authors has been particularly interested in the possible significance of the mothers' stress during pregnancy in the development of children's behavioural and psychiatric disorders (Huttunen 1971; Huttunen and Niskanen 1977).

The general system of the health care of pregnant mothers and growing children in Finland provides an exceptionally good set-up for the organization of a large prospective study of the development of children. These excellent conditions stimulated us in 1974 to start a major prospective study of the development of the approximately 5000 children born in Helsinki between 1 July 1975 and 30 June 1976. In our project special attention is paid to the role of the PBC and of the temperament of the children in the development of the children's behaviour. This epidemiological project is also closely associated with a simultaneous clinical trial of the use of family counselling in the prevention of children's psychiatric disorders (Arajärvi et al. 1977). This report is a description of the general outlines of our epidemiological project.

General setting for the study

In Finland, there is an excellent functioning network of maternal and well-baby clinics serving the general health-care of the pregnant mothers and growing children. Practically every pregnant mother and growing child (approximately 98 per cent) visit these small out-patient clinics several times during pregnancy and childhood. In these clinics the condition of the pregnant mothers and growing children are continuously recorded and taken care of by midwives and nurses. Most of the pregnant mothers contact these maternal clinics during the first trimester of their pregnancy. In our project, these small out-patient clinics were used to contact the mothers and children, to deliver the questionnaires to the parents, and to get information from the records of these clinics. In the City of Helsinki there are 30 maternal clinics and 38 well-baby clinics serving a population of 500 000 inhabitants.

In Helsinki, approximately 5000 children are born every year. The great majority of these children (about 95 per cent) are delivered in the two big central obstetrical clinics of the city, the University Obstetrical Clinic and the Midwives' Institute. Both of these clinics keep similar excellent and detailed records of all the complications and events of the delivery and of the neonatal condition of the child. In our project, we are using these hospital records as the source of the data concerning the pregnancy, the delivery and the neonatal period.

Finnish registers useful to this longitudinal project

In Finland, there is a central population register using a social security number as the identification code. The social security number is based on the birth date, and all the other available registers are arranged according to the social security number or the birth date. In our country, there is not a central register for psychiatric diseases or suicides, but these data can be obtained from the other available registers. The Social Insurance Institution of the State has the computerized records of all persons who receive social security benefits for illnesses, get invalid pensions for any somatic or psychiatric diseases, or continuously use the free-of-charge drugs for major disabling chronic somatic or psychiatric illnesses. The State Medical Board keeps a central register of all the admissions and discharges of the somatic and psychiatric hospitals in the country.

There is also a central birth and death register, which includes the medical reason of the death and the mode of death (e.g. suicide). Finland is divided into districts of psychiatric health care, each of which has a central psychiatric hospital with detailed hospital registers. The City of Helsinki forms one district of this kind. Furthermore, there is a central register for criminality. All of these above registers are in principle available for research purposes, but permission has to be applied for from the appropriate authorities. Those gaining access to the registers have to guarantee the protection of the anonymity of the people under investigation. It is evident that the existent registers provide a good opportunity for the careful follow-up of the children under study.

Administration and funding of the project

The project is funded by the Academy of Finland. The project is divided into two separate parts, the epidemiological part and the trial of family counselling for the prevention of children's psychiatric disorders. Professor Terttu Arajärvi of the Department of Child Psychiatry is the director of the whole project and the director and co-ordinator of the family counselling project. Dr Matti O. Huttunen of the Department of Psychiatry serves as the co-ordinator and director of the epidemiological part of the project. The available funds are quite limited and this has resulted in the slow pace of the coding and analysis of the already available basic data.

In 1974 during the preliminary stage of the project we were also given financial support from the State Medical Board of Finland. The project has also been given financial and consultation aid by Dr Sarnoff Mednick from Denmark, and by Drs Alexander Thomas and Stella Chess from the United States.

Definition of the sample

Our basic sample of children is defined as follows: all children who were born between 1 July 1975 and 30 June 1976 in the two above-mentioned central obstetrical clinics of Helsinki (approximately 95 per cent of all the children born in Helsinki) and whose mother was living in the City of Helsinki at the time of the delivery. The total number of the children is about 5000–5500; the exact number is not yet available. Most of the mothers of these children were contacted during the first trimester of their pregnancy when they visited the maternal out-patient clinics. Similarly, when the mothers visited the well-baby clinics they were given the questionnaire concerning the temperament of the children as these children reached the age of 6 to 8 months.

By the definition of our sample we have detailed data of the delivery and neonatal condition of all the children of our cohort. The obstetrical records also include detailed information about the course of the pregnancy.

The recovery and availability of all the other data has depended upon the motivation of the children's parents to fill out the various questionnaires (see below). The data on the temperament characteristics of some children may be missing due to the fact that their parents had moved out of the City before the child had reached the age of 6 to 8 months. This loss of some of the temperament data results from the fact that the temperament questionnaire was delivered to the mothers by the nurses of the well-baby clinics.

The epidemiological follow-up of the sample is intended to cover all the children of the basic cohort. At the moment, we plan to monitor the temperament of the children and the general conditions of the child and the family, as the children of our sample reach the age of 5 to 6 years. Depending on the availability of funds, this re-examination will either be limited to the children and families living in Helsinki at that time or an effort will be made to follow-up all the children of the basic cohort.

Assessment of the cohort

The following data is presently available from all or part of the children of our cohort:

(1) *Complete data of the delivery and neonatal condition of the children.* These data have been obtained from the detailed hospital registers of the two central obstetrical clinics, in which the children of our cohort were born. These hospital records also include detailed data on the course of the pregnancy, on the use of drugs during the pregnancy, on the possible previous pregnancies of the mother, and on the medical and gynecological history of the mother. A complete list of these PBC data is presented in Table 8.1. This data is available for all the children of our basic cohort.

(2) *Data on the social, physical, and psychological condition of the parents at the time of the delivery.* When the mothers of our cohort children made their first visit to the out-patient maternal clinics, they were given a structured questionnaire. This questionnaire was designed to obtain information concerning the general history and social conditions of the parents, including the professional and social status of the parents, housing and working conditions, and information regarding the possible presence of somatic or psychiatric diseases in the parents and their relatives. The recovery of this questionnaire is estimated to be 80 per cent.

(3) *Data on the occurrence of minor infections, psychological and somatic stress, panic states, depression, and insomnia during the pregnancy.* When the mothers of our cohort children first visited the maternal out-patient clinics, they were given a 12-piece set of simple questionnaires (see Table 8.2) and were asked to fill out one questionnaire for each clinic visit during pregnancy. The purpose of these questionnaires was to obtain some information on the occurrence and exact timing of the above-mentioned events which may affect the delivery or development of the child. The recovery of these questionnaires is estimated to be 50 per cent.

(4) *Medical data of the children who needed special paediatric hospital care during the neonatal period.* The records of the paediatric hospitals were used to register the medical details (laboratory examinations, etc.) of all the children of the cohort who needed special paediatric attention during the neonatal period.

(5) *Data on the general condition of the child and family during the first six months of the child's life.* The nurses of the well-baby clinics were able to interview approximately 3300 of the mothers of the cohort children in order to get this information.

(6) *Data on the temperament of the children at the age of 6 to 8 months.* When the children of our cohort reached the age of 6 months, the nurses of the well-baby clinics delivered to the mothers a structured questionnaire requesting information on the temperament of their children. Based on the research by Thomas *et al.* (1968), Carey developed a temperament questionnaire (Carey

TABLE 8.1

Pregnancy and birth complications—List of data recorded from the structured hospital records

---

I Medical history of the mother
   mother's previous somatic and psychiatric illnesses
   illnesses in the relatives of the mother
   mother's gynaecological diseases
   menstrual history of the mother
II Previous pregnancies of the mother
   the number and year of previous pregnancies and deliveries
   the sex and birth weight of previous children
   the duration of the previous deliveries
   the list of the complications of previous pregnancies
III History of the present pregnancy
   estimated time of delivery
   list of symptoms and diseases during pregnancy (includes 21 items)
   list and time of medication during pregnancy
IV Prenatal medical condition of the mother
   weight and length
   weight increase during the pregnancy
   blood group and Rhesus antibodies
   blood pressure, heart size, pulse, temperature
   presence of protein and glucose in the urine
   estimation of the amount of bleeding
   foetal heart sounds
   measures of the pelvis

V Data of the delivery
   duration of the delivery
   quality of the contractions
   time of rupture of the membranes
   quantity, quality, and color of the amniotic fluid
   condition and measures of the placenta(s) and umbilical cord
   manner of birth (presentation, assistance, section, etc.)
VI Medication during the delivery
   list, dosage, time of medication
VII Condition of the child(ren) in hospital
   time of birth
   exact time of onset of respiration
   Apgar points at 1 and 5 min
   weight, length, sex, measures of skull
   malformations
   medical condition of the neonatal child
   laboratory findings (glucose, bilirubin, pH, Ca, urine)
   list of symptoms (pulse, temperature, color, crying, etc.) (24 items)
VIII Medication and treatments of the neonatal child
   drugs, vitamins, transfusions, X-rays, etc.
IX Postnatal condition of the mother
   list of complications

TABLE 8.2

Rating scale of somatic and psychic stress during pregnancy

Name ——————— Date ——— Social Security no. ———————

1. Have you had any of the following symptoms during the past month?
   1. fever   2. sore throat   3. running nose
   4. coughing   5. muscle pains   6. ear ache
   7. headache   8. diarrhoea   9. malaise

2. When did the above symptoms start?
   1. 0–1 weeks ago   2. 1–2 weeks ago   3. 2–3 weeks ago
   4. 3–5 weeks ago

3. How long did the above symptoms last?
   1. 1–3 days   2. 3–7 days   3. more than 7 days

4. Have you been somatically stressed (e.g. heavy homework, travels, etc.)?
   1. no   2. somewhat   3. a lot

5. Have you experienced psychic stress (e.g. worried, depressed, anxious, fearful, etc.)?
   1. no   2. somewhat   3. a lot

6. How have you been sleeping?
   1. worse than usual 2. as usual   3. better than usual

7. Have you been frightened, experienced a strong affection or a panic reaction?
   1. no   2. yes

8. When did this happen?
   1. 0–1 weeks ago   2. 1–2 weeks ago   3. 2–3 weeks ago
   4. 3–5 weeks ago

9. Has your mood changed from the time before pregnancy?
   1. no   2. somewhat   3. a lot

10. Have you been tired?
    1. no   2. somewhat   3. a lot

11. Have you been restless or nervous?
    1. no   2. somewhat   3. a lot

12. Has your mood been unstable or capricious?
    1. no   2. somewhat   3. a lot

13. Have you been depressed?
    1. no   2. somewhat   3. a lot

14. Do you smoke?
    1. no   2. more than 5   3. only occasionally
                          cigarettes per   or less than 5
                          day   cigarettes per day

1970). In our study we used a modification of this original questionnaire and included more examples of the child's behaviour to help the mother in her choices. The Finnish modification of Carey's questionnaire can be obtained from the authors. In a preliminary study of 300 mothers this modification of Carey's questionnaire was shown to yield a distribution of the different temperaments similar to that in the original study (Huttunen *et al.* 1977). The recovery of this questionnaire is estimated to be 50 per cent.

Background information

At the present moment we do not have any information on the grandparents or other relatives of the children. We have available the social security number of the father and mother. The data we have include some soft data on the medical and psychiatric history of the mother and father, as well as their parents. In principle, using the available registers it would be possible to obtain the information concerning, for example, the presence of major psychiatric diseases in the parents and grandparents of the children. However, this monitoring would, of course, need substantial extra funding that is not presently available.

Status of the data

Most of the data is still in raw form. We are currently working on the coding and punching of the data, which will probably be completed during 1977. The pace of the coding, punching, and taping of the available data is somewhat slowed by the lack of sufficient funding.

Future plans

Our aim is to re-examine and to follow-up the cohort every five years. It is our purpose to monitor the temperament of the cohort children at the age of 5 to 6 years using a questionnaire developed by Thomas and Chess. At the same time the parents of the children will be asked to fill out a structured questionnaire concerning the general conditions of the child and the family. Originally, we had plans to measure the galvanic skin response (GSR) and the response of the heart rate to auditory stimuli in a large sample of our cohort children. Due to the lack of available funds we have had to postpone the monitoring of these psychophysiological characteristics of the children. We do have the necessary instruments available, however, and plan to do these measurements at least among selected groups of the children. These plans include the measurement of the GSR and the heart rate response among the children with difficult PBCs and difficult temperaments.

General outline of the trial of family counselling for the prevention of children's psychiatric disorders

The epidemiological study of the described large cohort of children is closely associated with a simultaneous clinical trial of family counselling for the prevention of children's psychiatric disorders. This project of family counselling is described in more detail elsewhere (Arajärvi *et al.* 1977).

In this project we selected every eighth child coming to the eight districts of the well-baby clinics, covering approximately 1600 families of the larger epidemiological cohort. The final group used for family counselling consisted of 170 families, since 23 families refused to participate in the study, two children were treated in children's homes, and one child had died. The parents of these 170 families were interviewed by a psychiatric nurse 3 to 6 times during the first six months of the child's life. The purpose of these interviews was to get an estimation of the risk status of these 170 families before dividing them into the index counselling group and the control group. The families were divided into four groups of different estimated risk status and the counselling and control groups were designed to consist of an equal number of families. In defining the risk status of the families we used a rating scale of the various risk factors (see Table 8.3). Group I consisted of the families with 0 points, group II of the families with 1 to 13 points, group III of the families with 13 to 20 points, and group IV of the families with over 21 points on this simple rating scale. In our group of 170 families there were 58 families with 0 points, 83 families with 1–13 points, 17 families with 14–20 points and 12 families with more than 20 points on this rating scale. When making this family diagnosis we used the material obtained from the interviews of the parents as well as the information obtained from the hospital records and questionnaires. After the family diagnosis of risk status was done the group of 170 families was divided into two groups, the index counselling group and the control group. The index group of 85 families will receive regular family counselling for five years, and the other group of 85 families will serve as a control group. The families of the control group will not be met by our research group for the next five years, but these families can naturally use the general existent health care system for their possible mental health problems.

TABLE 8.3

Rating scale of the risk factors in the child and the family

I. Somatic and psychic risk factors

1. Mode of interaction between the family members

Risk factor	Score of the factor	
	mild	severe
Lack of mother or father		8
Deviant attitude of the mother towards the child	5	8
Deviant attitude of the father towards the child	5	8
Deviant attitude of the siblings towards the newborn		2
Initial insecurity of the mother with the child		1
Initial insecurity of the father with the child		1
Difficulties in the mother's own childhood	2	4
Difficulties in the father's own childhood	2	4
Deviant interaction of the parents	2	3
Deviant interaction of the adults living in the family	3	5

2. Health of the members of the family

Risk factor	Score of the factor		
	Psychic disorder	Somatic or psychic illness	
		mild	severe
Illness of the newborn		1	3
Somatic illness of the mother			2
Somatic illness of the father			2
Psychiatric disorder or illness of the mother	4	7	10
Psychiatric disorder of illness of the father	4	7	10
Somatic illness of the siblings		1	2
Psychiatric disorder or illness of the siblings	1	2	4
Death or severe illness of a close relative			1

II. Socio-economic status of the family

Risk factor	Score of the factor	
	mild	severe
Change of the caretaker of the child		2
Difficulties in housing	1	3
Economical difficulties		3

The family counselling will be done by three psychiatric nurses, who will visit the families one to three times per three months. Our idea is to test the hypothesis that simple family counselling can improve the interaction between the child and his parents, and thus prevent the development of psychiatric disorders in the child by decreasing the parents' unnecessary fears concerning the development and behaviour of the child.

After five years our aim is to study the children and the family dynamics of both the index and control families. At the same time we will be recording the temperament and the problems of the children of the large basic cohort using simple questionnaires. The data obtained from the 170 families of the prevention programme will then be compared with the data obtained from the large cohort of children.

Special advantages of the project

The exceptional conditions provided by the Finnish health care system and the health and population registers give this project some special advantages over a number of other projects of this kind. The existent network of the well-baby clinics and the presence of only two major obstetrical clinics in Helsinki has made it possible to collect detailed information on the PBCs and temperament characteristics of a very large number of children unselected in relation to their genetic risk for behavioural disorders. The number of children in the sample will make it possible to get reliable data on the aetiological importance of PBCs, e.g. in schizophrenia and asocial behaviour.

At the moment, there is no knowledge of the possible importance of different temperament characteristics in the aetiology of adult psychiatric disorders. Neither is there any knowledge about the role of PBCs in the aetiology of the different inborn temperaments of the children. This project will bring some answers to these questions, even if the temperament data obtained with the present simple questionnaires is considered as relatively soft data.

The simultaneous clinical trial of preventive family counselling among a subsample of the basic cohort does provide an additional advantage, as the comparison of the epidemiological results with the clinical experiences during counselling may provide interesting views on the interaction of biological factors, family dynamics, and social factors in the aetiology of psychiatric disorders.

9. Chronic somatic morbidity, psychiatric disorders, and psychosocial adaptation in children and youth: a 20-year follow-up cohort study of children born in Helsinki in 1955 (Finland)

GUSTAV AMNELL

Aims and scope of the study

The aim of the study is to follow up a given child population from birth to adulthood in order to elucidate a number of important medical, psychic, and social aspects of the cohort members' lives and development. The amount of data that can be obtained from an investigation of this kind is almost infinite. Therefore, the aims must be limited so as to prevent over-loading. The specific aims of this study are as follows:

(1) To estimate the frequency of certain chronic somatic diseases and disabling disorders in childhood and to investigate the age-dependence of these states, variations of their incidence and prevalence, and their relevance to adaptation to adult life;

(2) To investigate the frequency of psychiatric treatment contacts, i.e. children's visits to psychiatric clinics or psychiatric child guidance centres for examination or treatment, and the bearing of such contacts upon the subsequent mental health of the individuals;

(3) To investigate the correlation between social child care and later social adaptation and psychological health;

(4) To investigate somatic and psychological morbidity in relation to social adaptation in youth;

(5) To investigate the relevance of pre-, peri-, and postnatal factors to morbidity in childhood and youth and to social adaptation at the end of adolescence.

In addition, the study has the special aim of providing material for reference or comparison for possible further enquiry into the importance of so-called maternal heart volume control for preventing prematurity and sequelae of prematurity. This topic has been discussed by Räihä (1964, 1968), Räihä and Kauppinen (1963), and Kauppinen (1967). The investigation is planned to continue until the cohort members have reached the age of 20, but in principle it can be carried even further if the economic prerequisites are secured.

The population investigated—the cohort

The population or cohort selected for the investigation consisted of all the 6789 children born in Helsinki in 1955 to mothers living permanently in the city at the time of delivery. Helsinki, the capital of Finland, had 403 970 inhabitants in 1955. At that time, maternity health centres were already well organized in the city and the frequency of visits to municipal guidance centres was approximately 95 per cent. The deliveries took place at some of the six maternity hospitals in the city. There were no actual deliveries at home. The cohort is 7·7 per cent of the 89 740 children born in Finland in 1955, but it is representative only of a population of pregnant mothers living in Helsinki. The material is typically urban.

Out of the 6789 cohort children 3504 (51·6 per cent) were male and 3283 (48·4 per cent) female. In two cases the sex could not be determined. There were 208 (3·1 per cent) twins among these children, which makes a total of 6685 mothers. Out of these 6685 mothers, 6250 (93·6 per cent) were married, 421 (6·3 per cent)

unmarried, and eight (0·1 per cent) widowed or divorced. The civil status of six mothers was unknown. Mothers below the age of 30 comprised 68·4 per cent of the total. The mothers were divided into social groups according to the professions of their husbands. The social groups were determined according to the classification used by the statistical bureau of the city of Helsinki. Thus, 23·8 per cent of the married mothers belonged to social group I, 20·6 per cent to social group II, 37·7 per cent to social group III and 13·4 per cent to social group IV. Four mothers (0·1 per cent) were married to invalids, and 4·4 per cent of the mothers were married to students. These data on the mothers concern the time of delivery.

Method of the study

Methodologically, the study is a cohort investigation. The population or cohort is clearly defined and delimited. Those selected for the population investigation were all the children with a weight at birth of 600 g or more, born in 1955 at one of the six maternity hospitals in Helsinki to mothers who gave this city as their place of residence at the time of the birth of the child. The investigation is longitudinal and the follow-up extends from the time of delivery to the twentieth year of life of the cohort members. The cases observed are clearly defined. According to the definition given by MacMahon and Pugh (1970) the investigation is partially retrospective. The implications of all the data are, however, prospective in that they are based upon case-book entries made simultaneously with the events they describe.

Practical procedure

The work involved in the investigation was started in Spring, 1955. The *first phase* of the work consisted of identifying the index children, i.e. of compiling a birth register. This was done by making an inventory of the 1955 records of the six maternity hospitals in the city. Information on the child's date of birth, sex, weight at birth, neonatal status, and where the child went after discharge, as well as data concerning the mother's age, civil status, parish, and register authority were filed and transferred to so-called primary cards.

The *second phase* was the tracing of the children, i.e. finding out their domiciles and addresses. The cohort children were 10 and 11 years of age when this phase was started, and consequently most of the addresses reported in the delivery journals were out of date. In 1965, the creation of a computerized central population register was initiated in Finland, but until 1970 this register was too deficient to be of any use in tracing. The investigation staff had to employ conventional tracing methods. The Helsinki register of children of school age proved to be the best source. In Finland the municipalities are obliged to keep registers of all children of compulsory school age, and the register of the city of Helsinki is rather accurate. The rest of the cohort (35 per cent) was traced by means of enquiries to the address agency of the Helsinki police office. After the inventory of the Helsinki address agency, about 15 per cent of the cohort children were still untraced. The remainder were traced through enquiries to various local address agencies in

Finland and to the Finnish parish in Stockholm, which registers Finnish people resident in Sweden. The tracing was time-consuming and laborious, because it had to be done manually.

The *third phase* of the work consisted of establishing the children's state of health during the first follow-up period from birth to 31 May 1969. When the first part of the follow-up period expired, the children had normally finished their seventh school year, which in Finnish conditions also meant that practically all the children who were to continue their education had moved on from elementary school to secondary grammar school. This was the predominant rationale of selecting 31 May 1969 as the date of expiration of the first follow-up period.

The aim of what is here called follow-up work was to identify those children who had, or had had, some of those diseases which the investigation was concerned with. These children were identified primarily by means of their school health records. In Finland, child health centres and school health services are well organized and co-ordinated. In 1962, the year the cohort children started school, a new system using cumulative health records was introduced (Hultin 1973). The idea of the new record was to allow a follow-up of the child from birth until school-leaving. In principle, the information concerning the cohort children ought to have been transferred, in 1962, from the old health records to the new cumulative ones. In fact, some interesting data from the time before school age seems to have been omitted. Anyway, the children had gone to school for seven years when the first follow-up period expired, and it is thus probable that all graver diseases and defects had been entered into the health records. According to Hultin and Paavilainen (1967) only 3·5 per cent of all Finnish children born in 1956 had not been examined by physicians. During the first school year, 1·1 per cent of the children in Helsinki and 2·6 per cent of the children in Uusimaa, the administrative province where Helsinki is situated, had not undergone medical examinations. Consequently, the school health records may be regarded as a reliable source for the identification of all more serious diseases during the entire follow-up period and of other diseases that had begun after the year 1962. It is, however, probable that certain milder diseases of a temporary nature that the children had suffered from before school have not been carried over to the new cumulative records. This is true, in the first place, of asthma, certain skin affections, temporary convulsions, and passing behavioural disorders. In cases where information could not be obtained from the health records, an enquiry was sent to the parents. Information on the health condition of the children was obtained from the health records in 94 per cent of the cases and in 6 per cent of the cases from the parents.

The *fourth phase* of the work consisted of two additional inventories. In order to determine the frequency within the cohort of psychiatric examination or treatment contacts, the archives of all the thirty-nine psychiatric guidance clinics working in the country at that time and those of the psychiatric children's hospitals in Helsinki were searched. In order to establish child welfare measures concerning the cohort, the archives of the child welfare office in Helsinki and those of the child welfare boards of municipalities to which cohort children had moved were examined.

In the *fifth phase* of the work, clinical data concerning children known to have, or have had, any of the diseases relevant to the investigation were collected. These data were gathered from the archives of different hospitals, polyclinics, psychiatric guidance clinics, and, occasionally, from individual doctors. Information on causes of death were obtained from the register of death at the Central Statistical Office in Finland.

The *sixth phase* of the work consisted of collecting pregnancy and delivery information for the cohort children. This information was obtained from the children's delivery journals.

All data were coded and stored on punch cards and magnetic tape. The *statistical processing* was done at the data-processing centre of the University of Helsinki by means of a Burroughs 6700 computer using statistical program packets planned for this device. Significance was tested by means of statistical standard tests (t- and X^2-tests). The differences between the various groups were analyzed by means of discrimination analysis. Three significance levels were given: very significant ($p<0·001$), significant ($p<0·01$), and nearly significant ($p<0·05$).

The clinical data concerning the first follow-up period were obtained from journals of various hospitals, polyclinics, and guidance centres. No clinical examinations, tests, or interviews were made. The results of the first follow-up phase have been described by Amnell (1974). At present, work is proceeding on the second follow-up phase, spanning the time to 31 December 1975, when all cohort members had reached the age of twenty years. Accordingly, the results to be reported in the following section concern the first follow-up period, i.e. the time from the birth of the cohort children to 31 May, 1969. The work was started at the II Paediatric Clinic at the University of Helsinki under the guidance of the then chief of the clinic, Professor Carl-Eric Räihä. From 1970 onwards, the investigation has been carried out at the Department of Public Health Science of the University of Helsinki, whose chief, Professor Ilari Rantasalo, has given it active support. The investigation is lead by the reader in public health science Gustav Amnell, M.D. Participating in the second follow-up phase are Fredrik Almqvist, M.D., Klaus Winell, M.D., and Leif Martelin, M.D.

Results

Follow-up results

On expiration of the follow-up period, 31 May, 1969, 307 (4·5 per cent) of the cohort children had died, clinical data on the state of health had been obtained regarding 6170 (90·9 per cent), and 312 (4·6 per cent) were untraced. Of the 6170 children whose health data were known 6101 had been followed up before 31 May, 1969, whereas 69 had dropped out earlier. Out of these 69, 39 were healthy and 30 had, or had had, some of the diseases relevant to the investigation. To sum up, 6408 children, 307 of whom were dead and 6101 alive, had been followed up before 31 May, 1969. The total follow-up percentage as of 31 May, 1969, was 94·4 per cent.

Of the 381 children lost to follow-up before 31 May 1969, 197 (51·7 per cent) had already dropped out in the first year. The drop-out during the first year was 2·9 per cent of the whole cohort as against 0·1 to 0·3 per cent per annum in the following years. For 312 of these 389 lost to the follow-up, health data were lacking completely and in 69 cases health data had been obtained. The 312 whose health data and addresses could not be found were brought together into a group called untraced children. Some of these children might turn up in the second phase.

Data of pregnancy, delivery, and the neonatal stage

Pregnancy. There were 3040 (45·5 per cent) primiparous mothers and 3641 (54·5 per cent) multiparous. Previously the multiparous mothers had borne a total of 6616 children, i.e. 1·8 children per mother. The previous stillborn rate was 1·4 per cent, the previous 0–7 days mortality was 1·7 per cent, and the total previous perinatal mortality was 3·2 per cent. There were 1157 (17·8 per cent) of the mothers who had previously had one or several miscarriages. Most of the cohort mothers (97·3 per cent) had visited either maternity health centres or doctors during pregnancy; 2·7 per cent had visited neither maternity health centres nor doctors; 2·0 per cent of the married and 12·3 per cent of the unmarried mothers belonged to this group ($p < 0·001$). In 1955, 95·2 per cent of all childbearers in Finland were enlisted in maternity health centres (Hultin 1973).

The frequency of toxaemia was 9·0 per cent among all mothers, 8·4 per cent among the married ones, and 15·0 per cent among the unmarried ($p < 0·05$). Placenta praevia occurred in 41 cases (0·6 per cent), ablatio placentae in 47 cases (0·7 per cent), anomalies of uterus in four cases (0·1 per cent), and leiomyoma in eleven cases (0·2 per cent). Because information on vaginal bleeding was unreliable, it was excluded from further treatment. Urinary tract infections had occurred in 1·7 per cent, active tuberculosis in 0·3 per cent, and seropositive lues in 0·1 per cent of the cases. Not a single mother had gonorrhoea. In a more recent Finnish study (Hartikainen 1973) the frequency of diagnosed urinary tract infections was reported to be 8·4 per cent, which shows that as far as the cohort is concerned, only the manifest urinary tract infections had been entered into the delivery journals. Because the obstetric data were collected retrospectively, the investigation excluded all acute infections that had not been entered into the journals in a reliable way, as a matter of routine.

The were 58 (0·9 per cent) of the mothers who had symptoms of organic heart disease, 17 (0·3 per cent) suffered from diabetes mellitus, and one mother from tyre toxicosis.

Labour and delivery. In 67·4 per cent of the cases labour had started spontaneously, in 29·2 per cent amniotomy was carried out, in 0·7 per cent amniotomy was combined with oxitocic induction, in 0·9 per cent only oxitocic induction was used and in 1·8 per cent (120 cases) Caesarean section was done prior to labour.

Delivery occurred spontaneously in 76·2 per cent of the cases, forceps were used in 2·0 per cent, vacuum extraction in 0·1 per cent, and uterine-stimulant drugs in 13·0 per cent of the cases. In 390 cases (5·8 per cent) Caesarean section was made, which means that section was done in 270 cases in labour.

Disproportion between foetus and pelvis occurred in 2·8 per cent. Hartikainen's (1973) Finnish sample from 1966 gives 1·3 per cent as the corresponding figure. The lower frequency in this sample, which is younger by eleven years, seems to depend upon the lower frequency of rachitic pelves.

The neonatal period. In 130 (1·9 per cent) of the cases children were stillborn, and 6659 (98·1 per cent) were born alive. Of the children born alive 40 (0·6 per cent) died at the maternity hospital, 6078 were discharged as healthy, 295 (4·4 per cent) were sent to neonatal clinics for further treatment, 5 (0·1 per cent) to other clinics, 52 (0·8 per cent) to children's homes, 186 (2·8 per cent) to mothers' homes (homes for single-mothers and children), and 3 children were adopted directly from the maternity hospital. There were 441 (6·5 per cent) of the children born prematurely, i.e. having a birthweight of 600–2500 g.

Entries in delivery journals on the children's neonatal status were generally scarce and of questionable value. Notwithstanding, data on incubator care, asphyxia, icterus, neonatal convulsions, birth injuries, and malformation were collected. Data on malformations concerned all the children; other neonatal data were for the 6659 children who were born alive. Of these children 305 (5·3 per cent) had entries on asphyxia without incubator care. In 1955 the Apgar score was not yet in use. Ninety-three children (1·6 per cent) had had incubator care, but the indications for incubator care did not appear from the journals. Mild icterus occurred in 10·0 per cent of the cases, grave icterus without immunization in 0·1 per cent, and icterus with Rh-immunization in 0·3 per cent. Only 5 (0·1 per cent) of the children were recorded for neonatal convulsions. The number was probably greater, but then the children had been sent to neonatal clinics without mention of the convulsions in the delivery journals.

Care in paediatric neonatal clinics. In 1955 there were four hospitals with paediatric wards in Helsinki. All of them also cared for newborns. In 1955, paediatric care in maternity hospitals was not yet organized, but small prematures and new-borns with complications were, as a rule, sent to some of these hospitals. There were 295 (4·4 per cent) of the live-births of the cohort who were looked after in some of these neonatal wards; 59 (20 per cent) of these infants were twins and 180 (61·0 per cent) had a birthweight of 600–2500 g. This means that 180 (49·7 per cent) of the 362 live-born prematures of the cohort were taken care of in a neonatal ward. Of the children, 74 died in neonatal wards.

Division of the subjects

On the basis of the facts received concerning the state of health of the children, the cohort was divided into the following groups:

(1) Healthy children;
(2) Children with congenital or acquired defects (mental retardation and subnormality, malformations, neurological diseases and sequelae, and defects of the senses), henceforth called handicapped children;
(3) Children with certain psychosomatic and internal diseases, who will be referred to as children with other diseases;
(4) Somatically healthy children who had been in for psychiatric treatment or examination;
(5) Untraced children.

Table 9.1 shows the division of the cohort into these groups.

TABLE 9.1

Division of the cohort into main groups (31 May 1969)

| Group | Total | | Living and traced |
	N	per cent	per cent
Healthy	4735	69·7	76·7
Handicapped	536	7·9	8·7
Other diseases	310	4·6	5·0
Psychiatric cases	589	8·7	9·6
Dead	307	4·5	—
Untraced	312	4·6	—

Clinical data

The clinical data summarized here concern mental retardation, mental subnormality, malformations, neuromuscular disorders, defects of the sense organs, psychosomatic and internal diseases, and psychiatric treatment contacts. The sum total in the groups to be described in this chapter is greater than indicated by Table 9.1, because several children have more than one handicap or disease.

Mental retardation and mental subnormality

There were 65 children (32 boys and 33 girls) who were mentally retarded (IQ 0–67). Of these, 56 children were alive on completion of the follow-up period on 31 May 1969. Nine (13·8 per cent) of the mentally retarded children had died. Six of the deceased suffered from Down's syndrome, one from hydrocephalus, and two from cerebral palsy (CP). Forty-two (64·6 per cent) of the children had manifest clinical signs of organic injury (central nervous system (CNS) injury, malformations, or defects of the senses), while 23 (35·4 per cent) lacked diagnosed organic injuries. Ten (15·4 per cent) of the 65 children had, or had had, epileptic seizures, 8 (12·3 per cent) had been born prematurely.

There were 231 (137 boys and 94 girls), who were classified as mentally subnormal (IQ 68–89). One of them had died during the follow-up period, 47 (20·3 per cent) of them had signs of organic injury, and 184 (79·7 per cent) were 'aclinical'. Nine (3·9 per cent) of them suffered, or had suffered, from epileptic seizures, and 8·2 per cent had been born prematurely.

All mentally retarded and mentally subnormal children had been tested.

Malformations

There were 111 of the 536 children in the handicap group, and 74 of the dead children, who had diagnosed malformations. Out of these 185 children 99 (53·5 per cent) were male and 86 (46·5 per cent) female. Of the 226 cohort children who died perinatally, there were 43 (19·0 per cent) with verified malformations; there were 31 (38·3 per cent) of the 81 cohort children who died after the perinatal period who had verified malformations. It is seen that 74 (40 per cent) of the 185 children had died during the follow-up period. Of the 111 living children with malformations 29 (26·1 per cent) belonged to the mentally retarded or mentally subnormal groups, and 18·9 per cent of the malformed children were premature. Table 9.2 shows the occurrence of malformations in the groups perinat-ally dead (PN), later dead (LD), mentally retarded (MR), mentally subnormal (MSN), and normally intelligent (NI). Incidence figures are included in Table 9.2 but the epidemiology of malformations is also exposed later on.

Neuromuscular disorders

There were 135 children who had signs of neurological sequelae or neuromuscular diseases. Of these children 126 were alive and 9 had died. The number 135 does not include those perinatally dead children who had neurological diagnoses according to ICD XV (certain causes of perinatal morbidity and mortality).

All the 135 children had been examined by specialists, paediatricians, neurologists, or child psychiatrists. Therefore the diagnoses can be regarded as reliable. The diagnoses given in the text are

TABLE 9.2

Malformations in the group perinatally dead, later dead, mentally retarded, mentally subnormal, and normally intelligent

Malformation	PN	LD	MR	MSN	NI	Total N	per cent	Incidence per thousand
Anencephalus	5					5	2·7	0·7
Hydrocephalus	10	3	1			14	7·7	2·1
Hydrocephalus + meningomyelocele	1					1	0·5	0·1
Diastematomyeli					2	2	1·1	0·3
Microcephalus		1				1	0·5	0·1
Cerebri alii	2					2	1·1	0·3
Monstrum	6					6	3·2	0·9
Neurofibromatosis					1	1	0·5	0·1
Syndroma Down		6	5			11	6·0	1·7
Anophthalmus		1				1	0·5	0·1
Coloboma		1		1		2	1·1	0·3
Naeves permagna retinae					1	1	0·5	0·1
Cataracta					1	1	0·5	0·1
Maleformationes auris			1		5	6	3·2	0·9
Maleformationes cordis	7	11	2	1	16	37	20·3	5·8
Hypoplasia pulmonis	2					2	1·1	0·3
Palatoschisis	1	2	1	1	3	8	4·3	1·2
Atresia oesophagi	1	1				2	1·1	0·3
Atresia intestini	1	1				2	1·1	0·3
Atresia ductus biliaris		1				1	0·5	0·1
Morbus Hinschprung		1				1	0·5	0·1
Duplicatio jejuni					1	1	0·5	0·1
Diverticulum Meckelii					1	1	0·5	0·1
Hypospadia	1	2	2		2	7	3·9	2·0
Maleformationes renis	2	2			6	10	5·5	1·6
Pes equino-varus	2			1	7	10	5·5	1·6
Luxatio coxae				1	19	20	10·8	3·3
Syndactylia				3	3	6	3·2	0·9
Polydactylia				1	2	3	1·6	0·5
Pectus excavatum			1		2	3	1·6	0·5
Pectus carinatum					2	2	1·1	0·3
Chondrodystrophia				2		2	1·1	0·3
Ossium et musculorum aliae	1				4	5	2·7	0·7
Syndroma Klinefelter				1		1	0·5	0·1
Turner				1		1	0·5	0·1
Waardenburg				1		1	0·5	0·1
Alport					1	1	0·5	0·1
Fructosuria					1	1	0·5	0·1
Defectus coagulationis					1	1	0·5	0·1
Fistula branchialis					1	1	0·5	0·1
Maleformatio multiplex	1					1	0·5	0·1
Totals	43	31	15	14	82	185	100·0	

PN perinatally dead; LD later dead; MR mentally retarded; MSN mentally subnormal; NI normally intelligent.

based upon entries in the clinical journals of the children. The neurological states have been divided into the following diagnostic groups: CP syndrome, MBD syndrome, epilepsy as only symptom, and other neuromuscular states.

CP syndrome. There were 38 children (28·1 per cent of the 135) (17 boys and 21 girls) who had a CP syndrome. Of these, 28 children were spastics, 7 dyskinetics and 3 had ataxia. Ten (26·3 per cent) had or had had epileptic seizures. Four, all of them athetotics, had diagnosed grave hearing impairment. Four had verified post-natal aetiology, and the remaining 34 had a probable pre- or perinatal aetiology. Two of these children were malformed (one hypospadias plus diplegia and one Turner's syndrome plus hemi-plegia). Of the the living children with CP, 28 had an IQ over 90, 6 were mentally subnormal, and 12 were mentally retarded. Thirteen (34·2 per cent) of the children with CP syndrome were premature.

MBD syndrome. Seventeen children (12 boys and 5 girls) i.e. 12·6 per cent of the 135 children with neourological injuries, had an MBD syndrome. All of them were clumsy, 2 suffered from epilepsy, 5 from squint, 1 from nystagmus, 1 from hearing impairment, and 1 from sequelae of Erb's palsy. Twelve of the children had an IQ over 90 and 5 below 90. Not a single one of the 17 children had a verified postnatal aetiology. Six (35·3 per cent) of the children with an MBD syndrome were premature.

Epilepsy as only symptom. There were 55 children (12·6 per cent of the 135 children with neurological disorders) (31 boys and 24 girls) who had epilepsy as their only symptom. Six of the children had died, 36 (73·5 per cent of the 49 living children) had normal intelligence, 9 (18·4 per cent) were mentally subnormal, and 4 (8·2 per cent) were mentally retarded. Two of the 49 epileptic children had a verified postnatal aetiology. Of the remaining children, one suffered from progressive myoclonic epilepsy, whereas the aetiol-ogy of the others was unknown. Seven (14·3 per cent) were prema-ture

Of the 49 living children 25 had actual epilepsy, defined as epilepsy under active treatment during the three years preceding the expiration of the follow-up period. All these 25 children were looked after by specialists.

Other neuromuscular states. Of the 135 children with neurological disorders, 25 (18·5 per cent) belonged to this group. Sixteen were boys and 9 were girls. Nine of the 25 children suffered from flaccid paralysis due to diseases of the spinal cord, 9 from late effects of brain injury, 4 from peripheral paralysis, and 2 from Duchenne's muscular dystrophy.

One child suffering from SSPE (subacute sclerosing encephalitis) had died. Out of the 24 living children, 19 (79·2 per cent) had normal intelligence, 4 (16·7 per cent) were mentally subnormal, and one child was mentally retarded. Out of the 9 flaccid paralyses 8 were sequelae from polio and one was caused by diastomatomyelia. Six of the 9 late effects had resulted from cerebral infections, 2 from operated cerebral tumours, and one from a cerebral contusion. Out of the 4 peripheral paralyses 2 were congenital facial paralyses, one was a result of Erb's paralysis, and one was caused by a complicated radius fracture with radial paralysis. Not a single one of these children had epilepsy and none was premature.

Defects of sense organs

Squint, eye defects, and vision impairment. Of the 536 living chil-dren in the handicap group 101 (18·9 per cent) had one or more eye affections; 34 (33·7 per cent) of the 101 children had one or several additional handicaps. All children with verified eye disorders had been examined by ophthalmologists.

There were 84 children who had squint, 7 had unilateral am-blyopia without specified aetiological diagnosis, and 5 had malfor-mations of the eyes.

Only one child, a boy with double anopthalmus, was totally blind. Three children suffered from grave vision impairment (two myopia-magna and one nystagmus). There were 31 children with mono-ocular amblyopia, combined with squint in 21 cases. In seven cases the cause of the amblyopia was unknown and in three cases amblyopia was combined with malformations.

Hearing impairment. There were 38 (7·1 per cent of the 536 living children in the handicap group), 22 boys and 16 girls, who had diagnosed grave hearing impairment. In 36 cases, the diagnosis had been verified by audiologists. Twenty-two (57·9 per cent) of the 38 had one or more additional handicaps, 4 of the children were completely deaf in both ears, 4 were deaf in one ear, and 30 had various degrees of hearing impairment. The hearing impairment of 5 of the children was combined with malformations of the ears, 3 with other malformations, 6 with neurological disorders. Thirty of these children were of normal intelligence and 8 had an IQ below 90. Aetiologically the 38 children with hearing impairment fell into the following groups: 10 with prenatal aetiology (6 Rh-immunization, 4 prematurity with complications); 2 with postnatal aetiology; and 16 with hearing impairment without explicit aetiological speci-fication. Five of the 38 children with hearing impairment were premature.

Other diseases

There were 359 children who suffered, or had suffered, from psychosomatic or internal diseases; 49 (13·6 per cent of the 359 children) also had handicap states. Of these 359 children, 191 (52·3 per cent) were boys, and 178 (46·8 per cent) were girls. There were 220 children who had, or had had, skin affections of an atopic or allergic nature, 75 only asthma; 12 of the children with skin affec-tions also had diagnosed asthma. Nine children had psoriasis, 28 'migraine', 12 diabetes mellitus, 7 rheumatoid arthritis, 5 duodenal ulcer, and 2 thyreotoxicosis. One child suffered from ulcerative colitis.

Psychiatric treatment contacts

Our term 'psychiatric treatment contact' refers to examination or treatment contacts and should not be associated with psychic dis-ease. The method used in the investigation does not give reliable information on the actual psychiatric morbidity in the cohort. The psychiatric morbidity is probably greater than what could be deduced from the frequency of psychiatric treatment contacts.

Of the 6111 living children followed up, 1006 (16·5 per cent) had had one or several psychiatric treatment contacts during the follow-up period. Moreover, 4 of the 307 children who died had undergone psychiatric examination; 629 (62·5 per cent) of the children with psychiatric treatment contacts were boys and 377 (37·4 per cent) were girls. There were 368 (68·7 per cent) of the handicapped children and 49 (15·8 per cent) of the children with any of the other diseases who had one or more psychiatric treat-ment contacts.

Most of the treatment contacts (72·1 per cent) had taken place at psychiatric guidance clinics for children and young people. In 12·1 per cent of the cases the children had seen school medical officers, and in 2·6 per cent of the cases they had gone to private practi-tioners. In addition, 113 (11·2 per cent) of the 1006 children had been treated at psychiatric children's hospitals and 20 at paediatric hospitals. During the follow-up period, 2·2 per cent of all the living cohort children who were followed up had been treated at hospitals on psychiatric indications.

Epidemiological results

Mortality

Out of 6789 children of the cohort, 307 (4·5 per cent) had died when the follow-up was completed on 31 May 1969, and 130 (42·3 per cent) were stillborn. Table 9.3 shows the various mortality rates, the size of the risk population, and the number of the dead.

TABLE 9.3

Mortality rates, risk population, and the number of dead

Mortality	Risk population	N	per cent
Total	6789	307	4·5
Male	3504	178	5·1
Female	3283	127	3·9
Stillbirth	6789	130	1·9
Perinatal	6789	226	3·3
Neonatal	6659	110	1·7
Post-neonatal	6659	33	0·5
Infant	6659	143	2·1
Later	6659	34	0·5

Thirteen (0·2 per cent of the 6659 live-born children) were killed in accidents. The case-fatality rate within the cohort cannot be calculated because the total number of accidents is unknown. Seven of the children followed up had malignant neoplasmas, and six (85·7 per cent) of them died.

Malformations

There were 185 (of the 6408 children who were followed up) who had verified malformations. This gives a total incidence of 2·9 per cent. Of these, 91 (45·5 per cent) of the malformations were already diagnosed at the maternity hospitals and 109 later on. Figure 9.1 shows the annual detection rates of diagnosed and verified malformations. Table 9.4 shows total incidence, case-fatality rate and point prevalence on 31 May 1969 for malformations divided into main groups.

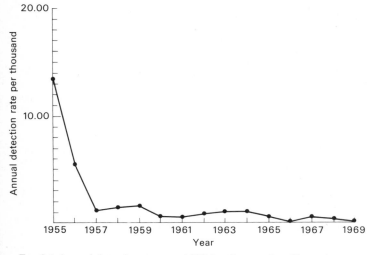

FIG. 9.1 Annual detection rate per 1000 for diagnosed malformations.

Disorders of the neuromuscular system

There were 135 (2·1 per cent of the 6408 children who were followed up) who had diagnosed neuromuscular disorders; 83 (61·5 per cent) of these had been diagnosed before 1962. Table 9.5 shows total incidence, case-fatality rate, and point prevalence on 31 May 1969 for neuromuscular disorders. Total incidence for Duchenne's muscular dystrophy was 0.3 per thousand. The total incidence for epileptic convulsions was 10·5 per thousand and the point prevalence on 31 May 1969 for 'actual' epilepsy was 6·1 per thousand.

TABLE 9.4

Total incidence, case-fatality rate, and point prevalence on 31 May 1969 for malformations divided into main groups

Malformation groups	Incidence N	per thousand	Case-fatality N	per cent	Prevalence per thousand
Central nervous system	32	4·7	28	87·5	0·6
Down's syndrome	11	1·7	26	54·4	0·8
Eyes	5	0·8	0	0	0·8
Ears	6	0·9	0	0	1·0
Circulatory system	37	5·8	18	48·6	3·1
Cleft palate	8	1·2	3	37·5	0·8
Other digestive system	8	1·2	6	75·0	0·3
Genito-urinary system	17	2·6	7	41·2	1·6
Dislocation of hip	20	3·3	0	0	3·3
Bones and muscles	31	4·8	3	9·7	4·6
Other†	10	1·6	3	30·10	1·5
Total	185	2·9	74	40·0	18·4

† Other: 2 with pulmonary hypoplasia, 1 each Klinefelter's, Turner's, Waardenburg's, Alport's syndrome, fructosuria, coagulation defect, bronchial fistula, multiple malformations.

TABLE 9.5

Total incidence, case-fatality rate, and point prevalence on 31 May 1969 for neuromuscular disorders

Disorder	Total incidence N	per thousand	Case-fatality N	per cent	Prevalence per thousand
CP	38	5·9	2	5·3	5·9
MBD	17	2·6	0	0	2·9
Epilepsy as only symptom	55	8·9	6	10·9	8·0
Other	25	3·9	1	4·0	3·9
Total	135	21·3	9	6·7	20·7

Mental retardation and mental subnormality

Of the 6408 children followed-up, 65 (1·0 per cent) had an IQ between 0 and 67, 154 (2·4 per cent) had an IQ between 68 and 85, and 77 (1·2 per cent) had an IQ between 86 and 89. The children with an IQ between 0 and 85 belong to the group 'mental retardation', according to ICD VIII. The epidemiological data concern these 219 children. Figure 9.2 shows the annual detection ratio for mental retardation and mental subnormality.

Table 9.6 shows the total incidence, case-fatality rate, and point prevalence for mental retardation and mental subnormality.

The point prevalence on 31 May 1969 for IQ less than 20 was 1·5 per thousand; for IQ 20–35, 1·2 per thousand; for IQ 36–51, 1·3 per thousand; for IQ 52–57, 1·3 per thousand; for IQ 58–67, 3·9 per thousand; and for IQ 68–75, 6·9 per thousand. The prevalence for 'borderline-intelligence' (IQ 86–89) on 31 May 1969 was 12·5 per thousand.

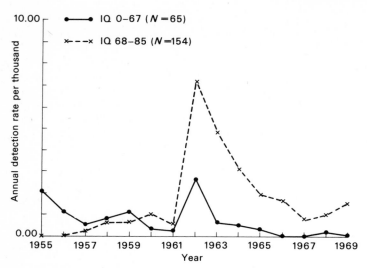

FIG. 9.2. Annual detection rate per 1000 for mental retardation and mental subnormality.

TABLE 9.6

Total incidence, case-fatality rate, and point prevalence on 31 May 1969 for mental retardation and mental subnormality

	Total incidence		Case-fatality		
IQ-group	N	per thousand	N	per cent	Prevalence per thousand
0–67	65	10·1	9	13·8	9·2
68–85	154	24·0	0	0	25·2
Total	219	34·1	9	4·1	34·4

Disorders of sense organs

Only one of all the 6408 children followed up was totally blind. The incidence for total amaurosis was 0·2 per thousand. Three other children had grave vision impairment. This means that disabling eye defects occurred with a total incidence of 0·6 per thousand and with a point prevalence (310569) of 0·7 per thousand. The prevalence on 31 May 1969 for diagnosed squint was 13·8 per thousand. The total incidence for grave hearing impairment was 5·9 per thousand and the point prevalence on 31 May 1969 was 6·2 per thousand.

Other diseases

There were 359 (5·6 per cent of the 6408 children followed up) who suffered or had suffered from diagnosed psychosomatic or internal diseases. Table 9.7 gives the total incidence and the point prevalence, on 31 May 1969, for those psychosomatic and internal diseases that were diagnosed in a reliable way.

For asthma and supposedly atopic and allergic skin diseases only the total frequencies are given. Because these diseases were registered in a deficient way and the diagnoses in many cases were not verified, reliable incidence and prevalence figures cannot be supplied. The total frequency of asthma was 12·3 per thousand and that of skin diseases 38·0 per thousand. 'Migraine' was registered in a frequency of 4·6 per thousand.

School attendance and the school on 31 May 1969

Finnish children normally begin school in the year they reach the age of seven. For the cohort children, the normal date of beginning school was 1 September 1962. Children who are not sufficiently mature for starting school, or who are otherwise retarded in their development, may get a respite. As a rule, only those children of this age whose development has been gravely impaired, are totally exempted from school. On the other hand, children may be allowed to start school one year earlier, if after a psychological maturity test they have been found to be ready for it.

TABLE 9.7

Total incidence† and point prevalence on 31 May 1969 for reliably diagnosed psychosomatic and internal diseases

	Total incidence			
Disease	N	per thousand	N	Prevalence per thousand
Diabetes mellitus	12	1·9	12	2·0
Rheumatoid arthritis	7	1·1	7	1·1
Duodenal ulcer	5	0·8	0	0
Ulcerative colitis	1	0·2	1	0·2
Tyrotoxicosis	2	0·3	0	0
Psoriasis	9	1·5	9	1·5
Total	36	5·8	29	4·7

† Total incidences in Table 9.7 are calculated from the number of children who survived the perinatal stage and were followed up (N = 6182).

Data on the commencement of school were obtained concerning 6111 of the living children who had been followed up until 1 September 1962. Of these children 95·5 per cent were in the first form of primary school, 2·3 per cent were in the second form of primary school, 1·7 per cent (105) had received a respite, and 0·4 per cent (23) were exempted. Six children were in a class for the deaf and one child in a remedial class.

On expiration of the follow-up period on 31 May 1969, 74·8 per cent of the children were in secondary schools, 22·1 per cent in primary schools, 2·5 per cent in special schools, and 0·5 per cent of the children were exempted.

Child welfare within the cohort

According to the Finnish Child Welfare act, those children who, owing to their parents' death, infirmity, or incapability of taking care of their children, are deprived of necessary care, shall be granted help from the communal social welfare board. In accordance with this act, physically sick, physically impaired, or socially maladjusted children who cannot be adequately looked after by their own parents, are also granted help from the social authorities in the municipality where they live. In addition, illegitimate children are followed up, and, if it be considered necessary, their mothers receive help and guidance in matters concerning the children's care and education.

During the follow-up period, 844 (12·8 per cent) of the 6563 cohort children who survived the perinatal period had been in touch with child welfare authorities and received help of various kinds. Table 9.8 shows the nature of contacts with child welfare authorities. The contacts have been divided into the following categories:

(1) *Illegitimacy only*, meaning that the child has been in touch with child welfare authorities only formally, as provided by law, for no other reason than its illegitimate birth;

(2) *Social assistance only*, meaning that child welfare authorities have helped the parents or the children in various ways without taking the child into custody;

(3) *Custody*, meaning that the child welfare authorities have taken charge of the child and, in most cases, provided for care in some children's home or foster home;

TABLE 9.8

Nature of child welfare contacts within various groups of the cohort

Child welfare contacts	Healthy children in				Children with other diseases		Children with psychiatric treatment contacts		Handicapped children		Untraced and drop-outs		Later dead		Total	
	Secondary schools		Primary schools													
	N	per cent	N	per cent	N	per cent	N	per cent	N	per cent	N	per cent	N	per cent	N	per cent
None	3617	94·1	677	81·4	280	90·3	427	72·5	374	69·9	286	77·2	58	71·6	5719	87·2
Illegitimacy	70	1·8	30	3·6	8	2·6	19	3·2	13	2·4	23	6·2	9	11·1	172	2·6
Social assistance	45	1·2	24	2·9	2	0·6	7	1·2	6	1·1	3	0·8	3	3·7	90	1·4
Custody	67	1·7	49	5·9	12	3·9	57	9·7	98	18·3	29	7·8	11	13·6	323	4·9
Protective education	28	0·7	46	5·5	4	1·3	66	11·2	41	7·7	2	0·5	0	0	187	2·8
Adoption	18	0·5	6	0·7	4	1·3	13	2·2	3	0·6	28	7·5	0	0	72	1·1
Total	3845		832		310		589		535		371		81		6563	

(4) *Protective education*, meaning that the child, due to its social behaviour, needed special care, either approved school or protective supervision;

(5) *Adoption*, meaning that the child got substitute parents who legally acknowledged the child as their own.

Of the 6563 children, 511 (7·8 per cent) had been looked after in a children's home or a foster home.

Discussion

In what follows, only some of the most important results from the first follow-up period will be discussed. The investigation is still going on, and we shall probably be able to publish the results of the second phase of the follow-up within three or four years. In connection with these communications, we shall have occasion to return to the first follow-up period with further details.

Pregnancy, delivery, and neonatal data

Information on pregnancy, delivery, and the neonatal stage was collected from the delivery journals more than ten years after the children were born. This meant that some important data from this time were scarce, or not available at all. In case of a prospective plan, data concerning the mothers' social conditions and conditions of work, their state of health, smoking habits, etc., could have been collected in a more adequate way. Here, the time factor was decisive for the decision to select a cohort from 1955. A 'genuine' prospective investigation could have been thought to reach the stage of the present one in 1986–7, at the earliest. However, the existing pre- and perinatal data do give quite a lot of valuable information. Without entering into a detailed analysis, it can be said that but for the frequency of induced deliveries and the frequency of deliveries whose second phase had a duration of more than 30 min, the pregnancy and delivery data of the cohort do not differ in any remarkable way from those given in the Finnish investigation by Hartikainen (1973).

Mortality

The perinatal mortality in the cohort was 33·2 per thousand as against 31·8 per thousand in the whole country. In Tampere, the next biggest city in Finland (109 903 inhabitants in 1955), perinatal mortality in 1955 was 33·3 per thousand (Hulkko *et al.* 1973). The perinatal mortality in the cohort was thus of the same magnitude as in the city most similar to Helsinki, and somewhat higher than in the whole country. The infant mortality in the cohort (21·4 per thousand) was lower than in the whole country (29·7 per thousand); the same was true of maternal mortality, which in the cohort was only 0·29 per thousand as compared with 1·05 per thousand for the whole country. The slightly greater perinatal

mortality in the cohort, in comparison with that in the whole country, is explained, in the first place, by the fact that the cohort is a typically urban one. Mothers in big cities are more exposed to the risk of prenatal complications than mothers living in the country. The reason why infant and maternal mortality in the cohort was smaller than in the whole country was probably that in 1955 medical care in Helsinki was still better organized than in the rest of Finland.

Malformations

The total incidence of verified malformations in the cohort was 2·9 per cent. Now, it is generally known that data on incidence and prevalence of malformations vary considerably in different investigations. Saxén and Rapola (1969) refer to five investigations in which what is reported to be the total incidence of malformations varies between 2·3 and 10·1 per cent. There are many reasons for this state of affairs, but they will not concern us here. In the two comprehensive Finnish epidemiological investigations on malformations which have been done up to now, total incidence are given as 2·8 per cent (Klemetti 1966) and 3·3 per cent (Hakosalo 1973). Hakosalo's materials are from the time of an influenza epidemic ('the Asian flu'). The total incidence for malformations in the cohort is intermediate between the incidence figures of the two previous Finnish investigations. (Details will not be described in this context.) There is, however, a probability that all graver malformations in the cohort have been traced but that a great number of the milder ones (equinovarus, luxatio coxae, hare lip, etc.) and some of those that are usually diagnosed later in life (certain malformations of interior organs) were not detected. Therefore, the total incidence of the cohort, 2·9 per cent, should be understood to represent a minimum number of malformations among the children who were traced. The prevalence of malformations on 31 May 1969 was 1·8 per cent, which shows the great lethality (40·0 per cent) in malformations.

Disorders of the neuromuscular system

The total incidence for neurological diseases among the cohort children who were followed up was 2·1 per cent. This number does not include children who died perinatally from neurological injuries. This incidence must be considered minimal. It is probable that a great deal of the so-called aclinical mentally retarded children would have been found to suffer from neurological sequelae (i.e mild cerebral disorder syndromes), had they been examined clinically. The figure 2·1 per cent includes several types of neurological disorders. As far as total incidence is concerned, it is difficult to make comparisons with other studies, because diagnostic criteria and investigation methods often differ from each other. Comparisons of specific neurological states can be made more easily.

The incidence in the cohort for cerebral palsy (CP) was 5·9 per thousand. The same incidence was established by Levin *et al.* (1949) in connection with the so-called Schenectady investigation. The incidence 5·9 per thousand is the greatest hitherto reported in the literature.

On 31 May 1969, the prevalence for CP in the cohort was 5·9 per thousand. According to Tuuteri *et al.* (1967), the prevalence for CP in Finland between the ages of 3 to 17 years was 2·0 per thousand, a figure which tallies with that given by Goldberg *et al.* (1973) as the average incidence for CP syndromes. It is an interesting question whether the high CP figure in the cohort is reliable, accidental, or a result of too broad diagnostic criteria.

The chances are that the figure is reliable. The diagnostic criteria agree with commonly accepted criteria of CP syndrome and the diagnoses had been made by experienced specialists.

Among the cohort children, the number of milder CP cases was greater than those given in previous investigations. This is probably due to the intensiveness of tracing in this study.

The prevalence in the cohort for the so-called minimal brain damaged (*MBD*) syndrome was 2·9 per thousand. This must be regarded as a minimum figure. Comparisons with other studies cannot be made, because it is impossible to count the actual occurrence of MBD on the basis of epidemiological investigations without contemporaneous exact clinical estimation of all the children of the population.

The total incidence for *epileptic convulsions* in the cohort was 10·5 per thousand and the prevalence for actual convulsions on 31 May 1969 was 6·1 per thousand. These figures do not include neonatal convulsions, febrile convulsions, and breath-holding spells. The figures of the cohort are comparable to those reported by Rutter (1970c) (7·2 per thousand in the age group of 9 to 12 years), Pond *et al.* (1960) (7·9 per thousand in the age group of 5 to 14 years), and Cooper (1965) (8·2 per thousand at the age of 15 years). On the other hand, the figures of the cohort are considerably greater than those reported by Sillanpää (1973) in his investigation from the district of the Turku central hospital, which is situated in Western Finland. Probably Sillanpää traced only the gravest cases.

The total incidence for mentally retarded and mentally subnormal children (IQ 0–85) was 34·2 per thousand. There is no way of comparing the cohort's figure with the results of other Finnish investigations prior to the present one, because there are no previous measurements of the incidence for mental retardation and mental subnormality. The prevalence figures, however, can be compared. The prevalence in the cohort on 31 May 1969, corresponding to the age group 13–14 years, was 34·4 per thousand for the whole group, IQ 0–85. Again, these figures cannot be compared with any information given in previous Finnish investigations, because none of them embraced the whole of this intelligence range. In a previous study (Amnell 1966), the prevalence for IQ 0–75 in the age group 10–14 years was 9·1 per thousand. The corresponding prevalence figure for the cohort was 16·1 per thousand, or nearly twice as much. It is a case in point that the figure 16·1 per thousand for IQ 0–75 remains low in comparison with corresponding figures in a number of carefully prepared clinico-epidemiological studies made in England and Sweden: Birch *et al.* (1970) found a prevalence of 27·4 per thousand for IQ 0–75 in the age group 8–10 years among children in Aberdeen; Rutter (1970c) found a prevalence of 25·3 per thousand for IQ 0–70 in the Isle of Wight study comprising children aged 5–14 years; and Åkesson (1961) established a prevalence of 37·2 per thousand for IQ 0–68 in the age group 10–15 years in southern Sweden. The number of cohort children with IQ 0–75 would probably have turned out to be much greater if another screening method had been used in connection with tests.

The frequency of squint among the cohort children is low in comparison with the figures reported in the literature; only 13·8 per thousand of the cohort children had diagnosed squint. Davie *et al.*

(1972) found squint in more than 3 per cent of the children in the '1956 cohort' material.

Psychiatric treatment contacts

The data that were collected about the psychiatric treatment contacts of the cohort children tell nothing about the actual psychiatric morbidity in the cohort, but only show to what extent the children had been examined on psychiatric indications. A more reliable picture of the psychiatric morbidity can only be obtained by means of a combined clinico-epidemiological investigation of a sufficiently large, unselected child population. The cohort meets the demand as far as the population is concerned, but as no clinical investigations were made, the study does not give any information on the incidence and prevalence for psychiatric disorders among the children followed up.

Each sixth child, i.e. 16·5 per cent of the living children who were followed up, had had one or several psychiatric treatment contacts during the follow-up period; 62·5 per cent of these children were boys, which agrees with previous investigations (Rutter 1970c).

Of the children in the handicap group 68·7 per cent had had one or several psychiatric treatment contacts. The fact that such a great number of these children had had psychiatric treatment contacts certainly is connected to some extent with the great need for psychiatric evaluation in solving schooling and habilitation problems of handicapped children, but it probably also reflects a greater prevalence for psychiatric disorders among children with handicaps. In the Isle of Wight study, Rutter (1970c) found, among children with 'neuro-epileptic' symptoms, a fivefold frequency (34·3 per cent) of psychic disorders as compared with somatically healthy children.

Child welfare within the cohort

Of the cohort children who survived the perinatal stage 12·9 per cent had received some form of help or care from child welfare authorities. The investigation clearly showed that disease of the child combined with low social status of the parents increases the need for child welfare measures. The number of children born illegitimately was also significantly greater among the child welfare children.

Comparison between the various clinical groups in regard to pre- and perinatal factors

The statistical analysis showed that in both groups of *healthy children* there were less pre- and perinatal complications than among the children who died and the handicapped children, a logical result. There were also no significant differences in relation to the groups of untraced children and children with other diseases, which was expected due to the method of grouping the children. The number of pre- or perinatally injured children among the untraced cohort members is expected to be small, since, to be sure, if a child with a handicap remains in the country, he is likely to be discovered by some welfare authority. There is, then, a strong probability that most of the children with graver handicaps were identified. There were, however, certain differences between the healthy children and those children who had been treated or examined psychiatrically. This point will be discussed later on. Particularly in the group of healthy secondary school children the number of unmarried mothers was small, the number of mothers from the higher social groups was great, and it was also the case that a great number of the mothers had been private patients at the maternity hospitals. Accordingly, health and success at school at the age of 13–14 years was correlated with the mother's social situation during pregnancy.

The group of untraced children was marked chiefly by the great number of unmarried mothers. The children with psychiatric treatment contacts differed from the group of healthy secondary school children with regard to certain pre- and perinatal variables. The frequency of previous miscarriages among mothers of children with psychiatric treatment contacts was higher than among mothers of the healthy secondary school children ($p < 0.05$). The import of this connection has not been analysed, but it seems to point to an aetiological relation between miscarriage and psychiatric disorders of the following child. In the group of children with psychiatric treatment contacts, the frequency of anomalous foetal positions was somewhat higher than in the group of healthy secondary school children ($p < 0.05$). The same was true of the occurrence of anomalous amniotic fluid and complications of the umbilical cord ($p < 0.05$). The birthweight within the group of children with psychiatric treatment contacts was significantly lower than in the group of healthy secondary school children ($p < 0.001$). These differences may indicate that the group of children with psychiatric treatment contacts contains a number of children with undiagnosed pre- or perinatally conditioned cerebral disorder syndromes. This supposition can be verified only by means of a clinical investigation of the children in the psychiatric group.

The results obtained from the statistical analysis of the relation between perinatal mortality and pre- and perinatal variables differ from those previously reported in the literature only in respect to the importance of toxaemia (Baird and Thomson, 1969). The significance of toxaemia depends upon the age and the parity of the mothers. The number of toxaemic mothers of perinatally dead cohort children was so small ($N = 29$) that a statistical analysis was not carried out.

The number of unmarried mothers in the three large groups of handicapped children (malformations, neurological disorders of a pre- or perinatal nature, and aclinical mental retardation) was significantly greater ($p < 0.001$) than in the group of healthy secondary school children. The same was true of the social groups, because in the handicap groups, the number of mothers belonging to social groups III and IV was significantly greater than in the group of healthy secondary school children. The correlation between prenatal social factors and disabling diseases and defects of children is well substantiated in the literature, but it is most complex and often difficult to interpret (Birch et al. 1970; Montagu 1971; Richards et al. 1972; Pilling 1973). It is an interesting fact that the group with aclinical mental retardation did not differ from the group of healthy primary school children in respect to the mothers' civil status, social group, and age. Of the biological pre- and perinatal variables, only the birthweight and the intrapartum complications were of greater relevance. The following figures illustrate the significance of prematurity: 66·4 per cent of the infants who died perinatally were prematures, and 11·0 per cent of the living children in the various handicap groups were prematures, as compared to 3·5 per cent of the healthy secondary school children and 4·1 per cent of the healthy elementary school children. The frequency of prematurity in the different clinical groups are as follows:

Percent of prematures per group

Group	Percent
Healthy secondary school children	3·1
Healthy elementary school children	4·1
Entire cohort	6·5
Mentally subnormal (IQ 68–85)	8·2
Mentally retarded (IQ 0–67)	12·3
Hearing impairment	13·1
Epilepsy as only symptom	14·3
Malformed	18·9
CP	34·2
MBD	35·3
Dead perinatally	66·4

Continued research—follow-up until 31 December 1975

The second follow-up period of the investigation spans 31 May 1969 to 31 December 1975 and comprises the life of the cohort members from 14–21 years, i.e. puberty and adolescence. The *aim* of the second follow-up period is manifold:

(1) To give a descriptive epidemiological picture of disabling and chronic somatic diseases, mortality, psychiatric disorders, and social maladjustment (abuse of alcohol and narcotics, vagrancy, and registered criminality) during this period;

(2) To illustrate the correlation between conditions in youth and previous events in the lives of the cohort members, i.e. to analyse the links between pre-, peri-, and postnatal factors, and morbidity to social adaptation and adult life;

(3) To make a follow-up of the various clinical groups from the first follow-up period to see how these groups passed through puberty and adolescence and in what way they adapted themselves to 'adult' society.

If the second follow-up proves successful, it will be possible to illustrate several interesting specific problems, such as the following: What does it mean to be handicapped in childhood? How do children's handicaps affect the children's families? How many of the handicapped children are totally disabled as young grown-ups? How many of the handicapped children adapted themselves to society and learned a trade? What is the relevance to later prognosis of having been psychiatrically examined as a child? How do children who were born illegitimately progress in life? How well do children who spent their youth in children's homes and foster homes adjust later? How do prematures and twins manage?

The method used will be the same as that of the first follow-up, but now the investigation is truly prospective, in MacMahon and Pugh's (1970) sense. Furthermore, the tracing of cohort members and the recording of data has been simplified and made more efficient thanks to a considerable improvement in recent years of the Finnish official registers. The tracing has been made possible by the Finnish population register which has furnished us with information on the cohort members' names, children, if any, and addresses as of 1 January 1976. These personal data are confidential and have been received from the population register upon special application. The information from the population register renders it possible to identify the cohort members anew and determine their domiciles in Finland. This also simplifies the collecting of so-called clinical data and enables us to make personal contacts with the cohort members. Some of the cohort members, of course, had to be traced from the police address agencies. The so-called clinical data were collected from the following registers: data on causes of death, from the death register; data on psychiatric diseases and psychiatric treatment, from the districts of mental health services; data on registered criminality, from the criminal records; data on chronic disabling diseases, from the pension department; and data on social maladjustment, from the social welfare boards. In addition, the medical department of the armed forces will supply us with health data on the male cohort members who have done their military service. A large part of this work has already been done.

The investigation includes a postal interview. Forms have been sent to all cohort members. The interview consists partly of an enquiry, composed especially for this investigation, and partly of Cornell's Medical Index. Up to now, the enquiry has been answered by about 75 per cent of the cohort members.

If resources allow, we shall carry out a number of intensive studies of particular groups, such as handicapped, illegitimate children, and a selection of those classified as healthy. These intensive studies are planned to include personal contacts with the cohort members concerned.

The financing of the investigation

Initially, the investigation was financed by a number of private funds, Signe and Arne Gyllenberg's fund according the major part of the grants. From 1972, the investigation has been sponsored primarily by the Academy of Finland, but also by Signe and Arne Gyllenberg's fund and the Finnish–Norwegian Medical Fund.

Summary

The aim of the study is to follow up a given child population from birth to adult age in order to elucidate a number of important medical, psychic, and social aspects of the cohort members' lives and development. The study gives descriptive epidemiological data concerning disabling somatic diseases, psychic disorders, and social maladjustment in childhood and youth, and also illustrates the relevance of pre-, peri-, and postnatal factors to morbidity and the process of adaptation during adolescence.

Methodologically, the study is a cohort investigation. The population or cohort is clearly defined and delimited and consists of all the 6789 children born in Helsinki in 1955 to mothers permanently resident in the city at the time of delivery. The study is longitudinal and the follow-up period expands from the time of delivery to the twentieth year of the cohort members (1975). All data were collected in a prospective way.

The first follow-up phase spans the period from birth to 31 May 1969 when the cohort members were 13 and 14 years old. The results of the analysis of the first follow-up period were published in 1974. They have been summarized in this article. Work on the second follow-up phase is being carried out now and the first publications from this phase can be expected in two or three years.

The cohort members were traced with the aid of various school, address, and population registers. Data on the dead were obtained from the death register; data on the state of health and on diseases in school age from the school health service, hospitals, and out-patient clinics. Information on social child welfare was provided by child welfare authorities. In connection with the second follow-up the archives of the social insurance institute, the army, and the criminal register could also be used as sources. In 1976, an enquiry form, including the Cornell Medical Index, was dispatched to all cohort members.

As of 31 May 1969, 6408 children (6101 living and 307 dead) amounting to 94.4 per cent of the 6789 cohort children had been traced. Of the living children 76·7 per cent were healthy, while 23·7 per cent belonged to one or more of the clinical groups. The incidence for malformation was 29·0 per thousand, for neuromuscular disorders 21·3 per thousand, for mental retardation (IQ 0–67) 10·1 per thousand, for mental subnormality (IQ 68–85) 24·00 per thousand, for disabling eye disorders 0·6 per thousand, for grave hearing impairment 6·0 per thousand, for diabetes mellitus 2·0 per thousand, for rheumatiod arthritis 1·1 per thousand, and for ulcerous colitis 0.2 per thousand. Of the children who were followed up 16·5 per cent had been examined or treated psychiatrically and 12·8 per cent had been in touch with social child welfare and received some form of assistance.

The discrimination analysis clearly showed that the healthy secondary school children differed from those who died and the handicapped children mainly in respect of three social variables: the mothers' social group and marital status in 1955, whether or not the mother was a private patient in the maternity hospital, and a biological variable, the infant's birthweight. Infants who had died perinatally, those who died later, and handicapped children were more often found to be children of unmarried mothers or of mothers from social groups III and IV than the healthy secondary school children. An interesting fact was that in respect to these social variables, the aclinically mentally retarded group did not differ from healthy elementary school children. The following figures illustrate the significance of prematurity: 66·4 per cent of the infants who died perinatally and 11·0 per cent of the living handicapped children were born prematurely, as compared to 3·5 per cent of the healthy secondary school children and 4·1 per cent of the healthy elementary school children; 35·3 per cent of the children with MBD and 34·2 per cent of the children with CP were born prematurely.

10. The medical birth registry of Norway

TOR BJERKEDAL

In Norway midwives and physicians attending delivery of a foetus of 16-weeks gestation or more are by law requested to issue a report. This report is called *Medical registration of birth* (Mellbye 1967). A new report form for use in the registration scheme was introduced in 1967. A detailed listing of the content of the form is given in Table 10.1. The reason for requesting all this information is:

(1) To provide a basis for detailed analyses of causes of disease and death in pregnancy, of stillbirths, and of diseases and death among infants, so that new knowledge can promote further prevention;

(2) To obtain a registration of newborns with congenital malformations and of infants at risk of developing functional disorders, so that these children can be closely observed, and, when in need, be given early treatment;

(3) To make available data for a system of early detection of changes in incidence of certain malformations, so that, if these should occur with an increased frequency, studies of causation could be promoted.

The registration system

Medical registration of birth is issued in four copies. Two of the copies are forwarded on the ninth day after birth to local health authorities to give those on the local level in charge of the infant health care programme information of importance in the follow-up of the newborn infant. The original copy is collected nationally for central processing and analyses. Since December 1969 Professor Tor Bjerkedal has been in charge of the central handling of the

TABLE 10·1

Content of form presently used for medical registration of birth in Norway

About the newborn:
1. Whether livebirth or stillbirth.
2. Birthday, month, and year.
3. Hour of day.
4. Whether a single birth, twins, triplets, or quadruplets.
5. Sex, boy or girl.
6. Last name, and given name (only for livebirths).
7. Place of birth, name and address of maternity clinic or maternity home, district.
8a. For livebirths, signs of asphyxia.
8b. Apgar score after 1 and 5 minutes.
9. For livebirths and stillbirths, signs of congenital malformation, of birth injury, or disease. If so, indicate which.
10a. Length of newborn.
10b. Circumference of the head.
11. Birth weight.
12. For deaths within 24 hours, how many hours/minutes life lasted.
13. For stillbirths, whether death occurred before labour or during delivery.
14. Cause of death and whether autopsy has been performed.

About the father:
15. Last name and all given names.
16. Birthday, month, and year.
17. District of residence.

About the mother:
18. Last name, all given names, and maiden name.
19. Birthday, month, year, and person number, thus asking for the complete national identification number.
20. Residence, mailing address and district.
21. Marital status, whether unmarried, married, widow, separated, or divorced.
22. Year of marriage for those married.
23. Number of previous births, total livebirths, stillbirths, number of livebirths still alive.
24. Whether the mother is related to the father, in which case the relationship should be stated.
25. Health before pregnancy. If not normal, illnesses should be specified.
26. First day of last menstrual period.
27. Health during pregnancy. If not normal, complications should be specified.

About relatives:
28. Whether any serious, inheritable diseases exist in the family. If yes, the disease should be named and the relative identified.

About the delivery:
29. Whether induced or not.
30. Interventions performed. If yes, type of intervention should be specified, and information given on whether physician or midwife performed the intervention.
31. Complications occurring. If yes, details should be given.
32. Whether any pathology was noted with respect to amniotic fluid, placenta, or umbilical cord. If yes, condition should be specified.
33. The form has to be signed by the midwife and attending physician, giving place and date.

medical registration of birth reports and the utilization of the material provided by these reports. The work has been carried out at the Institute of Hygiene and Social Medicine, University of Bergen. This arrangement came into effect through an agreement between the responsible governmental institutions involved, namely the Directorate of Health Services and the Central Bureau of Statistics.

The registry

In order to facilitate the analysis of the material and to provide a basis for longitudinal follow-up studies, a computer-based file system was established in 1970 under the name *Medical birth registry of Norway*. The Registry includes all births (of 16-weeks gestation and more) since 1 January 1967 to mothers registered as residents of Norway by the Central Population Register, Central Bureau of Statistics. All information given on the medical birth registration forms, except for names and home addresses, is transferred to the computer file. The medical conditions of the mother and newborn are coded according to the Norwegian version of the ICD (8th revision) with a few additional codes.

Live births are identified by the 11-digit national identification number. This ID number is given to all Norwegian residents shortly after birth by the Central Bureau of Statistics. It is automatically transferred on a monthly basis to the *Medical birth registry*, using the mother's ID number as the link.

The national ID number provides for automatic linkage to the Central Population Register. In this way updating of the *Medical birth registry* with respect to names and home addresses is done quarterly. The national ID number is also used in linking to the *Medical birth registry* the official information on death among residents of Norway. This information is provided by the Central Bureau of Statistics on a yearly basis. It makes possible a current yearly follow-up study of births with respect to death and causes of death.

At present no other linkage to other national registers, such as the cancer register and psychosis register, is done on a routine basis. There is a great need, however, to link the information available from the medical birth registration to information on the development and health of infants and children. Pilot studies are underway to create data files with health information on all one year old and four year old children with residence in one county (Rogaland). Moreover, a data file containing the results of health examinations of children entering first grade of elementary school is being established in another area of Norway (Bergen). With these additional files, population-based follow-up studies on development and health of children would be possible.

Ethical considerations

The need to secure confidentiality in a system of central collection, handling, and storage of person-identifiable medical information is a continuous concern. A careful selection of personnel on the grounds of high moral standards and experience in the field of medicine is probably the most important issue. Strict rules must exist and must be enforced to leave no uncertainty in anyone's mind as to the way data are handled, used, and stored, whether original reports or after computerization. No person-identifiable information is given to a third party without written consent from the Director General of the Norwegian Health Services who ultimately is the responsible person. Summarized, tabular, or other not person-identifiable information may upon request be provided by the Director of the Registry.

Use of data

A system of monitoring birth defects and other conditions of the newborn has been in operation on a monthly basis since 1971. The system has disclosed apparent epidemic increases in congenital dislocation of the hip and anomalies of the limbs, caused by changes in registration practice. An increase in the registration of anomalies of the urogenital system that started in the autumn of 1972 has been investigated by a nationwide case-control study (Bjerkedal and Bakketeig 1975b). The material from this study is presently finalized for detailed analyses.

Some descriptive and analytical aspects brought out by the material for the years 1967–8 have been published (Bjerkedal and Bakketeig 1972) as well as some statistics for the five-year period 1967–71 (Bjerkedal and Bakketeig 1975a). Consequences of some chronic diseases of the mother for outcome of pregnancy have been studied (Bahna and Bjerkedal 1972; Bjerkedal and Bahna 1973; Bahna and Bjerkedal 1974; and Bjerkedal *et al*. 1975a). Moreover, outcome of pregnancy has been related to obstetric practices (Bjerkedal *et al*. 1975b). At present, studies on the epidemiology of prematurity, especially as it relates to siblings, are under way. Also under study at present are the relations between occupations of parents and such pregnancy outcomes as stillbirth, perinatal death, prematurity, and malformations. A special problem encountered in utilizing the material relates to the fact that the *Medical birth registry* has no formal status within the Norwegian Health Services. The activity is supported by the Directorate of Health Services which covers only a part of the cost. The main support is provided indirectly by the Institute of Hygiene and Social Medicine, University of Bergen, which houses the activity and allows the use of its computer facilities.

This lack of formal status means in effect that there is no guarantee of long-term funding of the project, and thus no permanent staffing is possible; the activities are carried out by personnel paid on a temporary basis. To improve utilization, the *Medical birth registry* must become a part of the Norwegian Health Services with a staff of its own.

The potentialities of the Registry in the following areas should be recognized:

(1) In monitoring not only birth defects but also the development and health of the child population and the health of pregnant women;
(2) In evaluation of obstetric care and preventive health services in infancy, including evaluation of antenatal and perinatal care, as well as mother and child health programmes in general;
(3) In allocation of resources and distribution of available health services to mother and child;
(4) In helping to establish and maintain local handicap registers making it possible to develop primary health care services based on an active case finding approach;
(5) In providing norms and standards for use in mother and child health programmes;
(6) In organizing the collection of additional data relevant to the study of causation of ill health and functional disorders among children.

These potentialities of the Registry all stem from the fact that the data system allows linkage of observations of identifiable individuals over long periods of time, thus encouraging longitudinal research.

11. Longitudinal studies in Aberdeen, Scotland
A. Overview

BARBARA THOMPSON

There are three major longitudinal projects at different stages in progress being carried out by staff in the Institute of Medical Sociology, University of Aberdeen (Director, Professor Raymond Illsley):

The Aberdeen maternity and neonatal data bank. This is currently being established to provide social, obstetric, and fertility-related gynaecological events from 1948 for a defined population. Fertility profiles will be constructed and maintained in future on an ongoing basis. The technical organization and development of this Bank is the day-to-day responsibility of Mr M. L. Samphier. Dr Barbara Thompson (a member of the sociological team since the Data Bank's inception) has general direction and is a principal user together with Professor Raymond Illsley and medical colleagues.

The Aberdeen child development survey is funded for 3 years 1976–9. The principal researchers are Professor Raymond Illsley and Dr Fiona Wilson.

The Aberdeen delinquency study ended in March 1977 when Dr David May's grant ended and he moved to other research employment. No further follow-up is envisaged.

The history and details of the projects are described below. Certain factors such as confidentiality are common to all projects.

Confidentiality

Staff. All staff of whatever grade, working on these projects are appointed by the Director. They are issued an individual copy of the MRC booklet *Responsibility in the use of medical information for research* for which they sign. Permanent ancillary staff include three clerical workers, one computer operator, and three technician/programmers.

Data gathering. All extraction and processing of data is done by designated, trained staff. Initial access is obtained by a scientific worker who identifies staff who will actually undertake the work.

Raw data. Whenever possible identification numbers only are used. The use of names and addresses is carefully controlled and has to be fully justified for a temporary period and specific purpose only. All raw data sheets etc. are treated as strictly confidential and kept under lock and key. The senior clerical supervisor makes frequent checks on the security and confidentiality arrangements throughout the Institute in order to ensure that standards are maintained.

Computerized data. Access to data is through M. L. Samphier via the principal research worker on any specific project, or direct to him by medical colleagues for individual research projects.

B. The Aberdeen maternity and neonatal data bank

MICHAEL L. SAMPHIER and BARBARA THOMPSON

Technical development

The Aberdeen Maternity and Neonatal Data Bank has been in existence since the late 1940s, and is recognized internationally as unique in both its scope and character. This reputation derives from a fortuitous combination of the skill and foresight of Sir Dugald Baird (1974) and his colleagues of the Medical Research Council (MRC) at the Obstetric Medicine Research Unit, and the remarkable stability of Aberdeen and its population over the post-war period.

Until Aberdeen became the centre of North Sea oil development in the early 1970s the population remained fairly stable at 180 000 to 190 000. The city comprised a well defined, compact urban area with no large suburbs, the nearest large town, Dundee, being some 70 miles distant. Aberdeen had long been the administrative and medical centre for the northeast of Scotland, but the establishment of the National Health Service (NHS) in 1948 permitted a considerable degree of unification of obstetric care focused on the Aberdeen Maternity Hospital (AMH). Within a short period the hospital was providing antenatal and maternity services for more than 85 per cent of all pregnant women in the city. Facilities for domiciliary confinements were available under the NHS, with midwives and general practitioners working in close co-operation with hospital staff. A diminishing number of women were delivered as private patients in nursing homes. Records on non-hospital births were integrated into the hospital records system. Thus since 1948 a comprehensive library of obstetric and neonatal case records for all Aberdeen city births has been available, and this has been the foundation of the data bank.

The MRC team led by Sir Dugald Baird included staff with clinical, epidemiological, statistical, and sociological expertise. Together they instituted a system of routine data collection, recording clinical and social details of all legitimate singleton births occurring to women resident in the city of Aberdeen. The population so defined, subsequently referred to as the city population, constituted the base population for statistical purposes. However, about half of the deliveries occurring in the Maternity Hospital are to women resident outside the city boundary but in the northeast region, for whom Aberdeen consultants provide a specialist service. Most of these come from the rural catchment area, but a proportion are referred to Aberdeen from throughout the northeast region for specialist care. Certain data were collected for these women to yield limited information on a hospital population.

This system had the simple objective of providing high quality research data. The initial work, using the city data, was directed at the identification of high risk groups of women and the elucidation of the differential morbidity patterns associated with variations in physical and social conditions of pregnant women and neonates. Similarly the hospital data were used to provide clinical information on the aetiology of the more uncommon obstetric conditions. This in turn made for a more informed evaluation of management techniques for such cases. The success of the application of what would now be termed a data base concept was amply demonstrated by the marked improvements in maternal and infant morbidity rates, well in advance of comparable urban areas in Britain, by a stream of publications, and by the establishment of an enduring academic

and clinical reputation which has continued under Professor Ian MacGillivray who was appointed to the Chair of Obstetrics and Gynaecology on Sir Dugald Baird's retirement in 1965.

In the first instance the *Research Records* system involved the transcription of data from maternity case notes on to Cope-Chat (edge punched) cards. This was performed for a short period by the hospital records staff and subsequently by a specially trained group of clerical staff under the supervision of clinicians. The Cope-Chat card was, and indeed still is, popular with medical staff. It provides a concise summary of the case, has space for further annotation, and is amenable to simple sorting procedures. Further, it is highly portable and sorting does not require special machinery (a knitting needle will suffice).

However, with the almost total decline of the domiciliary service, the closing of private nursing homes, and the increase in hospital deliveries (which included a few private patients) to around 5000 per annum, and as the limitations of the system were more fully appreciated, it became clear that an alternative method of data storage was needed—one that would facilitate faster sorting and retrieval of information. Accordingly in 1958 a Hollerith card (a standard 80-column IBM or Tab card) record was introduced for City cases, using the existing Cope-Chat card as a transcription sheet. The relevant data for the period 1948–58 were also punched on to Hollerith cards. At this stage the data base comprised a Cope-Chat card for all hospital deliveries from 1948 on. A sub-set of these, the previously defined City population which included the few domiciliary confinements, were also on punched cards.

With the development of research interests an increasing amount of data was coded and punched on to these cards. Since the system was based on card-sorting techniques, binary punching was used extensively to contain the data within a single card record format. (Binary punching is the technique of recording more than one numeric value per card column. Each of the twelve punch sites on a column may be used to signify a binary value (yes/no, present/absent) by the punch/no punch state. In this way several hundred binary items may be recorded in one 80-column card. For normal computer usage a single card will contain a maximum of 80 alpha-numeric characters.) In 1967 the data base was reviewed in detail and a new three-card Hollerith format was adopted partly to accommodate the ever increasing clinical detail and partly in anticipation of future computerization of the system. At that time computing resources were not available and three additional Hollerith machines were purchased (a high speed sorter, reproducing, and collating machines). It was also decided to extend the Hollerith card subset to include illegitimate and multiple births, and to widen the geographical boundary to include women resident in the developing suburban housing on the periphery of the city. Thus from 1967 Hollerith cards were punched for all deliveries occurring to women resident in Aberdeen city and suburbs.

Unfortunately the changes introduced in 1967 were less successful than had been expected. The three-card record format did not eliminate all the binary punching, and the problem of matching card sets further complicated the subsequent task of transferring these data to computer files. Similarly the three-card record proved almost totally unworkable from the practical point of view. The Hollerith machines purchased, and indeed any others available at the time, were essentially business machines, and lacked the flexibility needed for a research establishment. True, they could be set up to do the most complex manipulation, but the setting up proved to be a major research project in itself.

This situation was exacerbated by a progressive change in research interests away from traditional epidemiology. For a period the data contained in the Hollerith records were either inappropriate or inaccessible, and a majority of research questions were satisfied by reference to the manual Cope-Chat records which were still being maintained for the hospital population.

During 1971 the whole system was again subject to review, and it was agreed that the data base was deficient in four major respects. First, the system was organized around individual pregnancy episodes while the focus of obstetric research was shifting to the analysis of complete obstetric histories. Second, there was an unacceptable delay between the occurrence of an obstetric event in the hospital and the appearance of the coded data. (Basic statistics were always twelve to eighteen months out of date. Clinicians interested in operational research required more immediate data for monitoring innovations in patient management.) Third, there was a problem of linking obstetric and neonatal data. These were on separate Hollerith files and had proved exceptionally difficult to match and collate. Finally, most gynaecological events relative to fertility (spontaneous and therapeutic abortions, ectopic pregnancies, sterilization, etc.) occurred in other Aberdeen hospitals and were recorded in a completely independent system of Cope-Chat cards.

It was therefore decided to establish a research group within the MRC Medical Sociology Unit to investigate the possibilities of computerizing and otherwise improving the data base. This group, working in close collaboration with members of the Departments of Obstetrics and Child Health, initially concentrated on the technical problems of translating the binary punched Hollerith cards to computer tape files, the analysis of potential user requirements, and the documentation of the existing system. Subsequently resources were directed towards the design of a suitable data retrieval system, and the establishment of a common core of data for all deliveries and fertility-related gynaecological events.

A major factor in the planning of the project has been the somewhat atypical characteristics of obstetric medicine and maternity care. Most maternity patients are in fact quite normal and require only the routine monitoring of their progress. The case notes from which data are extracted range from the relatively brief notes of the uncomplicated pregnancy and delivery to the lengthy documentation of a small proportion of very complex cases. Second, there is a strong emphasis on a patient's total fertility history both by the clinician in his management of a patient and by the researcher investigating the aetiology of complications.

The general problems confronting the research group were therefore quite well defined, and nine major objectives or focal points were identified. These are detailed below. (It should be noted that the order of presentation does not denote order of priority.)

The phasing out of Hollerith files and equipment

When the question of computerization was first raised it was suggested that one of the most difficult obstacles would be the conversion of the Hollerith card files. As noted above many of the cards were binary punched rendering them unsuitable for normal computer input. The problem was further complicated by the fact that a variety of techniques had been used to compress the data. Moreover, formats had been changed from time to time. Our first objective was therefore to devise a general system for disentangling any given binary card format.

The problem was not difficult to solve. A two-stage process was adopted. The first was a machine code program which read the data cards without attempting to convert punching combinations into alpha-numeric characters. This provided us with a tape file containing binary card images in which the punch pattern on each data card was recorded. The second stage was a Fortran program to decode the binary punch pattern, differentiate the various data items, allocate integer codes, and to re-organize the data into an acceptable format. An innovation which afforded simplicity and economy was the utilization of a single binary punched card to pass data to the program concerning the original Hollerith format (Samphier 1975).

The practical task of translating the 100 000 cards was beset by unfortunate technical disasters and complicated by inordinately lengthy processing times. Nevertheless after some delay the vast bulk of these Hollerith card records was transferred to sequential tape files. To complete the initial computerization, programs for the generation of contingency tables, for descriptive statistics, and for conducting file searches were written.

The reconstruction of patient histories

The base data files contain records of individual pregnancy events, with no automatic method of linking the successive events occurring to one woman. The next stage of development of the data bank was the generation of fertility profiles for each woman represented in the population, including, where appropriate, live and still births, spontaneous and therapeutic abortions, and sterilization procedures. With the exception of the small proportion of out-migrants all these data are available from the medical records of the Aberdeen Maternity or General Hospitals.

As a first step in achieving this objective we have concentrated on linking the records of live and still births already on tape, and constructing profiles with dummy entries for missing events. This has been complicated by the case numbering system formerly in use in the Maternity Hospital. Until 1972 when a Unit Numbering System (a scheme long established in all other Aberdeen general hospital departments whereby an individual patient is always identified by the same reference number) was adopted, antenatal patients were allocated an A.M.H. number on first admission during any pregnancy which ran in sequence from 1–n commencing on the first of January each year. Thus a woman who has three pregnancies will have three different case reference numbers. The situation is further complicated by the fact that the AMH number may refer to the year prior to the birth event. Consequently within an annual series of births the case reference numbers may be of either the current or the previous year's sequence.

The problems of linking pregnancy records vary with the period in which events occurred. The simplest case is the woman who has a first pregnancy on or after 1 January 1972. This and all subsequent obstetric case records should bear her unique Unit Number. Records of events occurring between 1967 and 1971 although having different AMH numbers do include key linkage information such as date of birth and initial letter of Christian names, maiden name and surname. A fairly high rate of linkage was possible by matching records on these key data alone. Pre-1967 records do not have as much key information and are therefore more difficult to match. As a fallback there was a manual index file which cross-referenced all case records.

Extension of the data base

Early in the development of the project it was agreed that substantial resources should be devoted to extending the data base in several ways. (The Medical Research Council provided funds for six full-time clerical/technical staff for a three-year period.) The objective has been to eliminate the major deficiences of the old system. A massive data collection exercise has been mounted to achieve a minimum core of demographic, social, and clinical data for all records falling within a new Aberdeen District population definition, applied consistently from 1948 onwards. Aberdeen District is a new local government area which coincides almost exactly with the old City plus Suburbs area used for the period 1967–75. This new population boundary was chosen for three reasons. Prospectively it is the simplest one to use given the coincidence of local government and health authority responsibility. Retrospectively there was a minimum of extra obstetric case records to be included for the 1967–75 period. Finally, and perhaps more importantly, the District boundary encompasses a natural urban population group.

Clerical staff have been employed to collect the following data:

(a) Supplementary demographic, social, and clinical (DSC) data for obstetric records already on file;
(b) A basic set of DSC data for records previously excluded from the Hollerith subset, i.e. some illegitimate and multiple pregnancies, and non-City residents now included within the District;
(c) A basic set of DSC data for a small number of domiciliary confinements that occurred outside the old City boundary, but which are now included within the District;
(d) Basic demographic and clinical data for all relevant gynaecological events occurring to women of child-bearing age resident within the District boundary.

Upon completion of this exercise the data base will contain consistent minimum data on all obstetric and almost all fertility-related gynaecological events occurring to women resident in the district boundary. (A very few gynaecological events to private patients may be excluded.)

The addition of these supplementary data has also simplified the reconstruction of patient histories, since it will now be possible to match records accurately on a wider range of key variables, viz. patient's date of birth and marriage, maiden name, etc.

The vast wealth of clinical data already on file will also be contained within the data base, but obviously it will not be available for the total District population.

The assessment of user requirements and the design of an appropriate file structure

Data base design is always problematic, but in administrative and commercial applications there are, in theory at least, a set of basic management objectives. In contrast a purely research data base of the type we have must be an open-ended system. It is impossible to specify in advance all the types of data structures that will be requested by research staff. We have had to work with a very general brief: to design and implement a data base structure that will effectively satisfy anticipated research demands, a system that is flexible enough to satisfy simultaneously widely divergent usage patterns, and rapid changes therein, and a system that can be operated within available resources. Further, this data base structure should be such as to demonstrate the usefulness or otherwise of this type of socio-medical data system.

Four categories of user have been identified:

(a) Medical staff from the collaborating departments engaged on epidemiological, aetiological, and operational research;
(b) Staff at the Institute of Medical Sociology conducting demographic analyses, and studies of patient management, service provision, and medical intervention;
(c) Medical staff in the collaborating departments requiring summary data for patient management;
(d) Other data systems—notably Scottish Home and Health Department, Information Services Division, and Grampian Regional Health Authority, Research and Intelligence Unit.

Disregarding for the moment other data systems (see below) we

have reached the following general conclusions about the current and expected pattern of usage:

(1) Research users typically require access to only fragments of case records for subsets of the total population. Both the subsets and fragments vary between users and over time. Thus it is impractical to adopt conventional data base record chains;
(2) Users who wish to examine an entire case record almost invariably require access to the original case document. The data base can only serve to identify records of potential interest to those users;
(3) The exception to (2) above is the clinician who requires a brief summary of previous obstetric history for patient management. This potential demand is given low priority in devising an optimum file structure since the data base is primarily research-oriented. Our investigations suggest that a clinical data base would have a radically different structure in order to satisfy clinical demands efficiently.

We have therefore concentrated on designing a file which will both satisfy the random and selective pattern of usage, and work efficiently within the environment of a general purpose university machine.

As part of our assessment of user demand we have been monitoring the uses of the current sequential tape version of the AMH data. An analysis of 1164 tape passes, over a nine-month period, indicated that, on average, researchers required information from less than 25 per cent of the total records on file. Moreover only 3–7 per cent of the data contained within these records were utilized. In these circumstances sequential file structures involve the unnecessary processing of over 90 per cent of the data. Some form of random access is clearly an essential requisite. Bearing in mind the low rate of data utilization we began investigating the possibilities of total random access to individual data items rather than individual case records.

The technique adopted is that of file inversion, which is best described by means of a simple example. Suppose we have 20 patient records each containing 10 items of data—sex, age, marital status, etc. Conventionally these data would be stored as a sequence of records on punched cards or magnetic tape. Each data record would contain the ten data items for one patient. In order to compute say the age distribution for our 20 patients, it would be necessary to read 20 data records in order to extract the age from each one. The inverted form of this file would contain only ten records—one for each item of data recorded for each patient. The age record would therefore hold 20 patient ages, and in order to compute the age distribution for our 20 patients it is only necessary to read one data record. Similarly to generate an age × sex contingency table only two data records are required.

This example illustrates the principal advantage of the inverted file—data are stored in a manner which fits the predominant pattern of usage, and in a way that minimizes the volume of data that has to be read before the computation can begin. Obviously this basic structure has to be considerably elaborated to cope with hundreds of thousands of more complex records. Nevertheless, the end result is a far more compact, fast, and flexible data file.

Much of the maternity and neonatal data we record is of the dichotomous type—male/female, yes/no, present/absent, etc. With a modified form of inverted file it is possible to store only the yes, present, or positive data, with a corresponding saving in space otherwise taken up by null data.

The present sequential files contain over 15 million data items relating to more than 59 000 pregnancy events. The rate of growth is 600 000 data items per annum. However, using an inverted file to store only the positive information the file size is reduced to 2·5 million data items, with a growth rate of 125 000 items per annum.

Allowing extra space for directories and pointers, and accounting for the further reduction of data when records are merged on to a single profile for each woman, the basic file size is cut by over 80 per cent.

Four additional advantages follow with this type of file structure:

(1) The file may be extended and updated frequently without continual housekeeping exercises to optimize storage efficiency;
(2) Additional data from special studies may be temporarily appended;
(3) When the total space requirements of the file exceed the available storage, infrequently used items can be archived to a separate reserve volume;
(4) Programs for data retrieval and analysis are efficient and compact, and fit well into the University machine environment.

Design of data vet procedures

With the old data system, transcribed Cope-Chat cards were returned with the corresponding case notes to the clinician in charge of the patient. He was expected to check the transcription and coding of the notes with particular reference to items requiring some degree of clinical assessment. This imposed a heavy workload on the medical staff, and was one of the principal reasons for the delays in record processing. We are therefore concerned to devise methods of auto-checking the internal consistency of records. Some work has already been done in this field, but largely with reference to general medical records bearing far less detailed information, e.g. by the Scottish Home and Health Department Information Services Unit.

Some of the data can be assessed directly in terms of the logical interrelationship of variables. The detailed clinical data however are not, in the main, amenable to such procedures. It is hoped as an alternative to generate a series of probability ratings for the various interrelationships based on the existing data which have been verified by clinicians. This would be coupled with a sample check done manually. The program would incorporate a feedback system allowing for changes in probability ratings if and when the population characteristics change.

Data monitor

Many clinicians have expressed an interest in having available regular statistical summaries of the information within the data bank. Two types of summaries are envisaged, a general review of the maternity and neonatal services, and specific indices relating to individual research interests. These would probably be produced on a rolling quarterly basis, with each summary containing statistics for the preceding twelve months. Such material would be of greatest value if the figures were never more than three months out of date. Similarly an automatic flagging system to indicate unusual changes in statistics would be desirable (linked to the data vet procedure as noted above).

An important reason for including this service is its relevance to all medical staff irrespective of their research activities. Those who are not engaged on epidemiological work will still see a useful result from the departmental investment in the research records system.

Reorganization of data collection and coding

Under the Aberdeen Maternity service every pregnant woman who will be delivered in the Maternity Hospital attends the hospital ante-natal clinic at least once in early pregnancy. In preparation for this visit record staff initiated a case note on which were entered basic socio-demographic details and data from the preliminary interview with the patient. The Cope-Chat cards were prepared after delivery and together with the case notes were sent to the research records clerks who transcribed and coded the data. Clinicians were then expected to check the transcription of their own cases, a task they undertook with varying degrees of enthusiasm. When an entire year's deliveries had been checked and punched, marginal totals were computed and cross-checked against administrative records for gross accuracy. Only then were the Hollerith cards added to the main data bank files. Consequently there was a delay of twelve to eighteen months in this process.

A number of innovations have been proposed, and some implemented, to speed up this process:

(1) Cope-Chat cards have been dispensed with in favour of a new transcription/punching form;
(2) Coded data are keyed direct to magnetic tape using a Honeywell keytape machine;
(3) Maternity profiles will be updated in a two-stage process. Data collected at the first antenatal visit will be added to the data base within seven days. This will alert the system to a new pregnancy event, allow cross-referencing with existing data and permit feedback to the antenatal clinic staff. This procedure is designed primarily to fit the regime adopted for women resident in Aberdeen City who attend the antenatal clinic for clerking one week prior to their first clinical examination. By following this seven-day cycle it may be possible to provide clinicians with a synopsis of previous history derived from the data base and to alert research staff to cases of potential interest. The remaining data on the pregnancy outcome will be added, via the data vet procedures immediately after delivery, probably in monthly batches. In particular, data items which require clinical verification will be flagged until they are checked;
(4) Automatic coding of literal descriptions of occupations, diseases, medical complications, and residence has been adopted. This eliminates time-consuming manual coding;
(5) Scottish Home and Health Department statistics (SMR/2) are extracted from the data base files and returned in magnetic tape format.

Cross-linkage of mothers, daughters, and sisters

The data base has been operating for almost 30 years, and spans two generations of mothers. With the stability of the Aberdeen population there is now a large body of data suitable for intergenerational analysis. Once the individual profiles are completed there should be sufficient material to enable some family linkages to be made. In establishing mother–daughter links implicit sister–sister links are also created. Further work is required however to assess the problems of associating any sisters not born in Aberdeen.

Intercommunication with other hospital information systems

In Aberdeen there are a number of medical record projects at various stages of development (see for example Hall et al. 1973). It has been planned from the outset that where appropriate (see below) it should be possible for us to exchange data with these systems. We are particularly keen to maintain links with both the local and Scottish Research and Intelligence Units. As noted above, from 1976 routine statistical data on each maternity patient will be returned to the Scottish Home and Health Department direct in magnetic tape form.

Research

The special features and advantages of the Aberdeen Maternity and Neonatal Data Bank for research purposes are:

1. It relates to the total population of a clearly defined administrative geographical area;
2. A single obstetric/gynaecological unit and the initial sociological team have collaborated throughout;
3. All medical and sociological data used have been recorded contemporaneously;
4. There is a large core of families permanently resident in the district, which allows familial studies:
    (a) Sisters and sisters-in-law are included;
    (b) A second generation of childbearing is covered.
5. Certain total subpopulations are accumulating, e.g. twins of known zygosity, since blood has been tested for all twins born in Aberdeen since 1968.

Throughout the past 30 years the obstetric and gynaecological data banks which until now were completely separate, have been used extensively for a wide range of medical and sociological research. They have also served as a sampling frame for many empirical studies. A selection of the hundreds of publications related to use of the data banks in the various stages of development is available from the authors. It clearly indicates the inevitable change in research priorities and interests over the years.

The appointment of sociologists as members of a Department of Obstetrics and Gynaecology was a pioneer venture. Initially research was clinically oriented with a sociological component largely determined by obstetricians. Thus in the 1950s attention was concentrated on the contribution of sociological factors to obstetric performance, i.e. social obstetrics with a focus on perinatal mortality. Social selection factors in physical manifestations (e.g. height and physical condition) and in social characteristics (e.g. age, parity, social class, marital status) were studied and groups at high risk to complications of pregnancy and delivery or to abnormalities or death of the foetus were identified. A major interest developed in the relevance of obstetric and social factors in the aetiology of child functioning which led to a combined study of mental subnormality in the community. This in turn highlighted the need to study low-birthweight babies (less than, or equal to, 2500 g) and the necessity to delineate subgroups of particular clinical or aetiological significance and to attempt a sociological explanation for the observed differences in the development and achievement of low-birthweight babies (see The Aberdeen Child Development Survey). In this context the relevance of being able to study siblings has particular significance.

Although it was laborious to link pregnancy events of individual women or to identify family members in the old record system, this was done manually for many projects, e.g. familial patterns in pre-eclampsia (Adams and Finlayson 1961), fertility profiles and family spacing (Thompson and Illsley 1969). The maintenance of ongoing data on pregnancy outcomes and fertility regulation was particularly laborious (Thompson and Aitken-Swan 1973).

The maintenance of combined social and medical data has allowed sociologists to study many aspects of behaviour, e.g. the timing of antenatal clinic attendance in relation to social and marital status (Illsley 1956; McKinlay 1970). A continuing interest has been in the changes in sexual behaviour and fertility regulation which became a major focus of research in the 1960s as rapid changes occurred in sexual mores (Illsley and Gill 1968a, b). In addition, innovations such as those in contraception and in techniques of abortion and sterilization occurred. The timing of these can be identified in the data bank but in addition changes in local organization, policy, or staff are known. These factors can all be used to interpret results of data analysis. Although abortion had been performed in Aberdeen before the Abortion Act of 1967, this new legislation focused national attention on Aberdeen experience and a major study was undertaken which included an epidemiological analysis supplemented by mulitdisciplinary empirical research (Horobin 1973). Although the data bank may identify differential treatment of subgroups with certain social classifications, e.g. single or lower social class, this is only the beginning since other types of research are required to account for the patterns found if the mechanism by which this is manifest is to be understood (Aitken-Swan 1977; MacIntyre 1977).

In recent years, research output has been relatively limited since efforts have been concentrated on the establishment of the data bank rather than on laborious intensive manual extraction of data. However, research that is ongoing, recently begun, or already planned using the data bank includes: the epidemiology of pregnancies and fertility control; fertility profiles of women having low-birthweight babies; the outcome of pregnancies in 120 girls aged under 16 years and their subsequent reproductive experience; social and medical trends in sterilization; failed sterilization in relation to technique used and the outcome of subsequent pregnancies; the demographic implications of sterilization using cohort analysis; familial studies of pre-eclamptic toxaemia; the obstetric experience of twin sisters of known zygosity in an attempt to study genetic factors in reproductive performance; predictive values of indications for diabetes in pregnancy and the relevance of these in patient management; lipid metabolism in subsequent pregnancies, etc.

A major study is focusing on the consequences of different patterns of childbearing at various ages with particular reference to early and late reproducers and the changes that have occurred over time among subgroups of the population. The major problem to be investigated is the impact of number of pregnancies and the spacing of pregnancy events by age at marriage and age at entering the reproductive cycle on the health of the mother and the growth and development of the child. More specifically the study will examine these health-related problems for the mother and the child in terms of the changes that have taken place over the past 25 years in regard to age at first pregnancy, age at marriage, illegitimate births, spacing patterns, fertility span, and family size. Also to be examined are the changes that have occurred in pregnancy complications, the general health condition of the mother and of the child at birth at each pregnancy number in relation to previous pregnancy experiences, and the changes that have taken place in regard to voluntary abortions and sterilization. The study will determine at what stage in the reproductive cycle and under what life conditions women are likely to resort to abortions or sterilizations to avoid an additional birth or to prevent future pregnancy events. The impact of marital dissolution and remarriage on number of births and the spacing of births will also be investigated. Each of these questions will be examined in terms of socio-economic status groups and the wife's social mobility through marriage. The study will be extended to familial and generational comparisons.

The list of obstetric and gynaecological items included in the data bank is available from the authors. As already explained, details may not be complete for certain subsets of the population, e.g. medical data will be minimal and social data incomplete for domiciliary confinements. Also certain information, e.g. smoking, was not recorded in all years. For neonates admitted to the special nursery at the Maternity Hospital since 1966 additional information is available from the authors.

C. The Aberdeen child development survey

RAYMOND ILLSLEY and FIONA WILSON

The Aberdeen Child Development Survey was initiated in 1962 as part of a research programme sponsored by the American Association for the Aid of Crippled Children, in co-operation with the Obstetric Medicine Research Unit (now the Institute of Medical Sociology) in Aberdeen. Two projects were planned; one of these was a reading survey (R.S.) and the other was a study of handicapped children in Special Schools.

It was believed that poor reading might be a sensitive indicator not only of general educational functioning, but also of other forms of malfunctioning. The survey was therefore designed to investigate the extent to which reading handicaps might be caused by biological factors, social factors, or a complex interaction between the two.

It was decided to survey five complete school year groups. A number of siblings and twins were thus included. Although this creates some analytic difficulties, these are outweighed by the advantages of having full data on several members of the same family.

In December 1962 with the co-operation of the city of Aberdeen Education Committee and of the heads of the independent schools in the city, all children in classes primary III–VII in city schools were given a battery of reading tests and provided demographic information about themselves. Because of United States interests and collaboration both British and American tests were administered. These were:

Primary III
Metropolitan Achievement Test (M.A.T.) P. II battery
  1. Word knowledge
  2. Word discrimination
  3. Reading: sentences
National Foundation for Educational Research (N.F.E.R.) Sentence Reading Test 1.
Primary IV and V
M.A.T. Elementary Battery
  1. Word knowledge
  2. Word discrimination
  3. Reading
N.F.E.R. Sentence Reading Test I.
Primary VI and VII
M.A.T. Intermediate Battery
  1. Word knowledge
  2. Reading
N.F.E.R. NS6 Reading Test.

As many children as possible from special schools were tested on the primary III battery, and if the older ones obtained reasonable scores they were retested on the battery appropriate to their age group.

Nearly all children in normal city schools were included, the only exceptions being long-term absentees (approximately 0·1 per cent) who had still not returned to school by February 1963. However the following three groups of children escaped testing:

(i) Those regarded as untestable due to mental or physical handicap;
(ii) Those educated at schools outside the city but with parents or guardians resident in Aberdeen;

(iii) Those at homes or institutions outside of Aberdeen, including blind children.

Each child who took the tests also filled in a *Form A*, under the guidance of a teacher, giving name, address, school, class, date of birth, father's job and employer, and names of older and of younger siblings. The same information was obtained for all children who escaped testing.

Each school provided attendance records for the children, covering the previous two years. Scores were collected at the same time, and at later times as they became availble, for each child on the various group tests routinely taken by all children in state schools and by some independent schools. These tests were as follows:

7+ The Moray House Picture Intelligence Test was used to screen for mental handicap and was normally taken by each child within six months of his seventh birthday.
9+ The Schonell and Adams Essential Intelligence Test was used to screen for poor readers within six months of a child's ninth birthday.
11+ This is a battery of Moray House Tests—two verbal reasoning, one arithmetic, and one English—upon the results of which allocation of secondary school places depended. A teacher's estimate was available for each child based on a combined, weighted, and standardized estimate of his performance on the two attainment tests. Children normally took the exam when aged eleven or twelve.

Approximately 14 000 children were surveyed in 1962; of these 86 per cent had been born in Aberdeen so that obstetric and social information collected during the mother's pregnancy or at the time of the child's birth was available.

The information which was collected from these records included not only the usual parameters of birth (weight, length of gestation, pregnancy number, mother's age, and father's occupation, etc.) and a list of the complications (pre-eclampsia, ante-partum haemorrhage, type of delivery, and reason for Caesarian section, etc.), but also (for first births) such information as the father's age, the mother's education and occupation, her father's occupation, and her age at marriage. Illegitimate and adopted children were identified from official records.

The second stage of information collection started in July 1963, i.e. at the end of the same school year as the main reading survey. At this time information from school medical records was transcribed. Each child is usually examined at first entry to school at approximately five years of age, and again at around ages nine and twelve. Only the information on the five-year examination is complete. It included height and weight measurements, results of vision and audiometry testing, and laterality. There is also a record of major illnesses and disorders and of emotional, behavioural, or familial difficulties. There is also a list of all Aberdeen schools attended and dates of entry to them.

The final data collection took place in March 1964, 1½ school years after the original survey. All classes in normal schools (excluding two private schools) which contained children in the original study were included. The children completed a sociometric form, giving the names of the three other children in the class whom they liked best, and also listing all their previous schools and giving their home address.

The class teachers filled in a Scale B for each child. This is a questionnaire which is intended to screen for minor behaviour disorders. It was designed by Dr Michael Rutter and this administration served as a pilot for his Isle of Wight study. The teachers were also asked to name the children in the class who were best at sports, tidiest, untidiest, most helpful, and the worst tell-tales. They were also asked to state whether the children were seated according to ability, choice, etc., and to fill in a Scale P for the most disturbed child in the class. The latter also compiled by Dr Rutter was a questionnaire designed to study more serious behavioural abnormalities than Scale B.

Scales B and P were completed for children in special schools and institutions. The records of the psychiatric and child guidance clinics were checked for any reference to survey children.

The populations

Because of the nature of the data collection a number of subpopulations can be identified within the reading survey. These can be identified in two ways: first by presence or absence in the study at the two major survey times, i.e. 1962 and 1964; and secondly by whether they were in the city or the school population.

The city population is defined by date of birth—born October 1950 to September 1955; and by residence of parents, guardians, or legally responsible authority in Aberdeen. This population is incomplete in so far as possibly as many as 700 children who fitted these criteria may have been one class above or below the survey classes. However it is complete with respect to children in special schools or in schools or institutions outside of Aberdeen.

The school population includes those in primary III–VII in 1962, or in equivalent primary or secondary classes in 1964, in normal state or independent schools in Aberdeen City. It is a complete population.

The numbers in each population and the overlap between populations is shown in Table 11.1.

TABLE 11.1

Numbers of children in the city population, the school population or both

	1964 both city and school pops.	City pop. 1964 only	School pop. only	Not surveyed in 1964	Total children
1962					
Both city and school pops.	12 757	20	36	401	13 214
City pop. only	8	192	0	99	299
School pop. only	31	0	474	55	560
Not surveyed in 1962	365	12	488	—	865
Total children	13 161	224	998	555	14 938

The figure 488 for children who were not surveyed in 1962 and who were in the school population only in 1964, is made up largely of children who were outside the prescribed age range but happened to be in a class containing a few survey children in 1964. Many of the other children who were not included both in 1962 and 1964 were migrants and as such are not randomly distributed throughout the social class spectrum. (For a description of the characteristics of Aberdeen in- and out-migrants see Illsley *et al.* 1963.) The social characteristics of the out-migrants are, of course, directly determinable from the information collected on them in 1962.

The family survey

More detailed information was collected on a 1 in 5 random sample of the R.S. population by interviewing the mothers or mother substitutes of the children. Approximately 10 per cent of the sample refused or were otherwise unavailable for interview, but since all other data was collected through the schools, the general characteristics of these lost subjects are documented.

The interview topics included the child's health both past and present; the mother's attitude towards her child's schooling and her ambitions for the child; the spare time activities of parents and children; contact with relatives; the parents' education, occupations, and family backgrounds; and housing. Each mother also filled in a Scale A, which was directly equivalent to the Scale B completed by teachers. A detailed pregnancy history for each of the mothers in the Family Survey (F.S.) was collated from maternity hospital records. The data from both the R.S. and the F.S. are available on computer tape.

Research projects and current status

Many investigators have postulated a causal relationship between complications of pregnancy and labour and later malfunctioning in children. While some relationships are well documented and proven, others remain conjectural. Major difficulties in the establishment of cause and effect have stemmed from the use of small, biased or ill-documented populations, inadequate recording of the presumed cause (i.e. complications of pregnancy and labour), insufficient measures of later malfunctioning, lack of knowledge about how social conditions affect development between birth and the identification of childhood disorder, and the unknown weight to be attached to genetic factors (Illsley 1967b). Two research strategies were adopted: on the one hand we identified children in the community with known and measured types and degrees of malfunctioning (e.g. mental subnormality) and compared their obstetric origins and social characteristics with those of the population from which they were drawn; on the other hand, we identified possible causal conditions (e.g. pre-eclampsia, low birthweight) and studied the resulting children to determine which conditions were associated with later malfunctioning. The size of the population and the availability of social data on the children and their families enabled us to control, at least partially, for pseudo-correlations.

Intensive study of children with defined levels of mental subnormality (Birch *et al.* 1970) revealed an even distribution across social classes of children with severe subnormality, but a massive clustering of children with mild subnormality in the lowest social classes. Prevalence of mental subnormality of all degrees was ten times as frequent in social class V as in the non-manual section of the population; in families where several adverse environmental factors occurred in combination it was 30 times as frequent. Clinical signs of neurological damage were evident in 49 per cent of the mentally subnormal population. The incidence of such signs however fell with decreasing social class from 100 per cent in the non-manual group to 29 per cent in social class V. Where environmental conditions are favourable, therefore, mental subnormality rarely occurs without neurological damage. Low rates of subnormality in the upper social groups could have derived from a true relative scarcity of such cases or as an artefact of less complete ascertainment of mild mental handicap in families better able to protect themselves from the stigmatization that attaches to mental subnormality. While some evidence of the latter was found, the true differences between classes remains substantial.

Many obstetric complications occurred more frequently in the mentally subnormal group than in the total population. Most of this overrepresentation derives from the low social class composition of the mentally subnormal group. Three conditions, severe pre-eclampsia, twin pregnancy, and low birthweight occurred more frequently after controlling for social class and parity. Signs of neurological damage were present in nearly all cases of severe pre-eclampsia and twin pregnancy (which frequently occurred together and in combination with other potentially damaging factors). Low birthweight alone showed no excess of neurological damage. The association between neurological signs and obstetric complications applied only in the lowest classes and the imputation of cause and effect is made more difficult in these classes by the fact that siblings deriving from straightforward pregnancies often had similarly low levels of functioning. Our general estimate is that obstetric factors may have been causative agents in approximately 10 per cent of the mentally subnormal children.

Study of defined pregnancy conditions in the total population again emphasizes the close relationship between obstetric performance, development and socio-cultural factors. Children whose birth was characterized by Caesarean section or forceps delivery had a higher mean IQ score than the general population, and their superiority was closely related to their higher socio-economic status. Breech deliveries (low social class, low birthweight) had a low mean score, but so too did their siblings delivered by the vertex. Similar results were found for ante-partum haemorrhage. Indeed high scores are characteristic of certain groups noted for a high incidence of complications—primiparae and elderly mothers—and again the pattern of scores reflects a socio-economic pattern (Illsley 1966, 1967a). Detailed studies of each pregnancy complication continue, with use being made of both obstetric and sociological approaches; the availability of data on siblings is proving to be particularly valuable.

Analysis of the data has given rise to a number of further investigations. Priority, however was given to the problem of low birthweight. Numerically this is the largest category; children of less than 6 lbs accounted for 32·6 per cent of our mentally subnormal population compared with 11·5 per cent in the total population of births. Subsequent analysis (Illsley and Hart, unpublished) demonstrated moreover that low birthweight is of increasing relative importance. In Britain as a whole, the rate of low birthweight (2500 g or less) has shown no tendency to fall, despite its being associated with the characteristic poverty syndrome of low social class, short maternal stature, and high parity for age. Perinatal death, very similarly associated, has fallen sharply over that period. Low-birthweight babies now constitute almost three-quarters of perinatal deaths in Aberdeen. There is moreover some evidence that in Aberdeen the rate of low birthweight began to climb in the late-1960s. New factors may have emerged in post-war years to counteract improvements in living conditions. On the other hand, the possibility requires investigation that with falling birth rates those groups prone to low birthweight may not be lowering their fertility *pari passu* and that therefore they form a constant volume but an increasing proportion of a falling birth population.

Such problems were the starting point of a joint study by the Unit and the Department of Child Health. Previous studies had suffered from two principal defects on the clinical side—failure to classify the heterogeneous group of low-birthweight infants and lack of recorded clinical and bio-chemical information potentially relevant to long-term physical and intellectual development. The present study of low-birthweight babies and a control group of heavier babies matched for social class, parity, maternal height and smoking, and the sex of the child includes a detailed standard neo-natal examination, repeated clinical and biochemical examinations in the first week of life and a follow-up clinic at 40 weeks post-partum. The sociological study has aimed to identify the socio-cultural characteristics of the family into which the child was born, and

additionally to document the specific experiences of each child during the child-rearing period up to 18 months. Whilst the data are currently being analysed one finding is already evident. Despite the close matching described, the socio-economic characteristics of the family, and therefore child-rearing patterns, are strikingly different in study and control populations. It is not therefore surprising that the later growth of such children should also be clearly differentiated. The sociological data now demand further analysis and interpretation; cross-tabulation against the paediatric findings should reveal how far such results apply across the whole population of low-birthweight infants or how far they result from the special features of clinically definable subgroups.

The R.S. data-bank established for the conduct of these studies is being exploited in various ways. Screening for asthma, for example, revealed a prevalence rate of 4·8 per cent, much higher in boys than in girls and higher also in large families and lower social classes (Dawson *et al.* 1969). Within classes asthmatic children had higher IQ scores than their peers. This may possibly be a consequence of the differential environment and activity imposed by the condition itself. A further analysis focused on family size and position in family as influences on development (Oldman *et al.* 1971). An attempt was made to differentiate between two alternative models of explanation of the negative correlation of family size and achievement, the one postulating a direct and the other, an indirect association. There was a slight tendency for older children to perform better than their younger siblings on achievement tests at age 11 and this was most marked in two-child families, especially when the younger child was a girl. While this suggests some direct effect of family structure, there was evidence that different lifestyles, indicated by such variables as family planning practices, were more strongly associated with test scores.

A retrospective epidemiological study of twinning has been followed up by zygosity-testing of all surviving twin pairs born in Aberdeen in the period 1950–65 (608 pairs). The unit's interest stems from the associations of twin pregnancy with later malfunctioning noted earlier, but it forms part of a wider comparative study with twinning in Nigeria where the twinning rate is considerably higher than in Britain. The higher Nigerian rate applies only in dyzygotic twins.

These studies emphasize the multi-factorial nature of problems of development frequently attributed to birth conditions. They also underline the paucity of reliable data on parameters clearly relevant to development and functioning. In particular we are aware of the difficulty in specifying how social factors influence development.

Other studies recently initiated include:

(a) An investigation of the relationship between birthweight, a variety of obstetric factors, and later physical and educational development;

(b) A study of the correlations between a number of ecological factors, derived from the 1961 National Census data, and some information concerning the staffing of schools and school performance;

(c) An enquiry into the school performance and behaviour of a small group of girls who had an outcome of pregnancy before their sixteenth birthday;

(d) A comparative study in collaboration with the Polish Academy of Sciences (Professor M. Sokolowska), since some sociological and educational data from the R.S. are similar to those collected independently for the school population in Warsaw.

D. The Aberdeen delinquency study

DAVID R. MAY

The Aberdeen delinquency study is a retrospective longitudinal project; that is, the research was not planned *ab initio* as a prospective, ongoing study of delinquents, but rather, existing record files were used in order to simulate a longitudinal design.

Confusion still surrounds the use by criminologists of the term longitudinal research, and this term is all too frequently applied to work otherwise widely disparate in terms of objectives, design and procedure. Minimally, however, the design should exhibit three features:

(1) The sample should be defined independently of the dependent variable; that is, it must be a sample of normal children defined other than in terms of contact with the law-enforcement system;

(2) Data-collection should be carried out at repeated intervals;

(3) The procedures for data-collection should ensure that basic data relating to the independent variables are collected prior to the onset of delinquency.

The promise of such a design is fourfold:

(1) It facilitates causal analysis. By incorporating a sequential model, a longitudinal design promises 'a solution to the problem of causal order, at least in principle' (Hirschi and Selvin 1967). Such a promise, if realized, would have an extremely valuable predictive pay-off.

(2) It enables an accurate measure to be made of the incidence of delinquency. Cross-sectional studies, because of their need to maximize the dependent variable, risk seriously distorting the problem of delinquency. Using a sample of normal children and a longitudinal design it becomes possible to assess accurately the life-chances of becoming delinquent.

(3) Because it is concerned with development over time the longitudinal study promises to shed much light on the structure of delinquent careers, and the possible association between early onset and adult recidivism, a matter on which the present evidence is much more confused.

(4) Longitudinal studies promise to avoid the problem endemic to most cross-sectional retrospective studies, of data contaminated by the sample's prior involvement with the law-enforcement system.

The Aberdeen study incorporates the three basic features of longitudinal research as outlined above, yet its significance lies not so much in the longitudinal design, but rather in the size and nature of the population studied, and in the quality of the data collected. Indeed, in terms of the mode of analysis adopted (excepting possibly the analysis of delinquent careers) and the presentation of results, it more closely resembles a cross-sectional study, although this is not to say that in either respect it departs markedly from the conventional use of a longitudinal study in criminology.

In so far as the Aberdeen study is concerned this practice is justified by virtue of the fact that its primary concern is not with the aetiology of delinquency. It is axiomatic to the theoretical assumptions that inform the work that such a concern cannot usefully be pursued in this manner. Causal analysis is therefore eschewed for the more limited, but equally more viable task of *describing in as precise and detailed terms as the data permit the kind of children identified and labelled delinquent by a particular organization of criminal justice. The organization in question is that which operated in the city of Aberdeen throughout the 1960s and early 1970s.*

Formulation and development

The Aberdeen delinquency study is a product of the epidemiological work carried out in the 1950s and early-1960s by the MRC Medical Sociology Unit in Aberdeen. The study population is that brought into being by the 1962 Reading Survey, slightly modified to facilitate the identification of the delinquents, so that in this instance it is limited to all children born between 1 January 1951 and 31 December 1954 (inclusive) whose parents or guardians were resident in the city of Aberdeen on 31 December 1962.

The development and structure of the Reading Survey have been fully described in Part C of this chapter. It may, however, be worthwhile to identify the particular strengths of this work for the study of delinquency. These are as follows:

(1) Altogether 11 004 children constitute the study population. This clearly produces a sizeable delinquent sample and permits analysis of some complexity to be carried out.

(2) The population, which forms at one and the same time both a sampling frame and a control group, was virtually complete within the limits of the age and residence criteria employed. It was not stratified in any way. The Aberdeen sample possesses a high generalizability factor. Of course, it is restricted to one Scottish city, but even this can be construed as an advantage given that the principal concern was not with delinquent behaviour as such, but with the operation of a particular system of law enforcement.

(3) The population includes a roughly equal number of males and females. This permits an analysis of ordinary female delinquency (that is, girls who have simply been referred to court, and not institutionalized). No other British study, and few American ones, have been in a position to achieve this.

(4) The socio-demographic data were collected at a time preceding for the most part the onset of delinquency in the population (see Fig. 11.1). Thus, the problems of data contamination have largely been avoided.

(5) With the exception of the data relating to IQ tests and school attendance the socio-demographic data used in the analysis were not collected for routine administrative purposes, but specifically for research purposes, by staff trained in research techniques, and under close supervision. As with all survey data, such supervision could not entirely eliminate idiosyncratic approaches to both the collection and processing of the data, and problems of meaning inevitably arose. These however, were not of the same order as would likely be encountered by research projects that rely heavily on extant administrative data, or on the data-collecting activities of non-research staff. The Aberdeen data therefore possess a high degree of reliability.

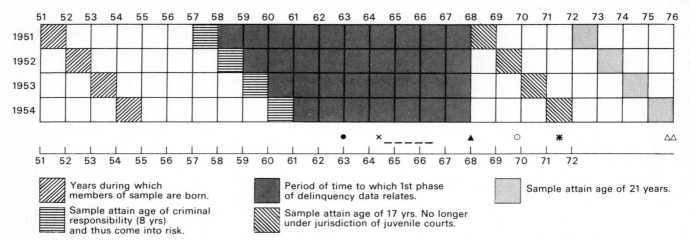

FIG. 11.1 The data collection process: (●) 31 December 1962 reading survey—collection of the main body of socio-demographic data; (×) March 1964—sociometric testing and teachers' assessment of behavioural disorders; (▲) 31 December 1967—collection of the delinquency data— 1st stage; (○) November 1969—creation of the new social work departments under the provisions of the *Social work (Scotland) act 1968*; (*) 15 April 1971—introduction of children's panels under the provisions of the *Social work (Scotland) act 1968*; (---) May 1964–March 1966–'the family interview'—the 1 in 5 sample; (△△) December 1975—collection of delinquency data—2nd stage.

Study of delinquents and delinquency in Scotland, apart from Ferguson's (1952) work on Glasgow school-leavers, had been relatively neglected and therefore in 1967 the Scottish Home and Health Department agreed to finance an examination of delinquency in Aberdeen based on the Reading Survey population.

Operationalizing delinquency and identifying the delinquents

The kinds of problems that the study was to investigate were largely determined by the availability of the data. Equally practical considerations influenced the operational definition of delinquency that was finally employed.

Initially, we had hoped to adopt as wide a definition of delinquency as possible, in furtherance of our general interests in the processes of social control, but prompted also by a dissatisfaction with court records as indicators of antisocial conduct. There were a number of agencies (e.g. probation, child care, school welfare, child guidance) that handled, on a more or less routine basis, children whose behaviour could easily have resulted in a court appearance. Unfortunately, it was soon apparent that recording practices in these agencies were so unsystematic, even idiosyncratic, as to render their files useless for comparative purposes. Certainly any attempt to identify a sample of problem children passing through these agencies on a retrospective basis, as was initially envisaged, was not possible.

In the end ambition was sacrificed for reliability. The Nominal Index of the Aberdeen City Police proved to be the most reliable, comprehensive, and usable mechanism for the identification of problem children, and it was on the basis of this system that delinquency in the study was defined. So far two separate searches of the Nominal Index file have been carried out. The first identified all children in the population born from 1 January 1951 to 31 December 1954 (inclusive) whose parents or guardians were resident in the city on 31 December 1962 to have made a court appearance prior to 1 January 1968. A subsequent search was made towards the close of 1975 and a court appearance record for the same population up to the age of 21 years was established.

Information relating to court appearances was either detailed on the Nominal Index record itself, or else was contained in a Criminal Records Office (CRO) file which could be easily traced from the Nominal Index. Additional relevant information that was obtained at the same time for each separate court appearance included:

Date of appearance;
The court in which the appearance was made;
The number and type of offences listed on the charge sheet;
The method of disposal ordered by the court.

Note that the criteria for inclusion in the delinquency sample was the fact of court appearance. Most criminological studies work with court-based samples of one kind or another on the assumption that such a sample is more or less representative of the delinquent population as a whole, or at least is representative of the more serious or real delinquent population. No such assumption is made here. Indeed the use of the term delinquent or delinquency in the project is meant to imply no more than children or children's behaviour formally dealt with by police or courts irrespective of its nature.

From the data available to the present study (no more than a bald legal description of the offence) it was simply not possible to differentiate between offences in terms of seriousness. Accordingly, the sample of juveniles identified from police records includes all those children in the population who made a court appearance regardless of the reasons for, or the outcome of, that appearance. This means that the delinquency sample includes a small number of juveniles who were referred to court but whose cases were subsequently deserted or they themselves found not guilty.

The formal structure of law enforcement

The legal basis on which the formal structure of juvenile justice rested throughout the 1960s was the *Children and young persons (Scotland) act of 1937*, supplemented by the *Children's act of 1948* and the *Criminal justice (Scotland) act of 1949*. The 1937 Act was essentially a consolidating measure which substantially re-enacted the provisions of the *Children and young persons (Scotland) act of 1932*. These statutes provided for special courts, special rules of procedure, and special provisions for punishment in dealing with offenders under the age of 17 years.

The 1937 Act gave local authorities the power to establish under a directive from the Secretary of State specially constituted Courts of Summary Jurisdiction for the purpose, *inter alia*, of hearing charges against children (persons under the age of 14 years) and young persons (persons who have attained the age of 14 years but are under 17 years of age). Aberdeen adopted this system. These courts were presided over by three justices of the peace (lay persons) chosen from a panel of specially qualified justices, who were felt to have some particular skill or experience in handling problem children.

Under the provisions of the 1937 Act the age of criminal responsibility in Scotland stood at eight years and remained so until the introduction of the *1968 Social Work (Scotland) Act* brought about sweeping changes in the whole notion of criminal responsibility in respect to juveniles. Thus, during the period under review it was conclusively presumed that no child under the age of eight years could be guilty of an offence. But the juvenile courts were not only empowered to deal with children who had committed offences. In line with their welfare orientation the juvenile courts had jurisdiction over juveniles whose behaviour and/or situation gave rise to a more general concern: juveniles who persistently refused to attend school; children or young persons felt to be exposed to moral danger or in some way regarded as being in need of care and protection; refractory juveniles who were deemed to be beyond the control of their parents or guardians. These juveniles constituted a small percentage of those making an appearance in court. Referral was seldom a result of police action. Rather, it more likely followed an initiative from the education authorities or a social work agency, such as the Child Care Department. In these cases children under the age of eight years could be referred to court, but even so such referrals were rare.

In Scottish law the right to prosecute in criminal cases is usually conferred on the Lord Advocate and the public officials under him who prosecute in the public interest. In practice this means that in the Courts of Summary Jurisdiction the right of prosecution rests with a number of public prosecutors, unlike the situation in England and Wales where it is in the hands of the police. In every court there is an official whose duty it is to prosecute all offences competent to be dealt with by that court. In the Sheriff Court he is known as the Procurator-Fiscal; in the Justice of the Peace Court, the Justice of the Peace Fiscal; and in the Burgh and Police Courts, the Burgh Prosecutor. The right of private prosecution is recognized, but it is one that is rarely exercised. There is a third class of prosecutor. Certain statutes confer upon specified officials the right to prosecute in respect of contraventions of their provision, thus for example, officials acting for local education authorities are on occasion seen prosecuting in the juvenile courts. But approximately 95 per cent of cases dealt with by the juvenile courts were police-initiated; that is, the juvenile concerned was accused of a violation of the criminal law, and the case was brought to court by the appropriate public prosecutor.

The organization of juvenile justice in Scotland throughout the 1960s assumed, in terms of its officially expressed ideology at least, a fairly overt welfare orientation. In dealing with juvenile offenders the principle of individualized justice was assumed to have primacy, and the courts were expected to operate on the basis of a set of criteria, in no way clearly specified, but certainly recognized as being more all-embracing than one that recognizes the offence itself as the only relevant factor. This principle, and the welfare orientation which underlies it, found concrete expression in courtroom procedure, in which relative informality prevailed, ritualism was reduced to a minimum, and which recognized the importance of probation officers and the need for comprehensive and carefully documented background reports.

These features were certainly all embodied in the daily practice of the Aberdeen Special J.P. Juvenile Court, which throughout the period under review appears to have extended and strengthened its jurisdiction over juvenile offenders. In 1959 it was dealing with a little under three-quarters (72 per cent) of all police-initiated juvenile cases. By 1967 this figure had risen to nearer 90 per cent.

Over the nine-year period (1959–67) the number of juveniles appearing before the J.P. Juvenile Court had increased by 68 per cent, while the number dealt with by the Sheriff (Juvenile) Court, the other principal juvenile court in the city, declined by 92 per cent.

The implementation of Part III of the *1968 Social Work (Scotland) Act* in April 1971 completely restructured the organization of juvenile justice in Scotland (Grant 1971). The processing of delinquent children up to the age of 16 was, with certain exceptions, removed from the ambit of the criminal law, and transferred to the Children's Hearings. The corollary of this was that the jurisdiction of the adult courts was extended to cover offenders from the age of 16, whereas previously it had applied only from the age of 17 onwards. The impact of these changes on the Aberdeen project was, however, minimal. By the time that the reforms were introduced most of the population at risk had passed into the jurisdiction of the adult courts, and of the minority who might have been brought before a Children's Hearing none was in fact so dealt with.

Jurisdiction over adult offenders is in practice shared by two courts, the Sheriff Court and the Burgh or Police Courts. A very small numer of cases (less than 0·2 per cent) are dealt with by the High Court. The Sheriff Court, which in Aberdeen hears approximately two-thirds of all adult cases, is presided over by a professional magistracy. It exercises both solemn and summary criminal jurisdiction, and therefore the Sheriff sits with or without a jury. The solemn jurisdiction of the Sheriff is limited by the fact that he can only impose a maximum sentence of two year's imprisonment. The Sheriff Court has summary jurisdiction in all common law offences, except murder, rape, incest, and wilful fire-raising, and in all statutory offences unless expressly or implicitly excluded. The Sheriff also exercises a concurrent jurisdiction with every other court within his sheriffdom in regard to all offences competent for trial in such courts. The remaining one-third of adult cases are tried in the Burgh Court. These courts are presided over by a lay magistracy, known as Baillies. They have only summary jurisdiction and limited powers of punishment (Gordon 1972).

As an alternative to court appearance, the Aberdeen City Police operated a Formal Warning System, officially reserved for first offenders and relatively trivial offences. Between one-half and two-thirds of all persons warned are juveniles. Up to a third of all police-identified juvenile offenders might be dealt with in this way in any one year. During the 1960s, however, there was a decline in the use of the Warning system, which was not arrested until the end of the decade. While the fact of a warning might be included in the Nominal Index record, it could not be assumed that this would always be the case, and it was highly unlikely that offenders who had received a warning, but had never made a court appearance, would be recorded in the Nominal Index record. Systematic recording of warnings was reserved for a separate book. Unfortunately, records here did not go back beyond 1964, so it was impossible to identify children in receipt of a warning on the same basis as those who had appeared in court. For this reason although all the available data relating to warnings were collected, they were kept separate from the court appearance data, and only a preliminary analysis of the material was made.

The offence typology

The adequacy of the concept juvenile delinquency as an analytic tool has come under attack from many quarters (e.g., Wootton 1959; Deutscher 1962). A juvenile may be brought to court for many disparate forms of behaviour—from acts involving serious damage to public and private property, to staying out late at nights, from persistent truancy to sexual precocity. To assume, as do many delinquency studies, by implication at least, that delinquency in this event constitutes a meaningful behavioural category, or that those to whom the term is applied have necessarily anything more in common than the experience of court appearance, may be misleading in the extreme.

Reliance on legal categories, which are the usual data available from police or court records, may well conceal important variations in the referral routes taken by particular groups appearing at court. Some sociologists have gone even further and suggested that there may well be wide discrepancies between the behaviour which initially prompted intervention and the legal categories used at a later stage of the law enforcement process (Sudnow 1965; Cicourel 1968). This is not to argue that no relationship between the two exists, but that it is problematic, and in the absence of data as to the specific nature of the relationship, should not be simply assumed.

The task of constructing scientifically meaningful typologies of delinquent behaviour is particularly important if one is concerned with the aetiology of that behaviour. The aim of the Aberdeen study was not to study aetiology of delinquent behaviour; rather, the concern was with the working of a particular law enforcement system over a particular period of time, and with the consequences of that system for the kinds of children identified and labelled delinquent. Thus, an offence-specific analysis assumes far less importance; the crucial point is that law enforcement agencies have been moved to bring the child to court, not the form in which this referral is accounted for.

Yet an offence typology can still bring more precision to the analysis than would otherwise have been the case, and its construction is warranted on these grounds alone. However, the offence data immediately available from police records were very limited indeed, consisting of little more than a terse, legal description of the offence, based apparently on the classifications used in the annual publications of *Criminal Statistics*. With such limited information it was not possible to organize the data in any qualitative sense. For example, in the case of property vandalism it was rarely possible from the data available to distinguish between minor acts of malicious mischief and more serious damage to property.

From data contained in the Nominal Index and C.R.O. files nine rather arbitrary, but roughly homogeneous, offence categories were derived. In an attempt to inject some element of comparability into Scottish delinquency studies the offence classification adopted by Shields and Duncan (1964) in their survey of the State of Crime in Scotland was followed as far as possible.

The nine offence categories created cover the whole range of behaviour for which a juvenile could be referred to court. They are as follows:

(1) Theft (except of motor vehicle) and reset;
(2) Breaking and entering lock-fast premises including cars;
(3) Vandalism;
(4) Breach of the peace, including actual and potential personal violence except for sexual offences;
(5) Motoring offences including theft of vehicle;
(6) Juvenile status offences—This category covers offence behaviour which applies only to juveniles, including welfare provisions, which are directed mainly at the younger children, especially care and protection proceedings, and also non-attendance at school, and those offences which apply most immediately to the older children, such as drinking under age, possession of an air-gun under age, etc.,
(7) Sexual offences;
(8) Frauds;
(9) Other minor offences:
offences relating to pedal-cycles
playing football in the street
making annoying telephone calls
false fire-alarms

making false statements to the police
contravention of the game laws.
Also included are the few recorded instances of Breach of a Probation/Supervision Order.

Sample mortality

The problem of sample attrition is not nearly so acute with retrospective longitudinal studies, especially in the Aberdeen case where the analysis was carried out on the basis of existing data and no personal contact with any sample members was required. All the socio-demographic data used in the Aberdeen delinquency study were collected in 1962 and 1964 prior to the establishment of the project. Data relating to court appearances were taken directly from police records.

The analysis was carried out on a population that was in existence in December 1962. It is quite likely that there were significant changes in the composition of that population over the years with which the delinquency research was concerned, 1959–75. Research into the effects of differential migration suggests that the Aberdeen population was a relatively stable one; roughly 85 per cent of children born in Aberdeen would still be residing there five years later (Illsley *et al.* 1963). Out-migration shows a clear social class gradient from 10 per cent of Social Class V to a little over 50 per cent of Social Class I. In-migration is even more sharply skewed toward the upper social groups.

Roughly 90 per cent of the study population were known to have been born in Aberdeen. In the 15 months elapsing between the two survey dates (December 1962 and March 1964), the only period for which an accurate figure is possible, 3·5 per cent of the original cohort seems to have moved out of the city. If this rate of out-migration had persisted throughout the period under examination then by 1968, the year in which the first sweep of police records was made, there would have been roughly a 14 per cent sample loss. However, this assumption cannot be made, if for no other reason than that the evidence suggests that the growing prosperity of Aberdeen in the late-1960s and early-1970s led to a reversal in the population trends that had characterized an earlier period.

More important than the attrition rate among the population at large was the problem of obtaining complete coverage of all relevant court appearances. For this we were wholly dependent on the recording procedures adopted by the Aberdeen city police. In the period immediately preceding our first data sweep the day-to-day business of producing and maintaining the actual written record was the responsibility of a uniform sergeant in charge of a small, mixed police/civilian records office team. The sergeant was in turn answerable to a uniform superintendent who supervised all clerical tasks within the force. Individual records were generated or, as the case may be, brought up to date, from the court lists sent over regularly to police headquarters.

The police have a long tradition of maintaining records of all cases passing through their hands, both for their own internal purposes as well as to meet government requirements. On the whole it appeared that the recording by the police of offenders they had officially dealt with was fairly comprehensive.

It was the usual practice to record details of all court appearances. There were occasional exceptions to this rule, but usually only involving the most trivial of cases, and even then only when the offender in question was not already known to the police (e.g. a first offender charged with riding a pedal cycle without lights). It is, however, interesting to note that this practice can produce its own distortions. If the pedal-cycle offender, or a member of his family, was already known to the police, or it was suspected that he was the kind likely to get into future trouble, then there is a greater chance that the offence will be included and retained within the records system.

The Nominal Index was also subject to continuous weeding out by Records Office staff as pressure on storage space built up. Records of first offenders dealt with for relatively trivial offences who had not subsequently come to the notice of the police (usually a period of 10 years free from further police involvement was demanded) were removed and destroyed.

At the time of our initial data sweep in 1968 the city police office had enjoyed a long period of relative stability, but all that was to change in the succeeding years. In April 1971 with the introduction of Part III of the Social Work (Scotland) Act responsibility for the maintenance of juvenile records passed to the Reporter to the Children's Hearing. It is doubtful, however, whether this had any major impact on police recording practice since the police continued for their own purposes to maintain a record of juvenile crime. Changes in premises and amalgamation of record systems also occurred.

It is difficult to establish whether the period of change, together with the general idiosyncrasies in police recording practices discussed above had any marked effect on our ability to identify those children in the population who had made a court appearance during the period under review. However, by conducting two separate sweeps of police records, in 1968 and again in 1975, and by comparing our results, we were able to arrive at some estimate of the loss. We were reassured to find that for children who had remained in Aberdeen and had appeared in city courts the number appeared to be very small. Of the 856 children identified by us from police records in 1968, only 20 (2 per cent) were not picked up again in 1975. This group was not distinguished in any particular way from those whose records were present on both occasions. Fourteen of the 20 had made only one court appearance in the period up to 1975, but this was not markedly out of line with the general pattern of delinquent appearances. Given the way that we were led to believe that police recording practices operated, we would have expected a greater number of missing records, showing many more common features. As it was it seems likely that our failure to trace certain records was random and not due to any systematic distortions in police recording practices.

The careful search procedures adopted yielded a high identification rate, and it seems likely that the delinquent sample includes, with very few exceptions, all those children in the study population who made a court appearance during the period under review. Any distortion that might have crept in is likely to be in the direction of understating the delinquent activities of three groups:

(1) Middle-class children, because of their higher rates of geographic mobility;
(2) Other rootless, or highly mobile groups. These are likely to be found at the very bottom of the social class scale;
(3) Children, who although normally resident in Aberdeen throughout the period, committed offences in other police areas.

The problem of mobility is one that assumes greater importance in the post-juvenile period. In theory, any involvement with police or courts outside of Aberdeen by any person normally resident in the city should have been reported to the Aberdeen police, and we did come across one or two cases of this kind. But in practice this was unlikely to happen except where serious offences were concerned.

The 1968 juvenile delinquency survey—some results

The Aberdeen delinquency project falls naturally into two parts following on the two separate data-collecting exercises. The analysis of the 1968 data has been completed and fully reported in May (1975a). Parts of that analysis have also appeared elsewhere (May 1973, 1975b, 1977). The results are briefly summarized below.

Of the 5654 boys in the population, 730 (12·9 per cent) had made a court appearance during the period under review. It was estimated that this would produce a court appearance rate of 17 per cent by the age of 16. Only 126 (2·3 per cent) of the 5350 girls appeared at court during the same period, giving an estimated court appearance rate of 3·5 per cent by the 16th birthday. Throughout males and females were separately analysed. Despite the difference in the size of the problem, female delinquents revealed much the same socio-demographic profile as the males (May 1977).

The analysis was organized around three groups of variables: social class, family structure, and school and school behaviour. The most significant finding to emerge was the association between official delinquency and what one might call social disadvantage. On each of the variables examined the tendency was for the delinquent to be concentrated towards the bottom end of the scale, where court appearance rates were considerably higher than the city average. This tendency is quite clearly illustrated in Table 11.2, where we have listed some of the factors found to be associated with delinquency: council housing; lower social class; large families; illegitimacy; low IQ; and unstable and low status employment.

TABLE 11.2

Some factors associated with court appearance

	No. of delinquents with attribute as a per cent of total delinquents (N = 730)	Delinquency rate per cent for boys	
		With attribute	Without attribute
Father's occupational status			
Lower-manual/working class (semi/unskilled/ unemployed)	36·2	21·9	9·7
Fishworker	13·7	26·9	11·9
Trawler deckhand	9·7	31·6	12·1
Unemployed	8·6	34·2	12·2
Residence			
In area of predominantly council housing	79·3	15·3	8·1
Inter-war tenements + post-war council. Phase I	30·8	22·6	10·8
Inter-war tenements	19·6	27·8	11·4
Family structure			
5 or more children in family	20·1	24·8	10·3
Illegitimate	7·6	24·1	13·2
School and school performance			
Attends 'high delinquency' school (Northern schools; schools on Phase I council estates; R.C. schools; central city schools)	54·7	17·9	9·7
Attends 'Northern' schools	20·0	20·7	11·8
Low IQ (<90)	23·6	29·2	11·0
Irregular school attendance	10·1	17·1	12·6
School behaviour 'problem' (Score of 9+ on 'Teachers' questionnaire)	21·8	27·9	11·2

Our findings further suggest that the more pronounced the disadvantage becomes the greater the risk of making a court appearance. Thus, while boys residing in areas of predominantly council housing have a delinquency rate that, at 15 per 100 boys at risk, is almost 20 per cent higher than the city average, boys living in the original slum clearance schemes of the Inter-War Tenements have a rate of court appearance that is more than double the city average (28 per 100 boys at risk). Similarly with father's occupation: boys of the lower manual working-class (i.e. boys with fathers in semi-skilled, or unskilled jobs, or who are unemployed) have a delinquency rate of 22 per 100 boys at risk, but dealing just with those boys whose fathers were unemployed the delinquency rate increases to 34 per 100 boys at risk.

Finally, the analysis also suggests that disadvantage has what appears to be a cumulative effect on delinquency rates. So as disadvantage is added to disadvantage the risk of making a court appearance correspondingly increases. For example while children from large families and children from lower working class homes have, separately, above average delinquency rates, lower working-class children from large families have a higher rate than either. So also with lower class children living in low status areas, who have higher delinquency rates than either lower class children in general or all children residing in low status areas.

This raises two important questions. First, in what way is cumulative social disadvantage related to delinquency rates? Is it, as has been suggested above, simply a matter of each additional disadvantage being reflected in higher delinquency rates? Second, is it possible to identify, in terms of the variables considered, particular subgroups in the population that are highly vulnerable to court appearance?

The kind of analysis that these questions give rise to is fraught with difficulties. Not only is there the problem of how precisely to define the disadvantages to be considered (e.g. should we deal with council house residence or residence in the Inter-War Tenements, with the lower working-class or just the unemployed?), but the equally difficult problem of determining in what precise order cumulative disadvantage is to be considered? A combination of low IQ and large family may be more significantly related to delinquency than, say, council house residence, lower working class, large family, and low IQ. Even with a limited number of factors the number of possible combinations is extremely large, and the number of permutations enormous.

Different analyses were attempted using a large number of factors in various combinations. The one which proved the most fruitful is set out in Fig. 11.2. It was soon apparent that to attempt to control for more than a half-dozen factors at any one time simply reduced the at risk population to virtual insignificance. In the event, five major controlling factors were chosen because (a) they each separately embraced over one-fifth of the at risk population, and (b) they were each separately associated with court appearance.

The method of analysis was simple. It was to take each of the factors in turn and progressively to dichotomize the population at risk until eventually, a sub-group of the total population had been defined which revealed very high rates of court appearance. The most productive way to attempt this analysis was to take the factors in order of their separate relationship with delinquency. Thus, the 5654 boys in the total population at risk were first of all dichotomized on the factor of family size. Altogether 1020 came from families of five or more children (in Fig. 11.2 the number in the population with the attribute in question is given in the rectangular boxes; the number without the attribute in the corresponding circle). This group of 1020 boys were then dichotomized on the basis of whether or not their fathers held semi-skilled or unskilled manual jobs or were employed in 1962. This process was continued until we were left with a group of 183 boys who came from large families, were lower working class, had mothers who held manual jobs prior to marriage, attended high delinquency schools, and lived in areas of predominantly council housing.

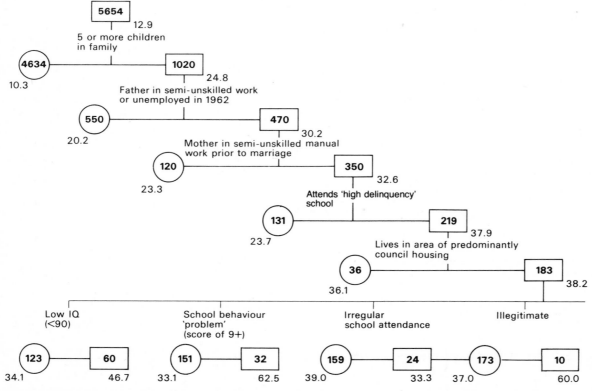

Fig. 11.2. The effect of cumulative social disadvantage on delinquency rates. Number in rectangular boxes = number of boys with attribute; number in circles = number of boys without attribute; figures outside boxes = delinquency rates (per cent).

Less than 10 per cent of all delinquents and just over 3 per cent of the male population at risk had all five attributes. More importantly, although the delinquency rate for this group was 38·2 per cent, three times the city average, this still means that a majority of the boys in the group had not in fact made a court appearance during the period under review. Furthermore, the tendency is for the delinquency rate to increase at a slower rate with each additional attribute. So, while taking those boys who come from large families in itself produces a doubling of the delinquency rate, from 12·9 to 24·8 per cent, it requires the addition of a further three attributes to boost that latter figure by 50 per cent. The discriminatory power of additional attributes is also markedly reduced. Boys from large families have a delinquency rate that is two and one-half times as great as boys from families of less than five children, 24·8 compared with 10·3 per cent. When the boys are dichotomized on council house residence (after controlling for the other four attributes) there is virtually no difference in the delinquency rates of the two groups.

This decline in discriminatory power is clearly a reflection of the extent to which not only the five control attributes, but also the various elements of social disadvantage are interrelated. While 18 per cent of the population at risk come from large families, 46 per cent of boys from large families are lower working class, 64 per cent have mothers who had held a manual job prior to marriage, 55 per cent attend the high delinquency schools, and 83 per cent live in areas of predominantly council housing.

As Figure 11.2 shows, it is possible to boost predictive ability by adding to the five control attributes a further attribute which on its own is highly correlated with court appearance. Thus, 62 per cent of boys who were identified as school problems, and who also possess the five attributes already discussed, made a court appearance. So too did 60 per cent of illegitimates who were similarly disadvantaged. This, however, still leaves a wide margin of error, and in any event with these two groups we are dealing with 20 and 6 delinquents respectively out of a total delinquent population of 730. Moreover, simply adding on further disadvantages does not automatically increase predictive ability. For example, boys who after controlling for the five main disadvantages are also irregular attenders at school, have a lower delinquency rate than the good attenders.

Calculating a social disadvantage score for all 5654 boys at risk in the population further illustrates the equivocal nature of the relationship between delinquency and social disadvantage. It has to be admitted that this was a somewhat arbitrary exercise. From the many factors that could have been used for this purpose we chose eight which were considered to reflect a socially disadvantageous position. All were used in the previous analysis. They were:

(1) Residence in an area of predominantly council housing;
(2) Mother having held a manual job prior to marriage;
(3) Attendance at a high delinquency primary school (i.e. those schools serving the northern and central areas of the city, schools on the immediately post-war council estates, and Roman Catholic schools);
(4) Father in a semi-skilled or unskilled job or unemployed;
(5) One of a family of five or more children;
(6) IQ below 90;
(7) Identified as a behavioural problem at school (i.e. with a score of 9+ on the Teachers' Questionnaire);
(8) Irregular school attendance.

A score of 1 was allotted for each of the above attributes, making a maximum possible score of 8. The results of the analysis are set out in Table 11.3.

This first of all shows a clear association between delinquency and social disadvantage: the more delinquent, the higher the social disadvantage score. This, however, is hardly surprising given that

Table 11.3

The relationship of delinquency to social disadvantages

Social disadvantage score	Non-delinquents	Delinquents	Recidivists
0–3	82·9	53·3	39·8
4 or more	17·1	46·7	60·2
N	4924	730	247
Mean score	2·1	3·4	3·8

| | Social disadvantage score | |
	0–3	4 or more
Non-delinquents	91·3	71·3
Delinquents	8·7	28·7
N	4473	1181
(Recidivists as a per cent of delinquents	(25·3)	(43·7)

each component of the social disadvantage score is itself separately associated with the risk of court appearance. The proportion of non-delinquents with a low social disadvantage score (less than 4) is twice the proportion of recidivists, 83 per cent compared with 40 per cent, while the proportion of recidivists with a high score (greater than 3) is more than three times the proportion of non-delinquents, 60 per cent compared with 17 per cent.

The corollary of this is that the higher the social disadvantage score, the more likely one is to be delinquent. Only 9 per cent of those boys with a low score are delinquent compared with 29 per cent of those with a high score. Furthermore, nearly half (44 per cent) of the high-scoring delinquents are recidivists compared with only one-quarter (25 per cent) of the low-scoring delinquents.

Of those boys who had a nil social disadvantage score (one in eight of all boys at risk) only 2 per cent were delinquent. Yet more than half (53 per cent) of the delinquents, and two-fifths (40 per cent) of the recidivists were in the low-scoring category (less than 4). The mean delinquent score of 3·4 was only 1·3 points higher than the mean non-delinquent score. Finally, despite the acknowledged association between delinquency and a high social disadvantage score, it was still the case that high-scorers were twice as likely to be non-delinquent as to be delinquent. In fact, the number of non-delinquent boys who had a score of 4 or more ($N = 842$) was greater than the total number of boys making a court appearance ($N = 730$).

Two points emerge from the above analysis. First, while there is a clear association between social disadvantage and delinquency, the latter phenomenon is in no way accounted for by the former. A majority of delinquents are, it would seem, hardly any more socially disadvantaged than non-delinquents. Secondly, in terms of the variables examined, we are unlikely to be able to identify subgroups in the population which reveal anything approaching a 100 per cent risk of making a court appearance. It would seem that the best we could hope for would be a predictive ability of around 50–75 per cent, and this could only be achieved in respect to numerically insignificant groups in the total delinquent population.

The follow-up study

One of the deficiencies of the first stage analysis is that it examined delinquency in the year 1968 when the children in the sample were aged only 13–17 years and therefore just reaching the peak of their involvement with the criminal justice system. The data on juvenile court appearances are accordingly incomplete, severely restricting the analysis of delinquent careers. More disturbing was the knowledge that the data further understated middle class and female delinquency, and thus detracted from one of the major strengths of the research design. Although the procedures adopted to estimate the full extent of juvenile court involvement proved, in the event, remarkably accurate, nevertheless a more extensive follow-up of delinquency was indicated.

A more important reason for undertaking further data collection was that it promised an answer to an enduring problem in criminology, where the evidence remains still tenuous and confused. Public concern with juvenile delinquency is prompted as much by what it is thought to signify for future conduct as the present problems it causes for society. The belief persists that a life of crime invariably has its roots in the juvenile period, yet studies of persistent adult offenders (e.g. Hammond and Chayen 1963; West 1963) have shown that a substantial minority at least have no police records as juveniles. This, however, may be more a reflection on the state of record-keeping than an accurate description of behavioural patterns. What is clearly needed is a prospective study of delinquent careers. In recent years West and Farrington (1977) and Wolfgang (1973) have made important contributions here, but the Aberdeen project is the first British study to examine the pattern of delinquent careers over both the juvenile and early-adult periods in a complete birth cohort, albeit confined to one Scottish city.

In the closing months of 1975 a further search of the Grampian police records was made, and all those in the previously defined population who had made a court appearance by their 21st birthday were identified. The procedures adopted were the same as in the previous data sweep. The search was restricted to the Nominal Index and the associated C.R.O. files. The data obtained were therefore equivalent to the data collected in 1968 and could be handled in the same way.

Of course, the longer a longitudinal study is extended, the more acute becomes the problem of sample attrition. One would expect that a significant proportion of the population at risk would by 1975 have moved out of Aberdeen, particularly as they reached young adulthood, and thus be lost to the study. No attempt was made to trace these individuals, to establish whether they had made court appearances outside of Aberdeen (except in so far as this could be ascertained through the Aberdeen police records), or even to estimate the size of the problem. On the other hand, the large number of delinquents identified suggests that it may not be such a sizeable problem as one had initially feared.

The additional data have been transferred to computer and merged with the existing files. Preliminary analysis began in 1977. As yet no work has been done on the females, and only the most superficial analysis of the males. Of the 5654 males at risk, more than 2000 (40 per cent) made at least one court appearance prior to their 21st birthday, 22 per cent of the at risk population made a juvenile court appearance, and 33 per cent appeared between the ages of 17 and 21. Of course, much of the court involvement appears fairly superficial; 43 per cent of those males identified made only one appearance during the period under review, and two-thirds of those making an adult court appearance were charged with a motoring offence (although this does not rule out the possibility of other charges). However, more than 1000 of the males who appeared at court (21 per cent of the at risk population) were never charged with a motoring offence.

It is intended that the analysis will follow the pattern established in the initial report (May 1975b), centering on three groups of variables: socio-economic status (father's occupation, residence, chronic unemployment, the fishing community); family structure (family size and birth order, fatherlessness, illegitimacy); and school and school performance (school attended, teachers' identification of problem behaviour, IQ, truancy, and school absenteeism). Close attention will be paid to the pattern of delinquent careers over the period to establish the relationship between juvenile offending (and specifically early onset of delinquency) and the delinquency of early adulthood.

The Aberdeen delinquency study does not pretend to explore the concomitants of delinquency. It seeks rather to throw some light, first on the pattern of official delinquent activity, and secondly on the social origins of those who become involved with our criminal justice system. To draw attention to the differences in orientation and theoretical underpinning between the Aberdeen study and the usual surveys of delinquency might seem to be making a rather fine point. In outward appearance at least it appears a distinction, without a difference. After all in terms of the kind of data employed, the questions examined, mode of analysis used, presentation of the material, and even the sort of results obtained, there would seem to be little to differentiate this study from numerous other surveys of the epidemiology of delinquency. Nevertheless, we believe it to be a crucial distinction with important implications for the selection of data and for any interpretation that might be imposed on the findings.

12. Longitudinal studies in Romania

A. The physical and neuropsychic development of children aged 0–3 years in relation to certain social and familial factors

IRINA CHIRIAC, ELENA ARBORE, and A. CHITU

Introduction

In view of the responsiveness of the infant organism to the family environment, a longitudinal study was carried out of a group of children aged 0–3 years who were brought up in different conditions with regard to familial environment, in an urban area.

This study is a synthesis of results obtained in a longitudinal study of 123 children, 66 boys and 57 girls, aged 0, 1, 2, and 3 years. In order to ascertain the psychosomatic characteristics of the children, an age-adjusted methodology was prepared and used for the somatometric and neuropsychic examination. The information on family living conditions was obtained by the house-to-house survey technique, conducted at the birth of the child and repeated yearly.

Analysis of the results obtained showed certain characteristics relating to the stages of physical development and made it possible to establish evolutional features regarding neuropsychic development; it also provided some information on the relationships between socio-familial factors and the psychosomatic development of the children in the first three years of life.

Physical development

Analysis of the material obtained from a study of 24 somatic parameters enabled the following observations to be made. The dynamics of physical development indicated the continuation of the growth process at a rate that diminishes with age and is non-uniform for the various parts of the body. Thus, at 3 years we noted a fourfold increase in weight, a twofold increase in height, and a twofold increase in plantar length compared with figures recorded at birth; between 0 and 3 years there was an intense rate of growth of the lower limbs and hands, together with a marked development with regard to size of head, thorax, and pelvis. At the same time, in relation to all the parameters studied there was a decrease in the rate of growth as the children became older.

During the first three years of life there is a change in the corporal habitus; this is evidenced by a gradual change in the conformation of the young child (large head, cylindrical thorax, short limbs), who begins to acquire the morphological features of the preschool child (relatively smaller head, flatter thorax, longer limbs), due in large part to the fact that the rate of growth is higher for volume parameters during the first year, while increasing for length parameters in the second and third years of life.

An important feature is the fact that from the third year onwards morphological differences are observed in relation to the sex of the children. Thus, girls show a relatively slower somatic development than boys in respect of most of the parameters studied, these differences being less evident at birth and gaining in significance as age increases. A slight change is also noted in the conformation of girls in comparison with boys, subcutaneous adipose tissue being more developed and the thighs larger (significant differences at 2 and 3 years), thus determining the approach towards the classic female conformation.

Neuropsychic development

The dynamics of neuropsychic development were studied by means of specific tests for monthly age groups between 1 and 12 months and three-monthly groups between 15 and 36 months, in relation to four areas of behaviour: motor, cognitive, verbal, and socio-affective. This study was aimed at establishing orientational indicators for assessing the normality of physical development of children aged 1–36 months in relation to chronological age for each of the behavioural fields concerned.

The development of motor behaviour during the first three years of life provides evidence of maturation and the acquisition and gradual improvement of static and dynamic co-ordination, both at the level of general motivity and at the level of segmentary motivity.

At this age cognitive behaviour becomes increasingly complex; this is shown by certain activities requiring differentiated reactions of manipulation, recognition, identification of dimensions, reproduction, and spatial orientation. Consequently, cognitive behaviour in the younger child up to the age of 36 months creates the possibility for adaptation based on gradual and ontogenetically realized acquisitions.

Verbal behaviour is marked by gradual acquisitions of increasing complexity, allowing the use of meaningful words and grammatical structure of language from the age of 1 year onwards.

Socio-affective behaviour holds an important place in the mental evaluation of the child, marking each stage in development by specific features in relation to the gradual differentiation of affec-tive reactions, and the gradual acquisition of a large number of habits on the basis of which the child becomes more independent but at the same time more co-operative in his environment; he begins to show marked preferences vis-à-vis those around him, and even opposition towards adults.

The mental development characteristics ascertained in respect of children aged 1–36 months allow diagnoses to be made of mental normality, advance, or retardation for each chronological age, as well as a longitudinal study of development by behavioural areas, by providing evidence of the specific age characteristics at the level of the four types of behaviour.

This analytical presentation of mental development between 1 and 36 months, carried out by the methodology for assessing the degree of normality of development at the various ages, provides an objective tool for assessing mental characteristics, the prevention of anomalies in mental development, such as retardation, and the forecasting of the child's subsequent mental development. Thus, apart from its importance from the scientific point of view, this new complex instrument of knowledge, which may be applied in a field that has received little study in Romania, constitutes a practical contribution of great value to specialists responsible for the care of young children.

It follows from this that there is a need to interpret the degree of neuro-psychic development taking into account factors other than age, namely, birthweight, nutritional status (eutrophy, dystrophy), and sex, which determine differentiation trends at certain ages, and also specific dynamics.

Relationship between psychosomatic development and socio-familial factors

Analysis of the changes in receptivity of the infant organism subjected to the influence of living conditions in the family has shown both a variability in the intensity of effect of social factors on the organism of children, and responses of a varying dimension in relation to sex, age, and the somatic or mental field of development.

The psychosomatic development of children aged 0–3 years is influenced by and differs according to the social gradient of the family environment factors. This difference becomes more pronounced with age and is directly proportional to the intensity of effect of the environmental factors. In the field of somatic development, the clear difference in height according to the social gradient of the social factors studied provides compelling evidence of the close relations existing between the organism and the environment at this age. In the field of neuropsychic development there is a clear accentuation of the influence of the environment according to the children's age, starting at 18 months, an age at which this field of development has been less affected in comparison with somatic development. The sensitivity of the infant organism to the effects of the social environment differs according to sex, the male organism being earlier and more strongly influenced from the somatic point of view, while that of the girls being correspondingly influenced from the neuropsychic angle.

In the first years of life the way the developing organism responds differs from one year to another, indicating a particular flexibility and capacity to adapt which develops continuously. From one year to another there is a change in the succession of environmental factors studied in relation to the extent of their effect on the organism; thus, as the child increases in age, certain factors assume increasing importance, while the child becomes less and less receptive to the influence of other factors.

While we have noted in the initial period of life a closer link between the child's somatic development and 'paternal' factors (occupation and educational level of the father and housing conditions), in children aged 3 years the influence of maternal social factors takes the fore: occupation and educational level of the mother. In the neuropsychic development of the young child of $1\frac{1}{2}$ – 2 years, special importance attaches to the occupations and educational levels of the two parents; other social factors, except for the size of the family, have less influence on the child's mental state. Similarly, the child aged 0–3 years is relatively more receptive to the influence of social factors from the angle of the development of motor behaviour and language than it is in the field of the development of the cognitive and affective functions.

The results of this study show the importance and usefulness of obtaining knowledge concerning the characteristics of physical and neuropsychic development of young children and the variability of their receptiveness to the effect of factors of family environment in providing a scientific basis for medical, educational, and social measures aimed at promoting the health of the younger generation and ensuring its harmonious psychosomatic development and adequate social integration.

B. Research on changes in the level of physical development of children and young people (0–18 years) in Romania, 1950–71

G. TANASESCU, IRINA CHIRIAC, and ELENA STANCIULESCU

Introduction

Systematic research on the height and weight levels of successive cohorts of children and adolescents has shown that, in all the developed countries, there is an increase in height and weight from one generation to another, together with an earlier maturation in young people and a shortening of the period of biological childhood. It has been demonstrated that this phenomenon has important medical and social consequences, manifested as a dynamic series of significant changes in human biomorphosis and pathomorphosis which, in its intensity and development, faithfully reflects the influence of differentiated living conditions of human communities and changes in their standard of living over a period of time.

In view of the profound economic and social changes and accelerated pace of economic and cultural development characteristic of the new stages in our country's historical development, it has become necessary to ascertain scientifically the changes occurring in the physical development of children and adolescents, who are the direct beneficiaries of the positive changes in the population's living standard.

To this end, in the very first years of the establishment of socialism, research was initiated on broad sections of the population, representative as regards the diversity and variability of living conditions characteristic for urban and rural dwellers and as regards the special geographical features of these conditions.

In 1950 the study group of 125 300 subjects was set up; this represented some 3 per cent of the country's population aged 3–18 years at that time. In order to know the trends in the level of physical development of the young population after 1950, a reflection of the favourable influence of socialism in our country, the study of the height and weight development of children and young persons was repeated, with the 0–3 year age group also being included in the study. The number of observations thus increased to some 310 000 subjects (approximately 6·5 per cent of the population between 0 and 18 years of age in 1957).

In 1964, the third repeat of the study on the physical development of children and young persons aged 0–18 years in Romania was done. We examined 340 171 children and young people between the ages of 0 and 18 years. Of these, 132 907 subjects lived in urban areas and 207 264 in rural areas.

In 1971, approximately 325 000 children and adolescents aged 0–18 years were examined. There were 160 000 children and adolescents from rural localities and 143 000 from urban areas. A group of some 21 000 subjects living in recently urbanized localities was studied as a comparative group.

The research programme provides for the implementation of the fifth study in 1978, using the same arrangement of centres and research areas.

Methods

So as to ensure the representative nature of the data at a national level, account was taken of three methodological requirements.

(1) Selection of rural and urban research areas, taking account of the different physical environment and socio-economic conditions of the population and the delimitation of certain territorial areas differentiated from the point of view of these conditions;

(2) The establishment of research samples at the level of study centres and areas, so as to be able to give the results a general value in respect of the urban population and the rural population, and similarly in respect of the study towns and areas;

(3) The observance of certain conditions which would ensure rigorous uniformity in the collection of data (uniform technique for the examination of subjects, using standardized and strictly controlled equipment), and the statistical and mathematical analysis of data.

Methodological criteria were laid down in 1950 when a preliminary study was conducted. These criteria formed the basis of the general research framework and operational techniques. The criteria are:

(a) A large amount of statistical information was analysed concerning the country's geoclimatic, economic, socio-cultural, demographic, and health characteristics. In view of the territorial diversity of these characteristics, 11 study areas covering the whole country were established.

For each of these territorial areas research centres were set up, each covering 3–4 rural areas that were the most representative both for the entire region and in respect of certain aspects of the living conditions that were typical for a given area. These research centres, set out in a network throughout the country, included 100 centres in rural areas (about 356 villages). One or more representative towns were designated for each area studied, making a total of 25 urban localities. In the analysis of the 1971 data, account was taken of a comparative population group living in 16 previously rural localities which had been recently urbanized.

(b) It was established that in rural communities the entire population of children and adolescents born in a given community should be examined, whereas in the sample urban centres the examination should cover only subjects born in and permanently resident in the respective locality.

(c) In each study centre the clinical and somatometric examination of subjects was carried out by a paediatrician or a school physician. The examination technique was made uniform, thus ensuring central control.

The technical controller decided not to include in the somatometric examination those subjects with acute illnesses, with acute deformities of the body or limbs, chronic patients with severe nutritional and developmental disturbances, and those who presented developmental disorders resulting from endocrinal diseases. The research was conducted simultaneously in all the areas set up throughout the country, during the months of May and June. The activity of the teams was controlled and directed by specialists of the Institute of Hygiene throughout the duration of the research.

Analysis of anthropometric data—height, weight, thoracic circumference, cranial circumference—was carried out on age groups according to number of months of age for children aged up to 1 year, according to a three-month period for children between 1 and 3 years of age, and by year for subjects aged between 4 and 18 years. Data were also recorded and analysed concerning the development of secondary sexual characteristics and the age of onset of the menarche, the development of temporary teeth and permanent teeth, and the characteristics of nutrition during the first year of life.

Results

The analysis of the results shows the positive influence of the socio-economic progress of the country during recent decades on the physical development of the young population.

1. Regarding children aged 0–3 years, comparison between the data obtained in 1971 and that for 1957 (first transversal study for this age group) shows that in the period 1957–71 the average values for height of boys living in urban areas have increased, with maximal values of increase of 2·3 cm at the age of 3 years, the corresponding values for girls being 2·5 cm at the same age. In the same period the average weight increased by some 0·62 kg for boys and by 0·72 kg for girls (at age of 3 years). In rural localities the increases in the average height and weight levels for the period concerned were, respectively, 2·2 cm and 0·57–0·58 kg at age 3 years.

2. A comparison of the data obtained in 1971 with that obtained in 1950 and in the intermediate stages of the study showed an obvious improvement in the physical development at all ages in both urban and rural areas and in all parts of the country. Compared with the height levels for the year 1950, boys aged 15 years in urban areas examined in 1971 were, on the average, 10 cm taller, while girls aged 12 years were, on the average, 7·8 cm taller. During the same period the average weight increased by 9·3 kg in boys aged 15 years and by 6·5 kg in girls aged 12 years. In 1971, the average height and weight of children and adolescents in rural areas was at all ages significantly higher than in 1950. Increase in height during this period was 7·8 cm in boys of 15 years and 5·9 cm in girls of 13 years, and the weight increase was 6·6 kg in boys of 15 years and 4·7 kg in girls of 14 years.

Important changes have also been noted in the chronology of the commencement of rapid prepubertal growth and the onset of puberty; these are reflected in the first and second transections of the height increase curves for girls and boys. In the 1971 study, the first transection of growth curves occurred at the age of 10 years, i.e. some eight months earlier than in 1950. In the same period, the second transection of the two sexes' growth curves occurs at lower ages (13 years 5 months), i.e. almost 1 year 3 months earlier than in 1950 (14 years 8 months).

The average age of the menarche, calculated for urban areas, is 13 ± 1 year, a lower age than that emerging from the 1961 study (13 years 3 months ± 1 year). Variability in the age of the menarche is clearly dependent on the living conditions of the population.

Research carried out in the context of this study programme has supplied a considerable amount of scientific information on physical development, pubertal maturation, and dentition. This information has been used in paediatric work and in establishing certain State measures for the promotion of health and for the improvement of education.

13. Construction, use, and utility of developmental scales for the first year of life (Belgium)

WILLIAM DE COSTER and GILBERT CLINCKE

Introduction

Few will dispute the importance of an early assessment of development for the prevention and treatment of developmental disorders. However, once assessment methods come up for discussion, feelings of discomfort are common experience. Paediatricians say that psychologists examine only a limited set of behavioural events when using their 'objective' tests, that they devote insufficient attention to organic, somatic, and environmental antecedents. Psychologists believe that without a minimum of carefully standardized tests and appropriate norms, a significant assessment becomes impossible. Although there is a substratum of truth in both points of view, they usually end up in a perhaps pleasurable polemic, which does not bring us nearer to a solution. Given this fact, we feel that the three following remarks are important for the kind of research that should be done in this area.

In the first place, it is a question whether existing developmental tests are in fact 'objective' and sufficiently standardized. We should not forget that they originated to a large extent from a paediatric tradition of careful behavioural observation. These observations were put into test items, which obtained the right to exist in the item pool without further empirical test. We have always thought that in the construction of objective, standardized tests, item selection should be based on empirical research. In the second place, appropriate norms do not exist for Belgium and the Netherlands (Kalverboer 1973). In the third place, developmental neurology still seems to be in the initial stage concerning the standardization of methods and techniques. Even the link between neurological development and behavioural development is not that clear.

A direct link exists between our research project and the first two points above. The general aim was to construct a more technical valid test, based on existing and new items, as well as to establish norms for the population of Ghent.

The use of developmental scales (infant tests)

Infant tests are used in two different settings. The first one is a diagnostic setting. The examiner wants to know how a child has developed relative to his peers. This is achieved by comparison between the number of items passed by the child and the average number of items passed by same age peers from the same population. (In many cases, the raw scores are transformed to a DQ or another index. However, we prefer to work with the raw scores.) To do that, the examiner must have at his disposal the norms gathered from an appropriate sample.

The second one is a research setting. Here the aim is to compare the average development of two groups of children drawn from different populations or having received different treatment in a research experiment. Norms are not required since group means can be directly compared.

From an economic point of view, as well as on principle, any test should be usable in both settings. It is the responsibility of the constructor to see that problems originating from both settings are sufficiently dealt with. This has often been neglected in the past.

Problems in using infant tests

The problems came to our attention in a research setting, where the participation of several examiners could not be avoided. In these projects, the Bühler–Hetzer test and the Bayley Scales were administered, but extensive use of other scales as well as use in a diagnostic setting confirmed our suspicion.

Most important was the fact that although examiners used the same set of instructions, their scoring resulted in large differences in group means for the same groups. This could be attributed to lack of effort and precision on the part of the examiners. However, closer examination of scales and items revealed the true origins of the problem. Nearly all scales are suffering more or less from one or more of the following shortcomings:

1. Incomplete and obscure instructions;
2. Incomplete and unclear standards to score items;
3. Little attention for physical circumstances which could influence the elicitation of specific responses;
4. Incomplete item series to investigate evolution of specific responses and ways of functioning;
5. Arbitrary subdivision of items into subscales;
6. Lack of empirical standards to select or eliminate items.

It is evident that under these circumstances the value and reliability of developmental scales as research instruments is very limited. In the light of these facts, one can easily understand why some test constructors put such emphasis on the training of new users. In our opinion, proper administration should be possible for any psychologist after reading the manual. Training is certainly useful in a research setting in order to reduce systematic error.

We already mentioned the absence of any norms for the Belgian population. This is a very serious problem. Several authors (Falmagne 1959; Parkin and Warren 1969; Kilbride 1969) have repeatedly warned against the use of foreign norms because of the considerable difference that can exist between these and local norms. As norms also tend to change over time, they will demand our permanent attention. The whole project can be seen as an attempt to solve some of these problems.

Construction of an infant test

The following topics will be discussed separately in this paper; the item pool, the research design, the sample, administration of the item pool, item selection, and evaluation.

It is clear that the follow-up method cannot be used for the construction of a developmental test, because of possible test–retest effects. Nevertheless, we feel that this project is important for the follow-up method and especially for the kind of research reported on in the following papers: De Coster et al. 1977; De Coster et al., in press; and De Coster et al. 1976. In our opinion, significant follow-up research can only be done when it works with objective, standardized, and reliable scales and tests. As long as these requirements are not met, results of follow-up research will be questionable and inconclusive.

The item pool. It was decided not to start with a time-consuming observation of behavioural events, since the most important responses are covered by existing tests and scales. The main problem was to elicit and score these responses in a proper way. Therefore we started to look at the items of the following developmental scales: 'Bayley Scales of Infant Development' (Bayley 1969a,b), 'Kleinkindertests' of Bühler and Hetzer (1953), 'Gesell Developmental Schedules' (Gesell and Amatruda (1954), 'The Abilities of Babies' of Griffiths (1970), 'Ring and Peg Test of Behavior Development' of Banham (1964), and the 'Denver Developmental Screening Test' of Frankenberg and Dodd (1967).

All items which required questioning of the parents were eliminated as our aim was not to administer a memory test for the parents nor to obtain socially desirable answers. All remaining items which could be passed by children between 3 and 9 months of age were put together and compared with each other. Similar items were retained only once, and a number of new items were added to the pool. Instructions to elicit a response, position of the examiner, undesirable physical circumstances for administration, scoring standards, etc. were examined and discussed by several persons. This was done for each item. As a result, most of the items got new and more precise instructions as well as new scoring standards. Items were eliminated when no agreement could be reached on these matters.

Different examiners tried out the resulting item pool on several groups of children at different age levels. Each item was discussed again on the basis of the results and the experience from this pilot study. After the last modifications were made the item pool contained 197 items suited for the age levels between 3 and 9 months.

The research design. An $A \times B \times (C \times S)$ repeated measures design, with factors examiner (A), sex of subject (B), items (C), and subjects (S) was chosen. Sex is a fixed factor while all others are random. With this design an internal consistency estimation (see Winer 1962) and the evaluation of the item selection became possible. Administrations were planned at the 7 age levels between 3 and 9 months of age, 3 and 9 months included. It was decided to examine 80 children (40 boys and 40 girls) at each age level. Four examiners were available. Children were randomly assigned to examiners, with the restriction that each examiner had to examine equal numbers of boys and girls at each age level. A total number of 560 children was needed to carry out the project. An analysis of variance, an internal consistency estimation, and an item selection was planned at each of the age levels.

The samples. One of our aims was to establish norms for the population of Ghent. Therefore, the 560 children had to be a representative sample from that population. The easiest way to reach such a large group of very young children is to visit day-care centres and institutions and examine the residents. However, these children form a selective sample in the Belgian situation and in consequence, we had to drop this method. The best way to get a representative sample is to draw a random sample from the population. This can only be done when one has access to all population data. We were very fortunate to be in that situation, as the local administration provided us with all birth registration lists. A random sample of 560 children (280 boys and 280 girls) with Belgian nationality was drawn from these lists. The children were randomly assigned to examiners and age level of examination.

In advance, it was decided to replace certain categories of children. As can be seen in Table 13.1, 14·8 per cent of the original sample was replaced at random for those reasons. This cannot be

TABLE 13.1

Categories with the number of children which were replaced at random in the sample

Hospitalized, sick, and severely physically handicapped children	18
Moved out of the described population before examination date, including children of boatmen	48
Adoptions and adjudications	10
Deceased	7
Total	83

regarded as true drop-out. As can be seen in Table 13.2 true drop-out is restricted to the number of children not examined due to any kind of refusal by the parents. We were amazed at the low 1·6 per cent true drop-out rate, since 20 per cent or even more is not unusual. We can only find a reason for this in the way introductions and appointments were made. A brief description will give an idea about the procedure.

TABLE 13.2

True drop-out in the original sample

Refusal by the parents	6
Absent after two appointments	3
Total	9

All 560 appointments were made by a staff social nurse. She visited the parents three weeks before the theoretical examination date. She introduced herself as belonging to the university, inquired about the baby, and explained the purpose of the project and the way in which the baby was selected to participate. Then, permission was asked to examine the baby. If the parents agreed, date, hour, and place of examination were fixed. The parents were told that a letter would follow one week before examination to remind them of the appointment. The letter contained a telephone number where the nurse could be reached. The parents were asked to inform the nurse in case of difficulties so that a new appointment could be made. Weekly the nurse passed the appointments to the examiners. Soon, it became clear that the person who made the appointments played a central role in the project. It struck us how quickly persons got informed by informal roads. After the first few weeks a lot of people who were asked to participate already knew what this was all about. We can only conclude that the person who made the appointments and the way in which it was done was responsible for the small amount of drop-out.

Administration of the item pool. All children were examined at home in the presence of the mother or the usual caretaker. Each examiner was instructed to administer as many items as possible and to go as far as possible in the elicitation of responses.

We tried to examine each child as closely as possible to the theoretical examination date. In 85 per cent of the cases this was done within four days before or after the theoretical date. The

remaining 15 per cent were done within seven days before or after the theoretical date.

Item selection and evaluation. The rules and standards used for item selection bear upon the problems we mentioned earlier in the paper. First, we created a base-line condition at each age level. All items which did not discriminate (passed by less than 5 per cent or more than 95 per cent) were eliminated. Analyses of variances and internal consistency estimations were carried out with the remaining items. This base-line condition was later used as a reference point for the evaluation of the two selections to come.

The first real item selection was based on the correlation between item and total score. Items with a not significant ($\alpha = 0.05$) item–total correlation were eliminated. This was done to cancel out the items on which examiners scored by chance and to make the pool more homogeneous. After the analyses of variance and the estimations of the internal consistency were carried out, the evaluation of the first selection became possible. The aim was to eliminate essentially unreliable items. Consequently, we decided to consider the selection as effective when the estimation of the internal consistency after the first selection was at least as high as in the base-line condition, despite the reduction of items. As can be seen in Table 13.3, all estimations increased by 0·01 except at the 6-month level where there was no change. This means that the effectiveness standard for the first selection was met.

TABLE 13.3

Estimations of internal consistency

Age level (months)	BL	S1	S2	RL
3	0·91	0·92	0·90	0·87
4	0·90	0·91	0·88	0·86
5	0·92	0·93	0·92	0·88
6	0·95	0·95	0·94	0·93
7	0·92	0·93	0·92	0·89
8	0·91	0·92	0·91	0·88
9	0·90	0·91	0·88	0·86

Note: BL = base-line; S1 = after the first selection; S2 = after the second selection; RL = base-line with reduced test length.

The second selection bears upon the uniformity with which the examiners interpret the instructions, administer the items, and score the elicited responses. As we said before, this is a major problem associated with developmental scales. It results in strong examiner–item interactions. The question arises where these effects can be seen at the item level. A simple calculation of the examiner difficulty for each item gives us the necessary information. The variance of these data for each item is called the examiner variance. As subjects were randomly assigned to examiners, examiner variance is expected to be zero for each item. There are two reasons why the expectation does not come out in reality. In the first place, there is always a possible effect of sampling error. In the second place, interactions between examiners and items produce a considerable amount of examiner variance at the item level. Since we used random assignment in our design, we can expect that the sampling error was very small. Therefore, we can say that a high examiner variance is an indication of strong examiner–item interactions. As it was our aim to reduce these interactions, we decided to base the second selection on the examiner variances.

At each age level, 20 per cent of the remaining items were eliminated. These were the items with the highest examiner variances. The 20 per cent is of course an arbitrary choice. Evaluation of the result of such a selection is an absolute necessity. We decided to consider such a selection as effective and useful when the following standards were met:

1. The estimation of the internal consistency after the second selection should be at least as high as the estimation of the internal consistency in the base-line condition, but calculated for a test length reduced by the number of eliminated items in the selections. Formulas can be found in Nunnally (1967).
2. The variance component of the examiner–item interaction (σ^2_{AC}) has to be smaller after the second selection than in the base–line condition.

Table 13.3 shows us that the internal consistency was higher on each age level after the second selection than was expected on the basis of the reduction of the test length. This means that relatively more unreliable items were eliminated by our selection and that the second selection was effective in regard to the first standard.

The reader may be amazed by the fact that we did not use the significance of the examiner–item interaction ($A \times C$) effect as our second evaluation standard. Significance of the $A \times C$ effect was useless in this situation because of the sensitivity of the design which made the smallest F-value very significant. The only way to get an idea of the effects the selections produced, was to follow the evolution of the variance component, which can be seen in Fig. 13.1. The decrease caused by the selections is very clear. At all age levels the variance component was smaller after the second selection than in the base-line condition, and the second evaluation standard was met.

We can conclude that the two selections were very effective since all standards were met, and the desired effects were reached. The result was a more homogeneous test that was less subject to examiner–item interaction. Besides the specific standards to evaluate the item selection, other data are available to get an idea of how successful the construction actually was.

Tests should discriminate well between subjects. Since our item selection was designed to reduce error variance a better discrimination should be the result. This means that the variance component of the subject effect ($\sigma^2_{S/AB}$) should be higher after selection than in the base-line condition. Figure 13.2 shows that this was the case at all age levels.

Examiner effect (A) as a main effect was another thing to avoid as an undesired error source. Our analyses of variance revealed only one significant A effect ($F = 3\cdot38$, $p < 0\cdot05$) at the 4-month level. We think this is probably a result of sampling error, for the following reasons:

1. We may expect the effect to occur at other age levels as well, since the examiners were the same and examinations were not carried out in age blocs. This is not the case.
2. We may expect that a main examiner effect should have a negative impact on the variance component of the examiner–item interaction. This is not the case in our data. The component is the third smallest of all at the 4-month level.

Our conclusion is of course an interpretation and we want to stress that only cross-validation can be conclusive in this matter. We think we have proved that by using this method of construction, developmental scales become more reliable and better standardized. This cannot be the end of the research. We want to see this result confirmed by cross-validation research. Another research topic is of course the investigation of the possibility of dividing the remaining items into subscales. In our opinion this subdivision must be based on empirical research. We also intend to extend the test to later ages by using the same method of construction.

Continuity of items across the age levels

It is clear that our method of selecting items poses a problem of continuity. We did not mention this before, because it was our main purpose to show how item selection based on empirical research can lead to better scales. Nevertheless, continuity is a problem to be solved before the test can be used properly. The problem originates from two different sources. The first source is the nature of the test and the second source is the procedure for the selection of items. As to the nature of the test, items are eliminated because they are age-specific. This happens at age levels where the responses occur for the first time or at age levels where all subjects have the

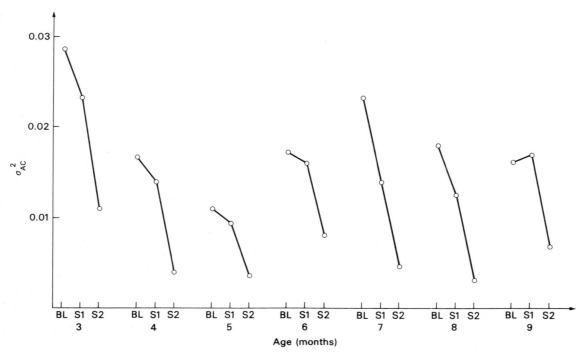

FIG. 13.1. Evolution of the variance component of examiner–item interaction, σ^2_{AC}, at each age level: BL=basal level; S_1=after first selection; S_2=after second selection.

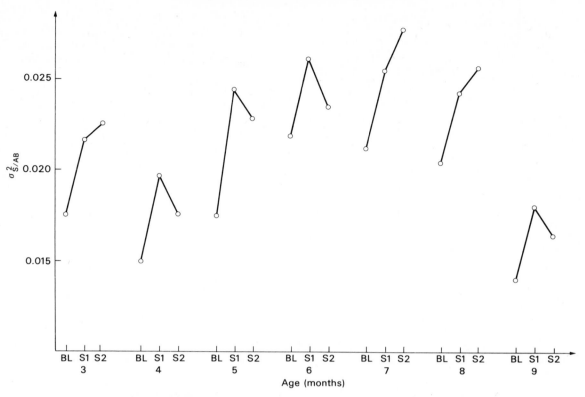

$\sigma^2_{S/AB}$

FIG. 13.2. Evolution of the variance component of the subject affect, $\sigma^2_{S/AB}$, at each level: BL=basal level; S_1 after first selection; S_2=after second selection.

appropriate responses. We are speaking about the items that were eliminated for the establishment of the base-line condition. This elimination had nothing to do with an attempt to reduce error variance. It is a standard frequently used for the construction of achievement tests, but of less importance for a developmental scale. If all subjects pass the item at a certain age level, the item is scored positive on later ages and kept in the pool, where it still may be useful to detect developmental retardation. Items which were eliminated because less than 5 per cent of the subjects passed it, can also be kept in the pool. They are useful to detect advanced development. The problem of continuity originating from this source was solved by adding these items to the pool. This was admissible, because these items do not have a negative effect upon the reliability of the test. One exception was made. Items on which no evolution could be seen across the age levels were not allowed in the pool. This kind of item gives us no information at all about the development of the response involved.

The second source is the procedure for item selection. The selection was carried out at each age level. Due to the arbitrary standards, items were eliminated at certain age levels but not at others. The elimination causing the gap was either due to a not significant item–total correlation or to a high examiner variance. In these cases, continuity can be retrieved by either eliminating the item at all age levels or by adding it again to the pool at the age level where it had disappeared for one of the two reasons we just mentioned. Now, the problem was to find a decision rule.

When we looked at the items where discontinuity occurred for one or more reasons, we found two clearly different categories. The first category was formed by items with one gap at a certain age level and hardly ever a second one. The second category was formed by items with at least three gaps. The decision rule we used was based on these facts. It is clear that the items in the second category are very strong sources of error. These items were eliminated at all age levels. For the first category continuity was retrieved by maintaining the items at all age levels. It is clear that

the discontinuity for these items was to a large extent caused by the arbitrary standards and not by proper shortcomings.

After the continuity was retrieved by application of the decision rules, we estimated the internal consistency once again and it appeared not to be negatively affected. The estimations were at the same level as after the second selection. This means that the decision rules we used are effective and can be further applied in the future.

Utility of developmental scales

Standardization, reliability, etc. are very important for the utility of developmental tests and scales. These have been the weak points and it was our main purpose to do something about this in our project. In our opinion, however, poor construction is not always to blame when developmental scales prove to be of limited use in certain situations. For example, take the conclusion that infant tests are poor predictors of later scores on intelligence tests (Bayley 1955; Knobloch and Pasamanick 1962; Elkind 1967). Technical shortcomings of a test can of course reduce the predictive value of a scale. But there is more. From Appleton *et al.'s* (1975) discussion of this problem we can deduce which assumptions are implicit in expecting an infant test to be a good predictor. The assumptions were:

(1) Intelligence is a unitary function;
(2) This function grows constantly;
(3) This growth is constant for each person at any period of development.

We know very well that these assumptions are not met. Hence, the lack of predictive value is more the result of unrealistic expectations than a result of shortcomings in the construction of infant tests. This does not mean that we believe early development to be unimportant for intelligence. It only means that developmental scales, whatever the qualities they have, are not sufficient to predict later scores on intelligence tests.

Appleton et al. (1975; p. 156) give a good example:

For example, form recognition must develop before a child can learn to read. But, since reading involves many other skills, we cannot predict success in reading on the basis of skill at form recognition. However, we can predict that if a child is not able to recognize forms, reading will not be learned.

We believe that developmental scales have an alarm function in a diagnostic setting. Retarded development is an indication that something went wrong. The causes of the retardation cannot be found in the test results, although they can point out the direction to search in. We must warn against conclusions based on a single administration of an infant test. Follow-up research has to be done to see to what degree a measured retardation level remains constant over time. In general, we can say that quite a lot of empirical research has to be done before we will know all about the utility of infant scales. This project is presented as a first step to more research and better understanding of these scales.

Acknowledgements

The authors are indebted to all persons who have collaborated in this research project, which was sponsored by the Fonds voor Fundamenteel Collectief Onderzoek. The authors wish to thank especially M. C. Dutoit, A. Goethals, T. Monsecour, J. Lerou, and K. Verheyden for their invaluable co-operation. The authors are also indebted to Dr A. Vandierendonck for critical comments on the manuscript.

14. A Danish birth cohort: a longitudinal prospective study of infants with transient neurological symptoms

BIRGITTE R. MEDNICK, NIELS M. MICHELSEN, BENGT ZACHAU-CHRISTIANSEN, and ÅGE L. VILLUMSEN

This chapter describes a 12-year follow-up study of a group of infants who in the neonatal period presented transient neurological signs which, if longer lasting, have been shown to be correlated with later brain damage symptomatology. The subjects' status at follow-up are evaluated in terms of their neurological, intellectual, and personality–social functioning. The experimental and control subjects of the study were all drawn from the subject pool of a Danish Perinatal Project. A short description of the latter provides the background for the study to be reported in this chapter.

Description of the Danish Prospective Perinatal Project

In September 1959 a Danish Prospective Perinatal Project was begun at the maternity departments of the State University hospital (Rigshospitalet) in Copenhagen. All deliveries (over 20 weeks gestation) which took place in this hospital between September 1959 and December 1961 were included in this project.

The following summarized procedures were employed in the study: The pregnant women were contacted and examined before delivery, and when possible, early in pregnancy. They were again contacted during attendance at the hospital's antenatal clinic.

In order to evaluate and code the social, general medical, and obstetric histories of the women in as uniform a manner as possible, the same physician did all the prenatal examinations. In addition to an obstetrician, midwives and midwife trainees were present in the delivery room and assisted in collecting the data describing the deliveries and the status of the neonates and the mothers immediately after birth. In all cases where the general condition permitted, the live-born infants were again systematically examined on the first and fifth day after delivery by one of three paediatricians. The first and the fifth day examinations included a physical examination and a thorough neurological assessment of the infants. Upon discharge from the hospital the mothers or guardians of the infants received a self-completion questionnaire concerning the infants' developmental progress during the first year of life. Information concerning attendance to infant health examinations, intercurrent diseases, admission to hospitals and other institutions, and records of immunizations were also obtained. As the children reached their first birthday, the mothers were asked to bring them to the paediatric out-patient department of the State University Hospital for a special developmental examination. A study team of three paediatricians systematically carried out these follow-up examinations of the total group of surviving infants. Great effort was made to include all surviving infants in the one-year follow-up. In cases where the parents were not able to bring the child to the hospital, home visits were arranged. Records of all hospitalizations of the infants during the first year were obtained from the files of the respective hospitals. All information obtained prior to, during or after the birth of the children as well as the data from the one year follow-up was precoded and is presently available on tape. The total number of deliveries included on the data tape is 9125.

The third and fourth authors of this chapter took part in the original data collection on the project and have published extensively on the results of the data analyses of the pre-, peri-, neonatal, and first year data of the sample (Zachau-Christiansen 1972; Zachau-Christiansen and Ross 1974; Villumsen 1970). In addition, Zachau-Christiansen has been responsible for the continuation of the project after the one year follow-up; in this capacity, over the last 18 years, he has effected extensive additional data collection pertaining to the whole sample as well as to specially selected subgroups.

Zachau-Christiansen has, over the years, encouraged and assisted many investigators in carrying out studies following up groups of subjects selected from the total sample according to special sets of criteria. The study to be reported in the present paper constitutes one such instance of a follow-up of a subgroup from the original birth cohort.

11-year follow-up of infants with transient neonatal signs

Of the 9125 individual births included on the data tape 7407 infants had birth weights over 2500 g. Of these 305 (4·12 per cent) showed one or more of a group of symptoms which, if persistent in the first period of life, have been shown to be correlated with increased rates of reliable signs of brain damage or neurological deviance later in life (Prechtl 1965; Thorn 1968; Amiel-Tison 1969; Drillien 1972). These symptoms include: convulsions, jitteriness, cyanosis, respiratory distress, restlessness, frog position, and limpness. In 90 of the 305 cases the children's conditions were serious or persistent enough to warrant transfer to other hospital departments or to institutions. In 215 cases (130 males and 85 females) the symptoms were not observed again after the fifth day. On the eighth day after birth this latter group of infants and their mothers were discharged to their homes. This policy was based on the assumption that such *transient* symptoms have no negative aftermaths. As far as we could ascertain this is not an uncommon clinical practice. It was the purpose of the present study to empirically examine whether the hypothesis, that these kinds of transient symptoms are benign, can be supported. The study compares the functioning of an experimental group consisting of pre-adolescents who neonatally evidenced transient neurological symptoms (TNS) with that of a matched control group. It is hypothesized that the experimental subjects will show relatively higher rates of abnormality within at least one of the areas of intellectual, personality–social, or neurological functioning.

Previous research

The rationale for hypothesizing increased levels of neurological deviance in the experimental group may be found in the follow-up studies referred to above. The results of these studies uniformly showed that children, in whom longer lasting neurological signs were observed in the neonatal period, presented higher frequencies of neurological impairment at follow-up. It seems a possibility that in spite of the fact that the neurological signs in our subjects were of a transient nature, they may still have been manifestations of a certain degree of CNS damage or dysfunction which may be found to have some impact on the later neurological functioning of the subjects. As pointed out by Windle (1969), Hewett (1973), and Kinsbourne (1973) the growth process is such that only rather gross neurological deficits or deficits of certain categories will show up in younger children. It seems likely that neonatal signs if only transiently present will tend to have more subtle types of long-term correlates. Such correlates are likely not to be observable until an older age when more highly organized behaviour patterns can be demanded and the subjects' performance on these can be evaluated.

Only one of the previously reported studies following up subjects with neonatal neurological deviance has examined the intellectual and social functioning of the subjects. Thorn (1968) reports findings of increased rates of intellectual and personality–social problems among her subjects. However, indirect support for the hypothesis that neonatal neurological signs are related to later intellectual and personality–social functioning may be found in studies following up cases with known pre- and perinatal complications (Benaron *et al.* 1960; Graham *et al.* 1962; Honzik *et al.* 1965; Rosenfeld and Bradley 1948; Schacter and Apgar 1959; Stechler 1964). In addition, retrospective studies suggest that children who present intellectual and/or personality–social impairment tend to have a history of elevated levels of perinatal difficulties (Lilienfeld *et al.* 1955; McNeil and Wiegerink 1971; McNeil *et al.* 1970; Pasamanick 1954). The intellectual difficulties which have been observed include perceptual–motor impairment, disorder of speech, memory, and thinking, and general failure to achieve academically. Further disorders of attention, tendency to perseveration, and intellectual immaturity have been reported to occur more frequently. The behavioural impairment characteristically includes hyperactivity, impulsiveness, sensitivity to stress, immaturity, and a wide range of other more or less disruptive

behaviour disorders. All of these symptoms may occur individually or in any possible combination.

Subjects

The 48 subjects (24 experimentals and 24 controls) of the present study were all drawn from the group of 7407 infants with birthweight over 2500 g who were included in the Danish Perinatal Study. It was decided to draw subjects only from among the mature deliveries so as not to be faced with the problem of having to consider the effects of prematurity in the follow-up data. The 215 maturely born infants who evidenced TNS were first divided according to sex. There were 130 males and 85 females. Then from each of the sex groups the *first* 12 consecutive deliveries, beginning 1 January 1960, in which the child met our selection criteria, were included in our experimental group. In addition to presence of TNS our criteria for selection were: (1) no congenital malformations; and (2) living in the vicinity of Copenhagen at the time of follow-up. (This last condition was instituted for practical purposes.) Table 14.1 describes the types and frequencies of the neonatal symptoms found in the experimental subjects.

The 24 experimental subjects were matched one to one with control subjects from the perinatal sample for age, sex, and social class. Table 14.2 describes the sample in terms of the matching variables age, sex, and social class.

TABLE 14.1

Frequencies of neonatal symptoms in experimental subjects

Symptoms	No. of cases
Jitteriness	9
Restlessness	8
Cyanosis, respiratory distress	8
Convulsions	5
Frog-position	5
Limpness	3

Note: This listing is restricted to neonatal symptoms which have been shown to be related to later signs of brain damage in previous research. A symptom is listed if it appeared on day 1 and/or 5.

TABLE 14.2

Characteristics of experimental and control groups

	Experimental	Control
Number of females	12	12
Number of males	12	12
Mean age in years at follow-up	11·25	11·02
Age range	10–11·90 years	10–12·20 years
Mean social class†	2·33	2·66

† Social class was determined by Svalastoga's scale (Svalastoga 1959). This scale runs from 0 (low) to 6 (high). It was developed specifically for use in Denmark.

Procedures

In the beginning of 1972 the 48 subjects were invited in for a day of intensive examination by a social worker who visited them in their homes. None of the invited subjects refused to participate.

Evaluation of neurological functioning

In addition to an intensive neurological examination, a test of motor impairment (Stott 1966) was also administered to the 48 subjects. In addition, data from the one year follow-up were utilized in the analysis of the neurological data.

Follow-up neurological examination. The neurological examination to which the subjects of the present study were exposed at age 11 was constructed to yield two kinds of data:

(1) Data which would reveal deviance known to be related to structural or physiological abnormalities of the central nervous system;

(2) Data which would yield a functional description of the motoric abilities of each subject (a motoric image) without necessary relevance to CNS functioning.

The examination procedure consists partly of subtests known from traditional adult neurological examinations (Paine and Oppe 1966; Touwen and Prechtl 1970) and partly of subtests known from paediatric neurological examination procedures and motoric performance tests described in the literature (Rutter *et al.* 1970a; Bakwin 1968). The selection of the single test components to be included was based on the specific relevance of the items to the functioning of 11-year-old children. The order in which the tests were presented was largely similar to the sequence described by Touwen and Prechtl (1970). The duration of the examination was 1–2 h. The data obtained may be grouped in 12 categories. Table 14.3 gives a short description of each of these categories.

Data reduction

All of the neurological examinations were completed and coded by the second author. The coding resulted in several hundred coded items. Michelsen, who was uninformed of the group status of the subjects, reviewed each subject's record and evaluated his examination in terms of the seven syndromes originally described by Touwen and Prechtl (1970). These ratings of the seven neurological syndromes were then made the basis of the data analysis. The seven syndromes (which are not mutually exclusive) are:

(1) Hemisyndrome;
(2) Syndrome of associated movements;
(3) Syndrome of dyskinesia;
(4) Syndrome of developmental retardation;
(5) Syndrome of co-ordination difficulties;
(6) Syndrome of sensory disturbance;
(7) Syndrome of miscellaneous symptoms.

Each subject was also rated for each of the following diagnostic categories:

(1) Minor nervous dysfunction-diffuse;
(2) Minor nervous dysfunction-focal (a subject would receive one of the above two diagnoses if the symptoms presented were of a light and rather non-disabling nature; neurological 'soft signs' belong in this category);
(3) Traditional cerebral dysfunction-diffuse;
(4) Traditional cerebral dysfunction-focal.

'Hard' or classical neurological signs were required in a subject if he was to receive one of the latter two diagnoses. These four categories are mutually exclusive. If a subject received a positive rating in one of the four diagnostic categories, his rating in the other three was zero.

Every subject received a rating of 0–4 for each of the seven syndromes and for each of the four diagnostic categories. In the rating, the number as well as the kinds of relevant subtests which showed deviance was taken into account. The meaning of the five possible ratings can be stated as follows:

0 = Normal;
1 = Uncertain–slight abnormality;
2 = Certain–slight abnormality;
3 = Certain–abnormality of moderate severity;
4 = Certain–abnormality of high severity.

TABLE 14.3

Description of the 12 categories of tests included in the neurological examination

(1) Biological constitution and development: Height, weight, cranial circumference, secondary sexual development.

(2) Ordinary physical examination.

(3) Examination of posture and gait: Deviate postures (head—neck—trunk—upper extremities—lower extremities), balance on one foot, ordinary walking, walking on heel, toes, and inverted feet, jump on one leg.

(4) Traditional neurological examinations: Muscle wasting, power, tone, reflexes, (biceps, triceps, radialis, patellar, achilles, abdominal, acromioclavicular, plantar), contractures and abnormal spontaneous position, sensitivity (pain, temperature, pressure, touch, sensitivity of joint position, two points discrimination), cranial nerves (visual field, pupillary size, and reaction to lights, visual axes and movements, cornea reflex and facial sensitivity, mimic, facial musculature, audiometri, nystagmus, tongue movements, movements of the palate, voice, trapezius- and sternocleidomastoid functioning), co-ordination (finger–nose test, knee–heel test, diadochokinesia, dyskinesia, primitive reflexes, Romberg).

(5) Special sensitive functions: Gnosia: (graphesthesia, fingeragnosia, Kinsbourne's simultaneous touch and side touch, stereognosia), dyspraxia (sniff, nod and shake the head, brush teeth, hair and crumbs off something, dressing and undressing), orientation, and imitation (hand–chin, finger-imitation, right/left orientation on and outside own body).

(6) Examination of eyes: Cranial nerves, co-ordination, dominance, visual axes, convergence, visual acuity, ophthalmoskopia.

(7) Co-ordination: Static (balance, Romberg) dynamic (hopping, walking on heel, toe, and inverted feet, handling a ball), reciprocal co-ordination (Luria), diadochokinesia, clapping hands, dressing, undressing, tests of fine motor movement, simultaneous movements from the test of motor impairment (Stott *et al.*) finger opposition, oral–facial (closing one eye separately, eye-movements, movements of tongue, motor impersistance test) (Rutter *et al.* 1970a).

(8) Associated movements (mimic, diadochokinesia, reciprocal co-ordination, walking tests, Prechtl's and Fog's tests).

(9) Laterality: Eyes (Worth-4-lights, convergence), hands and feet (general preference, Stott *et al.*).

(10) Language: Pronunciation, precision of speech, syntax, level of abstraction.

(11) Minor physical–structural abnormalities as described by Waldrop and Halvorsen (1971).

(12) Tests of motor impairment (Stott 1966): Static co-ordination (balance tests), dynamic co-ordination of upper extremities (handling ball), fine motor movement and simultaneous movement of hands and fingers.

Evaluation of intellectual functioning

The following data from the follow-up examination were used to test the hypothesis of higher degree of intellectual impairment in the Experimental Group.

1. *Memory for Designs Test (MFD) (Graham and Kendall 1960).* On this test, widely used for diagnosing possible brain damage, a score of 101 or below is normal; scores between 102 and 106 indicate borderline conditions; and scores of 107 or above indicate brain damage. The score is corrected for IQ.

2. *Feffer's Role Taking Test (RTT) (Feffer 1959)*. The RTT measures the ability to decentre or to change perspective. It has been shown to be a reliable measure of the developmental level of a subject's cognitive functioning. Besides being dependent on higher cognitive processes, adequate performance on the test also depends on verbal competence and requires a certain degree of memory functioning. (Possible range of scores is 0–20, a high score signifies high level of functioning.)

3. *Selected subtests from the Wechsler Intelligence Scale for Children*—similarity, vocabulary, block design, object assembly, mazes.

4. *The 'teachers' judgement of intellectual functioning'*. This measure was obtained from a questionnaire which was filled out in each case by the teacher who knew the subject best. Only the relevant subset of the data obtained from this questionnaire was included in the present paper. Of the questionnaire items, 13 were judged to be relevant to the child's intellectual functioning. These items are concerned with the child's ability to concentrate; reading, arithmetic, and language performance; memory functioning; and whether or not he evidenced perseveration in his thinking. An overall score for intellectual functioning was developed by determining for each of the 13 relevant items whether the teacher's answer indicated no disturbance (score of 0), moderate disturbance (score of 1), or severe disturbance (score of 2). ('Don't know' answers were regarded as 'no disturbance' answers.) The disturbance scores for each individual's 13 items were then summed. The sum of these scores constitutes the score for 'teachers' judgement of intellectual functioning' (range 0–26). It was decided to use this type of overall score in the analyses of the questionnaire data because item-by-item analyses were found to be difficult to interpret due to the varying number of 'don't know' answers given by the teachers to the individual items.

Evaluation of social functioning

The following data from the follow-up examination were used to test the hypothesis of more impairment in the personality and social functioning on the part of our experimental subjects: (1) Vineland Social Maturity Scale (Doll 1953); (2) 'Teachers' judgement of personality and social functioning'; and (3) relevant information obtained from interviews carried out with the subjects themselves and with their parents. Only the latter two categories need further comments.

Teachers' judgement of personality and social functioning. This score was obtained by the same procedures as were described under 'teachers' judgement of intellectual functioning'. The individual items contributing to this score are concerned with whether or not the child seems hyperactive and further describe the child in terms of impulse control, maturity, independence, aggressiveness, and success in peer relations.

Interview data. The parent interview, developed at the Psychological Institute, is designed to provide a detailed description of the child and the atmosphere of his home. Information dealing with the child's tempermental characteristics, peer relations, maturity, psychosomatic symptoms, and whether or not he ever had been referred to a psychologist were included in the analyses relevant to the personality and social functioning of our subjects. The child interview was also originally developed as a general information-gathering tool to be used in different types of subject populations. Answers to questions dealing with adaptation in school, social relations, aggressiveness, anxiety, and perseveration in emotions were employed in the analyses of the personality and social functioning of the subjects.

Additional data set

Apart from analyses of the data described above which bear directly on the main hypotheses of the study, some additional categories of data were collected and analysed.

Life history data

The design of the present study should not be understood as suggesting that a simple cause–effect relationship is believed to exist between the neonatal and follow-up data. Clearly a variety of intermediary variables will have been influencing the development of the subjects during the time between the neonatal observations and the follow-up. Consequently, we can at best expect the neonatal symptoms in question to account for a limited proportion of the variance of the follow-up scores—if any. Care-giving patterns, SES, maturational rates, sibling position, physical health, intactness of family, temperamental factors, genetic endowment, and differential life experience are some of the possible intermediating variables influencing the results of the follow-up examination. The importance of many of these variables may only be adequately estimated through data obtained by continuous observation of the subjects. Unfortunately, we have no such observational data available. Other intermediary variables could not be taken into account due to insufficient sample size (e.g., sibling position). However, from the interviews, retrospective information was available concerning family constellation patterns, mother's work patterns, day-care experiences, and types of family stress (marital, economic, poor health, etc.). In addition, data on the biological development and constitution of the subjects were analysed. This category of data was obtained in connection with the neurological examination.

In view of the fact that other studies have reported differential long-term outcome after perinatal problems as a function of social class differences (Drillien 1964) the possible intermediary influence of SES in our data was assessed. Social class was determined by Svalastoga's scale (Svalastoga 1959). This scale was developed specifically for use in Denmark.

Pregnancy, delivery, neonatal, and one-year data

All information relevant to the pregnancy, delivery, neonatal, and one-year status of each subject was extracted from the files of the Danish Perinatal Project and scored according to a scoring system which yields an estimate of the severity of complication or deviance within each of six categories of data. In this manner, the several hundred data items available for each subject were reduced to the following six scores (serious attempts at factor and cluster analysis proved unsatisfactory):

(1) Pregnancy score;
(2) Delivery score;
(3) Neonatal physical status score;
(4) One-year neurological examination score;
(5) One-year physical examination score;
(6) One-year motoric development score.

This scoring system was developed at the Psychological Institute in Copenhagen by a collaboration of American and Danish obstetricians and paediatric neurologists. It assigns a weight (1–5) relative to the judged seriousness of every indication of deviance or complication within a given category of data. A subject's score for each data category is the sum of the total number of weights assigned to the relevant symptoms or complications. A more detailed description of these pre-, peri-, neonatal, and early developmental scales may be found in Mednick *et al.* (1971). Data on the pregnancies and deliveries were included in the data analysis due to the aetiological relationship which might exist between these variables and the TNS. The three groups of data from the one-year examination provide us with a chance to examine how well the experimental subjects had succeeded in recovering from or compensating for any neonatal disability. Further, the one-year data contribute toward filling the gap which exists in our knowledge about our subjects' development between the neonatal period and the follow-up at age 11.

Coding and data analyses

All the data collection done in this study as well as all scoring and coding of the collected data was done blindly. In the data analyses 2×2 factorial analyses of variance by group and sex were employed. In the analyses estimating the intermediating effect of social class, 2×2 factorial analyses of variance by group and SES were used.

Results

Neurological functioning

Since the variable sex evidenced no significant direct or interaction effects on the neurological examination, results related to this variable will not be reported so as not to complicate the presentation.

The evaluation of the subjects' performance in terms of the seven neurological syndrome ratings was based on their performance on the 12 subcategories of tests into which the complete neurological examination was divided (Table 14.3). Three of the categories described in Table 14.3 exercised only a limited influence on the syndrome scores. For this reason each subject's performance on each of these three categories of subtests was rated on the 0–4 scale described above and for each category the scores for the experimental and control groups were compared by ANOVA. The three categories of scores subjected to this analysis were:

(1) Biological constitution and development;
(2) Ordinary physical examination;
(3) Language.

No significant differences were found on these three tests.

The neurological syndrome ratings are presented in Table 14.4. As can be seen, the experimental group is worse than the controls

TABLE 14.4

Means and standard deviations by group for neurological syndrome ratings, diagnostic category ratings, and test of motor impairment

Hemisyndrome	Experimental group		Control group	
	Mean	SD	Mean	SD
	Neurological syndrome ratings			
Hemisyndrome	0·42	0·93	0·26	0·69
Syndrome of associated movements	1·33	1·31	0·13	0·34
Syndrome of dyskinesia	0·46	0·66	0·30	0·47
Syndrome of developmental retardation	0·50	0·83	0·00	0·00
Syndrome of co-ordination difficulties	2·66	1·20	1·52	0·95
Syndrome of sensory disturbance	1·12	1·07	0·74	0·75
Syndrome of miscellaneous symptoms	1·67	1·09	0·74	0·75
	Diagnostic category rating			
Minor nervous dysfunction diffuse	2·46	1·32	1·09	1·00
Minor nervous dysfunction focal	0·29	0·62	0·09	0·29
Traditional cerebral dysfunction diffuse	0·38	0·65	0·00	0·00
Traditional cerebral dysfunction focal	0·26	0·69	0·26	0·69
	Test of motor impairment			
	8·25	9·71	4·83	4·81

on all of the seven syndrome ratings. These differences reached significance on:

(1) Syndrome of associated movements ($F = 17·65$, 1,44 df, $p < 0·001$);
(2) Syndrome of co-ordination difficulties ($F = 13·50$, 1,44 df, $p < 0·001$);
(3) Syndrome of miscellaneous symptoms ($F = 11·10$, 1,44 df, $p < 0·001$).

The diagnostic category ratings are also presented in Table 14.4. As might be expected in a non-clinical population, almost none of the subjects in the groups evidenced minor nervous dysfunction-focal or traditional cerebral dysfunction (diffuse of focal). Fourteen subjects in the experimental group and one in the control group received ratings of three or above (certain abnormality of moderate or high severity) for the minor nervous dysfunction-diffuse category. The experimental–control group difference was highly significant ($F = 16·31$, 1,44 df, $p < 0·001$).

In any random sample one must expect to find a variety of minor neurological abnormalities, e.g. slight difficulty in co-ordination. In view of this, the number of subjects in each group who were considered by the neurologist as evidencing a certain neurological disturbance of at least moderate severity on any of the seven syndromes was determined (rating of '3' or above). A total of 17 experimental and two control subjects received a score indicating this degree of abnormality. On the test of motor impairment no significant difference was found between the groups.

Specific neonatal symptoms and symptomatology of 11-year-olds. Attempts were made to relate specific neonatal symptoms to neurological functioning at 11 years of age. No significant relationships were found; however, one almost significant relationship was noted. Six experimental subjects received a rating of four (the highest degree of abnormality) on minor nervous dysfunction-diffuse. They also received a rating of four on syndrome of co-ordination difficulties. Of these subjects, five had evidenced jitteriness in the neonatal period. Of the remaining 18 experimental subjects a total of four evidenced this neonatal symptom. This difference is just short of significance at the 0·05 level (Fisher exact test).

The analyses reported above are in support of the hypothesis that impaired neurological functioning at age 11 may be a correlate of the transient neonatal signs present in our subjects.

Intellectual functioning

Table 14.5 provides the means and standard deviations by group and sex for the data relevant to the intellectual functioning of the subjects. The MFD, the RTT, and the 'teachers' judgement of intellectual functioning' showed significant group differences. On the MFD the experimental group performed, as predicted, significantly worse than the control group ($F(1,44) = 4·76$, $p < 0·05$). The same pattern of results emerged from the analyses of the role-taking test (RTT), ($F(1,44) = 5·07$, $p < 0·05$). The analyses of the 'teachers' judgement of intellectual functioning' yielded a significant group difference ($F(1,44) = 7·29$, $p < 0·01$), as well as a significant interaction effect ($F(1,44) = 4·09$, $p < 0·05$). The teachers' judgements indicate that the experimental females are having more problems within the area of intellectual functioning than either the experimental males or both sexes of the control group. The subjects' scores on 'teachers' judgement of intellectual functioning' were examined individually in order to ascertain whether only one or two very extreme cases among the experimental females would be responsible for the very elevated mean score presented by this group. It was, however, discovered that six experimental females, or half the group, had obtained scores of 9 or above (possible range 0–26) whereas only two experimental males and no control subjects had obtained scores indicating this high degree of abnormality.

Analyses of the results obtained on the WISC revealed no group differences, neither on the three scale scores nor on any of the subtests. However, significant sex differences were found on all three scales. The females scored lower than the males (verbal scale: $F(1,44) = 6.92$, $p < 0.025$; performance scale: $F(1,44) = 4.66$, $p < 0.05$; full scale: $F(1,44) = 7.15$, $p < 0.025$). Within the experimental group no difference was found between the scores on the verbal and the performance scales. The same was true for the control group. It should be emphasized that the means for both groups on all three IQ scales show that the groups are of average IQ. The experimental females obtained the lowest mean IQ score, 99.75, and the control males the highest, 112.33. Attempts were made to relate specific neonatal symptoms with the scores obtained on the follow-up examination. No significant relationships were disclosed.

TABLE 14.5

Mean and standard deviations by group and sex on variables relating to the intellectual functioning of the subjects

	Experimental		Control	
	Mean	SD	Mean	SD
MFD:				
Males	102.58	4.06	101.75	3.57
Females	104.75	6.57	100.08	1.98
Total	103.67	5.45	100.92	2.95
RTT:				
Males	8.92	4.54	10.75	4.63
Females	8.25	4.85	12.63	4.88
Total	8.58	4.61	11.65	4.74
IQ verbal:				
Males	106.83	8.96	111.92	12.29
Females	102.75	12.41	98.17	12.86
Total	104.79	10.79	105.04	14.17
IQ performance:				
Males	108.67	11.87	110.67	16.34
Females	96.42	20.62	102.67	14.88
Total	102.54	17.60	106.67	15.82
IQ full scale:				
Males	108.41	10.59	112.23	13.76
Females	99.75	15.12	100.53	13.66
Total	104.08	13.51	106.33	14.74
Teachers' judgement of intellectual functioning:				
Males	3.92	3.16	3.08	2.24
Females	8.09	5.61	2.27	2.22
Total	6.00	4.56	2.69	2.23

Conclusion. In light of the fact that three group comparisons relevant to intellectual functioning yielded results in the predicted direction, one might consider the hypothesis of higher frequency of intellectual problems within the experimental group to be supported by the data.

Personality and social functioning

The analyses of the data relevant to the subjects' personality and social functioning yielded only two significant results. The experimental group was found to show a lower degree of social maturity or independence on the Vineland Social Maturity Test ($F(1,44) = 5.30$, $p < 0.05$). On an item from the child interview dealing with whether or not the child felt lonely, the experimental subjects admitted to significantly more loneliness than the controls

($F(1,44) = 6.07$, $p < 0.025$). Table 14.6 shows the means and standard deviations for the two variables described above which significantly distinguished the experimental group within the area of personality and social functioning. None of the other 17 analysed interview items showed any significant group or sex differences. The 'teachers' judgement of personality–social functioning' showed an almost significant group difference in the predicted direction ($F(1,44) = 3.92$).

TABLE 14.6

Means and standard deviations for the two variables which significantly differentiated between the groups on the personality–social dimension

	Experimental		Control	
	Mean	SD	Mean	SD
Vineland Social Maturity Test:				
Males	104.25	9.10	114.92	16.40
Females	104.08	12.25	109.91	9.70
Total	104.17	10.56	112.52	13.56
Child: I often play alone†				
Males	0.67	0.65	0.42	0.67
Females	1.00	0.74	0.33	0.49
Total	0.83	0.70	0.38	0.58

† Range of scores, 0–2.

Conclusion. Of the 20 comparisons made on the data relevant to the subjects' personality and social functioning, only two yielded significant group differences (of 0.05 and 0.025 levels, respectively). Maintaining 95 per cent confidence limits, one of these results is likely to have been significant by chance. In view of these considerations we must view the support given to the hypothesis of more personality–social problems among our experimental subjects to be weak.

Life history variables

Neither the biological development nor the environmental conditions of the subjects as mirrored by our data showed any significant differences in the group × sex analyses of variance. In the analyses by group and SES by which we attempted to evaluate the intermediating influence of SES on the follow-up data, only the MFD was significantly related to the SES of the subjects ($F(1,44) = 5.72$, $p < 0.05$). Children from lower SES background scored lower on the MFD. No interaction term proved significant.

Pregnancy, delivery, and neonatal physical status

Table 14.7 presents the means and standard deviations of the two groups on the scores describing the pregnancies, the delivery, and the neonatal physical examination. As can be seen from Table 14.7, the group difference on the pregnancy score was not significant. The experimental females, however, present a score which is noticeably higher than that of the experimental males, though this difference did not reach significance. With regard to delivery complications, a significant group effect was found. The experimental group suffered more delivery complications than the control group ($F(1,44) = 5.26$, $p < 0.05$).

As expected, the experimental group received a higher average abnormality score than the controls on the neonatal physical examination. The ANOVA for group difference on this variable yielded a highly significant F-value ($F(1,44) = 23.36$, $p < 0.001$). On this variable the experimental females again presented a higher degree of abnormality than the males. A test between the means of the experimental males and the experimental females yielded a value of 2.11 (46 df, $p < 0.05$).

TABLE 14.7

Means and standard deviations by group and sex for the pregnancy, delivery, and neonatal physical scores

| | Experimental | | Control | |
	Mean	SD	Mean	SD
Pregnancy complications:				
Males	4·50	3·40	4·40	2·94
Females	6·42	4·80	4·17	3·35
Total	5·46	4·18	4·29	3·09
Delivery:				
Males	8·92	3·87	4·92	2·99
Females	7·83	4·50	6·33	4·96
Total	8·38	4·15	5·63	4·07
Neonatal physical:				
Males	8·92	4·96	4·25	2·30
Females	12·75	3·77	5·67	5·18
Total	10·83	4·73	4·96	3·98

The one-year examination

The one-year examination included a physical and a neurological examination. A questionnaire which the mothers had been asked to fill out during the child's first year of life was also collected. This questionnaire, along with a few items from the physical examination, provided data for the score for one-year motor development. Table 14.8 presents the means and standard deviations for the groups on the one-year variables. The one-year motor development variable is the only one of the three variables in this category which presents significant differences between the groups. The experimental group performed worse on this measure ($F(1,44) = 16·26$, $p < 0·001$).

TABLE 14.8

Means and standard deviations by group and sex for the one-year examination

| | Experimental | | Control | |
	Mean	SD	Mean	SD
1-year physical:				
Males	8·17	5·02	7·42	4·50
Females	8·67	4·94	8·67	4·94
Total	8·42	4·88	8·04	4·28
1-year neurological:				
Males	0·92	1·24	0·92	1·31
Females	1·83	3·35	0·42	0·67
Total	1·38	2·52	0·67	1·05
1-year motor development:				
Males	3·09	2·98	0·73	1·00
Females	5·00	3·30	1·40	1·50
Total	4·09	3·23	1·04	1·28

Discussion

Neurological functioning

For several reasons, earlier published studies following up children with neonatal neurological symptomatology are difficult to compare with each other as well as with the present study:

(1) They have used different criteria for determining whether neurological sequelae were present or absent at follow-up;
(2) The duration of the neonatal deviance was seldom reported;

(3) In most cases the incidence rate of the selection criteria in the population, from which the index cases were drawn, was not reported;
(4) Most studies draw their subjects from hospital or clinic groups; only one of our subjects had ever been treated as a neurological patient. However, as a function of the last fact it seems a reasonable assumption that the experimental subjects of our study represented cases of less serious neonatal deviance than the majority of the subjects of the previous studies described in the literature.

As a consequence of this milder degree of neonatal symptoms on the part of our subjects, it would seem reasonable to expect either that a lower percentage of neurological sequelae would be found at follow-up in this study, or that whatever sequelae were found were of a different nature than those reported in previous studies. The percentage of the experimental group of this study receiving a score indicating 'certain neurological deviance of (at least) moderate severity' was found to be 70 per cent. This figure is not lower than the comparable figure in the studies by Prechtl (1965), Amiel-Tison (1969), and Thorn (1968) referred to above. The rate of sequelae reported in these studies range from approximately 50–75 per cent. It appears, however, that our subjects in comparison were suffering from different and less severe sequelae at follow-up. Almost all of the deviance found in our subjects belongs within the 'soft' sign category and would not have been observable in young children. As has been pointed out by other researchers, many of the symptoms considered abnormal, though 'soft' signs in 11-year-old children, such as lack of co-ordination or overflow movements, are considered normal in 4-year-olds (Kinsbourne 1973; Hewett 1973). Had our subjects for example been followed up at pre-school age, it seems likely that we would have found a rate of sequelae much lower than that reported by previous investigators.

An empirical finding relevant to this study has been reported by Rubin *et al.* (1973). In a follow-up of premature children, most of whom were neurologically deviant at birth, it was found that there was no significant difference in neurological functioning between prematures and normals at one year; there was however, significantly more neurological deviance in the premature group when the groups were examined again at seven years of age. From the data in Table 14.8 it may be concluded that the neurological development of the subjects in the present study seems to have followed the same path as that of the subjects in the study by Rubin *et al.* Our experimental subjects did not show any significant signs of neurological abnormality at one year. The notion of a latency effect in the correlates of certain types of neonatal neurological deviances was discussed by Drillien (1972). On the basis of her own work she hypothesized that relatively transient neonatal neurological symptoms, not observable at one year, may have long-term neurological and mental consequences. Our data yield support for this notion.

The finding of rather mild neurological deviance later in life on the part of our subjects should not be interpreted to mean that whatever symptoms they presented at follow-up probably have no clinical significance or have had no impact on their lives. The neurological impairment they presented is quite similar to the symptoms repeatedly reported as common in populations referred to child clinics because of different combinations of behaviour and/or intellectual problems frequently summarized in a diagnosis of MBD. The degree of similarity between our subjects and MBD patients described in the literature will be further attended to in the following two sections where the intellectual and personality–social functioning of the subjects will be discussed.

Intellectual functioning

Of the variables relevant to the intellectual functioning of the two groups, the MFD and the RTT yielded the most straightforward support for our hypothesis. Children with TNS evidenced poorer performance. With regard to the 'teachers' judgement of intellectual functioning', a more complicated picture presents itself. In view of the fact that the total scale score differentiated between the groups, it was deemed of interest to investigate which of the individual items of the scale were making the major contributions to this difference. Fisher's Exact Test was used for group comparisons on the individual items constituting the scale. The item-by-item analysis revealed that only items concerning distractability or lack of concentration significantly differentiated between the groups. The rest of the items (difficulties with reading, arithmetic, language or memory, and perseveration) did not yield significant group differences when analysed individually. The results uniformly tended to be in the direction of the experimental subjects performing worse.

With respect to IQ scores, the results of the present study clearly seem to demonstrate that, though some kind of later intellectual impairment may be correlated with TNS, an overall decrease in tested IQ is not to be counted among the reliable later correlates.

The reported findings of the males of both groups receiving higher scores on the WISC than the females is a puzzling result which the authors are most tempted to explain as a sampling artefact. However, the authors are familiar with a parallel result obtained on another, large sample of same-aged Danish subjects. In a yet unpublished study of 250 11-year-olds, Mednick and Schulsinger found that the males obtained significantly higher scores on the WISC. In view of this, an alternative explanation of the sex difference on the WISC may be that the Danish edition of this test tends to favour males when applied to this particular age group.

Personality and social functioning

As mentioned above, the support is weak for the hypothesis that personality–social problems are among the pre-adolescent correlates of TNS. The experimental group in this study was found to be a little immature and somewhat lonely. However, the behaviour disorders which are much more commonly cited as signs of brain damage in school-aged children, such as hyperactivity, impulsivity, unpredictability, and sensitivity to stress, etc., did not occur significantly more frequently in our experimental group. There are different ways one might try to explain this finding:

(1) It is possible that the initial trauma suffered by the experimental subjects in this study was too light or transient to be correlated with the types of sequelae mentioned above.

(2) Another related explanation is based on a rather common notion in the field (Bender 1949; Birch 1964; Bradley 1955; Ernhart et al. 1963; Hanvik et al. 1961; Willerman 1973). These researchers see the manifestation of brain damage in a child as resulting from a more or less unfortunate interaction between an organism which has suffered some degree of primary damage to the brain and the surrounding environment. The quality of the latter will heavily influence the outcome for the patient. The effects of a primary lesion may be successfully compensated for or significantly attenuated by the individual–environment interaction. It follows that the less severe the primary trauma was, the more unfortunate environmental agents must be involved in producing a symptom picture of a certain severity. With regard to the relative absence of personality–social deviances found in the present study, one could imagine that very unfortunate combinations of strength of primary symptoms and unfortunate interactive agents were not present in our experimental group.

(3) Finally, it should be added that many of the earlier studies examining the psychological and behavioural functioning of children diagnosed as having brain damage were done with subjects who were actually initially selected on the basis of behaviour disturbance. The subjects were often clinic populations referred for

such disturbance. Despite the fact that such studies may provide a somewhat unrepresentative picture of the range of symptoms which might be observed in children with brain damage, our expectations with regard to the experimental group were to some extent based on such studies. It seems obvious that children whose personality and social problems go in the direction of increased loneliness and immaturity (such as our experimental group) will have a smaller chance of being referred to a clinic than children with disruptive behaviour disorders, unless their intellectual functioning is profoundly disturbed.

With regard to the absence of the hyperactivity syndrome among the experimental group, a few remarks may be in order. Hyperactivity is often cited as one of the cardinal symptoms of brain damage in children though it has been demonstrated (Birch 1964) that the frequency of hyperactivity among children with known brain damage has been vastly overestimated. We would, however, have expected a somewhat higher incidence rate of this disorder among our experimental group. One reason for the lack of this finding may be ascribed to another bias which has been influencing the results of earlier research on clinic populations. The subjects of these studies have been predominantly males. Wender (1971) cites the incidence rate of hyperactivity as four to 10 times as high for males as for females. Since the number of males and females in the present study was predetermined to be equal and it further turned out that the females showed more signs of impairment at follow-up, the deviances observed in this study would naturally be different from deviances observed in male-dominated samples. The impairments found in the present study may be more characteristic of female subjects. Again, it is possible that the neonatal symptoms in our experimental group were too short-lived to be correlated with later hyperactivity. Only more research which employs severity ratings of peri- and neonatal factors can illuminate this question.

Sex differences

The data of the present study tend to show the experimental females to be in a worse condition than the males. The females had (according to their teachers) significantly more intellectual problems and showed on several other follow-up variables a tendency to score lower than the males. On the early life variables a similar pattern of results emerges. On the score for neonatal physical status the experimental females scored significantly worse than the males and with regard to pregnancy complications and one-year motor developmental score, there was a noticeable—though non-significant—tendency in the same direction.

At first sight this pattern of results seems surprising in the light of the well-established greater vulnerability on the part of male foetuses, infants, and older children (Maccoby and Jacklin 1974). However, when one considers the sampling method applied in this study together with this increased male vulnerability, a probable explanation of the sex differences in our data suggests itself. The 215 infants from among whom our experimental group was chosen consisted of 130 males and 85 females. From previous research (Maccoby and Jacklin 1974; Mednick et al. 1971) we know that males in general have a lower tolerance of pre- and perinatal stress than do females. It is therefore likely that the 85 females would have to have been more severely traumatized or affected than the males in order to be detected as showing symptoms in the new-born period. Most likely some of the 130 males were as severely traumatized as the average of the 85 females, but the variance in degree of traumatization is likely to have been much greater in the male group as compared with the females. Since we deliberately chose an equal number of subjects from each sex group, we should according to this line of thinking, expect our female subjects to have been exposed to more traumatizing pre- or perinatal events. The tendency of the female experimental subjects to have had worse prenatal periods and to do worse on the neonatal physical examination points in this direction. The poorer performance of the females on the follow-up measures may then be seen as a correlate of more severe early traumatization.

Conclusions

Certain neonatal symptoms, which when persistent in the new-born period have been shown to be correlated with presence of brain damage signs later in life, have measurable negative correlates in later neurological, intellectual (and maybe to a lesser degree personality–social) functioning even when only transiently present in the new-born. In the interpretation of the data one should, however, bear in mind that we have not been able to control for many of the important mediating variables which may potentially be influencing the results of the follow-up examination.

One might also mention one strength of this study residing in the fact that the subjects stem from a well-defined birth cohort. The experimental group was chosen so as to be representative of mature-born infants with the transient symptoms in question. This fact increases our confidence in the generalizability of the reported findings.

Acknowledgements

The Danish Perinatal Study was carried out under the guidance of professors P. Plum and D. Trolle. In addition professors E. Rydberg, E. Brandstrup, and F. Fuchs provided expertise and support in the planning phase as well as during the data collection phase.

The research presented in this paper was supported by grant MH 19225 from the National Institute of Mental Health, Center for Studies of Crime and Delinquency.

15. Studies in epidemiology of mental disorder, population genetics, and record linkage in Iceland: a brief outline

TÓMAS HELGASON

Several research projects are combined under this heading. The main object of all of these studies is to identify aetiological clues to mental disorders and deviant behaviour, and to identify persons who eventually might have an increased risk of developing such disorders.

The first studies we conducted included a study of the prevalence of treated mental disorders in Iceland in 1953 (T. Helgason 1954), and a study of the expectancy of mental disorders in the general population (T. Helgason 1964). The latter was based on a cohort of 5395 Icelanders born between 1895 and 1897 and alive in Iceland in 1910. This cohort has since been followed up (T. Helgason 1973) and will still be followed further. The drop-out rate from the cohort has been extremely small; there is less than 1 per cent on whom we have not succeeded in obtaining sufficient information. The main reason for the success of our follow-up is probably the unusual circumstances which are found in such a small population within a delimited geographical area with fairly good records of the main events in people's lives.

In 1965 the Genetic Committee of the University of Iceland was established on the initiative of the late Professor of pathology Niels Dungal, and Dr Sturla Fridriksson, geneticist. Other members of the committee are the present professor of pathology, the professor of psychiatry, the director of the Blood Bank, and the former director of the University Computer Centre. The aims of this committee are mainly to carry out studies in population genetics by using the unusual facilities available in Iceland for record linkage of various records of individual persons as well as linking individual persons into families. The main efforts of the Genetic Committee have so far been in transcribing on to punchcards all births records of people born from 1911 to 1952, as well as transcribing the census data from 1910 to punchcards and tracing the ancestors of those alive in 1910 back to 1840. The census data and all birth records after 1910 have been linked to the national registry or to the death records. Among other things the records contain information on multiple births from 1916 in Iceland, as well as information on cousin marriages and adoptions. A file of all known psychiatric patients has been established by collecting information on those who have been seen by a psychiatrist in Iceland from 1908 to the

present date, either on an out-patient basis or as in-patients. Various other registers were also in existence, although only the cancer register was directly available for computer record linkage with the national register. In order to facilitate the generation of computerized pedigrees which will eventually be developed, all marriage records have been transcribed to punchcards. These have in turn been linked to birth records in some pilot studies (e.g. first-cousin marriages). Data on achievement in elementary school from 1932 to 1969 have been punched on cards, and an attempt has also been made at linking those data with birth records and mental health records (T. Helgason 1976).

A central register of criminality is available. Research workers have gained access to this with permission from the state prosecutor and the Ministry of Justice. Extreme care is being taken in maintaining the confidentiality of information regarding individual persons or families. The registers are only available to authorized persons for research purposes. By linkage of the available records and those being collected various longitudinal studies in mental health and somatic health will be carried out.

An attempt has already been made to trace the children of the cohort born 1895–7 (T. Helgason 1964, 1973) as well as their spouses. The majority of children born within wedlock have been traced, but illegitimate children have not yet been traced. The mental health register will be examined for entries of the spouses and children of the probands of this cohort. A further study will be carried out with regard to their health and life experiences.

Studies related to the major projects which are under way include studies of first-cousin marriage families (see Chap. 42); of the incidence of treated alcoholics and the mortality of alcoholics who have been in treatment; of the incidence of hysteria (Stefánsson et al. 1976), and of the incidence of delirium tremens (Grímsson 1977). Other unrelated studies which will be used as base line data for longitudinal research are a social psychiatric and medical study of trawler-fishermen (T. Helgason et al. 1977); a study of drinking habits, and the prevalence of alcohol abuse, as well as self-reports on the prevalence of mental and emotional disorders evaluated from the Cornell Medical Health Questionnaire (Bergsveinsson 1974; T. Helgason 1975).

The problems encountered during these studies have mainly been related to funding, and even more so to staffing. Some of the data analyses, particulary those related to the study in population genetics, are very complicated due to the great mass of data involved and difficulties in developing effective computer-programs which make the data available for different sorts of linkage.

As most of the projects are longitudinal in scope, involving one or more generations, long-term analysis of mental health will be possible. Further, intergenerational comparisons will be possible. This is expected to contribute to the detection of families at risk of developing mental illness, and will probably also give some leads for necessary preventive measures. The longitudinal aspects of the studies also make them useful in evaluating prognoses and the general impact made by the various therapeutic and preventive measures undertaken. It would undoubtedly be of great value if there were contacts with other European longitudinal projects to attempt solutions of common problems in data-handling and research design.

Acknowledgements

The research of the Genetic Committee of the University of Iceland has been supported by grants from ERDA (Contract no. EY-76-C-02-3214) and the Eco-Science Panel of NATO. The study of trawler-fishermen has been supported by the Icelandic Science Fund. The studies related to alcohol were supported by the State council for alcohol prevention and the State fund for rehabilitation of alcoholics in Iceland.

b. Prospective school age cohort studies

16. Project Metropolitan: a longitudinal study of a Stockholm cohort (Sweden)

CARL-GUNNAR JANSON

The single most important asset of Swedish social sciences might well be the access to an extensive and reliable population registration system in the wide sense. It enables the researcher to keep track of a person literally from birth to death as long as the person stays within the country. Also, the registers and files of the system provide the researcher with a host of adequate data for various research projects. Admittedly, the prevailing attitude, at least among behavioural scientists, for a long time was to see secondary sources as second-rate sources. Here one can sense the superior effect of American sociology with its emphasis on interviewing and questionnaire studies. Thus, Swedish behavioural scientists may not have utilized the population registries to their full potential. Nevertheless, something of a Swedish longitudinal research tradition developed.

Of course, Swedish sociology and related social sciences are replete with cross-sectional studies, i.e. empirical studies providing sets of synchronic data. Especially when interview or questionnaire techniques are employed the tendency to aim at conditions at a given, fixed time or time period seems overwhelming. Such studies can build on well established and adequate research techniques and often give excellent data on the situation and time in question.

Frequently, however, interpretations in terms of processes and diachronic extrapolations to changes creep in more or less inevitably. For these purposes cross-sectional studies are less well suited, since it is awkward to reach for valid diachronic conclusions from synchronic data. Short-time effects in the first place can be revealed by the use of panel designs in surveys and by the before-and-after designs in experiments. Sometimes one tries to cover a longer period in surveys by asking retrospective questions to respondents of cross-sectional samples, e.g., in obtaining 'life histories', which now seem to be popular. This, though, is generally only second best, because of slips of memory and subconscious reorganization of events and courses that are invited by the procedure. Rather, to study long-time processes and effects, efficient extension of panels and schemes of continuous or intermittent, experimental or non-experimental, observation over longer periods are needed, i.e., the longitudinal elements should be strengthened. Especially in some fields the case for studies of individuals or other units over a period of time or at successive stages, i.e., for longitudinal studies, is

strong, since they can produce prospective data instead of retrospectives ones. Note that prospective and retrospective both refer to data which are connected to subsequent data in the analysis. Such data could build on evidence produced at the time they pertain to at the latest or at some later time. In the first case they are prospective; in the second they are retrospective. Note that according to this definition prospective data may be recorded at a much later time than they bear upon. Among such fields are those of developmental psychology and gerontology, socialization and deviance, diffusion and effects of communication, social change, demography and geographical mobility, and the field of social stratification and mobility.

Obviously, diachronic data are needed if one is to study change. By longitudinal, or cohort, studies, however, we usually refer to a special kind of empirical study involving diachronic data. First, we exclude diachronic studies that use their time-periods or points in time, i.e. their temporal units, as their analytical (statistical) units. Longitudinal studies use other kinds of analytical units, e.g. persons, families, or neighbourhoods, or categories of such entities. Second, the same analytical units are observed over time, and their characteristics are compared individually over time. Cross-sections of observations thus are made on related samples. If the same variable is observed diachronically the within-periods component of its variance can be partitioned into a between-units component and a residual component. Note, though, that a longitudinal study does not necessarily involve observing the same variable at more than one point in time, since the set of variables may well change over time. Third, a longitudinal study should cover a 'long' period of time, although what is considered a 'long' period of observation depends on the context. Whatever its length there should be continuous or intermittent observations referring to various parts of the period, not only at its beginning and end. Thus, although diachronic, panel studies, before-and-after experiments, and follow-up studies are not longitudinal, or cohort, studies as here understood: studies in which a set of units are followed by continuous or intermittent observations over a long period of time.

At least two kinds of analyses of longitudinal data can be distinguished. First there is the external type of analysis in which the whole cohort (or a given category of the cohort) at a specific time is the analytical unit. Variations to be investigated are those between different times of the same cohort, between different cohorts at the same time, or between different cohorts of the same age. If a category of the cohort is singled out, the variations refer to characteristics of that category only. Second there is the internal type of analysis in which differential changes of or differences between individuals or categories within a cohort are studied.

In the first kind of analysis findings will be expressed in terms of age, cohort, and period factors, and possibly their interactions. Here one faces an identification problem, because the three factors are connected by the formula

$$A = P - C; (A:\text{age}; P:\text{period}; \text{ and } C:\text{cohort}).$$

Hence each factor can be substituted by a given linear combination of the two others. The choice made between the factors on the basis of data requires some assumption or principle.

If there is but one value on one of the three factors, the two remaining factors will covary completely and thus cannot be distinguished. For instance, if observations are made in one period only, we have a cross-sectional analysis of age categories, which belong to different cohorts. With one cohort only, changes over time can be related to age or periods.

Thus, for external analysis of longitudinal studies it is essential in most respects to have more than one cohort. As a rule, however, even the full design with several cohorts and periods restricts data to a particular country, region, or community, limiting findings to conditions in that socio-ecological setting to be extended to more general conditions according to assumptions. Also, presumption of independence or near-independence of characteristics of periods and of cohorts may be dangerous at least as far as adjacent periods and cohorts are concerned. The degree of dependence may be no less for them than for cohorts or periods in various socio-ecological settings. Hence one could argue that parallel studies of one cohort, not necessarily the same one, in different, fairly widely separated socio-ecological settings may substitute for the study of several cohorts in the same area.

The internal longitudinal analysis does not require more than one cohort, although it must be kept in mind that with only one cohort overall changes for that cohort can be period, cohort, or age effects. For instance, a change over time in amount of variance accounted for in one variable by a given set of factors may be due to age or period or be specific to the cohort. To choose among these explanatory possibilities one must refer to evidence external to the cohort. Also, with only one cohort in a spatially-limited social system the problem of generalization of findings is even more difficult than with several cohorts of the same or various systems.

The relevance of longitudinal studies is essentially based on the quest for a time order of predominantly prospective data covering a 'long' process. For the fields of social sciences referred to above, except possibly demography, the proposed analysis will be internal rather than external.

Here is where Scandinavian social scientists can come in, through their access to an extensive and efficient population registration system. To the extent that this is a unique opportunity of research and that it is possible to generalize results beyond national borders, one may even, if somewhat pompously, claim an international reponsibility of the Scandinavians.

Focusing on Swedish conditions, one should point out that not only is the population registration system extensive and sufficiently accurate for many research purposes, but also it has been accessible for social researchers until quite recently through the Publicity Principle and special permissions granted. According to this principle, stated in the Constitution, all documents and proceedings of any authorities are open to the public unless the contrary is

explicitly stated. The public is denied access to official documents mainly for three reasons:

(1) State security and military considerations may require that a document is not made public;
(2) If a document is prepared within an official agency for internal use only, it is not public until the case it refers to is closed. However, this clause does not apply to a document that is received from an external source, be that another official agency, a private company, or a private person;
(3) Availabilty to the public of official documents is limited from considerations of personal integrity. Thus information that may be humiliating or dishonourable cannot be revealed about individuals.

This third reason is most important for social research. Because of it, the register run by the State Prison Board since 1900 on court sentences of felonies is not open to the public, nor are the Social Registers run by each municipality since 1937 (or in the biggest cities much earlier, e.g. in Stockholm from 1895) on dependency and Child Welfare Committee cases etc., and registers on prisoners, on cases of drunkenness, on alcohol addicts sent to special institutions, and on cases of venereal diseases. However, such hindrances imposed on publicity to protect personal integrity were often waived by the government and other proper state authorities to facilitate responsible research. Necessary conditions for a research project to be given the special privilege of having access to secret individual data were the non-commercial character of the project, a promise to make all reports in such a form that individuals or families cannot possibly be identified, and the good professional standing of the researcher and the project. That the researcher honoured his professional ethics and thus did not reveal individual data to unauthorized persons was taken as a matter of course. Access to non-public data appears to have been given without political bias. Project Metropolitan was given access to data on court sentences, police records, delivery records, draft board data, and social registers before the 1974 Data Law came into force.

There are several Swedish longitudinal projects in progress, some of which are described in this volume. The Stockholm branch of Project Metropolitan is one of them. Compared to the other studies included here it is somewhat more sociologically-oriented and relies heavily on data from registers and files. It was planned as part of a Scandinavian project. Working within the field of social stratification and mobility Kaare Svalastoga of Copenhagen reached the conclusion that prospective longitudinal studies were highly needed in that field. In the early 1960s he was pressing for such a study. In addition to the Scandinavian studies up to that time, such as Gunnar Boalt's Stockholm study and the Hallgren–Husén Malmoe study, Svalastoga was inspired in the first place by Douglas's study of a sample of the British cohort of 1946. This project had already begun in 1945. Later he was encouraged by other projects too, e.g. the start of Flanagan's American 'Project Talent' and Girod's Geneva project. It was realized, however, that a longitudinal project would contain many practical problems. For instance, there are the difficulties generated by the cohort member's moving between areas. A cohort by definition would refer to the population of an area at a given time. With the cohort under observation for any length of time some members will leave the area and the cohort will be dispersed over a larger territory than the defining area. If the dispersion is considerable, it will cause trouble for several reasons:

(1) Granted it is possible to keep track of cohort members, interviewing and the use of local or regional registers will be expensive and time-consuming;
(2) Environmental conditions will be increasingly heterogeneous and their variation probably systematically related to

various background and personal variables through selective forces. This might be theoretically challenging but will mean complications and would perhaps necessitate a larger sample than otherwise;

(3) The dispersion of the cohort will make its original area delimitation artificial, as one will not be observing what happens to a cohort of a specified population but what happens to a special, non-random sample of a more diffuse population of a wider but rather vaguely delimited area.

Naturally the amount of moving would depend on the period of observation, but if one includes adolescence and young adulthood until the occupational career is reasonably discernible, it seems one ought to reckon with rather much mobility. To some the whole country appeared to be the smallest practicable area unit. However, a national sample would be expensive and difficult to handle with the type of study Svalastoga had in mind.

He wanted a study covering the years from early school age to early middle life, a study involving all four Scandinavian countries, and dealing with inter-generational mobility and differential life chances in a wide sense. Such a jointly Scandinavian project seems to have been discussed as a serious possibility for the first time in 1960, at a Scandinavian sociological conference in Finland. There Gunnar Boalt pointed out that he had found 94 per cent of the boys in his Stockholm cohort still living in the city when they were approximately 24 years old. Thus it might be possible to keep a cohort geographically together for a considerable period of time by limiting the population to those who had grown up in the place with the country's presumably highest centrality, i.e., in the biggest metropolitan area of the country.

A committee was constituted for planning a Scandinavian longitudinal study. Svalastoga drafted a programme which was distributed in March, 1961. He outlined four main problem areas for the study. The first one was that of social mobility, especially inter-generational mobility, and the role played by education. The educational career of the children is determined to a considerable degree by their social background, and later their education is a main determinant of their social position. The second area concerned membership in groups and formal associations, and the third one conformity and deviance. Two kinds of deviations were distinguished: *positive deviation*, where the individual does more than expected, e.g. becomes a prize-winning athlete, a creative artist, or a moral guide; and *negative deviation* in the form of mental or physical disease, crime and delinquency, alcohol or drug addiction, social isolation, etc. Finally, mate selection, marital adjustment, and possible divorces in families of procreation belonged to the fourth field.

Variables as to behaviour within the four areas would make up a set of related variables, the variations of which could be partially accounted for by the subsystem of remaining variables of the same or previous dates. By using variables of previous periods only, prediction might be attempted. To increase statistical determination certain psychological variables ought to be included, e.g. mental abilities, adaptation to school, level of aspiration, vocational plans, interests, and some attitudes. Naturally such variables would themselves be interrelated and also would be possible as dependent variables. Another system of variables, mainly to be used as independent ones, would concern the child's family of orientation: its social, economic, political, and educational status; personal relations within the family; and interests, aspirations, and attitudes, e.g. to education, of parents. Of course, some variables of this set were necessary, if inter-generational mobility was to be measured. Finally the larger social enviroment of school, other non-familial training institutions, local community, etc. ought to be described.

A prospective approach was necessary, especially because special tests and variables on attitudes and opinions and data on groups were included in the design. The population to be studied was limited to boys, mainly because of boys' greater vocational variability and higher frequency of recorded deviance. Ideally the boys should be studied from their birth. On the other hand, as mentioned before, it was important to extend the period of observation up to an age when the boys have completed their education and their vocational careers are well under way. Furthermore, with an earlier upper age limit the part dealing with families of procreation would be seriously curtailed. Thus an observation period of 30 years would be needed. However, even a 20-year period is a long time for a project, especially if the project leaders themselves want to take part in the whole project. With an estimated maximum of 20 years at disposal the period from about 10 to around 30 years of age was chosen, though the advantages of beginning earlier, just before school, say, were understood and admitted. However, the lower limit of 10 years would be only approximate. It set the earliest possible time the boys and their parents could be contacted for questioning in person. Actually the first questionnaire study was later to be planned for the age of 12 or 13. On the other hand the boys and their families could well be studied by documentary methods from the day of the birth of the boy, and the parents even earlier.

The considerable length of the suggested study implied various complications. Some changes of staff would be unavoidable and probably would cause some changes of interests and orientation. In 20 years current theories and problems, variables and methods most likely would not be the same as when the project started. This made a very broad approach appropriate. Variables should be included, if they seemed to be of interest, just to be safe, even if one did not know exactly what to do with them at the time of observation. Obviously that is precisely how not to act according to the textbooks. Also, data were intended as a basis for various minor projects, which would contribute some additional data too.

After some delay, in October 1963, Svalastoga in co-operation with Natalie Rogoff-Ramsøy and Ørjar Øyen of Oslo, succeeded in arranging a meeting in Oslo. In addition to these people Gösta Carlsson and I attended. We decided to try to start the study in 1964. Svalastoga would be in charge in Copenhagen, Ramsøy and Øyen in Oslo, and I in Stockholm. As no Finnish delegate was present at the meeting, Helsinki had to be left out for the time being. Hopefully, a Finnish team would join the project later, but we realized that probably it would be only for a partial study.

One cohort, preferably the same, was to be studied in each city. Originally the intended cohort comprised the boys born in 1950. Now, as the project had been delayed, a change was made to the cohort of 1953. The four main areas were fixed as suggested in Svalastoga's programme. Within the frame of the project, however, there was to be allowance for local variations and additions according to fields of interest. For instance, Oslo was specially interested in the influence of the local community and peer groups on behaviour, and Stockholm wished to analyse juvenile delinquency and geographical mobility within the city. Also, we decided to study the metropolitan areas of the cities and not only the central cities, although this would complicate the collecting of data, since more local authorities and registers would be involved.

The project had to be financed in each country separately and, reasonably, for a few years or for smaller parts at a time. Also for planning purposes it was advisable to divide the project in parts. Obviously it was not possible to plan the whole project in detail, nor was there any point in doing so. In research planning, as in other planning, the longer the time span, the more room must be allowed for interventions of unexpected circumstances.

The main features of the project would be a questionnaire study at school and interviews with a sample of the mothers, both as soon as possible; questioning at the end of the period; possibly one or two interview or questionnaire sample studies in between; and continuous collecting of register data. Also it was decided that the local communities within the metropolitan areas should be described in special ecological studies. So, in 1964, Project Metropolitan began, not like ten but four little Indians.

To co-ordinate the ecological studies a meeting was held in Stockholm in July 1964. Here Helsinki was represented by Frank L. Sweetser of Boston University, who spent a year at the University of Helsinki. The study of Helsinki in 1960 was rapidly carried through by Sweetser (1968) and published separately, and the study of Stockholm was made part of a project on Swedish urban spatial structure at the National Institute of Building Research. The analysis of the 1960 structure was published in 1971 (Janson 1971; see also Janson 1976), and scores on eight dimensions were calculated for 244 area units of the Stockholm metropolitan area. Corresponding analyses for 1965 and 1970 are being prepared. In Oslo several variables were tabulated for the various local communities.

As to the main project, the Danish cohort was defined to comprise all boys born in 1953 in the city of Copenhagen and the three counties of Copenhagen, Frederiksborg, and Roskilde, regardless of the boy's residence in 1964. Copenhagen and the three counties together make up northeastern Zealand and include areas outside the Copenhagen metropolitan area. In 1960 their total population was 1 590 000 as against 1 220 000 for 'Greater Copenhagen'. The cohort of 1953 numbered 12 270 boys. They were listed from the 1953 registers on midwives' birth reports. This turned out to be a rather time-consuming procedure.

The questionnaire study at school was carried out in two steps in 1965. In May the major part was executed. It contained a mental test, constructed by Kjell Härnqvist (Professor of Education, University of Gothenburg; the test was designed for his longitudinal study, the Individual Statistics Project) and translated from Swedish, a test of creativity, sociometric questions, and questions on social aspirations. In the autumn the boys had tests in Danish and arithmetic and answered questions on their educational plans and social backgrounds. Both before and after the school study the Danish, Norwegian, and Swedish teams met for discussions and co-ordination.

In 1968 it was time for the family study, again after meetings with the Norwegian and Swedish teams. Almost 4000 mothers were interviewed about their and their spouse's education, occupation, and social background, and about relations within the family, plans and aspirations, etc. Together with the non-response cases they were a stratified sample, in which mothers of boys in the first and last deciles of the mental test distribution in the school study were over-represented.

Coding the extensive sets of data, putting them on cards and tape, and collecting data from registers kept the Danish team busy for the next few years. Svalastoga's main collaborators were Tom Rishøj, Erik Manniche, Erik Høgh, and Preben Wolf. After Svalastoga, Rishøj acted as director, later to be succeeded by Wolf. Contacts with the Stockholm study remain close.

In Stockholm the cohort was defined slightly differently. It was taken to comprise all boys born in 1953, regardless of where they were born, as long as they lived in the Stockholm area on 1 November 1963. Operationally that meant that the boys were listed in the 1964 population register for the area. The Stockholm metropolitan area was defined as Stockholm city and those surrounding municipalities which satisfied three criteria in 1960: held more than 50 per cent agglomerated population, had less than one-third of the population in agriculture, and had more than 15 per cent of the economically active population commuting to the central city. All 18 suburban municipalities and four municipalities of the outer suburban zone qualified. The population of the area was 1 130 000 in 1960. The number of boys in the cohort became 7719.

The first two years the Swedish project operated on grants from the Stockholm City Council and the Social Science Research Coun-

cil, but from 1966 the Tercentenary Fund of the Swedish Bank took over. On its first grant the school study was carried out in late spring, 1966. It had Härnqvist's test and other attitude scales taken over from the Individual Statistics Project, no creativity test, but evaluations of occupations, sociometric questions, and questions on school, leisure, and conception of the future. (My main collaborator during the first years was Lars Gustafsson, who left after the school study for political commitments, which made him an MP in the 1968 general election.)

In time for the school study the definition of the cohort was changed to also include the girls. With 7398 girls the total cohort became 15 117 cases. The family study came in spring, 1968, on a sample of 4021 mothers, with the same kind of stratification as in the Danish study. From then on all data have been taken from registers.

As in Copenhagen the research was found to involve more perspiration and less inspiration than we had reckoned with. It is an open question, which fortunately need not be answered, whether we would have started the project, had we had a more realistic conception of what we were getting ourselves into. Most of the time the project has been understaffed, not because the Tercentenary Fund has refused funding, but partly because I have had difficulties getting time to handle a faster moving project with more staff, and partly because the interest in the project has generally been small among sociology students and researchers. Hence large sets of challenging data lie waiting, while the staff works on its parts. We co-operate with Jackson Toby, Rutgers University. Parts of the study are linked to international projects run by him, one concerning juvenile delinquency and the other concerning the handling of delinquency cases. Another affiliated study is one run by Olof Fränden of Stockholm, on political socialization.

In Oslo the cohort was defined as in Stockholm. They tried to list its members through the school register, but got into serious trouble almost immediately. The conservative newspaper, the *Aftenposten*, attacked the project, which was depicted as an invasion of privacy. The ensuing debate went on heatedly in the press and over the radio, and was even carried to the parliament. The listing of cohort members had to be interrupted and the school study was postponed to let things cool off. For a while the Norwegian team thought of having the family study before the school study, but neither study materialized, and finally we had to face the sombre fact that the Norwegian branch of the project was out.

In Finland no one was ever found who was interested and naïve enough to take charge of the Finnish part. To some the future of Finnish rural society was more interesting. Others, given the 'theoretical' orientation of leading Finnish sociologists, must have found the prospects of collecting data for some twenty years too drab and empiricist. After some years even Svalastoga's optimism as to a Helsinki study ran dry. Clearly there would not be a Finnish Project Metropolitan, at least not this time. Then there were only two little Indians. The livelier of them is the Stockholmer, who is adequately fed by the Tercentenary Fund of the Swedish Bank. By now he has collected a substantial series of data sets. Their organization in time, as of March 1979, is summarized in Table 16.1. Data start from the very beginning. From delivery records at the hospitals we recorded complications during pregnancy and in delivery, together with length of pregnancy, and weight and height of the new-born baby. These data are available only for children who were born in the area. When those who were born outside the area, at home, or not at major hospitals are subtracted, records exist for some 12 000 deliveries.

For the whole cohort place of birth, parents' date of marriage and occupation in 1953 are known. (When a variable is said to be known or available from register data for the whole cohort or for a specific part of the cohort, it should be understood that data are missing for a certain (small) number of cases. There are always a remainder of

TABLE 16.1

Project Metropolitan's data (N = 15 117)

1953	Delivery records	Birth place, social class	Criminal record of		Social register (dependency and	Address
1954		of parents	family head		child welfare committee cases)	
1955						
1956						
1957						
1958						
1959						
1960	Census of population and housing					
1961						
1962						
1963	Definition of population	Family, income, social class			Exits	Address
1964						
1965						
1966	School study	Marks, sixth form		Police record		Address
1967						
1968	Family study N = 4021					Address head of family
1969		Marks, ninth form	Application for gymnasium and fackskola			
1970				Attendance and marks in gymnasium and fackskola		
1971	Draft board data (boys)	Income of head of family				
1972						Address head of family
1973						
1974		Income				
1975						Address
1976						
1977						
1983						

cases where usable register data are missing or would take more work to produce than one can spend on single cases out of a series of 15 000. For instance, relevant data on parent's occupation in 1953 are missing on some 600 cases including 400 who were born abroad.) If the member of the cohort has left his/her parish of birth, which often is the case, data and receiving parish are recorded. The occupation of the head of the family is coded in socio-economic categories. The family's record, if any, as a dependency case or as a Child Welfare Committee case is taken from the so-called social register of each municipality for the period 1953–72. In Stockholm City the handling of the cohort's delinquency cases between 13 and 16 years of age by the Child Welfare Committee was recorded from the social register.

From the 1960 Census of Population and Housing housing conditions, family composition, and some occupational and educational classifications of the head of the household are available for families within the area. Community scores on eight ecological dimensions also build on data from the 1960 census. The analysis of urban spatial structure in 1965 will give scores for that year too. For 1963, the year of definition of the cohort, parental occupation and assessed income, address, and family composition, including name and birth data of each member of the family, are known. The occupation of the head of the household has been coded in socio-economic categories.

The data of the school study, a new set of addresses, and most of the marks from sixth grade refer to 1966. Addresses and names of heads of families are also available for the end of next year, and

1968 has the family study for a sample of the cohort. The school study and the family study both have a non-response rate of about 9 per cent. Most marks of ninth grade of comprehensive school came in 1969, and the remainder in 1968 and 1970. In 1968–72 there were also applications to the three- or four-year courses (*gymnasium*) and the two-year courses (*fackskola*) of secondary school. Thus the plans expressed in 1966 in the school study could be checked with actual applications, although we did not ask about *fackskola* in 1966, since it was so new then that we feared not many of the pupils would have opinions about attending it. With the application to secondary school acceptance at *gymnasium* or *fackskola* was also recorded, and so were marks for completed secondary education, which data were received from the National Central Bureau of Statistics. Also included are police records between 1966 and 1971. Of the boys 1299 were known to the police for some delinquency after the age of fifteen. The criminal records of the heads of the families also are available. Of all persons searched for, 1858 were found in the files of the National Prison Board.

Draft board data from 1971 for boys comprise mental test scores and information on education, occupation, and medical status. Further additions to the data archives are addresses as of a given week of 1972 and assessed incomes of 1971 for those members of the cohort and those heads of families who still lived in the metropolitan area as of 1 November 1970. Addresses for cohort members as of a given week of 1975, this time together with assessed incomes of 1974 are also known. Exits (out-movings and deaths) from the cohort are recorded until 1 November 1970. Until then 444 girls and 503 boys, i.e. 6 per cent, had left the cohort. In September 1975, the number of exits had increased to 1543, i.e. 10 per cent.

All data except those on family composition in 1963 or on parental criminality and those from the 1960 census now are on tape. An interview study on mate selection and the first part of the occupational career was discussed for 1978 but was cancelled. We still plan to close the project's data collection by surveying the cohort in 1983. After the laborious and time-consuming excerpting of dependency and Child Welfare Committee cases was completed, we have only added a few items to the data archives, but the data-collecting activities are now resumed. Police records 1972–8, addresses in 1978, and assessed incomes of 1977 are being added to the files. New data series may also be gathered, although on a somewhat smaller scale than before.

The main reason for the hopefully temporary reduction of the data collecting activities of the project from 1976 are complications introduced by the Data Act of 1974 and mass-media debates on invasion of privacy. The Data Act applies to research data, if they are handled by computers and contain personal identifiers in a broad sense. For such registers on individuals permission by the Data Inspection Board is required. The project applied for permission to run its data registers in June 1974, and the board decided on the application in June 1976. The decision was to permit the project to run its present register. However, for new data the consent of the cohort members would be required in principle. This referred not only to interview and questionnaire studies, in which the co-operation of the respondents is obviously necessary, but also to the use of registers and files, public and non-public, although exceptions to this would be possible. If the board sticks to the stated principle, a survey to get the permission of the registered persons would thus be required before excerpts from a file could be taken.

This position taken by the Data Inspection Board brings the inherent conflict between the Data Act and the traditional publicity principle to a head, and, generally applied, virtually brings to an end the large-scale use of registers and files for research purposes, as far as computer-run, individually identifiable records are concerned. The present situation is somewhat disquieting both to the project specifically and to Swedish social sciences generally. For the time being the project will restrict its data collecting from registers and files to data for which the Data Inspection Board will waive the consent requirement or to which the Data Act does not apply, because they do not involve the computer or do not register individual identifications. It might be added that the non-response rate in interview studies could usually be brought down to, say, 10 per cent, but now it is often difficult to get the rate below 20 per cent. (A Data Inspection Board decision with effect from April 1977, is especially alarming. In following up an earlier research project on social deviance a research team wanted to collect register data on persons who were estimated to run a higher than average risk to be negatively deviant. The researchers did not consider it ethically defensible to tell the subjects why they were being studied, which it would be necessary to do if they were asked to consent to be studied. The Board agreed to this and drew the conclusion that as consent could not be obtained the personal file requested for the study could not be permitted under the Data Act. Thus, if the researchers continue with the project, they must not use computers.)

Fortunately, however, when the Data Act fell upon Swedish behavioral research, our project had reached a stage where a temporal reorganization was due, with less of the resources spent on data collecting and more of them directed towards preparing for analyses and carrying them out. Obviously the full potential of a longitudinal study cannot be realized before the whole period of observation has elapsed. However, for some parts shorter periods will do, and there is always the possibility of cross-sectional studies

of separate parts of the data. Thus far only few, mostly rather tentative analyses have been made within the project, partly from lack of time of the staff who are mostly involved in preparation of data, and because few competent outside researchers are interested, but also because some key variables were made ready for use only recently and others were still in preparation, being collected, coded, or checked.

At that time, although one would have wished for some additional data, say, on family composition, health, and various forms of deviance, all major series of data had been collected for the period of 1953–71. With the dependency and Child Welfare Committee cases on tape, the time had come to start the general analyses of educational careers and their social background. There were also various other preparations of data to be made, while we waited for an opportunity to carry the project further. Recently prospects have become somewhat less gloomy. A parliamentary commission with the task of examining the Data Act and its application reported in August 1978. It recommended that the Data Act be kept unchanged. Thus, it turned down, e.g. suggestions made by several social scientists that 'research registers' be exempt from the provision of approval by the Data Inspection Board and just be filed by the Board. However, the commission recommended some changes of policy. A gradual, if slight, change towards a more liberal policy as to research projects may be traced in decisions by the Board. Thus, it recently waived its earlier decision on Project Metropolitan and permitted the extension of police records to 1972–8 and the recording of new addresses and assessed incomes without the consent of the cohort members. We hope the Data Inspection Board will take a similar stand on other applications by the project.

In 1975 a report series was started, the volumes of which are sent out free of charge to interested parties as long as editions are limited to 300–400 copies. In 1975 four reports were issued. The first one is a presentation of the project, its background, and a short summary of some other Swedish longitudinal projects. Large sections of the present chapter are excerpts from this report. The second one is a description of the project's data archives, and the following two reports are code books of the school study and the family study, with separate frequencies for girls and boys. There were two more reports in 1976. Number five, by Peter Martens, deals with patterns of child rearing ideology. After a review of the literature of the field it presents a factor analysis of some questions on child rearing in the Family Study. This was the first report on an empirical study within the project, after the sample of tables in the first report. Marten's study however, is not longitudinal, as it uses data from the Family Study only. Number six in the report series, Kaare Svalastoga's 'Analytical strategy in sequential research. Project Metropolitan revisited', is essentially the paper presented at the Geneva meeting in December 1975, of the ISA Research Committee on Social Stratification. In 1977 there were two further reports. Report number seven ('The handling of juvenile delinquency cases') is part of an international project directed by Professor Jackson Toby, Rutgers University, New Brunswick, New Jersey, USA. The way juvenile delinquency cases are handled is studied in four cities in different countries. In Stockholm the cases were those of Project Metropolitan cohort members recorded with the Stockholm Child Welfare Committee from 1966 to the day the member reached the age of sixteen, in 1969. The statistical units are the Committee's decisions on treatment, 815 on 545 persons. The study tries to test a part of the labelling theory, interpreted to imply that youngsters in a low socio-economic position would receive harsher treatment and have their cases more thoroughly investigated, given the characteristics of the cases. The emerging picture gives little support to this version of the labelling theory. In 76 per cent of the cases the decision on treatment was to let the kind of treatment already in progress (none, supervision, etc.) continue. A series of multiple regression analyses were made with treatment change as dependent variable. Regressors were delinquency characteristics, delinquency characteristics plus descriptions of other problem behaviour, the same regressors plus some personal characteristics, and, finally, family-prolem variables were inserted. To each series in turn social class, minority status, and dependency were added. Three levels of treatment in progress were analysed separately. The proportion of variance accounted for differed between analyses, but with the most effective sets of regressors it was around or beyond 50 per cent. The increment in variance accounted for by the socio-economic variables were usually negligible. Corresponding results were found when different aspects of the extent of the investigation of the cases were used as the dependent variable.

In the next, i.e. eighth, report of the series ('Who were the young leftists?') Olof Frändén reports on one of his studies of political socialization. In 1971 he had pupils of secondary schools in the Stockholm area fill out questionnaires on political opinions. Most respondents were born in 1953 and the Project Metropolitan School Study files were searched for them. Testing several hypotheses Frändén mostly finds weak relations between attitudes and interests in 1966 on the one hand and political attitudes in 1971 on the other. The ninth report was published in 1978. It discusses various methodological problems of the longitudinal approach ('The longitudinal approach—problems and possibilities in the social sciences').

Two reports are forthcoming at the time of writing. In the tenth report Olof Dahlbäck analyses the educational process as a decision-making process, testing various hypotheses on the project's data ('Beslutsteoretiska aspekter på utbildningsprocessen', in Swedish with an English summary). Olof Frändén presents further notes on the young leftists in the eleventh report. Other studies in preparation include one on the 145 pairs of twins in the Metropolitan cohort. Of the pairs 95 are same-sexed. For most of them zygosity was taken from the Twin Registry at the Karolinska Institute. Another study deals with the desirability of occupations as evaluated by mothers in the Family Study and by cohort members in the School Study. Peter Martens continues his analyses of the child-rearing ideology, Olof Dahlbäck studies the differential development of intelligence in boys, and Helga Seibel looks at sex differences in educational and occupational aspirations. A longitudinal model of juvenile delinquency, presented in the ninth research report will be presented in more depth.

Finally, code books will be prepared for the project's data from registers and files in the same way as code books were made for the School Study and the Family Study in reports 2 and 3, respectively.

Hopefully, that will not be the end of the series, but rather the end of the beginning. There are four more years to go until 1983, the year the cohort members become 30. We hope to plod on, putting together data on our cohort, and slowly beginning to present a picture of the lives, conditions, and adventures of its members. Of course we will carefully protect our data and never reveal or publish anything from which a specific person or family may be identified, as the old professional ethical code commands and the new Data Act implies.

17. Project Metropolitan: a longitudinal study of 12 270 boys from the metropolitan area of Copenhagen, Denmark (1953–77)

ERIK HØGH and PREBEN WOLF

Introduction

Project Metropolitan was initiated by Professor K. Svalastoga of the Sociologisk Institut, University of Copenhagen. Professor Svalastoga acted as chairman of the project until 1976 with Tom Rishøj as project director up to April 1976. Since then the project has been carried on by a team of researchers consisting of Birthe Holten, Erik Høgh, Erik Manniche, Tom Rishøj, Gert Strande-Sørensen, Kaare Svalastoga, and Preben Wolf. The latter succeeded Svalastoga as chairman in 1976. Up to 1976 Project Metropolitan had partly been financed by the Danish National Scientific Foundation; since then parts of it have had financial support from the National Council for the Prevention of Crime and Delinquency.

Copenhagen (København) is the capital of Denmark. The metropolitan area consists of the municipalities of København, Frederiksberg, and Gentofte together with three adjacent counties (amter) of Copenhagen, Roskilde, and Frederiksborg with a total population of 1 768 000 inhabitants in 1975. In 1977 the whole area was known as the HT-area, named after the official public traffic organization, covering the area with a densely integrated traffic system.

The population of the HT-area or metropolitan area is just about 35 per cent of the total Danish population. Denmark today is a so-called welfare society with industrialized agricultural production, light industries, shipping trade, air transport, and an extensive commercial system. Denmark belongs to the EEC and the NATO alliance. At the same time it forms a part of the Scandinavian social system together with Norway and Sweden. A project parallel to Project Metropolitan in Denmark is going on under the same name in the metropolitan area of Stockholm, the capital of Sweden. The Swedish project is directed by Professor Carl-Gunnar Janson of Stockholm University, Department of Sociology, and it too concerns a birth cohort from 1953. The two projects co-operate.

According to official statistics 12 270 boys were born within the metropolitan area of Copenhagen during 1953. It was on the basis of those 12 270 boys that the Danish longitudinal study called Project Metropolitan was orginally founded. As of March 1977 it has been possible to identify 12 140 males (98·94 per cent of the 12 270 metropolitan boys) who according to official statistics were born in 1953. These males have been considered the basic birth cohort, and at intervals, have been the main target of research within the longitudinal project. This birth cohort will hereafter be referred to simply as the cohort. The specific relevance of this particular cohort has been discussed in previous publications (see for further information: Svalastoga 1976).

In 1977 the researchers of Project Metropolitan succeeded in identifying 11 540 living boys (94·05 per cent of the original birth cohort), and 600 (4·89 per cent) who had died before 1977. This adds up to 98·94 per cent of the cohort now being identified within the project. Deaths are continuously being registered as they occur.

Actual research based on the cohort began in 1965 with respect to birth data from 1953 and school data from 1965. Later studies were concentrated around the years 1966, 1968, 1975, and 1976. Most of this research has been concerned with the cohort as a whole. In addition to the cohort studies, research has been carried out on a 25 per cent random sample (hereafter referred to as the sample) drawn from the cohort.

Table 17.1 shows the major studies of the cohort which have been carried through up to now; the table presents information on the year of each study, the kinds of information obtained, whether the cohort or the sample was used, and the percentage of members for whom information has been obtained. All information concerning the cohort and the sample has now gone through the main processes of coding, and has been transferred from code sheets to punched cards and magnetic tape.

Table 17.1

Project Metropolitan: Years of concern for studies of the cohort (12 270 boys) or the sample (3833 boys) carried through from 1953 to 1977, kind of data sought, and percentage of respondents or members from which information was actually obtained

Year of concern	Kind of data	Total cohort	Sample	Per cent obtained from cohort $N = 12\,270$	from sample $N = 3833$
1953	Birth data	+	(+)	94·47	(−)
1965	School data I	+	(+)	77·73	(−)
1966	School data II	+	(+)	77·73	(−)
1968	Family data	−	+	—	82·29
1975	Demographic registration	+	(+)	94·05	(−)
1976	Crime and delinquency	+	(+)	94·05	N.A.

+   = Information available for the cohort and/or the sample.
(+) = Information available, but the sample comprised within the cohort.
−   = Information not sought for the cohort.
(−) = Information not sought for the sample apart from the cohort from which the sample was drawn.
N.A. = Not ascertained at present.

The data

Integration of data

Since the study of the boys' families in 1968 was based on a random sample (the sample) drawn from the cohort and consisting of 3154 respondents, it is now possible to establish two integrated files. One file, *the cohort file*, will comprise the original group of 12 270 boys of which up till now 11 591 have been studied. The second file contains the 3154 respondents of the sample (members of the sampled boys' families, usually the mothers of the boys). This file we shall refer to as *the family file*.

The cohort file contains an integration of the following kinds of information: birth data from 1953, school data from 1965 and from 1966, data from the official demographic registers as of 1975, and data on crime and delinquency from 1975–6. It must be remembered that the cohort always includes the family file.

The family file integrates the same birth data, demographic data, and data on crime and delinquency as are integrated in the cohort file, but school data is only from 1965; in addition this file includes all specific data on family conditions, relations, etc. from 1968. The information gathered will be catalogued in the next section of this chapter followed by a closer characterization of some of the major types of studies carried through within the context of the project as a whole.

In addition to the cohort and the sample, on which the longitudinal aspects of the project have to be based, a control sample has been drawn from the total Danish population and connected with Project Metropolitan. The control sample consists of 3852 Danish males and females randomly selected, and was drawn on a national basis in 1975. The control sample, among other things, contains

information similar to that of the metropolitan cohort and sample with respect to official demographic registrations and data concerning crime and delinquency.

Furthermore a number of ecological data have been gathered from the metropolitan area, mainly dating from the years around 1960. Thus it will be possible to study the interaction between cohort data concerning individuals and the ecological macrodata.

A catalogue of information obtained

Birth data from 1953. In Denmark births are entered into registers and birth certificates are made out with great care. When Project Metropolitan was finally started in 1965, its group of researchers began by studying and copying available information from such certificates and registers. In this way the following kinds of data have been obtained concerning 11 591 (94·47 per cent) of the total number of 12 270 boys born during that year within the area in question:

1. Date of birth.
2. Information concerning possible adoption.
3. Place of birth: Name of municipality.
4. Place of birth: Name of parish.
5–6. Permanent address 1953: Given as 3. and 4.
7. Place of birth: Medical service district.
8. Name of midwife.
9. Direct physical place of birth, such as in a clinic, a hospital, or at home.
10. Duration of birth measured in hours.
11. Whether single, twin, or multiple delivery.
12. Weight at birth measured in 100 g.
13. Height at birth measured in cm.
14. Mother's marital status.
15. Mother's age at delivery.
16. Father's social status at time of delivery.
17. Family name.
18. First name(s).

In 1965 about 5·5 per cent of the birth cohort had not been ascertained. The main reason for this defect has been found to be the number of deaths occuring from 1953 to 1965, of which not all had been identified or noted at the time of study in 1965. Category number 16 (father's social status) has been constructed on the basis of 23 occupational strata, all of them transformable to one or another of the recognized social class scales.

School data I 1965. In 1965 the members of the cohort were asked to fill in an elaborate questionnaire presented to them by their teachers during school hours in the class room together with their classmates; 9537 (77·7 per cent) of the cohort filled in the questionnaire while they were at school on a particular day in 1965. The questions below (19–56) comprised this questionnaire, thus covering data on the school system, peer popularity, father's social status, occupational preferences of boy, motivation for school attendance and education, leisure time activities, motivation for leisure time activities pursued or preferred, IQ, and creativity potential. The members of the cohort were approximately 12 years of age at the time of this questionnaire. The completed questionnaire yielded the following items of information:

19. Name of the school.
20. Whether the school was a private school or a municipal (public) school.
21. Form or grade of boy.
22. Father's occupation.
23. IQ-test (Härnquist). Range of scores 0–120.
24. IQ-test—verbal. Range of scores 0–40.
25. IQ-test—spatial. Range of scores 0–40.
26. IQ-test—inductive. Range of scores 0–40.

27. Creativity test (Mednick 1962). Range of scores 0–25.
28. Sociometric choices. Choice of 3 class-mates as companions in a given situation (travelling).
29. Choice of future occupation.
30. Reasons for having chosen a particular future occupation.
31. Whether respondent believes that he will reach a higher social or occupational level than that of his father.
32. Whether respondent is acquainted with anybody who has the occupation preferred by respondent.
33. Whether respondent has ever discussed his preferred choice of occupation with anybody.
34. Whether respondent is acquainted with anybody who does not like the occupation preferred by respondent.
35. When would respondent prefer to leave school.
36. Which school subjects does respondent like best.
37. How does he like to go to school.
38. How important is it, according to respondent's own opinion, to get high marks in school.
39. Is it necessary to do a lot of homework in order to get high marks in school.
40. What is done (how does one respond or react) if a teacher grumbles because one has not done one's homework.
41. The preferred leisure time activity.
42. Time spent daily on preferred leisure time activity.
43. Total amount of time spent on preferred leisure time activity.
44. How well (degree of eminence) is respondent able to do what he prefers to do during his leisure time.
45. How much does respondent read about what concerns his preferred leisure time activity.
46. Has respondent talked with people who are well informed about the kind of spare time activity which is preferred by him.
47. Membership of club or association etc. concerned with respondent's preferred spare time activity.
48. Attending of courses etc. concerning respondent's favourite leisure time activity.
49. If respondent would like to have more time available to pursue his preferred leisure time activity.
50. How does respondent view the prospects of moving away from home in order to study for a medical degree.
51. Would respondent want to become a doctor if it meant that he would have to wait longer before he could marry and have children.
52. Would respondent want to become a doctor if it meant that he would not be able to earn much money before the age of 25.
53. Would respondent want to become a doctor if it meant that he would have to go to school for another seven years before he could begin his medical studies.
54. 51 different occupations put in rank order by respondent according to his own preferences with regard to future jobs.
55. 33 leisure time interests put in rank order by respondent according to preference.
56. Last name of respondent.

School data II 1966. One year later, in 1966, the members of the cohort were asked to fill in another set of questions during school hours. Approximately the same number of respondents filled in the school questionnaires in 1966 as in 1965 (77·7 per cent). The information obtained was as follows:

57. Arithmetic test. Range of scores 0–9.
58. Danish language test (in writing). Range of scores 0–5.
59. Name of school.
60. Form or grade.
61. Father's occupation.

62. Structure of school classes, whether divided according to some academic criterion, or undivided.
63. Structure of respondent's particular class.
64. Whether the particular school class was classified as literary (theoretical) or not literary (practical) according to official educational criteria in use in Danish schools at the time of the study.

Some of the questions were answered by teachers concerning each of the boys.

Family data I and II 1968. In 1968 a random sample of 25 per cent of the original birth cohort (12 270 boys) was drawn, and the families of the boys in the sample were visited for personal interviews with the mothers or mother substitutes of the boys. This sample consists of three subsamples: a random sample comprising 3064 mothers of boys in the sample; a sample made up of the 10 per cent highest scoring boys on the IQ-test from the school data of 1965 (953 boys); and a sample comprised of the 10 per cent lowest scoring boys (953 boys). The three groups thus comprising the sample whose families were visited and whose mothers were interviewed add up to a total of 3833 families, after due corrections have been made for overlaps, deaths, etc. From this sample 3154 mothers (82·29 per cent) were actually interviewed.

The family survey has provided information about the following items:

65. Whether the person interviewed is the biological mother of the boy, stepmother, or mother substitute (e.g. grandmother or aunt).
66. Size of household.
67. Mother's marital status.
68. Father's age.
69. Father's place of birth.
70. Mother's age.
71. Mother's place of birth.
72. Time of marriage.
73. Place of marriage.
74. Place of residence since marriage.
75. Number of changes of address (removals) since marriage.
76. Number of children in family.
77. Boys in family in rank order according to age.
78. Girls in family in rank order according to age.
79. Boys in family in rank order according to school training (education).
80. Boys in family in rank order according to occupational training.
81. Mother's occupation.
82. Mother's place of work.
83. Size of mother's place of work.
84. Father's occupation.
85. Father's place of work.
86. Size of father's place of work.
87. Mother's school training (education).
88. Father's school training (education).
89. School training of mother's mother.
90. School training of mother's father.
91. School training of father's father.
92. School training of father's mother.
93. Mother's occupational training.
94. Father's occupational training.
95. Occupational training of mother's mother.
96. Occupational training of mother's father.
97. Occupational training of father's father.
98. Occupational training of father's mother.
99. Whether boy's grandparents are still alive.
100. Occupation of mother's father.

101. Occupation of father's father.
102. Size of residence.
103. Whether residence is owner-occupied or not.
104. Kind of residence (house, farm, flat, etc.).
105. Possession of durable consumer goods.
106. Possession of books.
107. Newspaper reading.
108. Reading of books.
109. Mother's memberships in associations, etc., and membership activities.
110. Father's membership in associations and membership activities.
111. Mother's participation in meetings, etc.
112. Father's participation in meetings, etc.
113. Degree of association with friends.
114. Political party allegiance and voting behaviour at the parliamentary election (*Folketingsvalg*) 22 Nov. 1966.
115. Party allegiance and voting behaviour at the parliamentary election (*Folketingsvalg*) 23 Jan. 1968.
116. Religious attitudes.
117. Mother's leisure time activities.
118. Father's leisure time activities.
119. Consciousness of social class.
120. Attitudes toward school attendance and education.
121. Whether boy has his own room or not.
122. Mother's height given in cm.
123. Father's height given in cm.
124. Boy's height given in cm.
125. Occupation of boy.
126. Boy's form or grade in school.
127. Kind of school.
128. Boy's work outside of school (other than school work).
129. Mother's evaluation of boy's school work.
130. Mother's estimation of boy's possibilities in passing examinations after ten years at school (realexamen) and/or after twelve years (*studenterexamen).*
131. Does father or mother help boy with his homework.
132. Mother's judgement concerning a suitable future occupation for boy.
133. Mother's actual suggestion of a future occupation for boy, chosen among 9 possible choices put before her.
134. Amount of interaction (being together) between boy, mother and/or father.
135. Co-operation between parents and boy with regard to boy's future opportunities.
136. Co-operation between parents and boy with regard to other matters.
137. Previous marital status of mother.
138. Previous marital status of father.
139. Whether mother has regretted her present marriage.
140. Mother's opinion of marriage as an institution.
141. Marital status of mother's parents.
142. Marital status of father's parents.
143. Mother's opinion concerning women working away from home.
144. Form of wedding ceremony at time of marriage (boy's parents).
145. Parent's mutual acquaintance before marriage.
146. Methods of birth control applied in family.
147. Distribution, spending, and control of family income.
148. Degree of equality between boy's parents.
149. Psychological climate in family, especially relations between boy and parents.
150. Principles of upbringing held and applied by boy's parents.
151. Time of day when the interview took place.
152. Whether boy had ever been victim of a criminal act.
153. Whether mother had ever been victim of a criminal act.

For every five families sampled an interview was attempted with the boy's father as well as with his mother. In the subsample thus obtained the fathers were asked to fill in a written questionnaire, which was less elaborate than the one on which the personal interviews with the mothers was based, although it contained identical or similar questions. The information obtained from interviewing the mothers has been filed as Family Data I, while information from the fathers' responses to the questionnaire has been filed as Family Data II. There were 401 fathers (40·3 per cent) who actually filled in the questionnaire.

Officially registered demographic data 1975. For 11 540 (94·05 per cent) of the original birth cohort of 12 270 boys a number of demographic data have been ascertained officially in 1975 through the appropriate public sources, as follows:

154. Present occupation of cohort member.
155. Marital status.
156. Form of wedding ceremony if married.
157. Membership of State Church.
158. Present residence.
159. Family name.
160. Time of marriage.

This data formed the basis of the study of crime and delinquency mentioned below, which was carried through from 1975 to 1976, when the boys were about 22 years old.

Data on crime and delinquency 1975–6. Of the 11 540 members of the cohort found in the official registers of Denmark in 1975, 4108 (35·6 per cent) have been registered by the police (Central Police Register in Copenhagen) for at least one punishable offence against the law up to January 1976. The information on crime and delinquency thus obtained concerning the cohort comprise data on the following items:

161. Year of first registered offence.
162. Police district where first registration was made.
163. Kinds of offences registered at first registration.
164. Name and place of court handling the first registered offence.
165. Decision or sentence made by prosecution and/or court concerning first registered offence.
166. Year of latest registered offence.
167. Police district where latest registration was made.
168. Kinds of offences registered at latest registration.
169. Name and place of court handling the latest registered offence.
170. Decision or sentence made by prosecution and/or court concerning latest registered offence.
171. Year of registration of most serious offence as measured by severity of sentence (decision).
172. Offence(s) registered in connection with most severe sentence (decision).
173. Name and place of court handling most serious offence registered.
174. Decision or sentence made by prosecution and/or court concerning most serious offence registered.
175. Offences and combinations of offences registered during the whole period of study for each person registered (up to January 1976 at the latest).
176. Total number of registrations per person during the whole period studied.
177. Whether boy has ever been registered as being taken care of by child welfare authorities.
178. Each offence or combination of offences noted by year of

registration in a perfect chronological order for each of the registered members of the cohort.

The study of registered crime and delinquency has been the latest major collection of data concerning the cohort, which had reached the age of about 23 in 1976 when the gathering of those data was completed. Thus the latest study of the cohort is a documentary study like the first one from 1965 concerning birth data from 1953.

The collection of data on registered crime and delinquency constitutes the first actual output of Project Metropolitan for which it is possible to utilize previously collected information as input, thus deriving the full advantage from the longitudinal research technique applied to a cohort.

The ecological study 1960. Based on available statistical information about each of the municipalities (parishes) and other local communities within the metropolitan area an ecological data register has been established in connection with the project. From this ecological register information on 70 variables or factors descriptive of the geographical area of the project are available. All the ecological factors stem from 1960 or thereabouts.

In order to establish an analytical instrument appropriate for the task and the computers available with regard to ecological material of Project Metropolitan, four elements or vectors have been selected from among the number of 70 factors:

179. Vector no. 1 is the general ecology vector, consisting of:
    1.1 and 1.2: Per cent single-family houses and per cent agricultural holdings in the area.
    1.3: Per cent workers in other than agricultural occupations (i.e. occupation of head of family).
    1.4: Per cent with an assessed income of 20 000 D.kr. or more per year.
    1.5: Per cent having property (capital) worth 100 000 D.kr. or more.
    1.6: Land value per hectare.
180. Vector no. 2 is the demographic vector, composed of:
    2.1: Per cent children under the age of 14 within the area.
    2.2: Per cent having reached the age of 65 or more.
    2.3: The male/female ratio of the area.
181. Vector no. 3 is the political vector, composed of;
    3.1: Size of poll (per cent voting) at parliamentary elections in the area.
    3.2: Per cent voting for socialist parties including the social-democratic party.
    3.3: The proportion of socialist party votes minus the social-democrats to the number of social-democrats in the area.

3.4: Per cent voting for the law on the preservation of nature when it was put to vote by referendum.
182. Vector no. 4 is the environmental or milieu vector, composed of:
    4.1: Number of burial mounds, round barrows (stone circles of the Bronze age), long barrows (of Neolithic age), dolmens, cairns, etc. found in the area.
    4.2: Number of houses in the area protected and scheduled as monuments of class A or B according to Danish law of preservation.
    4.3: Number of monuments and memorial tablets in the area.

Analytic orientation

Researchers involved in Project Metropolitan have been broadly oriented in their analytic directions. Kaare Svalastoga (1976) has suggested and described how a path analytic model could be used in analysing careers. Svalastoga's path model is composed of 56 variables of which 45 are predictor variables. Thirty-seven variables have to do with the boys of the cohort themselves, 11 with the mothers or the fathers of the boys, 6 with grandparents, and 2 with places of residence. The model contains 8 structural equations. In Svalastoga's own words: 'Thus, this will be a visit into the world of concrete reality approaches'. Several traditional analyses of the Markovian process type will be attempted with regard to social mobility and development of criminality. Since the cohort has been described over the period 1953–77 by 182 variables, it is in fact possible to correlate the actual observations with an enormous but still finite number of theoretically possible descriptive states. Methods of testing and analysing which are based on cybernetics and information theory will also be applied (for example, as discussed in Høgh 1976).

Project Metropolitan proceeds

The first phase of the collection of data will be closed in 1983 when the cohort has reached the age of 30. The corresponding first phase of analysis will then be concluded in 1987. From 1978 to 1983 information will be gathered with respect to the boys' marital relations and family of procreation, their employment and working conditions, politics and voting behaviour, consumer behaviour, mental health, and health conditions in general.

A bibliography of articles related to this research is available from the authors.

18. A mixed longitudinal interdisciplinary study of the growth and development of Dutch children

BIRTE PRAHL-ANDERSEN

Introduction

This paper provides a description of the mixed longitudinal, interdisciplinary study of the growth and development of Dutch children lately completed at the University of Nymegen, The Netherlands, under the direction of Professor Frans P. G. M. van der Linden and with the support of the Praeventiefonds (literally, funds for research in the prevention of disease). The design is of the mixed longitudinal, or linked cross-sectional, type, with overlapping cohorts. The original idea motivating the introduction of this class of designs was to 'accelerate' the classical longitudinal approach of collecting data for the estimation of age-specific norms, growth curves, growth rates, differential growth rates, etc., over a given period of time, but a number of additional benefits have been noted as these designs have been developed and applied (Prahl-Andersen *et al.* 1979).

Design of the study

In studying growth and developmental processes, variables other than simple chronological age must often be taken into account if we are to adequately characterize differences in the developmental patterns of the groups under consideration. Cohort, time-of-measurement, and learning (testing) effects may significantly interfere with our ability to directly study development if the traditional cross-sectional and longitudinal designs are used. Mixed longitudinal studies with well scheduled control groups, may better serve the scientific community in the design of studies dealing with the measurement of change.

In providing systematic treatment of an appropriate model from this point of view, Schaie developed a trifactorial model which isolates the contributions to developmental data of the three factors A = chronological age, C = cohort, and T = time of measurement (Schaie 1965). In this model, development D is viewed as a function of these variables, $D = f(A,C,T)$, in contrast with the traditional unifactorial designs which view development simply as a function of age, $D = f(A)$. Despite the obvious dependencies which exist between the three components of the trifactorial model (e.g., given an individual's age and cohort, time of measurement is determined), it is possible to isolate and study their effects. Depending on which of the three factors is viewed as being determined by the other two, we get particular cases of Schaie's model called, respectively, the cohort-sequential design; the time-sequential design; and the cross-sequential design. Which particular design is adopted in a given situation depends on the purposes of the investigation and the sets of *a priori* assumptions deemed most reasonable in that situation. For the purposes of the present discussion, the particular Schaie design actually used in the Nymegen Growth Study, namely Schaie's 'most efficient' design, is illustrated in Fig. 18.1

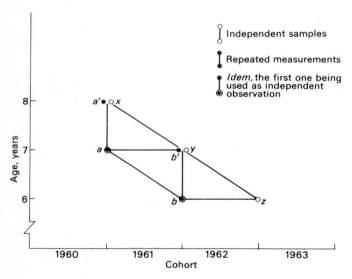

FIG. 18.1. Schaie's 'most efficient' design.

Interdisciplinary aspects of the study

The interdisciplinary approach to the study of normal growth and development of children has seldom been adopted, and the attempts that have been made have not been very successful. The main problems seem to be lack of communication, integration, and organization. Despite the original intentions, the problems are usually attacked within the traditions of the single disciplines.

In the Nymegen study an interdisciplinary approach is applied to some problems of normal growth and development of children. At the start of the study an analysis was made of the variables and the interaction of variables to be studied. This selection was made by a steering committee of highly skilled and educated specialists in the different disciplines included in the study. These were the medical, dental, sociomedical, and psychological disciplines. The development of interdisciplinarity is influenced by at least three main factors: development of society, development of individuals, and development of organization and communication. Also it should be noted that it is very seldom possible to start an interdisciplinary study right away. This approach requires a period of introduction and, because different disciplines often are organized differently, it also requires a compromise on the organizational level. Thus only after some time has been given to these processes can an interdisciplinary team be successful.

In this study the problems of communication and organization were solved by the establishment of a co-ordinating team with one member from each discipline, and a representative from the statistical consultation group. This team intercepted many problems that otherwise would have had to be solved by the steering committee (which as a matter of fact, became rather superfluous). The management of the funds and politics of employment were carried out separately by the administration of the dental school. The aim of the co-ordinating team was to distribute information, to preserve optimal communication, to anticipate and solve organizational problems, and to facilitate quick decision-making. Problems of a more general nature and of importance to all participating scientists were discussed in a few yearly meetings. The development of the scientific hypothesis and the interdisciplinary teamwork were promoted during retreats, two- or three-day workshops for the whole scientific group with consultants.

In this study the medical and dental disciplines represent the rational mind whereas the psychological and sociological disciplines represent more abstract and philosophical thinking. The first-mentioned disciplines usually apply direct measurements and, when studying development with sequential examinations, use the same measuring device; this is in contrast to the psychological and sociological disciplines which use indirect measurements and different measuring instruments. These observations call for a careful preparation and a patient coaching of the developing interdisciplinary teamwork.

The conduct of the Nymegen growth study

The Nymegen Growth Study was designed to provide information concerning the growth and development of Dutch children from 4 to 14 years of age. Six overlapping cohorts (generations of children) were studied for a five-year period, from February 1971 through February 1976.

In Nymegen approximately 2050 children could be considered for the study, meaning that their birth dates fitted the planned age ranges (4 to 9, 7 to 12, and 9 to 12 years of age) and the time intervals planned for examinations. On the basis of the distribution of the school vacation, four equally distributed periods of six weeks were chosen for examination. The time between two subsequent periods of examinations was long enough to enable the investigators to evaluate the data collected and store them in the computer. From municipality records a total of 900 children were selected at random and invited to participate in the study. In the letter of invitation the purpose of the study and a promise of free dental care for the duration of the study period was given. The parents of 486 children accepted this invitation. These families are referred to as participants, in contrast to the 414 non-participants who either did not answer or declined the invitation to participate in the study. The sex-specific sample sizes and the dates of birth for each of the six cohorts are given in Table 18.1

TABLE 18.1

Sample sizes and birth dates for the six cohorts comprising the Nymegen Growth Study

Cohort	Sex	Sample size	Birth date
1	M	39	Aug./Sept. 1961
	F	45	
2	M	36	Nov./Dec. 1961
	F	52	
3	M	47	Nov./Dec. 1963
	F	38	
4	M	39	Feb./Mar. 1964
	F	49	
5	M	37	Nov./Dec. 1966
	F	27	
6	M	34	Feb./Mar. 1967
	F	43	
Total	M	232	
	F	254	

Each examination period lasted five to six weeks and corresponded to the period of birth dates plus 3 and/or 6 months. The examination schedule is illustrated in Fig. 18.2. The horizontal axis gives the dates of examinations, the vertical axis the ages of the participants in the study. The cohorts 1 and 2 (Table 18.1) were examined four times a year, the cohorts 3 and 4 were examined twice a year to the age of 9 years then subsequently four times a year, and the cohorts 5 and 6 were examined twice a year.

The three socio-medical enquiries were carried out in 1972, 1974, and 1975. This part of the study was realized through interviews with the parents at their homes. The first socio-medical enquiry consisted of an extensive questionnaire which was presented to both participants and non-participants at home in order to check on the representativeness of the participating sample.

The T-points in Fig. 18.2 refer to the measurement schedule for control groups (approximately 20 boys and 20 girls), matched by age and sex with the study groups. These control groups were selected at random from children not so far addressed by the study and were included in order to test hypotheses concerning learning effects or possible effects of measurement on the study groups. It may be noted that the birth dates for each of the cohorts are not equally spaced along the age axis and consequently the amount of overlap between adjacent cohorts was not constant. This departure from the standard symmetrical mixed longitudinal design was due to pragmatic considerations.

As indicated in Fig. 18.2 a pilot study was conducted in 1970 to test the feasibility of the proposed measurement battery and number of children to be examined in one day. The result was that during each examination which took place in the morning, approximately 170 measurements were taken on each child. Twelve children a day were measured from 9 to 12 o'clock, totalling about 300 children during one examination period. Separate appointments were made for dental treatment. Demographic information and medical history for each of the children were collected at the start of the study. Only healthy, Caucasian children were incorporated in the study. The measurements consisted of a somatic and a psychological part with a time ration of 2:3, which meant that a child was subjected to psychological examination for one hour with half an hour for organizational problems.

A flow chart illustrating the ways in which these various kinds of data were recorded and processed is given in Fig. 18.3. This is presented to give an overview of the kinds of data being collected; a more

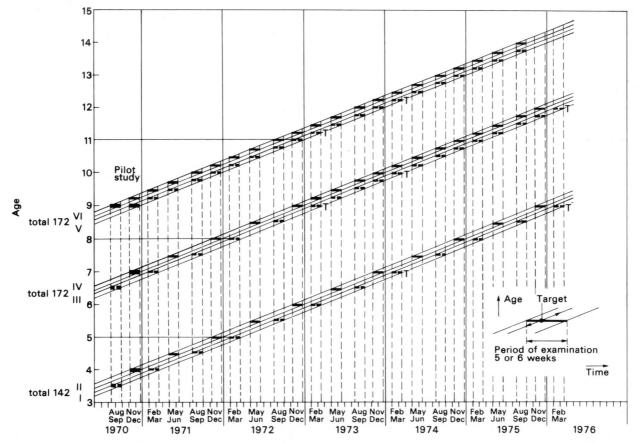

FIG. 18.2. Examination schedule.

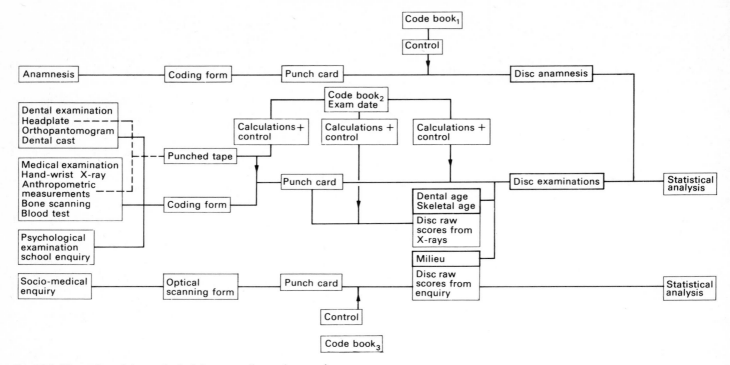

FIG. 18.3. Illustration of the method of data recording and processing.

detailed description of the definition of variables and data recording are presented elsewhere (Prahl-Andersen and Kowalski 1973).

The personnel necessary for the performance of the examinations were:

1. A physician;
2. A dentist;
3. Two dental assistants;
4. A psychologist;
5. An assistant to the psychologist;
6. An X-ray technician;
7. An assistant for the anthropological measurements;
8. A doctor's assistant;
9. A secretary.

The physician, the psychologist, and one of the dental assistants were active during the entire five-year period. This was thought to be important because the children became accustomed to these people and were possibly more comfortable.

The time between examinations was used for data processing and analysis. For this purpose a full time statistician and two half time programmers were employed.

It was felt that one of the main problems in a study containing a longitudinal component would be to keep the children in the study. Therefore, special attention was paid to public relations. The parents were asked to accompany the child at the first visit. During this visit the project was introduced and its purpose explained to the parents and children. Information on the procedures during the examinations was given in the form of a video tape shown on a television set. The authorities of the school the children attended were informed about the study, and permission was asked for leave of absence. Also, the local dentists and the municipal school dental and medical services were informed and asked for approval, as were the local physicians. The children were called in for examination by a letter which also contained an enquiry about past illness and possible start of menstruation. At appropriate times an enquiry was made about the name of the school the children were attending. The children brought this questionnaire with the answers at the time of examinations.

The children were picked up at their homes and brought back after the examinations; in this way the transportation was taken care of by the study. The schools which the children were attending were informed as to the time of the examination and the absence of the children from school. During the study psychological and medical advice was given to the parents, if wanted or felt necessary, in addition to the full dental care already mentioned. The children were invited to a yearly party, and a social photograph was taken at the start and at the end of the study and given to the parents. The control groups also had photographs taken and presented as an appreciation of their participation. Three booklets were composed during the five years with information on the study and the results; these booklets were presented to the parents and the school authorities.

At the end of the study, 121 children were under orthodontic treatment and all children except 7 had conservative dental treatment by the dentist connected to the study. This treatment was executed between examination periods. The result of these efforts was a drop-out rate of 12·4 per cent at the end of the study. The main reason for quitting the study was moving of the family to another part of The Netherlands. In some cases the children did come back to Nymegen for the examinations, in which case the study paid for transportation. The blood tests were experienced as being very unpleasant and caused some children to quit the study. In Table 18.2 the reasons for drop-out are shown. Much time and effort were put into the organization of the study, with special attention paid to public relations.

Data processing

The total measurement battery included approximately 150 different anthropometric, dental, and psychological quantities. In addition, a series of sociological inventories were taken in 1972, 1974, and 1975. Each family participating in the study filled out the questionnaires containing 2000 scores on 900 different items. When recoded and/or transformed data are added, the total number of measurements recorded per individual was up to 9200.

TABLE 18.2

Number of children who never missed an appointment, number of missing dates, and drop-outs

	Sample size	Complete series	One missing date	Two missing dates	Three missing dates	Four missing dates	Drop-out	Not Caucasian or seriously ill	Max. number of periods
Males									
1	39	24	7	—	1	—	7	—	20
2	36	20	6	2	—	—	6	2	20
3	47	33	2	—	—	—	8	4	16
4	39	23	5	3	1	2	3	2	16
5	37	28	3	1	1	—	2	2	10
6	34	23	1	—	—	—	8	2	10
Subtotal	232	151	24	6	3	2	34	12	
Females									
1	45	32	5	3	—	—	5	—	20
2	52	32	9	3	1	—	6	1	20
3	38	28	4	—	—	—	5	—	16
4	49	44	1	—	—	—	4	—	16
5	27	20	5	—	—	—	2	—	10
6	43	31	2	—	—	—	4	6	10
Subtotal	254	187	26	6	1	—	26	7	
Total	486	338	50	12	4	2	60	19	

Faced with the magnitude of the observation vectors and the fact that a very flexible updating system would be needed to accommodate the varying measurement and preprocessing schedules of the several disciplines involved in the study, it was all but mandatory that a study-specific system be developed (see Fig. 18.4).

None of the existing general packages was adequate to handle the special problems associated with the more complex structure of the mixed longitudinal design. The longitudinal sequences making up the design also required that special attention be paid to missing data; since several existing multivariate analysis programs operate only on complete sets of data, ignoring cases that contain any missing observations, we needed a special system that would allow us to update the observation vectors to include temporary estimated values at selected time points, along with some facility for monitoring the pattern of missing data points.

The system operates on the IBM 370/158 computer housed at U.R.C., the Computing Centre of the University of Nymegen. All files are permanently stored on disk and each data file has four back-up copies recorded on magnetic tape. (For further details see Van't Hof *et al*. 1977.) Data quality control is of special importance since mixed longitudinal data sets are comprised of linked longitudinal segments. Four programs were developed to deal with this problem (see Fig. 18.5). Data analysis strategies which incorporate formal procedures for assessing the impact of the age, cohort, time

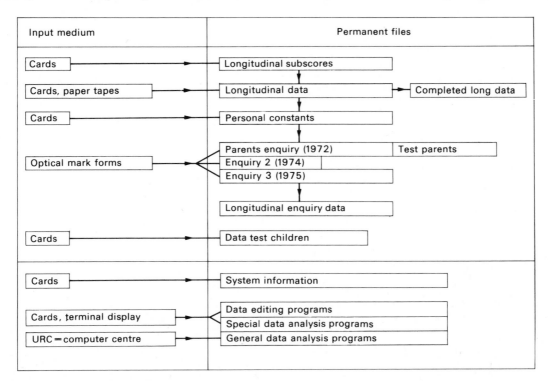

FIG. 18.4. A study-specific system for data processing.

of measurement, and/or testing effects, on developmental data, have been used as well as more traditional data analytic strategies (BMD, CLUSTAN, SPSS, etc.).

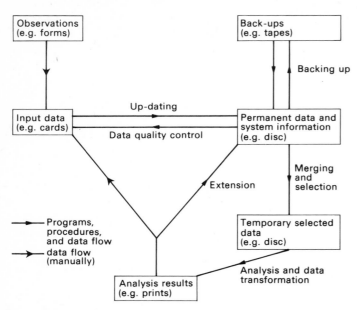

Fig. 18.5. Data analysis strategies.

Psychological development: problems and preliminary results

(Mönks *et al.* 1975)

The measurement of psychological development presents many difficulties. The first problem to be encountered in every statistical investigation is the procurement of a representative sample. In the context of the Nymegen Growth Study, this problem presents itself in two distinct ways, namely (1) only slightly more than one-half of the families randomly selected for inclusion in the study agreed to participate, and (2) some of the participants failed to actively continue in the study. In an attempt to assess the impact of non-participation on the representativeness of the sample, a concerted effort was made to obtain at least certain base-line information from the non-participating families in order to compare the attributes of this group with those of the participants. The problem of drop-outs, i.e., selective survival, has also long been recognized as a potentially important source of bias in longitudinal studies. We have been fortunate in this respect that only 12·4 per cent attrition has been realized. Nonetheless, the presence of missing data presents difficult data-analytic problems [Kowalski 1972 and Kowalski and Guire 1974], especially when the missing data points are not randomly distributed, and when we are reserving judgement on decisions like whether, in particular cases, certain missing data values can be estimated, as opposed to summarily excluding all cases containing missing data from the analysis. It should be mentioned in this connection that, owing to the mixed longitudinal structure of the study, cases presenting incomplete data may be of some value in cross-sectional comparisons even if they have to be excluded from the longitudinal component of the study.

Another problem in the assessment of psychological change, especially relevant in estimating differences between children of different ages, is that different instruments for measuring such parameters as intelligence, school achievement, etc. must often be used. Here the question of the correlation between instruments becomes critical, because when different instruments are used to assess the same variables at each age level, age differences are confounded with differences between the instruments. While every effort has been made to employ only standardized (directly comparable) test instruments, we have when changing instruments, administered both the old and new tests to a subsample of the children in order to check on this supposed comparability. Most of the correlations have been of the order of *r* = 0·70 to *r* = 0·80, attesting to definite relationships between these instruments, but signalling that considerable care should still be exercised in the interpretation of age differences estimated in this manner.

Of course, an even more fundamental problem involves the correlations between the same tests when administered to the same children, i.e., the reliability of the instruments. The correlations are computed from data obtained on the 150 children comprising the oldest cohorts (born August/September 1961 or November/December 1961) in the study. The periods refer to time of measurement, a difference of one period representing a three-month time difference. The correlations between the two forms of the test range between 0·56 and 0·77, while the test/retest correlations range from 0·64 to 0·75. Our results would tend to indicate that although the reliability diminishes with increasing time between the test and retest, it remains at a reasonably high level even after the passage of a year's time.

The fact that the one-year test/retest correlation coefficients for the verbal (number facility and spatial relations) subtests are substantial, each attaining the 1 per cent level of significance, lends some support to the hypothesis that there is a second-order general factor at work in addition to the primary mental abilities and, moreover, that these three subtests are not completely independent of one another. Some additional evidence of the existence of a second-order general factor of intelligence has been obtained. The fact that there is a fairly consistent proportion of the common variance in the IPAT and PMA measurements can be developed to provide such evidence; but the details of this argument will be postponed until we have had the opportunity to analyse all of the relevant data. In addition to the psychological measurements explicitly discussed above, the Nymegen Growth Study is also accumulating data on the relationship between role-taking and social intelligence; the validity of teacher evaluations; the development of achievement motivation and its relationship with school achievement, intelligence, and personality characteristics; child-rearing practices; and a number of interdisciplinary relationships, e.g., the relationship between dental hygiene practices and personality characteristics. The investigators intend to compare the longitudinal results with existing norms, most of which are based on cross-sectional findings, and would be happy to enter into collaborative studies contrasting results from Nymegen with those found in other populations.

The socio-medical enquiries

Information on the socio-cultural background of the participating children was collected through three enquiries in 1972, 1974, and 1975. The number of parents interviewed can be seen in Table 18.3. A system based on two elements was used for data collection: a standard optical mark reader form, and a thin cardboard overlay of the same size on which the questionnaire was printed. The question overlays are placed over the optical mark reader form;

Table 18.3

Number of parents participating in three enquiries (1972, 1974, and 1975) into the socio-cultural background of the participating children

Cohort	Enq. 1		Enq. 2		Enq. 3		Max. number	Birth date
	M	F	M	F	M	F		
Boys								
1	35	35			31	31	39	Aug./Sept. 1961
2	30	31	30	30	30	30	36	Nov./Dec. 1961
3	40	40			37	37	47	Nov./Dec. 1963
4	32	33	30	30	28	31	39	Febr./March 1964
5	31	32			28	31	37	Nov./Dec. 1966
6	25	26	23	23	22	23	34	Febr./March 1967
Girls								
7	38	38			37	37	45	Aug./Sept. 1961
8	48	49	42	45	42	44	52	Nov./Dec. 1961
9	30	31			28	30	38	Nov./Dec. 1963
10	37	37	36	37	39	42	49	Febr./March 1964
11	21	21			19	20	27	Nov./Dec. 1966
12	34	34	30	30	32	35	43	Febr./March 1967
Partic.	401	407	191	195	373	391	486	
Non-Partic.	170	181					185	
Total	571	588	191	195	373	391		

they are provided with cut-outs punched at those places where an answer can be given by means of a black line on the optical mark reader form underneath. With this method the data collection and data providing went very quick. The optical mark forms were read at a speed of 1000 forms per hour with 43 columns per card to be punched. Less than 1 per cent refused. Since recruitment into the study was based on an appeal for co-operation emphasizing the social value of the information gathered and an offer of free dental care for participants throughout the duration of the study, the importance of contrasting the groups with respect to such parameters as social milieu, health-related attitudes, and income was immediately apparent. Analysis of these data revealed that the lower class Dutch families were slightly underrepresented in the sample when contrasted with the economic stratification of the city of Nymegen. While the random sampling procedure itself did fairly represent this group, even an offer of free dental care did not induce a proportionate number of the lower class families to participate in the study. The questionnaires were factor analysed and the corresponding factor structures of the two groups (participants and nonparticipants) are currently being compared in an attempt to discover further characteristics of the group of participants which might limit the eventual generalization of the findings of the study to the entire Dutch population.

The further aspects of main interest investigated were:

1. Attitudes towards bringing up children and towards school;
2. Medical attitudes;
3. General attitudes, such as aspiration, alienations, etc.;
4. Relation man/woman;
5. Social background, cultural educational level, etc.;
6. Attitudes towards orthodontic treatment.

Summary

A harmonious growth and development of normal children is mainly dependent on somatic, psychological, and social well-being. Therefore, whenever development of children is to be studied it should be with an interdisciplinary approach and with a design that recognizes the important role of cohort, time-of-measurement, and testing effects in the study of change.

The design and methods are described for the Nymegen Growth Study, a mixed longitudinal and interdisciplinary study of growth and development of Dutch children from four to fourteen years of age. The study lasted from 1971 to 1976.

19. Project growth and health of teenagers: a mixed longitudinal study (the Netherlands)

H. C. G. KEMPER

Purpose

The purpose of this paper is to describe a so-called mixed longitudinal study of teenagers. This investigation has been set up to describe the course of the physical and mental development of teenagers and to study whether there is a period of deterioration in the health status of the growing population. The population studied consists of girls and boys of 12 and 13 years of age, pupils from two secondary schools around Amsterdam. The same children will be studied for four consecutive years. Physical and mental health are described in terms of body build, body composition, motor performance, personality traits, attitudes, and social interactions. In order to find explanations for the age changes in the above-mentioned variables, we simultaneously measured biological age, normal daily diet, and habitual physical activity.

The mixed longitudinal design

In developmental studies three main designs can be distinguished: a longitudinal approach, a cross-sectional approach, and a time-lag approach. While each of these three designs can be used to measure changes resulting from age, cohort, and time-of-measurement effects, those effects cannot be isolated. In view of these insufficiencies we compromised by setting up a mixed longitudinal study with four repeated measurements (1976, 1977, 1978, 1979) in two overlapping cohorts (1963 and 1964) (Fig. 19.1). Each of the 8 groups (G_1, G_2, G_3, G_4, G_5, G_6, G_7, and G_8) can be defined by the various combinations of the factors age (A), cohort (C), and time of measurement (T) (Van't Hof et al. 1976). In this system we have 8 equations with eleven parameters:

4 time-of-measurement effects (T_{76}, T_{77}, T_{78}, and T_{79});

5 age effects (A_{13}, A_{14}, A_{15}, A_{16}, and A_{17}); and
2 cohort effects (C_{64} and C_{65}).

As such, this system cannot be solved without imposing two additional assumptions:

(1) The sum of all time-of-measurement effects is zero;
(2) A one-year difference in birth does not cause cohort effects.

The advantage of this approach is that prior to the experiment it identifies all the possible effects present in the model and brings forward the assumptions necessary to set up the experiment.

So far we have omitted from consideration learning or test effects. Repeated measurements and treatment effects can bring about disturbing influences in longitudinal studies. These test effects can be separated when we select suitable control groups without repeated measurements. Therefore we performed a second mixed longitudinal study concurrently on a comparable school. In this school instead of repeated measurements, independent samples are taken at each of the four times of measurement. In this design, comparing data of the same cohorts from the two schools' test effects may appear to be combined with possible school effects. When the measurements are taken for the first time in both schools, school effects can be isolated (Kemper and Van't Hof 1978).

Subjects and methods

This mixed longitudinal study was carried out in two secondary schools: Pius X Lyceum (Amsterdam) and Ignatius College (Purmerend). The choice of both schools was not arbitrary but rather, was provided for organizational reasons. Therefore the population studied cannot be considered as an aselect sample of the teenage population in the Netherlands or Amsterdam.

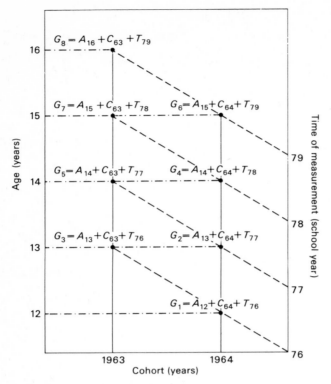

FIG. 19.1 The mixed longitudinal design in two cohorts (C_{63} and C_{64}) with four times of measurement (T_{76}, T_{77}, T_{78}, and T_{79}) gives five age groups (A_{12}, A_{13}, A_{14}, A_{15}, and A_{16}).

For practical reasons the two cohorts, 1963 and 1964, are defined as the pupils participating in the first and second forms of both schools during the school year 1976–7. In the first year we started with a total number of 325 boys and 340 girls. Pupils who stay in the course of the study remain in the same cohort, and in that way selective drop-out will not appear. All measurements take place in the course of the school year during regular school hours. Most of the measurements are performed in a mobile research unit (10×3, 5×2, 5 m) placed in the neighbourhood of the school.

The sample was contacted by the director of the schools. The purpose of the project was explained in an information booklet. In the course of the first year we organized school evenings for the pupils and their parents. On these occasions we presented a 16-mm colour film *Growing up fit*, which was especially made for this project, and discussed the objectives and methods of the project. A medical examination to determine the level of health of the pupils, insofar as this is measured by freedom from injury, ailment, abnormality, or disease, preceded the physiological and performance tests described below.

Physiological characteristics

In the following we summarize the measurements that are included:

(1) Body build and body composition by anthropometric measurements according to the International Biological Programme (Weiner and Lourie 1969): height and weight three times a year in order to make a better tracing of the height spurt, 3 circumferences, 4 skinfolds, and 4 diameters.

(2) Serum cholesterol in venous blood (Abell *et al.* 1952).

(3) Forced Expiratory Volume in one second related to the Vital Capacity (FEV%).

(4) Forward-backward bend of the thoracolumbar spine by means of an optical system (Snijders 1971).

(5) Skeletal maturity is determined by X-ray evaluation of the bones of wrist and hand by the TW II method (Tanner *et al.* 1975).

(6) 8 basic physical performance tests (Kemper and Verschuur 1977a). These tests have been selected as representing the more important and measurable aspects, for example: running speed (10×5 meter sprint), arm speed ($50 \times$ plate tapping), static arm strength (arm pull, Bettendorff dynamometer), explosive leg strength (standing high jump), muscular endurance of the arms (flexed arm hang), of trunk/leg (10 leg lifts), flexibility (sitting trunk forward flexion), and aerobic power (12 min run-walk endurance run).

(7) The capacity for performing maximum aerobic power is related to the capacity of the cardiovascular–respiratory systems to deliver oxygen to active tissue. Maximal aerobic power is measured with a direct method using a standard treadmill test. The speed of the treadmill is set to 8 km/h and after an accommodation period(3×2 min against a slope of 0, $2\frac{1}{2}$, and 5 per cent respectively), the slope is increased every 2 min by $2\frac{1}{2}$ per cent. The test is continued until exhaustion is reached. The test score is slated as the maximum oxygen uptake ($\dot{V}O_2$ max). It is measured directly by monitoring respiratory gas exchanges and pulmonary ventilation per min. Oxygen consumption (STPD) is determined by an Ergo-analyser (Mijnhardt B. V.) consisting of infrared CO_2 and paramagnetic O_2 analysers and a dry Parkinson–Cowan Volumeter (Kemper *et al.* 1976a).

Psychological characteristics

The primary objective is to collect data on a broad spectrum of the mental development of a teenage population measured as personality traits, achievement motivation, and attitudes. Moreover it is supposed that mental and physical development are very closely connected to each other. Statements of opinion about the psychological effects of exercise have been a part of the literature on psychosomatic relationships for many years. An examination of earlier research indicates that most of the studies have utilized research designs that do not readily lend themselves to interpretation in terms of cause-effect relationships (McLoy-Layman 1974). Use of more pre- and post-test types of studies and longitudinal studies with appropriate control groups can clarify the confusion about the relationship between physical and psychological characteristics of the same individual during adolescent growth. The questionnaires involved are:

(1) NPV-J, The Netherlands Personality Inventory, youth-version (Bücking *et al.* 1975).

(2) PMT-K, the Performance Motivation Test, children-version (Hermans 1971).

(3) Group coherence inventory, adapted according to the SAGS (Defares *et al.* 1970).

Educational characteristics

The set-up of this mixed longitudinal study was actuated by previous investigations in 12- and 13-year-old boys with the intention to acquire information about the effects of physical education, varied in work intensity (Kemper *et al.* 1971), and in frequency of the number of lessons a week (Kemper 1973; Kemper *et al.* 1976b). On the one hand we should therefore pay special attention to describing changes in teaching behaviour from the pupil's viewpoint, i.e., atttudes of the pupils towards physical education lessons. On the other hand and in conjunction with these everyday observations of pupils, videotaped lessons are taken during each school year. With the aid of a Physical Education Interaction Analysis System (PEIAS), the behaviour of the physical education teachers is systematically observed and coded in a number of social–emotional categories in real time (Tavecchio *et al.* 1976).

Daily food intake and habitual physical activity

Caloric input from food intake is regulated so as to correspond to caloric output from the amount of physical activity in a normal healthy organism. It is assumed that in most teenagers there is a dramatic fall in daily physical activity (motorized bicycles, for example, in the Netherlands are permitted from the age of 16). This goes with a change in daily food intake (snacks and alcohol).

In an interview with the pupils, completed with information from their mothers, a dietitian will measure the daily food intake by way of a cross-check method (Pekkarinen 1970). Reliability of the given quantities will be enhanced by asking the pupils, e.g. to grease butter bread and to indicate the sizes of potatoes, spoons, etc. used at home.

Because physical activity of teenagers is not only a matter of sports clubs and/or physical education, it is necessary to develop objective methods for the measurement of physical activity during spare time. The choice in our project is based on these subjoined demands: minimal influence on normal behaviour; continuous registration over a period of at least 24 hours; and applicable in large numbers of subjects. As to the measurement methods, we have chosen:

(1) Registration of heart rate during 48 hours with a portable 8-register heart beat integrator;
(2) Registration of vertical displacements of the body by means of pedometers worn from the waist. The restriction of this simple method is that neither intensity nor all kinds of physical activities (bicycling, rowing) can be registered (Kemper and Verschuur 1977b)

Aside from the observational methods we also use a question-naire interview, by which an estimate is made of the weekly time spent in various activities over the preceding months. The activities are differentiated on three levels: light (5–7 cal/min), moderate (7–10 cal/min), and heavy (greater than 10 cal/min).

Data analysis and results

Since this project started in August 1976, data collection is still in progress. All data are stored on punch cards for computer analysis. The project team consists of two physiologists, three psychologists, a dietitian, two computer experts, and a secretary.

Acknowledgements

This research project is performed in the Laboratory of Health Sciences (Prof. dr. R. L. Zielhuis) and the Laboratory of Psychophysiology (Prof. dr. P. Visser) of the University of Amsterdam. This investigation is supported by a grant from the Praeventiefonds and the Stichting voor Onderzoek van het Onderwijs in The Hague, The Netherlands (project number 0255).

20. Individual development and environment: a longitudinal study in Sweden

D. MAGNUSSON and A. DUNÉR

Introduction

The planning of the project started in 1964 and the first data collection took place during the spring semester of 1965. From its beginning, the project has been performed under the responsibility of the two authors of this report. In a monograph published in 1975, the purpose, the research strategy, the methodological problems, the groups of individuals studied, the methods for data collection and data treatment, the variables covered, and the main results of seven cross-sectional studies were presented (Magnusson *et al.* 1975; see also Magnusson 1978).

The problems

What importance for development do disturbances in behaviour of various kinds impose? Are there reasons to be concerned if a ten-year-old child is anxious, restless, or unruly, if he is unmotivated for his school work, etc.? To what extent is it possible to predict the later development of a child? We need to obtain answers to these kinds of questions, so that we can allocate resources in the most efficient ways whereby we can contribute towards improving the prospects of those children who run the risk of having a dismal future.

Important problems concerning children and their development and the obstacles which they meet along the way are difficult to study in a reliable manner. The difficulties in obtaining reliable answers are in fact problems of research strategy. It is only too easy to draw conclusions regarding the causes of problems by looking at conditions that are operating simultaneously and which may give rise to, for example, undesirable forms of behaviour on the part of pupils. A radical solution of problems often requires a knowledge of factors leading to the problem situation, factors which may have been at work for many years. It is necessary to follow the same group of individuals for long periods of life to be able to achieve such knowledge. Most researchers are busy getting fast answers to the many problems, following rapid changes of society. Often they do not take the time to consider the fact that they are working with problems which call for a longitudinal strategy. They attempt to elucidate the problems with data from one single occasion or too short a period of investigation. The shortcomings are often disguised by advanced experimental designs and statistical techniques.

During the school years all children have one part of their environment in common. At school there are possibilities of observing and, with limited resources, of obtaining essential information about a large sample of children under similar conditions. At the same time the school and the class comprise a part of the environment which plays an important role in the development of the children.

The relation between the individual and a social system may be viewed from two main standpoints. One of these is the agreement between the individual's behaviour and the demands that define his role in the system as judged from the viewpoint of the system. The other is the agreement between the individual's needs, motives, and evaluations on the one hand, and on the other the rewards he gains judged from his own viewpoint. The first of these aspects may be called the individual's *extrinsic* adjustment and the second his *intrinsic* or subjective adjustment. From the definitions given it follows (a) that the measures of extrinsic adjustment are to be found in reports and judgements by others, and (b) that the main direct measures of intrinsic adjustment are to be obtained in reports from the individual himself. Derived measures as indicators of intrinsic adjustment may be obtained from behavioural data and from reports and judgements by others.

The demand for a certain role behaviour may emanate in two ways: either from a production process in which the individual is involved, in which case it is then a question of what we usually call achievement; or from the social needs of members of a system, where it is then a question of a certain social behaviour or interaction. It should be observed that the individual's subjective adjustment in relation to a certain social system is dependent not only on his needs and the rewards he receives. Adjustment also concerns his expectations of need satisfaction in the relevant relationship.

In the study of children and their possibilities of developing into healthy and harmonious adults, it is of special interest to concentrate on children with problems of adjustment. Various indicators of intrinsic and extrinsic maladjustment and various ways children have of coping with problem situations should be considered with special interest.

Discrepancies between the demands made on an individual in a social system and the individual's behaviour elicit measures within the system, aimed at influencing the individual so that the discrepancies are reduced. In some cases, a modification of the demands may be possible. When the discrepancies exceed a certain level, the system expels the individual. At a place of work this means that the individual is dismissed. Transferring an individual to a less responsible position, which implies a change of role, or removing him to another subsystem, have similar implications. In some societies a drastic measure used is to take the individual into custody or isolate him in an institution. Viewed from another angle, such a measure may be regarded as an attempt to influence the individual so that he can later satisfy the demands of society.

Every step taken by a society which implies sanctions against an individual may be used as a criterion of what that society considers to be extrinsic adjustment. It may be more difficult to find equivalent criteria within social systems at lower levels, e.g. at places of work, since the sanctions there often do not have the same formal character.

When the discrepancy between the individual's intrinsic needs and the situational conditions exceeds a certain level, the individual may leave the system if that is possible. This deliberate act is an element in an active process of adjustment, adjustment by choice of system or role. It may be an indicator of a disturbed state of adjustment, but to ascertain this, it is necessary to know the underlying circumstances. If, for one reason or another, the individual considers it impossible to leave the system, and cannot affect his adjustment by influencing the external situation or by modifying his own intrinsic structure, we may expect this to affect his personality system or one or more of its subsystems. This can take the form of various symptoms which may be manifest or extrinsic behaviour, or

certain states or processes in the biological system. It may be added that phenomena which are symptoms according to some criteria may also be regarded as adjustment reactions. Change of work may be an indication of maladjustment but also an active step in a natural adjustment process.

The purpose of the project

In very general terms, the aim of the project is to study how an individual's life situation as an adult, as it can be described by others and as it is experienced by the individual himself, has its roots in a developmental process in which potential person factors interact with physical, social, and psychological factors in the environment. One element of the purpose of the project is to identify characteristics, types of behaviour or reactions which, alone or in combination with each other, or with certain environmental factors, indicate that an individual runs the risk of entering a state of prolonged and serious maladjustment. Another element is to investigate the role of environmental factors. An attempt is made to acquire knowledge of the causes of extrinsic and intrinsic maladjustment, thereby providing a basis for therapeutic and prophylactic measures from the school or other organs of society.

The general formulation of the purpose has been broken down into more specific terms to be useful for steering the planning and performance of the project. From the start, data collection and data treatment have been concentrated on a few problem areas, of which the main ones are the following:

(1) The predictive value of early indicators of possible maladjustment. Stability of single adjustment symptoms or patterns of symptoms, and sequences of changes (see Magnusson and Backteman, 1977a, b).
(2) The educational and vocational career and its impact on the life situation (see Dunér, 1978; Ekehammar, 1977, 1978).
(3) The developmental process underlying criminal behaviour and alcohol addiction (see Olofsson, 1971; Stattin, 1979).
(4) Norms and values and their role for the adult life situation (see Henrikson, 1973).
(5) Neglect, isolation, and rejection at an early age and their relation to the adult life situation (see Zettergren, 1978).

Research strategy

A number of requirements are to be fulfilled in order to attain the goals of the project.

Longitudinal approach

A group of children must be studied at reasonably short intervals for a long period of time and to adult age. This is a consequence of the viewpoint that individual adjustment is regarded as the result of an interaction process. Repeated measurements of the same variable or variables which are specially relevant for different age groups provide opportunities for drawing conclusions about causal relationships with a considerably greater degree of confidence than do single measurement studies.

Investigations aiming at mapping how adjustment disturbances arise are usually of the *ex post facto* type. They are concerned with groups of individuals who, according to certain criteria, are maladjusted—criminals, for example. The investigation groups are then studied in the current situation by psychological, psychiatric, medical, and other investigatory methods, as well as retrospectively, by interviews with the individual himself, interviews with people who know him, data from the registers of various institutions, and so on. Comparisons are made with corresponding data for a control group of normally adjusted persons matched in certain ways. Some of the weaknesses of this investigation design are:

1. Data describing the individual's state at the time he is chosen as a member of a group to be investigated, that is, just when he has shown distinct symptoms of maladjustment, will contain items that are effects of the adjustment disturbance we wish to study. These secondary phenomena may be consequences of the fact that the individual, on account of his primary adjustment disturbance, has been led into changing his lifestyle or has been affected by the reactions of his surroundings and the steps taken by society to remedy his disturbed adjustment. We must make serious attempts to obtain data which describe the person at the time at which the extrinsic maladjustment begins to appear, and earlier.

2. Registered data describing the individual and his situation before his maladjustment became manifest do not give, as a rule, a sufficient basis for analysing the background of the maladjustment.

3. Retrospective data suffer from lapses of memory and the like.

4. There is a risk for criterion contamination when retrospective data are collected. If, for example, we apply to a teacher or an employer for information on a person who has become a criminal, there is a risk that the individual's earlier behaviour will be interpreted in the light of knowledge about later behaviour.

The alternative to an *ex post facto* investigation is a longitudinal study. By collecting information at different points in time about a group of growing individuals, we can cover the aspects we consider relevant to the causes of adjustment disturbances, and we can avoid contamination by components that are secondary in relation to such disturbances. Since it may be assumed that the early development of an individual is of prime importance for the rise of adjustment disturbances later in life, such follow-up studies should be started as early as possible. Early studies may be concerned with a child's family situation, the parents' methods of upbringing, and so on. Later there will be opportunities of studying the child's own behaviour. The demand for the collection of data early in a person's life must be balanced against the costs and administrative problems connected with such a study, especially since the investigation group must be sizeable.

To arrive at inferences of causal relationships is a main goal of research. The most efficient method is the experimental method, applied in a closed system, where all external variables are excluded, or known and controlled. All problems, however, are not possible to study in a laboratory. If a problem of great public interest is translated to a form which is possible to treat experimentally, the relevance for the problems of society is often diminished or lost. Though the longitudinal study gives no safe, sure, or easy way to arrive at causal inferences, it is superior to cross-sectional, one-occasion studies in this regard.

Sample. The size of the group investigated should be sufficient to permit the division into reasonably large moderator subgroups for separate analyses. The purpose of the project does not in itself call for dividing the total group into subgroups in adult age on the basis of, for example, occupation or other criteria. Such far-reaching goals would have demanded such a large group size as to make our more immediate goals impossible to achieve. In carrying out the surveys involved in the project, great importance must be attached to minimizing drop-out rates.

Variables. A large number of variables must be measured. Account must be taken of the entire individual when studying his adjustment in a development process. This means studying his environment and the whole of his organism.

Flexibility in design. In certain problem areas our previous knowledge is inadequate, and in others available measuring methods are extremely expensive. These circumstances imply a need for different kinds of methods for various problems. Effectiveness in the use of available resources can be enhanced by approaching certain problems through a more intensive study of smaller groups of children at the same time as the majority of problems are studied in a larger group.

Successive age groups. Of decisive importance for the outcome of a longitudinal study are, among other things, the choice of problems, the formulation of hypotheses, the choice of techniques and instruments for data collection. Early mistakes in these respects usually cannot be revoked or compensated for later on and may have strong effects, sometimes disastrous, on the results. Since great costs in terms of money and personnel are invested and committed for a long period in a longitudinal project, it is important that the study be carefully prepared. One of the most effective ways of preparation is a pilot study in which:

(a) Preliminary results can be obtained and used as a basis for the choice of problems for further investigations and for the formulation of hypotheses;
(b) Methods and instruments for data collection and data treatment can be tested.

Only one age group is usually followed in longitudinal studies. Some problems are inherent in such a design. Changes in the macrosocial system may have specific effects on the group being investigated. With only one age group it is not possible to estimate the degree and extent of such influences, which are confounded by age effects. In the successive collection of data on a group of subjects, later results may be affected by the subject's earlier participation in responding to the instruments of measurement, the so-called panel effect. With only one age group at hand it is not possible to estimate this effect.

In view of these and other problems connected with the use of only one age group in a longitudinal study, the technique of *successive age groups* has been used in the current project. Two age groups have been followed, of which one has served as pilot group and the other one as main group.

Ethical considerations. In performing studies of the same individuals for a long period of time and in keeping records of many variables, it is necessary to have a spirit of co-operation and to make the persons in the investigation groups feel at ease. When formulating the items for the instruments of measurement, the integrity of the subjects must be respected. The fact that the subjects are children also calls for special ethical considerations. In data collection and data treatment, measures must be taken to ensure anonymity.

General survey

In the following the program and the ways in which the strategical considerations have been implemented will be described. However, it seems necessary to give a short overview before entering into details.

A cohort of approximately 1000 pupils who were born in 1955 and who were third-graders in the public school in Örebro during the school year 1964–5 is being followed up to adult age (the *main* group). The survey also includes a *pilot* group consisting of the Örebro pupils who were born in 1952 and who were sixth-graders in 1964–5; they are also being followed up to adulthood. Certain instrumental tests and pilot studies have been and are being carried out on this group. A pilot study was also made on pupils in Örebro who were eighth-graders in 1964–5, but this group has not been followed up any further. Table 20.1 provides a schematic illustration of the course of the project until 1975.

The data which have been collected for the studies may be classified into three groups:

(a) *Basic information* on total groups. Data have been collected on pupils at the ages of 10, 13, and 15 years, respectively (grades 3, 6, and 8) for the following main areas using the following main methods for data collection:

Area	Methods for data collection
Domestic background, domestic situation	Parental questionnaire
Intrinsic adjustment, satisfaction etc.	Pupil questionnaire
Classmate relationships	Sociometric methods
Extrinsic adjustment: behaviour	
in school	Teacher ratings
at home	Parental questionnaire
in society	Public records
Intelligence, knowledge	Tests and grades given on report cards
Attitudes and values	Semantic differential

(b) *Information concerning special problems* collected in the course of subprojects and applying to *total* groups, e.g.:

Area	Age	Methods for data collection
Norms	15	Situation inventory
Symptoms (girls)	15	Questionnaire
Criminality (boys)	16	Questionnaire, self-reported delinquency
Study and vocational decisions	13–19	Questionnaires Semantic differential
Goals, values in life	18	Questionnaire

(Note that school start is at age 7. Grades 1–9 are in comprehensive school. In grade 3 most children are 10, in grade 6 they are 13 and in grade 9 they are 16. Upper secondary school (gymnasium) has three grades, the students are 17–19 years old.)

(c) *Information concerning special problems* collected in the course of subprojects and concerning random samples from the total group (used when expensive methods are necessary), e.g.:

Area	Age	Methods for data collection
Social relations (N=90)	10–12	Interview etc.
Biological variables (N=225)	13–15	EEG, hormone analysis, ossification measurements, physical achievement capacity
Drop-out problems	16–17	Interview, questionnaire

Investigation groups

When the project started in 1964 it was possible to obtain full support from the local school authorities in Örebro, a town in central Sweden with about 100 000 inhabitants.

TABLE 20.1

Survey of the project 1965–75

Year	Pilot group born 1952	Main group born 1955
1965	Whole of grade 6 960 pupils	Whole of grade 3 1032 pupils
1966		Intensive survey of social relations, grade 4, 90 pupils
1968	Grade 9: The educational and vocational choice process	Grade 6: Total group survey The educational and vocational choice process
	Self-reported delinquency, boys	Medical examinations, random sample of 250 pupils
1969–70		Grade 8: The educational and vocational decision process. Norms and norm conflicts. Symptom load, girls. Ecological surveys. Intelligence measurement, standardized achievement tests. Ossification measurements, random sample, 250 pupils. Social relations
1971	Grade 3, upper sec.: The educational and vocational choice process Intelligence, creativity	Grade 9: Total group survey Follow-up from 1965. The educational and vocational choice process. Self-reported delinquency, boys
1972	Post-sec.: Educational and vocational choice (technical line only)	Grade 1, upper sec.: Upper secondary school questionnaire. Transition to new type of school. Random sample of all school-leavers from grade 1: interview
1973	Post-sec.: Employment and study conditions. Postal questionnaire to former upper sec. students	Grade 2, upper sec.: Educational and vocational choices 2-yr lines of upper sec. school. Values Leisure occupations
1974		Grade 3, upper sec.: Educational and vocational choice School experiences Values Leisure occupations Anxiety, situation test Personality test
1975	Post-sec.: Employment and study conditions. Pupils leaving school in 1968: Postal questionnaire	

To reiterate, three cohorts, children born in 1950, 1952, and 1955 respectively and attending the public schools in Örebro, are the investigation groups. Of these, the youngest group is our *main* group (denoted M), the middle group is a *pilot* group (denoted P). The oldest group served as a pilot group in the first years of the project.

When the first investigation was undertaken, in the spring of 1965, the numbers of pupils in the three grades were as follows:

Age 10, Grade 3 (M): $N = 1025$
Age 13, Grade 6 (P): $N = 960$
Age 15, Grade 8: $N = 1330$

Most of the children, about 88 per cent, had been born in 1955, 1952, and 1950, respectively; about 10 per cent had been born the year before these 'normal' years of birth for each grade; about 1 per cent were born the year after the year of birth for the majority in the grade, i.e. they were under-age. As the principles for judging school readiness were not changed between the years in which these groups started school, each of the grades, with the exceptions given below, comprised an age stratum of the whole population of Örebro.

The following categories were excluded from the groups.

1. Children with serious intellectual shortcomings, i.e. with an intellectual level corresponding to an IQ of 70 or lower. Such children are transferred to a special school during their first school year.
2. Children with grave physical handicaps, e.g. blindness.
3. Children with serious social adjustment disturbances, taken into custody by society and placed in foster homes or school homes outside Örebro.

Custody of the type mentioned in point 3 is extremely unusual with respect to children of nine years of age. Exclusion of this type has not affected the composition of the main group on the first investigation occasion to any great extent. It must be pointed out that there are very few private schools in Sweden. Children from all social groups attend the public school.

For a follow-up study to be meaningful, it is very important to have a group that will remain in the same environmental system during a long period. Örebro was chosen because it has a well-developed educational system and a diversified labour market, and should thereby offer families many opportunities. This stable pattern can be expected to continue when the children leave school and seek employment.

There is, however, always some migration, which over a long period may mean a considerable loss of subjects. It is also impossible to prevent drop-outs affecting the collection of data. Parents fail to reply to questionnaires, students may be absent on account of illness, truancy, or the like, when data are collected. A detailed account is given of how the project managed to obtain data from its follow-up groups and how these groups were reduced by people moving during the first years.

The period in compulsory school. First, the situation of the main group, which has been followed from grade 3, 1965, will be described. Of the children in this group, 88 per cent were born in 1955, i.e. they were about 10 years of age.

Table 20.2 shows the sizes of the groups that attended the different grades on the occasions when the total group investigations were performed on a large scale—1965, 1968, 1970, 1971, 1973, and 1974. It also shows how many of the students in the groups remained on separate occasions or for several of the total group investigations. The increasing numbers from grade 3 to grade 9 are explained by the fact that more pupils have moved to than from Örebro.

Long-term longitudinal studies of the main group can be made in

TABLE 20.2

Sizes of groups for which data exist for different grades and combinations of grades. Main group

Grades	Boys	Girls	Total
Total grade 3	515	510	1025
Total grade 6	543	557	1100
Total grade 8	600	590	1190
Total grade 9	609	578	1187
3, 6, and 8	421	440	861
3 and 6, not 8	31	27	58
3 and 6	452	467	919
6 and 8, not 3	81	65	146
6 and 8	502	505	1007
8, not 3 or 6	94	83	177
3 and 9	418	431	849
3 and 11	264	234	498
3 and 12	102	85	187
9 and 11	358	306	664
9 and 12	141	114	255
3, 6, 8, 9, 11, 12	101	85	186

the first place on total groups from any one single occasion and may then comprise total groups of 1025 students from grade 3 or 1100 from grade 6. The numbers are given for such combinations as 3, 6, not 8: the children present in grades 3 and 6 but not in grade 8 (58).

For most purposes, however, it will probably be most fruitful to start from a group that attended the nine-year public school in Örebro during the whole period of the investigation, for which data are available from all total group investigations. From grades 3 and 9, 849 students are registered, i.e. 83 per cent of the original group in grade 3. It must be regarded as satisfactory to be able to follow such a large part of a group over a period of six years in the same system. In some contexts, the follow-up group comprising students for whom information is available from grades 3 and 6 may be relevant. For these, there are 919 students, or 90 per cent of the original population. In the pilot group there was a somewhat larger drop-out during the period from grade 6 to 9. Table 20.3 shows that of the 960 pupils in grade 6 (children aged 13), 74 per cent or 709 were still in the Örebro schools when we made our investigations in 1968.

TABLE 20.3

Sizes of groups for which data are available for different grades. Pilot group, students born in 1952

Grades	Boys	Girls	Total
Total grade 6	486	474	960
Total grade 9	562	546	1108
Grades 6 and 9	387	403	709

The description given of the sizes of the groups refers to the total groups registered in the schools. Not all data are available for all individuals. Table 20.4 reports the number of individuals for whom data are available for each instrument. The number of drop-outs is quite acceptable in most cases and in some cases a uniquely high participation can be observed. Thus, for example, a reply frequency of between 96 and 98 per cent is reported for the extremely important questionnaires sent to parents. This is the maximum of what can be achieved when it is borne in mind that some families cannot be expected to answer such questionnaires on account of language difficulties, residing in other places for the moment, etc.

The period in or equivalent to upper secondary school (gymnasium). (Gymnasium = upper secondary school, or 3 years of education,

TABLE 20.4

Sizes of groups for which data are available from measurements with different instruments. Main group, grades 3, 6, and 8

| Instrument | Grade 3/65 | | | | Grade 6/68 | | | | Grade 8/70 | | | |
| | Boys | | Girls | | Boys | | Girls | | Boys | | Girls | |
	N	per cent	N	per cent	N	per cent	N	per cent	N	per cent	N	per cent
Parent questionnaire	501	97	492	96	536	98	542	97	—	—	—	—
Intelligence test	484	94	483	95	540	99	550	99	575	96	576	98
Achievement test	477	92	482	94	460	85	475	85	498†	83	497†	84
Sociometry	515	100	510	100	543	100	557	100	519	87	502	85
Teachers' ratings	475	92	490	96	540	99	557	100	585	98	545	92
Semantic differential	404	85	431	88	513	94	525	94	—	—	—	—
Student questionnaire	491	95	482	95	513	94	525	94	—	—	—	—
Creativity test	—	—	—	—	447	82	446	80	—	—	—	—
Vocational choice, questionnaire	—	—	—	—	522	96	526	95	539	90	529	90
Vocational differential	—	—	—	—	522	96	529	95	537	90	524	89
Interest form	—	—	—	—	522	96	529	95	—	—	—	—
Norm questionnaire	—	—	—	—	—	—	—	—	525	88	533	90
Symptom loading	—	—	—	—	—	—	—	—	—	—	520	88

† Refers to Swedish only.

10th, 11th, 12th grade. The student is usually 16 when he starts and 19 when he graduates.) The activities of the main group of 1187 students one year after completion of compulsory school are given in Table 20.5. They were 17 years of age at the time of this survey of their activities. The majority (77·1 per cent) continued their education directly at the gymnasium but many (11·4 per cent) dropped out during the first year for different reasons.

TABLE 20.5

The activities of the M-group one year after compulsory school

Activity	Total number	Per cent
Studies at high school	780	65·7
Drop-out from high school	135	11·4
Studies in the USA	4	0·3
Studies in other schools	4	0·3
Repeating grade 9	27	2·3
Employed	173	14·6
Unemployed	25	2·1
Migrated from Örebro	24	2·0
Dead	1	0·1
Not traced	14	1·2
Total	1187	100

The students from the main group attended upper secondary school with many students from a larger geographical region and of other ages. In the investigations, entire classes took part if the majority belonged to the original investigation group. Group members from other classes were assembled specially for the investigation. For some of the problems a larger part of the students took part in the investigations; for others we tried to test only members of the main group. These circumstances explain why the number of students varies from instrument to instrument. Table 20.6 gives the numbers of individuals for whom data are available for the instruments tested in the upper secondary school.

Postal questionnaire studies on the pupils after their graduation from upper secondary school have been undertaken in two cases. All students who were seniors in 1970–1 were requested to answer a questionnaire two years after leaving school. There were 415 of the 477 students who replied, or 87 per cent. The same group

answered a postal questionnaire in 1975, four years after leaving school, and on that occasion replies were registered for 435 individuals, making 91 per cent. Moreover, a group of students who did not intend to continue their education after grade 9 was asked to reply to a questionnaire seven years after leaving school. Out of 143 individuals 121 (85 per cent) answered.

These first follow-up studies in adult life indicate great possibilities for investigations of important problems.

TABLE 20.6

Sizes of groups for which data are available from investigations with different instruments. Secondary school (gymnasium)

Instrument	Grade	Boys	Girls	Total
Student questionnaire (drop-out investigation)	10	428	392	820
Student questionnaire†	11	152	145	297
Questionnaire, educational and vocational choice†	11	152	145	297
Leisure time activities	11	282	262	544
Life values	11	333	329	662
Student questionnaire	12	280	168	448
Educational and vocational choice	12	253	166	419
Leisure time activities	12	284	168	452
Life values	12	271	163	434
Anxiety inventory	12	275	165	440
Personality inventory	12	243	166	409

† Only for students who take 2-year study programmes in secondary school.

Groups for follow-up studies. In Sweden it is possible to follow any individual thanks to easily accessible registries. The intention has been to use the groups from the compulsory school period for follow-up studies into adult age. The subgroups which have continued their education directly by attending upper secondary school have been studied every year thereof. Most of the students continue studying directly, but some do interrupt their education and take a year or two for working, travelling, or doing whatever they want. Others take jobs not requiring skill or training and never take up further education. The size of the upper secondary school groups participating in data collections can be seen in Table 20.2. Some interesting follow-up studies will be performed on these subgroups.

The problem of loss of subjects. The harm done to the research by disappearance of subjects varies according to what is being investigated. For example, drop-out is a very serious problem in descriptions of a sociological character. In such cases, even small numbers of drop-outs, say 10 per cent, if biased, can lead to misleading conclusions. In the kind of questions of development with which this project is concerned, the loss of subjects is not that serious. If the children who migrate from Örebro to a large extent are extreme in a certain respect and we study a problem where this characteristic is relevant, the power of the study will diminish, rendering the conclusions less reliable but not biased.

Generalization. Admittedly, the studies are performed in one particular place, which is not entirely representative of Sweden in all respects. But the limitations which this imposes on generalizations should not be exaggerated. It may be that in a few special cases, the proportion of children displaying a particular behaviour pattern or answering a question in a particular way differs from what would be found in the population of Swedish children of the same age. However, surprisingly good agreement with respect to frequencies of certain answers has been found between the Örebro results and those from studies in recent years in other parts of the country, in some cases using the same instruments (see Bergman 1973a). The possibilities of generalizing to a Swedish population are probably quite good. This may be still more true of conclusions concerning explanations of behaviour, causal structures behind functions, and testing of theories and models.

Investigation methods and variables

The general survey of the project has given a first impression of the range of variables measured. Most of them have been measured with instruments that have been constructed for the express purpose of this study.

In Table 20.7 detailed information is given on the types of variables, types of instrument, and occasion. The variables are grouped into three categories:

    I. Basic individual variables;
    II. Individual adjustment variables;
    III. Environmental variables.

Basic individual variables

(a) *Psychological characteristics of the individual.* For some characteristics, which are clearly of importance for different aspects of adjustment to school, there are well-tested paper and pencil instruments that can be used on large groups of individuals. This is most obviously true of intellectual capacity. There are also tests to measure other types of cognitive functions, e.g., creative ability.

The above examples refer to aspects of an individual's capacity. Other psychological variables reflecting guiding mechanisms of importance to his adjustment—attitudes, values, standards, interests, etc.—may likewise be studied with the help of standardized, group-administered instruments. But here we are often concerned with variables that ought to be studied in greater detail with individually administered techniques, e.g., interview, if adequate knowledge is to be obtained.

(b) *Biological characteristics of the individual.* To obtain data describing aspects of an individual's neurophysiological and hormonic reaction pattern requires time-consuming and costly investigations. Other interesting measures of biological variables, such as the physical development of a growing individual, may be obtained by means of simple methods suitable for large scale studies.

Adjustment variables

(a) *Extrinsic adjustment variables.* Extrinsic adjustment in terms of achievement can be assessed through grades on report cards and results on achievement tests. Teachers may also make other evaluations to complement ordinary grades. A teacher's evalua-

TABLE 20.7

Survey of variables and methods. Main group

Type of variable	Total group investigation	Sample investigation	Investigation occasion
I. Basic individual variables			
A. Psychological characteristics			
1. General intellectual capacity	Objective tests		1965, 1968, 1970
2. Creative ability	Objective tests		1968, 1971
3. Aspiration level	Vocational questionnaires		1968, 1970, 1971, 1973, 1974
	Vocational differential		1968, 1970, 1971
	Teacher ratings		1965, 1968
4. Norms, attitudes, evaluations	Semantic differential technique		1965, 1968, 1971
	Student questionnaire, situations		1969
	Vocational questionnaire		1968, 1970, 1971, 1973, 1974
	Vocational differential		1968, 1970, 1971
	Student questionnaire, self-report delinquency		1971
	Student questionnaire		1971, 1973, 1974
5. Interests and activities	Student questionnaire		1968, 1971, 1973, 1974
6. Personality	Inventory		1973
B. Biological characteristics			
1. General physical capacity (working capacity)		Cycle ergometer test	1967
2. Neurophysiological situation		Electroencephalogram	1967
3. Hormonal excretion		Adrenaline – noradrenaline measures	1967
4. Biological age		Measures of ossification	1970

TABLE 20.7—*continued*

Type of variable	Total group investigation	Sample investigation	Investigation occasion
II. Adjustment variables			
A. Extrinsic adjustment			
1. Scholastic achievement	Objective tests		
a. Absolute achievement	Objective tests		1965, 1968, 1970
b. Achievement relative to the individual's capacity	Objective tests		1965, 1968
c. Grades			1965, 1968, 1971, 1973–4
2. Social behaviour			
a. Behaviour in relation to classmates	Peer ratings Sociometric methods		1965, 1968 1965, 1968, 1970
		Teacher interview	1966
b. Behaviour in classroom	Teacher ratings		1965, 1968, 1971
		Teacher interview	1966
c. Behaviour at home	Parent questionnaire		1965, 1968
d. Behaviour in society	Register data Student questionnaire		1967 1968, 1970, 1971
B. Intrinsic adjustment			
1. Experienced satisfaction of needs, etc.			1965, 1968, 1970
a. Total experience of school	Student questionnaire Vocational questionnaire		1971, 1972, 1973 1968, 1970, 1971, 1973, 1974
		Student interview	1966
b. Experience of school work	Student questionnaire		1965, 1968, 1970, 1971
		Student interview	1966
c. Experience of teacher contact		Student interview	1966
d. Experience of peer contact	Student questionnaire Student's ratings of own sociometric status		1965, 1968, 1971
		Student interview	1966
e. Experience of parent contact	Student questionnaire		1969, 1970, 1971
2. General emotional level (anxiety, uneasiness, depression, etc.)	Student questionnaire symptoms		1970
		Medical examination	1966
3. Experienced somatic symptoms	Student questionnaire		1965, 1968, 1971
		Medical examination	1966
4. Objective somatic situation		Medical examination Measures of adrenaline – noradrenaline	1966 1967
5. Symptoms in behaviour (disharmony, confidence, well-being, etc.)	Teacher ratings Parent questionnaire Peer ratings Student questionnaire symptoms		1965, 1968, 1971 1965, 1968 1965, 1968 1970
		Teacher interview Parent interview	1966 1966
III. Environmental variables			
A. School environment			
1. Teacher relations	Teacher ratings		1965, 1968, 1971
2. Peer personality	See individual variables		
3. Peer relations	Sociometric measures		1965, 1968, 1970
B. Home environment			
1. Economic situation of home, dwelling standard, etc.	Parent questionnaire		1965, 1968
2. Parents' educational level	Parent questionnaire		1965, 1968
3. Attitudes and norms of parents		Interviews	1966
C. External dwelling environment	Social ecological data		1969
D. Material standard of the school	Social ecological data		1969

tions may attempt to measure an individual's achievement in relation to his potential capacity. A more objective estimate of this relation can be obtained by comparing the student's actual achievement to his intellectual capacity as measured by intelligence tests. Both under-achievement and over-achievement in school work in relation to capacity may be regarded as signs of disturbed intrinsic adjustment. Over-achievement may be regarded as evidence of a compensatory effort in school work that may be impairing the all-round development of the personality, while under-achievement may be an indication of discomfort and disharmony in the school situation.

Measures of the aspect of a student's extrinsic adjustment concerned with social behaviour and interaction in the school situation may be gained through judgements by teachers and peers, sociometric choices of peers, etc. As far as such adjustment in the home is concerned, some information has been obtained by questionnaires, but important data, for example, about social relations in the family, have also been collected by personal interviews.

Adjustment to the macrosocial system may be studied in general by collecting data from social authorities and the police, or by questioning the student himself.

(b) *Intrinsic adjustment variables.* Information about a student's intrinsic adjustment to school, home, and society can best be obtained from the individual himself in interviews and conversation. In studies of large groups it is often necessary to work with statements by the students in written questionnaires, about experienced comfort and satisfaction, anxiety, etc., in the total school situation or in certain aspects of it, such as contacts with fellow students. Judging from theories about the emergence of symptoms in cases of lack of intrinsic adjustment, the question of somatic disturbances may also be relevant.

Another type of data relevant in this context is other people's observations of symptoms of intrinsic maladjustment in the individual. The line of demarcation between such data and data concerning extrinsic disturbances may be diffuse. Extrinsic adjustment disturbance is often regarded as a symptom of intrinsic maladjustment. Certain kinds of behaviour and reactions to which no great importance is ordinarily attached by other people may, perhaps, be classified as symptoms of intrinsic maladjustment to the prevailing situation.

Environmental variables

One of the principal aspects of a description of a social system is the contact pattern or general pattern of relations between the individuals in the system. Sociometric techniques can be used to map this aspect of the system.

Certain basic data, factors referring to families, which may be expected to serve as indicators of a student's environment in the home, may be collected by means of written questionnaires. However, many aspects of the microsocial system which are really important for an individual must be studied by individual techniques.

Register data

It has been possible to utilize data from central and local registers for the investigations and these possibilities will be used still more in the future studies of the groups in adult age.

(a) Population census has a long history in Sweden and the registers available today date back to the eighteenth century. They are now centralized, which makes it possible to obtain the address of any person living in Sweden at short notice. In the postal questionnaire studies performed thus far, all our subjects have been identified;

(b) From the Central Bureau of Statistics it will also be possible to ascertain information about taxed income, higher education, and civil status (Statistiska Centralbyrån);

(c) Local registers maintained by social welfare boards can be used for information on crimes and offences up to age 21, and the central, national Register of Criminal Offences for information on later criminality;

(d) From local registers of Child and Youth Guidance Clinics information can be obtained about all children treated at these clinics for psychological problems in childhood and adolescence;

(e) Registers are available covering the psychological and medical examinations of 18-year-old boys enlisting for military service (the Recruiting and Replacement Office of the Swedish Armed Forces);

(f) Information on income, number of days off the job because of illness, and occupation may be obtained from local public insurance offices (*Försäkringskassan*);

(g) A central register gives information on crimes in connection with alcohol abuse (*Riksskatteverket*);

(h) The National Board for Social and Health Problems keeps a register on young people who have had to serve a sentence in a home for juvenile delinquents (*Ungdomsvårdskola*).

There have been no problems so far in gaining access to the registers from which information is available. Register data will be used even more in the following-up of the subjects into adult age. No information on parents or older generations has been compiled from the registers.

Status of the data

Most data are punched and on tape. In some cases the material has been coded; in many cases new variables have been constructed from the raw data, e.g., after factor analyses, latent profile analyses, or other statistical methods for compressing data. Information which may be injurious to the individual if it should become public sometime in the future has not been stored on tape, e.g., register data.

Results

Only the individual reports and various publications can describe the results of the work of a decade (a publication list is available from the authors). To give an impression of the problems dealt with, some of the problem domains which have been studied hitherto can be listed:

(a) Norm and norm conflicts in adolescents;

(b) Delinquent behaviour in adolescent boys;

(c) Social adjustment in adolescent girls;

(d) The educational and vocational career (Dunér 1978; Ekehammar 1977a, b; 1978a, b);

(e) Intelligence, creativity, and development (Bergman 1973a, 1974);

(f) Social segregation in school classes and its effects;

(g) Intensive study of isolated and rejected children;

(h) Over-achieving children: what is the cost in a longer perspective? (Johansson *et al.* 1973; Bergman and Magnusson 1979; Magnusson 1977);

(i) Stability of behaviour, traits and other constructs (Magnusson and Backteman 1977);

(j) Methodological problems in longitudinal research (Bergman 1971; 1972a, b, c; 1973b; Magnusson, 1979; Olsson and Bergman 1973; 1977).

Results concerning problem domains (a–g) above are also presented in Magnusson *et al.* (1975).

The impact of the results which have emerged in this project is not easy to evaluate. In this type of research there is never a one-to-one relationship between results and action. The reports do seem to have stimulated great interest. Many persons in positions of leadership in society have commented that many of their decisions have been influenced by what they have learned from the project. Our reports have probably contributed to a new consciousness among school administrators in the National Board of Education that the schools are dealing with living, growing human beings, our future citizens, and that the whole school system in fact is in existence for the children's sake.

Pros and cons

Advantages of the longitudinal research design

A longitudinal study of the type represented by the research program offers a number of advantages. Besides the fact that it is the only possible design to obtain answers to many important problems (including stability of behaviour and traits, effects of factors in the individual and his environment for his development and for prediction of the outcome of his development), there are other advantages with a longitudinal study of this type:

(a) The data collected elucidate the original problems while at the same time serving as a base which can be used for the study of new problems which inevitably arise at various stages of societal development. An ongoing longitudinal project can answer questions in a short time, which otherwise had demanded research over several years. An example is the question of effects of social segregation in the school class. In 1970 measures were under consideration which would render the social economic status composition of classes more heterogeneous. The goal would be to give children better opportunities to learn from their peers and to become acquainted with the life style and mentality of other social classes. At that point, the project had data which made it possible to answer questions as to the effects of variations in social class composition upon achievement, attitudes, norms, educational and vocational choice, etc. Reports on these matters were presented within a few months, which can be compared to the approximately six years a special project would have demanded.

(b) In the course of a longitudinal project each data collection provides the basis for descriptions of a total group. These descriptions are of great interest for those working in the applied field. For example, our studies of norms, relation problems, crimes or offences, and attitudes during adolescence, have given psychologists, school and social workers as well as decision-makers information about total groups, rendering it possible for them to see the implication of behaviour in the special, extreme groups with whom they have to work. These may be the youngsters whom we notice most in public places or in the mass media and who tend to form our impression of young people in general. The professionals concerned with youngsters need to know what is really extreme and what is normal. Descriptions concerning many different aspects of development and covering several stages in development from age 10 to age 19 can be found in the list of reports and publications from the project.

(c) The broad scope of problems and, correspondingly, of the data collected has given the researchers possibilities for testing diversified ideas without taking too much time from the subjects. During their period in elementary and junior high school the classes spent the equivalent of 12 class periods with our investigation leaders, and in the high school about 4–7 class periods. Using fewer than 20 class periods for those who had the longest education, we obtained material which can be used for follow-up studies of a broad set of problems, both those which we formulated from the start and new ones.

(d) Much of the work has been done by undergraduates as part of their research training for a Bachelor's degree in psychology or by postgraduate students for their doctoral dissertations. It has been possible for them to study meaningful problems in a fruitful way which would have been impossible had they worked individually. The longitudinal approach calls for the solution of many problems in the collection and analyses of data, and this makes studies on development problems especially valuable in training of advanced students.

Practical problems

There are many problems met in the course of a longitudinal project.

(a) The most important one is the problem of funding the project in the long run. During the first eleven years, when the subjects of the main group were still in school, the project was funded by the Central Board of Education. Now it is funded by research councils to which applications were made for the study of specific problems. To run a longitudinal project, which preferably calls for maintaining the same trained staff, etc., while at the same time having to formulate specific problems and to depend on a number of small grants, is difficult and extremely time-consuming. What is needed are certain base resources, which would make it possible to plan more efficiently for longer periods instead of working with specific problem formulations just to obtain the money needed for the moment.

(b) What are described as advantages are also in certain respects problems. The interest in many relevant problems stimulated by societal debate has led us to use much of our limited resources for cross-sectional descriptions and other short-range studies, which have not been among the main problems. Those problems for which longitudinal data are necessary have not, until lately, been pursued to the degree they deserve.

(c) Another advantage which is not without its problems is the fact that the staff, to a considerable degree has consisted of students. By the time they have become quite familiar with the data and the routines of the project, they have also received their degrees and left the project for other tasks in society.

(d) The broad range of variables necessary for a longitudinal and, at the same time, interdisciplinary project results in such a great amount of data that automatic computers are a must. In Sweden today there is a national commission (*Datainspektionen*) which has been assigned the responsibility of inspecting all data registers on tape or punched cards to ascertain the personal integrity of all persons involved. Registers set up for research purposes must have this commission's permission to operate and must follow all of their regulations. It is possible that decisions by the commission will mean practical problems for the future endeavours of the project.

Ethical considerations

Within some branches of science, technical advancements have led to the development of research which can seriously harm humans, indeed even humanity. For example, in medicine, new possibilities have been opened to affect individuals in such ways as they would not always wish. Many experiments entail problems in weighing the usefulness of new knowledge against the harm or discomfort which the test persons must endure.

The realized need for setting rules or for formulating declarations of principles for research ethics, which has existed in the field of medicine for some decades, has spread to the behavioural sciences. Here it is not so often a matter of physical injury but of psychological injury. The encroachment of research upon personal integrity has come to take on a central role in the debate on ethics.

Awareness of ethical problems

It is of great significance that problems of ethics have come into public awareness and debate during recent years. It is also important that they be taken up at an early stage in the education of researchers and that researchers are continually reminded of them thereafter. Otherwise, researchers can become so enthralled by their research problems and theories that they go about trying to obtain needed information without considering what this may mean for the persons from whom they obtain it.

Internal contradiction

There is sometimes an internal contradiction between the expected usefulness of a given research project and the risks for unethical dealings which may arise during the collection of the data. In certain studies, it is necessary that the test persons be kept in the dark as to the researcher's intentions. This is diametrically opposed to the demand that a person's participation in a research project should be voluntary and should rest upon full information as to the implications of the study. In other cases, the investigation may be focused upon problems which call for intimate questions about relationships, thoughts, or feelings, or other matters which may cause the test person anxiety. In such cases, it can be difficult to decide what is best, since we live in a pluralistic society in which different groups have widely differing values. A researcher has his own system of values which may lead him, unknown to himself, to pose questions which hurt or injure the test person.

The researcher—the test person

Some decisions where one factor must be balanced against another, must be made in a manner that is satisfactory to both parties involved, the researcher and the test person. Otherwise, the research project cannot be expected to succeed. In the long run, it is imperative that the selected subjects are willing to participate and to give the researcher information in a spirit of trust. In so-called longitudinal research, the question of mutual trust assumes a singularly great importance. The very essence of this methodology is that one and the same group of people is followed over a relatively long period of time (so as to study them in certain aspects). Co-operation must be maintained over a considerable period of time, but this can never be established if the test persons do not find the experiment satisfying from the ethical standpoint. Such co-operation cannot arise of itself; it rests upon a number of measures which must be adapted to the prevailing circumstances. It may perhaps be of interest to describe some of the measures which we have carried out within the context of the project. During the more than ten years of the project's existence, matters having to do with ethics and mutual trust have occupied an essential part of the work invested in the project. At the start of the project in 1964, the debate on research ethics in the social sciences was still in its embryonic stages. Nonetheless, we were aware that if we wished to undertake a research project involving the same individuals for a number of years, we would have to be sure that no ethical encroachment could occur. In our country, the number of mishaps stemming from unethical practices of researchers in psychology or education has not been especially large. But there are in fact cases in which experiments originally designed to continue for quite some time have been called off abruptly after the first collection of data because the test persons (or their parents and teachers) found certain aspects of the investigations to be harmful or unethical. When designing longitudinal research, ethical rules must therefore be observed, not only as a matter of ethics but also of practical reality.

Information, provocation, and secrecy

The measures to be outlined here have purported to solve the problems of information, provocation, and secrecy.

Information must be given to all test subjects in order to help to motivate them to participate voluntarily. When an investigation assumes a broad design, in which the main part of the data collection takes place at school, the need for information also broadens. School personnel who are involved in some way must find out what is taking place in such a manner as to enable them to judge the intentions and implications of the investigation. A positive attitude on their part is a must. Since the project was initiated when the subjects were children, it was also necessary to give the parents information on what was happening at school.

The problem of provocation is especially crucial when investigations concern children. It is important to realize that differing opinions can prevail and to avoid such matters as can be experienced as negatively provocative, by either the children or their parents.

Secrecy must be guaranteed in two ways. For the one matter, it must be possible to promise the children that their responses to the questions and their achievement ratings as well will not be disclosed to anyone at school. They must be assured that the findings of the investigation will not affect their school situation. Secondly, the secrecy of the information which they offer must be guarded in a larger context, e.g., research reports should not contain information on individuals which would render it possible to identify them, and outsiders should not be able to search after, retrieve, or, even more importantly, take advantage of information on any single individual.

Ethical problems

A large part of the research effort within the project has been devoted to measures for dealing with the above-mentioned ethical problems in the best ways possible. Examples will be given of those measures which may be of special interest.

Reference group. One of the first local measures generated by the project was to create a work group, or, as such groups have now come to be called, a reference group. It has consisted of representatives from the Department of Education, the local school board, headmasters, heads of subject areas, all categories of teachers involved, parents, the school superintendent, and the school physician. The members of the group have been quite active and have felt a commitment to the project, reflected in a number of different valuable contributions. One of their tasks has been the very matter under discussion—to deal with ethical questions. During different stages of the preparatory work, which took place before every day's collection of data, this group studied all material carefully, including the instruments and individual questions on the questionnaires. The members of the reference group had various value systems and they were familiar with local conditions. Their viewpoints provided valuable information as to how the subjects would react to the questions, thereby avoiding otherwise unforeseeable ethical encroachments.

The reference group has also been of great service in other ways. It has put forth suggestions for additions more often than for deletions and has made many improvements in the wording, not least in the light of local conditions. The reference group deserves a large part of the credit for the fact that the work has continued almost friction-free for so many years.

The press. In research within the social sciences, there has been a tendency to view the press as an instance which should be avoided as long as an investigation is under execution. However, it is the duty of the press to keep the people informed as to what is happening in society. If a researcher is carrying out unethical research, the press by all rights should uncover the research and direct criticism toward it. This role of the press is especially valuable in cases where research is carried out in schools and children are the subjects to be tested. Children have a subordinate position in society and have difficulties in refusing to participate. It is always possible that the press, on the basis of erroneous information, may render damage to the project when there are, once everything is cleared up, no valid objections. Reality can be transformed as information is passed on from children to their friends, parents, and, finally, to a journalist. These circumstances could lead us to only one conclusion, namely that the local press should be well-informed before the investigation was started. During all of the data collection as the years went by, both of the local newspapers were given complete information on the instruments of investigation (the tests). Information was sent out to the pupils, parents, and teachers. All of the newspapers responded wholeheartedly to the trust placed in them by offering information to the public in such a way as to contribute positively to the execution of the project. This form of co-operation with the press should be regarded as self-evident in continued research of this type. It gives the newspapers an opportunity to maintain a continuous, well-informed appraisal of the various stages of the project. Ultimately, the press is then afforded better opportunities to spread information on the research as a whole and on the final results.

The design of the instruments. When the instruments of measurement are to be designed, one point of consideration is obviously the information needed for the problem posed, such as it is treated within the framework of a theory. Research ethics necessitate the consideration of two further points: in the first place, it must be asked whether it is ethical to measure a certain characteristic or to pose a certain question. Will it arouse anger, resentment, or anxiety; can it bring personal problems to the surface and thereby cause mental suffering? We have often refrained from collecting desired information out of such considerations. Second, it is important that the questions be worded in such a way that they are unequivocal and easily understood by everyone. Unclear wording can lead to misunderstandings and even unforeseen provocation. Our desire to study a group that was somewhat representative of its age, implying, for example, a significant variation in the ability to comprehend written text, has prompted us to devote a great deal of work to the design of various instruments. We had to make the text understandable even for those with reading difficulties.

Test leaders from the project. To ensure the pupils that neither their answers nor their achievement scores would come to the knowledge of the school personnel, we used the test leaders from the project to collect data. There was always at least one person from the project, often a teacher, on hand to talk to the pupil's teachers and give them information. Having test leaders from the project was also the best way to guarantee that the questions which the children could pose would be treated in the same fashion. In certain investigations, two leaders worked in every group so that they could treat individual pupil's questions thoroughly. All of these measures most certainly contributed to the low non-response rate which we experienced, despite the fact that we informed the pupils of their right not to answer.

Secrecy guarantee. It is important to be able to inform the partici-

pants as to how the data are stored. A system has been developed which renders it impracticable for outsiders to retrieve information on an individual participant. Various data, e.g., an individual's code number (different on every occasion), the information's location on the magnetic tape, a key matching the code numbers to their corresponding response alternatives, a key as to whether high numbers mean much or little of a characteristic, clues as to which tape the information is stored upon, are locked in different places, in strong-boxes or safe-deposit boxes, and in forms which are virtually impossible for an outsider to interpret. The personnel, who must of course have a security release to work with such material, have signed an extra contract whereby they are duty-bound not to release information on individuals in our specific study.

All channels of spreading information must be utilized. Apart from the measures described above, we have taken great pains to spread information in other ways as well. We sent written information to all parents, teachers, and headteachers whenever we were going to collect data, or hold meetings for parents or teachers, etc. To solve the information problem, it is imperative to use all possible channels and to take advantage of every opportunity.

Together, these measures have contributed to imparting in the pupils a profound trust toward the project. This trust has been documented in many ways. A good example can be seen from a data collection in the spring of 1975, the year during which the pupils in the pilot group celebrated their 24th birthday. Of the pupils who did not enter high school, 85 per cent answered a detailed questionnaire. It should be borne in mind that this was seven years after they had left school. Of those of their classmates who did graduate from high school, 91 per cent answered a similar questionnaire. Considering that the total group is a non-selected, fairly representative group of Swedish youths, these results are remarkable. The confidence in the researchers which this level of participation reflects can be worth noting in today's debate on the relationship between researcher and test subject in research in the social sciences.

Acknowledgement

Financial support for the project has been obtained from the Swedish National Board of Education, the Swedish Council for Social Science Research, the Office of the Chancellor of the Swedish Universities, and the Bank of Sweden Tercentenary Fund.

21. Isle of Wight and Inner London studies

MICHAEL RUTTER

The Isle of Wight studies began in 1964–5 with a series of epidemiological studies of educational, psychiatric, and physical disorders in 9- to 11-year-old children. These early studies, directed by Michael Rutter, Jack Tizard, and Kingsley Whitmore, were financed by the Department of Education and Science and the Foundation for Child Development (then the Association for the Aid of Crippled Children). The findings were fully reported in two books (Rutter *et al.* 1970a, b) and only brief details are included here.

The later series of studies, supported by grants from the Nuffield Foundation, Social Science Research Council, and the Foundation for Child Development, were concerned with four main developments from the first set of surveys. First, the same age cohort of children was re-examined in 1968 and 1969 when the children were

aged 14–15 and were in their last year of compulsory schooling. This study included two parts: (a) a follow-up study of children known to have educational or psychiatric problems at age 10 years, and (b) a new cross-sectional study of the total age group of Isle of Wight 14–15 year olds. The second development involved some new investigations of 5- and 7-year-old children. The 10-year-old surveys had suggested that many of the problems manifest at that age had their roots in early childhood, and the infant school studies were designed to investigate some aspects of this issue. The third development involved some pilot investigations into the prevention and treatment of reading difficulties. Fourthly, in order to determine how far the findings regarding Isle of Wight youngsters applied to children living in Inner London, a comparative study of the two areas was undertaken. The research strategies and findings of these various investigations were summarized in a report which brought together the work undertaken during the decade 1964–74 (Rutter *et al.* 1976a). Accordingly this chapter focuses specifically on the longitudinal studies which were included in the research programme.

In addition, the Inner London epidemiological work was extended in order to follow the same cohort of children (first studied in 1970 at age 10 years) through secondary school and into their first year of employment after leaving school. This longitudinal project, funded by the Department of Education and Science and the Inner London Education Authority, is also described in the present chapter.

The 1964–5 surveys on the Isle of Wight

Since Burt's (1925, 1937) monumental surveys of handicapping conditions in school children undertaken during and after the First World War there had been no comparable enquiries prior to the Isle of Wight studies. The 1964–5 surveys were carried out in part to determine how far the prevalence and pattern of handicaps had altered during the last half century in parallel with the marked changes in social and material conditions in this country. Three related surveys were carried out: in 1964 on intellectual and educational retardation in 9- to 11-year-old children, and in 1965 on psychiatric disorder and on physical handicap in 10- to 12-year-old children (i.e. the same age cohort).

In each survey mass screening methods were applied to the whole population (an N of approximately 3500) to pick out children who might have one or more of the conditions we were interested in. All children selected in this way, together with a randomly selected control group of children drawn from the general population, were then individually examined (an N of 492 in 1964 and, in 1965, 271 and 277 respectively for the psychiatric and physical disorder surveys). Further information was obtained from the teachers, parents, and the children themselves. On the basis of this information a number of children were diagnosed as having a handicapping condition. They were then compared with the control group. Because the surveys were concerned with children with several different types of handicap it was possible to estimate the number of children with multiple handicaps. However, each survey was conducted independently and all children were assessed without knowledge of which group they were in in order not to bias our findings.

Prevalence of handicaps in Isle of Wight children

Intellectual retardation (defined in terms of an IQ two standard deviations below the mean) was present in $2\frac{1}{2}$ per cent of the children. Severe retardation (equivalent to an IQ below 50) was present in about three children out of every 1000 and a third of these were mongols.

About 4 per cent of the children showed specific reading retardation (i.e. reading at least 28 months below the level predicted on the basis of age and IQ) and $6\frac{1}{2}$ per cent had general reading backwardness. These groups overlapped to some extent, so that altogether 8 per cent of the children in this age group showed severe intellectual or educational difficulties. Most of the children were not receiving any kind of special help although many needed it. Some 7 per cent of 10- to 12-year-old children showed a psychiatric disorder of sufficient severity to have caused social handicap. Most conditions had lasted at least three years at the time of the survey. Altogether $5\frac{1}{2}$ per cent of the children had a chronic physical disorder.

There was a substantial overlap between the different varieties of handicap. Even so, overall, one child in six had some form of chronic or recurrent handicap. This relatively high frequency of handicap means that for most children help must often be provided by general community services (e.g. the family doctor or school teacher) rather than by specialists in hospital clinics.

The studies produced many findings on the nature and patterning of handicapping disorders in children. These were described fully in Rutter *et al.* (1970b) and summarized in Rutter *et al.* (1976a). The particular importance of organic brain dysfunction as a causal factor in the genesis of psychiatric and educational difficulties was discussed in Rutter *et al.* (1970a) in the context of the epidemiological study of neurological disorders.

Isle of Wight—Inner London comparative study

Using the same epidemiological methods and the same two-stage procedures as those employed on the Isle of Wight, reading difficulties and psychiatric disorder were studied in 10-year-old children attending state schools in one Inner London borough (see Rutter *et al.* 1976a, for a summary of the main findings). It was found that behavioural deviance, psychiatric disorder, and specific reading retardation were all twice as common in London as in those children living on the Isle of Wight. For the purposes of this comparison children of immigrant parents were excluded (although they were studied in the same way, findings being reported in a parallel series of papers).

Quality control on all data is essential in any kind of epidemiological study but it is especially crucial when direct comparisons are made between surveys of two different areas. In all the Isle of Wight and Inner London studies a very high premium was placed on the development of reliable and valid instruments and on the maintenance of consistently high interview standards. The steps taken are discussed in Rutter *et al.* (1975a, 1976a) and Rutter (1977c).

Intervention studies on the Isle of Wight

So far in this chapter, the studies described have all been cross-sectional in design (although they formed the basis of subsequent longitudinal studies). However, there were many questions which emerged from the early epidemiological investigations which required a longitudinal strategy for their answer. The first of these concerned the efficacy of educational measures taken to prevent or relieve reading difficulties. Two extended pilot studies (described in Yule and Rigley 1969) were undertaken to evaluate (a) the efficacy of remedial teaching in secondary school, and (b) the value of in-service training in primary schools on the teaching of reading.

The remedial reading study

A remedial reading teacher was appointed to the project in 1967. All the poor readers previously studied were by then in their second and third years of secondary schooling. The remedial advisory teacher was assigned to two schools where he taught the poor readers in very small groups of three or four children. In two other schools, he acted as an adviser to volunteer teachers who took the children for reading. In two further schools, the poor readers received remedial help from teachers under an existing scheme, although those teachers were not especially qualified for the work. In the final two secondary schools, no special provision for remedial reading existed or was created. The ESN school was excluded from this study, and no poor readers attended either of the grammar schools.

Before the 'experiment' was undertaken, all the children were reassessed on their reading. Very few children had made any noticeable improvements in their reading by March 1967. The four groups of poor readers were found to be well-matched in terms of IQ, reading, and spelling ages.

The experiment lasted four school terms. The remedial teacher saw his group of 28 children in small groups on two or three occasions each week for a total of 1–1½ hours teaching per week. Teaching was carried out under far from ideal circumstances, there being no regular room available in which to teach. An eclectic approach was adopted, and children were taught through a variety of techniques, aimed primarily at improving their attitudes towards reading. In analysing the outcome of the intervention, changes in the rates at which the children were learning to read were looked at rather than merely the absolute levels attained. The analyses of covariance demonstrated that children taught by the remedial advisory teacher improved significantly more on the measure of comprehension of reading than children in any other group. From 1964 to 1967, they progressed at 0·3 months per month. During remedial teaching, they made progress at the rate of 1·3 months per month.

However, these statistically significant results pale into insignificance when the absolute attainment of the poor readers is compared with that of their normal peers. Overall, at the age of 14½ years, the poor readers were, on the average, reading at the 9½-year level. Whilst it is heartening to conclude that poor readers can respond to specialist teaching, it is necessary also to concede that such specialist help was both too little and too late.

This 'experiment' was an attempt to capitalize on a naturally occurring situation. There are many technical problems to be remembered, the biggest qualification being that we have no measure of teacher quality, nor do we have detailed measures of what was taught and by what method. Without satisfactory measures of these important variables, investigations such as these are bound to lead to equivocal conclusions.

In-service training

In the last decade, in-service training and teachers' centres have expanded enormously. However, they were in their infancy in 1967 when it was decided to evaluate a brief in-service course on the teaching of reading. Earlier studies had found that few teachers in junior schools had had intensive preparation for teaching reading skills. This was a deplorable state of affairs given that nationally about 50 per cent of 7-year-olds entered junior schools without basic skills of reading.

All children in first-year junior classes were tested on the Southgate Group Reading Test 1 in 1967. Twelve of their teachers were released from schools on three consecutive Fridays to attend the in-service training arranged by Mr L. Rigley. These 12 classes were matched with 12 control classes in terms of size, type, staffing ratio, and scores on the reading test. The teachers were given some lectures and seminars on the skills of reading, and they visited selected infants schools. Results could only be compared on 10 pairs, because of teacher mobility. At the beginning of the year, both groups of children were reading at the 7 years 3 months level. When retested at the end of the school year on the Southgate Group Reading Test 2, the children of the in-service-trained teachers were reading just above the 8-year level, whilst those in the control classes were reading just below the 7 year 11 month level. The difference just failed to gain statistical significance at the 0·05 level.

Nevertheless, given the brief nature of the intervention, the results are seen as very encouraging. Naturally, one wants to see if the effects can be replicated. Moreover, if this sort of effect can be obtained from three-days' training, what might be achieved with a longer course?

Infant school studies

Retrospective information obtained in the 10-year-old studies had suggested that many of the problems present in middle childhood could have been predicted at school entry. An extended pilot study

of infant school children was undertaken to begin an exploration of this possibility. Ideally such a study should have involved the development of satisfactory measuring instruments for use in infant schools before applying these instruments in a longitudinal predictive study. In addition, the prospective study should have continued until age 10 years. Unfortunately, time and resources did not permit either, but some leads were provided on follow-through from age 4 to 7 years.

Traditional school medical examinations have been called into question on a number of grounds. Principally, the reliability of the examinations has been found to be limited; secondly, the examinations paid too little attention to neuro-developmental aspects. An attempt was made to rectify this state of affairs, and a revised school medical examination, taking approximately 15 min to complete, was developed by Drs Martin Bax and Kingsley Whitmore (1973). All children starting school in 1967 on the Isle of Wight were given this new style examination.

The reliability of the examination was found to be satisfactory, particularly after a few items were revised. A number of substudies were carried out to establish the validity of the examination:

(i) During the first term, all the children were also given a large battery of psychological tests aimed at identifying children who would have difficulty with learning (see below). When the 10 per cent of children who performed worst on each assessment were compared, there was only a moderate degree of overlap. From this, it would appear that the two batteries are measuring different aspects of development.

(ii) The concurrent validity of the neuro-developmental examination was assessed by comparing the scores of children with incomprehensible speech, epilepsy, squint, undescended testicles, and asthma with the remainder. In each of the first four conditions, affected children had significantly higher scores than their normal peers. In the case of asthma, as expected, the scores of the affected and normal children were identical. Thus it appears that the examination has concurrent validity as a measure of neurological and developmental integrity. It is not greatly influenced by conditions which do not have a direct influence on central nervous system function.

(iii) All the children were the subjects of a number of follow-up studies. Over half the children whose neuro-developmental status indicated the likelihood of forthcoming difficulties did indeed show evidence of such difficulties some three to four years later. These children had either done badly in reading, had been identified by parents or teachers as having behavioural difficulties, or had been referred to the local educational psychologist on account of learning and/or behavioural difficulties. Fewer than 5 per cent of the children who were not identified on the initial medical examination were picked up in the follow-up studies. Thus it appears that this first attempt at improving the first school medical examination has been partially successful. However, it is recognized that by itself this is not sufficiently sensitive a predictor of later difficulties to warrant its use in isolation. In these first studies, it produced too many false negatives and false positives in relation to the number of true positive cases that it succeeded in identifying.

The earlier Isle of Wight studies of 8- to 10-year-olds strongly suggested that children who were identified as poor readers at that age had presented with histories of delays and deviations in a number of areas earlier in their school career. In particular, the literature on the early identification of children with learning disabilities suggested that difficulties in language and visual–motor co-ordination were strongly implicated.

Under the supervision of Professor J. Tizard and Mr W. Yule, a battery of 12 psychological tests was adapted and developed by Miss S. Butler. This battery was administered to all the children who entered school on the Isle of Wight in the autumn term

1967—some 440 children in all. The children were assessed on reading and arithmetic in both 1969 and 1970, to see how good the battery was at predicting later scholastic performance. Great attention was paid to establishing the reliability of all tests used. In summary, it was found that whereas the test battery score did correlate significantly with later reading scores, this was not sufficient for the purposes of making predictions in individual cases. This appears to be the general conclusion of all such studies so far. Early testing misclassifies many more children than it correctly identifies.

As noted earlier, there was only poor agreement with the independent medical examination. If anything, the psychological battery was slightly better in its predictions. However, the power of the psychological battery as a predictor is largely accounted for by the extent to which it reflects general intellectual ability. The original intention of the study had been to measure specific abilities particularly associated with learning to read. In common with subsequent investigations, it had to be concluded that better predictions could be obtained from using a well standardized test of general intelligence. These studies are reported in detail in Miss Butler's thesis for which she was awarded the degree of Ph.D.

The scales developed by Professor M. Rutter as screening devices in identifying behavioural and emotional disorder in older, junior school children have been very widely used in a number of studies. It was decided to adapt those scales for completion by parents and teachers of 5-year-olds. Although the adaptations were somewhat crude, the adapted scales clearly fill a much felt gap since already they have been used and developed by a number of other workers (Anderson 1973; Behar and Stringfield 1974).

The preliminary studies carried out so far on the sample of 440 children first identified at the age of four in 1967 show that behavioural ratings at age 5 years correlate significantly with reading attainment at age 7. Of the 37 poorest readers, 22 (or 59 per cent) were rated by their reception class teachers as showing poor concentration, compared with only 80 of the remaining 398 (i.e. 20 per cent) who turned out to be good readers. This suggests that temperamental characteristics evident by the age of 5 may, in part, underlie the later associations between poor reading and behavioural disorders.

The same sample was used to study enuresis (see Rutter *et al.* 1973). It was found that there was a slight *rise* in the prevalence of enuresis between 5 and 7 years of age due to a proportion of children who had gained bladder control during the pre-school years becoming wet again after starting school. This finding would only have emerged reliably from a longitudinal study.

Studies of adolescents on the Isle of Wight

The meaning of many of the findings from the cross-sectional surveys undertaken with youngsters in middle childhood depended to a considerable extent on what happened to the individuals and to their disorders over the succeeding years of development. As a result a systematic follow-through to the end of compulsory schooling (age 15 years at the time of the research) was planned.

Longitudinal studies are generally (and rightly) considered to be a very expensive type of research. However, the Isle of Wight study was actually quite cheap for several rather different reasons. First, the local authority concerned was relatively small (it dealt with a total population of about 100 000), had excellent links between the Health and Education departments, and was exceedingly co-operative. Its records were good and we had frequent informal contact with all of the key people. This made the job of tracing children very much easier than it would otherwise have been. Second, the study was run by people in full-time salaried positions with the Medical Research Council or London University so that

their time was provided as part of their required commitment to research. As a result, we managed with only one research officer (Mr L. Rigley) and a part-time secretary employed specifically for the study. Third, because the study was planned from an Institute with a responsibility for postgraduate training, we were able to call on a large group of experienced and well-trained ex-students for the fieldwork, knowing that they would be familiar with our methods of investigation. Each gave (for an honorarium) several weeks of full-time research on the Isle of Wight. This meant that we had a highly expert team of people to undertake the examinations. The cost was minimal because they were employed elsewhere and we needed to pay them only for the limited period during which they actually interviewed or tested children.

This method of working had the big advantage that it enabled us to see a very large number of children within a quite short period of time (and hence at the same age). During the most intensive period of data gathering we had up to 50 investigators all living in one hotel (more or less taken over for the period of the study) and going out each day to see parents or children. The children were all seen at school either in rooms loaned us for the purpose or in caravans parked in the school grounds for the duration of the study. Electroencephalographic recording (see below) was carried out in an old ambulance converted for the purpose and driven around from school to school.

Several different steps were taken to ensure that the measures taken on the children were comparable and maintained a high standard. First, all investigators either watched a videotape or sat in on an interview (or examinations) undertaken by one of the chief investigators. In subsequent studies we have found videotaped role-playing very effective in training but this was not included in the adolescent study. Second, each field worker was observed seeing children in a pilot sample until a satisfactory standard was reached. Third, throughout the fieldwork, sporadic interviews with children in the main sample were observed to ensure maintenance of standards. Fourth, every evening all fieldworkers met at the hotel with the project directors to discuss problems and to go over difficulties in coding. All workers had a mimeographed set of instructions on interviewing/testing and on coding, and addenda were issued from time to time to deal with new issues as they emerged. Fifth, each protocol was completed the same day with descriptive accounts as well as codings. These schedules were then systematically gone through within 24 hours by Philip Graham and Michael Rutter (for the psychiatric and medical measures) and by William Yule (for the psychological measures). Any errors or ambiguities were taken up immediately with the investigators concerned so that there was rapid corrective feedback. Sixth, reliability studies were undertaken for all new measures and the chief investigators met frequently to ensure that difficulties were dealt with in the same way by all concerned.

The success of such a large-scale longitudinal project with personal study of the sample is heavily dependent on extensive local co-operation. A variety of steps were taken to ensure this. First, we had made sure that everyone concerned had had good feedback on the results of the cross-sectional studies which formed the basis for the follow-through. Regular bulletins on all aspects of the research were provided to schools and to other interested parties. We had meetings with school teachers to discuss our findings more fully and also we met with Local Authority officials and with relevant committees of elected lay members. A meeting with the press was held and the study was reported in the local (as well as national) press. As a result, we were well known on the Island and people appreciated that we went to some effort to make sure that they knew what was going on.

Second, we had taken steps to ensure that the policy-makers and local authority executives knew about any results which carried implications for services. As a result, the Isle of Wight had employed a remedial teacher to help with the reading problems we had revealed in secondary schools, and the paediatric services had been partially remodelled to take account of some of the needs shown by our physical handicap survey. The impact on services, of course, was quite small but it helped that we were known to be concerned to do what we could to utilize research findings to improve what was provided for children and families in need.

In any study it is important to reduce losses to a minimum because non-responders are known to be often systematically different to those on whom information is obtained (as shown, for example, by our findings—see Cox *et al.* 1977). Population turnover in this age group was low on the Isle of Wight and, thanks to good records, there was little difficulty in tracing almost everyone who had left the Island. Total population coverage at the screening stage was virtually 100 per cent complete for teachers' questionnaires, as the teachers were very helpful and as we individually contacted all those who were late in returning forms. Coverage was almost as good in the case of psychological testing. Group tests were used in schools with the whole group concerned and repeat testings were provided to pick up all children absent on the first round. Contact with parents (for behavioural questionnaires) had to be by letter and inevitably the response rate was lower. Only about three-fifths of parents responded the first time to a letter and it was necessary to send out several reminders before some forms were returned. In this way, it was possible to reduce the non-response rate to only 12 per cent—an acceptable level. Because of the importance of the bias resulting from missing information a premium was placed on obtaining measures from several different sources whenever possible. By these means, there were almost no children upon whom we did not have some relevant information and in the great majority of cases information gathering was complete.

At the second stage of the follow-up study when subsamples were individually seen, a different form of contact was used. Letters were sent to all parents whose children were to be included in the intensive study. The letter briefly outlined the purposes of the investigation and the different types of study to be undertaken. No response was needed unless the parents did *not* wish their child to be interviewed and tested at school. A telephone number was given which people could call if they had any queries or reservations. This was manned continuously throughout the day and some parents did telephone with questions or special requests about testing. However, most did not respond and only very few (less than 1 per cent) refused permission for their children to be seen. The adolescents themselves were mostly keen to be seen and with very few exceptions their co-operation posed no problems.

In the letter to the parents they were told that someone from the study would be calling within the next few weeks to interview them. In most cases co-operation was good once personal contact had been made in the home and parents had been able to discuss the study and its aims. We had found previously that this method of contact was much more successful in gaining co-operation than was either a telephone call (it's much easier to refuse an unknown person whom you cannot see) or a letter offering a fixed appointment. Altogether, only 7·9 per cent of the parents could not be interviewed.

Follow-up of children with reading difficulties

In the 1964 survey of Isle of Wight children aged 9–11 years, 'reading backwardness' was defined as an attainment in reading accuracy or comprehension on the Neale test which was 2 years 4 months or more below the child's chronological age; 'reading retardation' was defined as an attainment on either reading accuracy or comprehension which was 2 years 4 months or more below the level predicted on the basis of the child's age and short WISC IQ (Yule 1967; Rutter *et al.* 1970b). Applying these definitions to the total

school population, 155 backward and 86 retarded readers were identified. The two groups overlapped considerably, and had no fewer than 76 children in common. In 1968 and 1969, when the children were aged 14 to 15 years, these two groups of poor readers were traced and individually tested, using the short WISC, the Neale Analysis of Reading Ability, the Schonell Spelling Test, and the Vernon Arithmetic–mathematics test (Yule 1973). A random sample of the general population ($N=184$) was similarly tested.

It was found that 56 per cent of all backward readers and 58 per cent of all retarded readers still had a reading attainment score more than two standard deviations below the general population control group mean. Only 4 per cent of the backward readers and 2½ per cent of the retarded readers had a reading accuracy score at the mean or above, and overall both groups of poor readers had average scores for the 9-year-old level. Thus, the majority of children who were found to have severe reading difficulties in their primary school continued to lag far behind in reading right to the end of their compulsory school days. Furthermore, at age 14–15 years they lagged even further behind in their spelling than they did in their reading. Their mathematics scores were well below those of the control group but, relatively speaking, mathematics was less impaired than reading.

In addition to the follow-up of poor readers, in 1968 and 1969 a total population survey of reading skills was undertaken in youngsters in their last year of compulsory schooling (i.e. aged 14–15 years). As in the earlier studies (Rutter *et al.* 1970b), a two-stage procedure was used to identify poor readers. The first stage consisted of testing all children on group tests of non-verbal intelligence (NFER Non-Verbal Test 3) and of reading (NFER test NS 6). All children who scored at least two standard deviations below the population mean, together with a randomly selected control group, were picked for individual testing, using the tests outlined above.

It was found that 6 per cent of adolescents scored at least two standard deviations below the population mean on the individually administered Neale test. This 6 per cent all had a reading accuracy score which was less than 9 years 1 month and were thus some six years behind in their reading. Reading retardation was defined, as before, in terms of a reading attainment at least two standard errors below that predicted on the basis of the child's general level of intelligence (on the WISC). Within this one year cohort, chronological age did not correlate with reading score and so was not included in the prediction equation. Using this definition, 4·8 per cent of the adolescents were found to have reading retardation. As these definitions include only very extreme levels of reading difficulty, it is evident that poor reading is still a very common problem even at the point children are able to leave school in mid-adolescence.

Because data were available on the same population at the age of 10 years, it was possible to determine how far reading difficulties at 14–15 years represented a continuation of problems already present in primary school. Of the 111 reading-retarded adolescents, 52 were identified as having reading retardation at the age of 10 years, a further 27 had been identified as backward readers in primary school, 13 had been selected at the age of 10 years as showing poor reading attainment on the group test (but fell just outside the group identified on individual testing), and 11 were newcomers to the Island and so had not been tested previously. Thus only eight youngsters with reading retardation in adolescence had not already shown severe reading difficulties in primary school. This small number merely reflects the sort of misclassification inevitable in the use of a particular cut-off point on any psychological test. It may be concluded that severe reading difficulties at the time of school leaving have almost always been present from primary school days.

The data from all the various Isle of Wight and London studies of children with reading difficulties were put together to see how far different diagnostic subgroups could be identified. The findings showed the importance of a distinction between *general reading backwardness* (i.e. low attainment in relation to age, regardless of intelligence) and *specific reading retardation* (i.e. a specific disability in reading not explicable in terms of the child's general intelligence). The two differed in terms of sex distribution, statistical properties, and clinical correlates (Rutter and Yule 1975). The differences certainly implied that the two types of reading disability had a somewhat different origin but it did not necessarily follow that these had any educational implications. Longitudinal data were needed to determine this, and the links between the 10-year-old and 15-year-old findings were utilized for this purpose (Yule 1973).

Initially (at the age of 10–11 years) the specifically retarded and generally backward groups were reading at about the same level, namely some 33 months on the average below the level in the general population control group. But, as implicit in the definition of the two groups, the average IQ of the reading-backward children was more than one standard deviation below that of the specifically retarded children. Nevertheless, as shown by the individual test findings at the age of 14–15 years, the specifically retarded children had made significantly less progress in reading during the four- to five-year follow-up period. They had also made less progress in spelling. In marked contrast to the findings for reading and spelling, just the opposite was found with respect to progress in arithmetic. On the arithmetic–maths test employed, the children with specific reading retardation had made more progress than the generally backward children (although both groups were performing below age level). In brief, the distinction between specific reading retardation did have educational implications of a particular kind. The next question clearly is: 'Do the two groups need different types of remedial help with their reading?' No data are available on this point but the findings suggest that the matter warrants investigation.

Follow-up of children with psychiatric disorder at 10 years

In 1965 the total population of children aged 10 and 11 years living on the Isle of Wight was surveyed and on the basis of individual study, about 6 or 7 per cent were diagnosed as having psychiatric disorder (Rutter *et al.* 1970b). In 1968 and 1969 the same total population was similarly surveyed when the children were 14–15 years old (Graham and Rutter 1973), and the original group of children with disorder was systematically followed up and studied in the same way. The outcome varied markedly according to the psychiatric diagnosis at the age of 10 years. Children with conduct disorders fared worst; three-quarters of them still showed disorder in adolescence. The disorders generally ran true to form in terms of diagnosis (the diagnoses at 14 years being made without knowledge of those at 10 years), but an appreciable minority of those with conduct disorders at 10–11 years showed emotional disturbance at 14–15 years. By contrast, children who had suffered from emotional disorders when younger never developed an antisocial problem. The outlook for children with emotional disturbance at 10–11 years was significantly better than for those with conduct disorders, but it was by no means uniformly good. Nearly half still had problems in adolescence, a rate more than double that in the general population. As might be expected, children with mixed emotional and conduct disorders had an intermediate outcome. No sex difference in outcome was found.

The most important prognostic factor with respect to the persistence or non-persistence of psychiatric disorder from 10 to 14 years was the diagnosis at age 10 years. Neither IQ nor reading attainment at the age of 10 years was of predictive value. On the whole, family disturbance was more marked in the group of youngsters with persistent disorders, but the only significant difference concerned whether or not the child had been in short-term care (of the Local Authority). In the group with non-persistent disorders only 8·7 per cent had been in care, compared with 32·8 per cent in the

group with disorders that had continued from 10 years to 14–15 years (Rutter *et al.* 1976b).

The findings are in generally good agreement with previous investigations in showing that, although psychosocial and educational variables are very important influences in the development of psychiatric problems, they are less critical in terms of the course of the problem once the disorder is established. Conduct disorders have a generally poor outcome with respect to both symptomatology and social impairment. Our own work shows this with respect to persistence of problems from middle childhood into adolescence, and other investigations have shown the same in terms of persistence into adult life (Robins 1966, 1972a). Emotional disorders proved less persistent, but even so nearly half the children continued to have problems. Other studies suggest that the long-term prognosis may be rather better.

Power *et al.* (1974) found that delinquents from discordant and disrupted homes were more likely to become recidivist than those from a cohesive home. The Isle of Wight findings with respect to the predictive importance of periods of short-term admission to children's homes or foster homes are in keeping with the results from Power's study in suggesting that family variables have some relationship to the course of child conduct disorders.

Although educational variables have a strong association with psychiatric disorder, and although educational failure or poor schooling may predispose to psychiatric problems, neither general intelligence nor scholastic attainment was of any predictive value regarding the persistence of emotional or behavioural disturbance. Whether this means that neither influence the course of psychiatric disorder, once it is established, or whether the negative finding simply reflects the fact that in the sample studied few children with scholastic failure improved over the course of the four-year follow-up cannot be determined from our data. It has sometimes been supposed that psychiatric disturbance in children frequently impairs intellectual test performance to a substantial degree. This may well occur in some children but our findings indicate that it is unlikely to be a common occurrence. Among the children who ceased to have psychiatric disorder during the follow-up period, the IQ remained constant at about 103 and among those who continued to show disorder it remained at about 102. The type of psychiatric disorder was unrelated to changes in IQ.

In addition to the follow-up study at age 15 years of children identified as having psychiatric disorder at age 10 years, there was a total cross-sectional survey of psychiatric disorder in adolescence. In 1968 and 1969, all 14- to 15-year-old children resident on the Isle of Wight were surveyed by means of parent and teacher questionnaires. All children with deviant scores on either questionnaire, together with all those who had been under psychiatric care or been before the courts in the previous years were studied intensively by means of interviews with parents, teachers and the adolescents themselves. A randomly chosen control group of 200 children was studied in the same way. In all cases, the interviewers were unaware of the reason for selection.

Considering only those children selected on the screening procedures and diagnosed on the basis of intensive individual study, 7·7 per cent of 14- to 15-year-olds showed a handicapping psychiatric disorder (Graham and Rutter 1973). Disorder was twice as common in boys as in girls, the sex difference being entirely due to the higher rate of conduct disorders and mixed disorders in males—a pattern closely similar to that evident at the age of 10–11 years. Emotional disorders were equally common in the two sexes and other diagnoses were uncommon.

Taking into account all available information, it was concluded that there was a slight rise in the rate of psychiatric disorder during early adolescence but the increase was only moderate (Rutter *et al.* 1976b). On the other hand, there were two marked differences in the type of disorders present at age 14 years compared to those manifest at the age of 10 years. First, depression was much more common in adolescence. At 10 years, there were only three children with a depressive condition, whereas at 14 years there were nine, plus another 26 with an affective disorder involving both anxiety and depression. This difference indicates the beginning of a shift to an adult pattern of psychiatric disorder. Secondly, at age 14 years there were 15 cases of school refusal whereas there had been none at the age of 10 years. In many cases the school refusal formed part of a more widespread anxiety state or affective disorder, but, in all, the reluctance to go to school constituted one of the main problems. The findings are in keeping with the clinical evidence that school refusal is most prevalent in early childhood and again at adolescence. In the younger children, the problem is more in keeping with normal developmental patterns and the prognosis is usually very good. In contrast, school refusal in adolescents is more often part of a widespread psychiatric disorder and the prognosis is considerably worse. Further findings are reported in Rutter (1979c).

Three-fifths of the psychiatric disorders evident at the age of 14 years had newly developed during early adolescence, but the remainder constituted continuations of conditions already present in the childhood years before the age of 10. These two groups differed sharply in a number of respects (Rutter *et al.* 1976b). First, whereas there was a marked preponderance of boys among the persistent cases, in the new cases the sex ratio was nearer equal. Second, the children with psychiatric disorders persisting from early and middle childhood tended to have marked reading and arithmetic difficulties. However, this was not so at all in the case of children with new disorders, whose scholastic attainments were closely similar to those in the general population. Third, with respect to all the variables measured, family difficulties were more strongly associated with psychiatric disorder arising in childhood than with disorder arising *de novo* in adolescence. Thus a third of the children with persistent disorders had been placed into the care of the local authority for short periods compared with only 8·3 per cent of those with new disorders. Almost two-fifths were not living with their two natural parents compared with less than a quarter of those with new conditions. In short, it appeared that the psychiatric problems arising for the first time during adolescence differed in several important respects from the problems beginning in earlier childhood.

Longitudinal data are particularly useful to sort out the timing of associations. Their value in this connection is illustrated by the findings on enuresis (Rutter *et al.* 1973). Associations between enuresis and behavioural deviance were examined in several different ways—by teacher questionnaire, parental questionnaire, and psychiatric appraisal. By all methods of assessment and at all ages there was a strong association between enuresis and behavioural deviance. However, this association was much stronger in girls than in boys and was probably more marked when day-time as well as night-time wetting was involved. So far as could be determined, the association with behavioural deviance was just as strong in the case of children who had never gained bladder control as in those who had achieved continence but later lost it. Behavioural deviance was three times as common in the children who had been enuretic at 9–10 years and who still wet at 14 years, as in those who gained bladder control between 9–10 years and 14 years.

A detailed examination of the pattern of associations indicated a stronger and more basic connection between enuresis and behavioural deviance than had previously been thought. Ten-year-old enuretic children who were also behaviourally deviant were less likely to become dry by 14 years than were 10-year-old enuretic children without behavioural difficulties. Conversely, behaviourally deviant enuretic children who became dry were more likely to lose their behavioural problems than those who remained wet. On the other hand, children who were dry at 14 years but who had been enuretic at the age of 10 years were more likely to show behavioural deviance at 14 years (i.e. when dry) than were youngsters who had gained bladder control before 9–10 years. Bed-wetting is a common disorder and the association with behavioural deviance in girls is strong. Further research is needed to determine the mechanisms involved.

An electroencephalographic (EEG) study of 14-year-olds was undertaken by Drs Fenton and Fenwick as part of the epidemiological studies of 14-year-olds (Fenwick *et al.* 1973; Fenton *et al.* 1973a, b, 1974; Maxwell *et al.* 1974). Resting bipolar recordings were performed on each youngster at school and the data were analysed by visual inspection and by auto power spectra computation. No association was found between EEG abnormalities (as determined visually) and either reading difficulty or psychiatric disorder. However, the mean power frequencies of less good readers were significantly greater than those for the better readers in the eyes-open situations, but not when the eyes were closed. The meaning of these differences remains uncertain, but Maxwell *et al.* (1974) have hypothesized that the increased power frequencies reflect inefficient brain functioning in terms of the use of more neurons than ideally required.

Overview of Isle of Wight studies

Throughout the entire period of the Isle of Wight project from 1964 to 1979, Michael Rutter and Jack Tizard remained as co-directors, with Philip Graham, Kingsley Whitmore, and William Yule jointly responsible as chief investigators for most of the studies. The investigations were initially planned when the directors were both members of the M.R.C. Social Psychiatry Research Unit, but the fact that the key people are now split between three separate Institutes of the University of London has not caused any major difficulties. Different investigators have taken prime responsibility for planning different aspects of the studies and this arrangement has generally worked very well in spite of the need for rather complex interdisciplinary collaboration. The only slight problems have come when there has been ambiguity about where the main responsibility lay.

Although not planned for this purpose, the project has been extremely valuable for both research and clinical training. The field workers have learned a great deal (as also we have) from seeing large numbers of normal children and from assessing handicapped children in their own environment away from the clinic. In addition, the project has provided good opportunities for people to learn epidemiological and longitudinal study techniques and strategies while working as members of a closely integrated research team. This has been taken advantage of by paediatricians, psychologists, and psychiatrists but, in retrospect, it is clear that we could have made greater use of training opportunities if the necessary studentships and fellowships had been available.

Despite quite tight restrictions on funding we have not been greatly troubled by budgetary difficulties at the stage of data collection. Inevitably there have been crises when there has been uncertainty about future funding but research grants have been received in time for advance planning and piloting of measures for nearly all aspects of the research. However, the long-term programmatic approach to the research issues has only been possible because initially the key people were in receipt of relatively long-term personal funding from either the Medical Research Council (Jack Tizard and Michael Rutter) or the Foundation for Child Development (Philip Graham and William Yule). Subsequently all four continued in tenured University posts which provided similar opportunities for programme planning.

The main headaches have concerned data analysis. The strength of the study has depended in large part on the possibility of linking epidemiological with longitudinal data, of linking screening information on the total population with much more intensive data on subsamples, and of bringing together psychometric, psychiatric, educational, and medical measures. However, therein have lain the difficulties. We have always lacked a computer programmer and it is now clear that a study of this size really requires someone with considerable experience in programming who can have the study as his main (or sole) responsibility. Although we have managed through our own skills in this area, or those of research assistants, it is not a very satisfactory way of doing things. As a result, although many of the data are on tape in a readily accessible form this is not so for all the earlier measures (which remain on punch cards which are less easily linked). The data are now all stored at the Institute of Psychiatry and whenever possible the original interview protocols have been retained. This has proved valuable on occasions when new research questions have meant going back to the raw data. Analyses are still continuing and further publications are in preparation. However, it is evident that we (like many others) originally underestimated the time needed for proper utilization of all the data. The phase when we have always been short of funds has been that of data analysis. As judged by our own experience, research grants given specifically for this purpose with well established studies would be very worthwhile.

Inner London studies

The Isle of Wight – Inner London comparative epidemiological study has already been mentioned. It started simply as a project to compare rates of disorder in two different geographical areas and to explore the *reasons* for any differences found (see Rutter *et al.* 1975b; Rutter and Quinton 1977, for a discussion of the findings on possible reasons). However, it also formed the basis for a longitudinal study which is still continuing; it is that aspect which will be described here.

The original study showed that rates of both behavioural deviance and reading retardation varied greatly from primary school to primary school. In some schools, rates of disorder were very high whereas in other rates were low. Two sorts of analyses suggested that these differences might represent the effect of a school influence on children's behaviour and attainments. First, the differences still remained even after controls had been introduced to take account of differences in the children's family background. Second, the school variation was systematically associated with characteristics of the school such as teacher turnover (see Rutter *et al.* 1975b). Both observations suggested that the school variation was not just an artefact of selective intake. On the other hand, in the absence of direct measures on the children's characteristics at the time they entered school any inference about a school effect would have to be speculative. A longitudinal study was needed to test the hypothesis that schools had a differential influence on children's development.

Follow-up into secondary school

Accordingly, it was decided to take the cohort of children studied at age 10 years and to follow their progress in secondary school. In this way it would be possible to look at *changes* in behaviour or attainment in relation to school characteristics. Because we had measures on what the children were like just prior to secondary transfer we could take account of any effects due to schools admitting different proportions of difficult or backward children.

This part of the study was funded by grants from the Inner London Education Authority and the Department of Education and Science to M.R., with Mrs Bridget Yule as the research worker who had prime responsibility for the study. As on the Isle of Wight, data collection was concentrated into a short period of time with maximum use of volunteers working on a short-term sessional

basis. Good co-operation from schools was maintained in the same way through regular school bulletins, frequent personal contact with both Headteachers and school clerical staff, and meetings to discuss findings with school teachers in all the schools concerned. Primary schools were able to provide us with details of which secondary school each child went to at age 11 years, and the tracing of children who moved home was mainly done through school records.

The data available on the sample at age 10 years included the Rutter B2 behavioural questionnaire completed by teachers (see Rutter 1967; Rutter *et al.* 1975a), reading attainment as assessed by the NFER group test SR1, and non-verbal intelligence as measured by the NFER group test NV5, together with certain social features (parental occupation and place of birth) and characteristics of the primary school attended (as indicated by statistical data such as that on teacher and pupil turnover).

At age 13 years (in 1973) the children were reassessed on comparable measures (the same teacher questionnaire B2, NFER Non Verbal Test 3 of the NFER group reading test NS6). In addition, the children's current absenteeism rate was noted by reference to school attendance registers. The children were widely scattered across some 100 secondary schools but vigorous efforts were made to trace and test every child, including those who had moved out of London. As luck would have it, this stage of the survey coincided with a period of exceptional difficulty for schools associated with considerable unrest among teachers. In spite of this we obtained data on over 90 per cent of the children. However, data were totally missing from one school with many cohort children and there were missing data on many children in another school. As this might have resulted in significant non-response bias the reading and behaviour survey was repeated in its entirety a year later when the children were aged 14 years. Because of the evidence that there was little change of IQ scores over 1 year at this age and in order to reduce the burden on schools, non-verbal IQ testing was carried out only for children who missed the 1973 survey. When it became apparent that retesting was needed, the findings showing a non-response bias (see Rutter 1977a, and Cox *et al.* 1977) were presented at one of our regular meetings with school teachers. They appreciated the need and as they were very concerned that the findings should present a true picture they readily agreed to the considerable extra work being asked of them.

In spite of continuing problems in London schools we received splendid co-operation from teachers for this second survey. In most cases teachers supervised the group testing themselves but in a few cases one of the research group did so and, in a few others, teachers from one of the other schools helped out. In order to ensure that absentees were tested, several repeat testings were held in each school to catch missing children whenever they returned. By these means reading scores were obtained on over 93 per cent of the children and behavioural questionnaires were available for virtually 100 per cent. Since 1970 we had had an informal advisory group of head teachers from local primary and secondary schools who met with the research team both to consider research planning and to note the service implications stemming from research findings. Not only was this group exceedingly helpful in working out what measures to use and how to collect them, but also they gave invaluable assistance in ensuring full co-operation from all their colleagues.

The marking of group tests and the scoring of behavioural questionnaires was done by paid volunteers (mostly colleagues in the Institute and teachers known to us) working over several weekends and supervised throughout by Bridget Yule. All scoring and marking was done a second time by a different worker in order to reduce error to a minimum. In addition to the behaviour and reading scores, delinquency records were obtained for all children up to age 14 years.

In the analyses which examined school variation attention was mainly focused on the 21 non-selective state schools which took most of the children. Although in theory the schools all served much the same part of Inner London and were non-selective in their intake, in practice some schools took a far higher proportion of difficult or backward children (as shown by our primary school measures) than others (see Rutter 1977a). Accordingly, it was necessary to take account of these intake differences when examining variations between schools. Both statistical regression and standardization procedures were used for this purpose (with closely similar results—see Rutter 1977a). The findings showed that marked differences between schools with respect to behaviour, attainment, attendance, and delinquency remained even after controlling for differences in intake (see Rutter 1977a; Rutter *et al*. 1979). Indeed, one of the schools with a superior academic record had one of the highest proportions of backward children at intake.

The results showed that the large variations in children's behaviour between secondary schools in Inner London could not be accounted for by the characteristics of the children (at least on our measures) at the time they entered secondary school. This could only have been found out through a longitudinal study.

Study of schools as social institutions

However, two further steps were required before school influences on children's development could be identified with any certainty. First, it was necessary to show that the variations were linked in a systematic way with demonstrable features of the school environment. This has been done in a detailed study funded by a grant from the Department of Education and Science to Professor Michael Rutter; with Miss Barbara Maughan (a social worker by training), Dr Peter Mortimore (an experienced teacher also trained as an educational psychologist). and Dr Janet Ouston (a developmental psychologist) as principal investigators.

The study has had several different objectives. In the first place, it has provided the opportunity to follow the same group of children through to age 16 years, which is now the point at which compulsory schooling comes to an end in Britain. This had enabled the delinquency figures to be updated with a coverage of the whole of the children's school years. As a result the data are complete in a way that they were not before (because much delinquency does not begin until after 14 years) and there are enough delinquents for a more satisfactory breakdown into types of offence and into once-only offenders and recidivists. Also, the educational findings have been greatly broadened by consideration of the public examination results ('CSE' and 'O' levels) at age 16 years. The findings again confirm the wide variation between schools.

The study also marked a shift from a focus on the individual as the object of study to an investigation of the school itself as a social institution. This necessitated taking measures on other different age groups of children to ensure that our longitudinal study cohort was representative of the school population as a whole. Such measures showed that, with a few minor exceptions, it was. In addition, various assessments were taken of children's behaviour in the school as a whole (these included measures of vandalism and of disruptive behaviour in classrooms and in the playground).

However, the main research investment during the last 5 years has been in the study of the school itself. The measures taken include standardized interviews with staff, pupil questionnaires, systematic time- and event-sampled observations in the classroom and elsewhere, administrative statistics, and a variety of more informal measures. One third-year class in each school was followed through an entire week's activity and a group of new entrants were observed during their first few days in class and again later in the school year. The findings show immense variations in ethos and practice between schools which are systematically associated with differences in children's behaviour and attainment

(Rutter *et al.* 1979). In this way it has been possible to identify school features which are likely to lead to the children gaining better scholastic attainments and showing a more normal behavioural adjustment.

Hopefully, the findings should have implications for educational policy. Nevertheless, it should be appreciated that another step is still necessary before firm conclusions can be drawn; that, too, requires a longitudinal design. The last step involves the *planned* alteration of school practice together with a prospective study to determine if the change in practice has indeed had the actual benefits that were hypothesized. This last piece of research has only recently begun.

Employment study

The final study to be described in this chapter is the latest follow-up of the cohort of children first studied in 1970 at age 10 years. The sample were first able to legally leave school in 1976 at age 16 years and the majority did in fact do so, although about one in five remained at school for at least a further year. The aim of this investigation, funded by the Department of Education and Science with Mrs Grace Gray as the principal investigator, is to study the first year of employment. The process of obtaining work and patterns (and levels) of employment and unemployment is being related to information on the secondary schools attended (from the study of schools as social institutions) and to individual data about the young people and their families obtained at age 10 years.

The sample consisted of the 300 or so young persons who were part of the intensive study in 1970 (and hence with detailed psychometric, psychiatric, and family data), together with about 70 individuals from each of the 12 secondary schools studied in detail—that is some 1000 people in all. Each person was personally interviewed at home (or at school for those still there) according to a pre-piloted standardized interview. A team of experienced interviewers (mostly consisting of psychologist and social work colleagues) have undertaken the interviewing on a sessional basis, as in the earlier Isle of Wight studies. All interviewers were thoroughly briefed by Mrs Grace Gray and all interview protocols and all codings were systematically checked by her.

The data concerning the young people who left school at age 16 years have been analysed and preliminary findings have been reported in Gray *et al.* (1980). Interviews are now nearly complete for those who left school at 17 or 18 years. All data are being maintained on either punchcards or tape, in a form available for linkage with any later follow-ups, should they take place. At present, the plan is to reassess employment (and possibly other aspects of functioning) in some 5 years time when it can be expected that most people will have settled on a career.

Impact of the London studies

Like the Isle of Wight studies, the epidemiological and longitudinal studies in London have been planned and carried out with the close collaboration of both local authority personnel and community workers (especially teachers). The informal advisory working group of research workers and teachers has been especially influential throughout the whole of the programme and has been very helpful in ensuring that both policy makers and the local community become aware of the relevant study findings. In addition to the regular meetings with schools described above, an open meeting for the general public was held as part of the local 'Mental Health Week' gatherings.

It is too early to assess the impact of most of the London studies as the longitudinal enquiries are still in progress. However, the earlier findings on the high rate of educational backwardness and problem behaviour in London schools played a part in the local authority deciding to set aside special funds for action projects to relieve these problems. As part of this programme, the authority seconded an experienced teacher (Veronica Wigley) to work with Dr Michael Berger and Mr William Yule in running workshops for primary school teachers on how teacher–child interaction in the classroom may be modified to reduce problem behaviour. The authority also funded the first part of the secondary school studies, indicating its concern to find ways of improving the situation in secondary schools.

In addition, the findings from both the Isle of Wight and London studies, especially those dealing with the prevalence and patterning of handicaps and those indicating the higher rate of disorder in metropolitan areas, have had some impact on governmental planning, as indicated by citation in various major reports such as those on reading difficulties (Bullock 1975), on child health services (Court 1976) and on scientific thinking, as indicated by references in textbooks and research papers.

Conclusion

Longitudinal studies in Britain are often thought of in terms of national enquiries following children from birth through childhood into adult life (see chapters 6 and 7). Such studies have obvious strengths but of necessity their focus is broad and their information gathering limited to data obtainable by questionnaire and standard examination or test. In contrast, the Isle of Wight and London studies have had a sharp focus; the longitudinal studies have generally been limited to periods of half a dozen years chosen for some specific purpose; and there has been an emphasis on the combination of total population coverage using screening measures with a much more detailed clinical study of selected subsamples. A great deal of effort has been spent on the development of reliable and valid measures and comparable standardized techniques have been used in each of the studies. As a result it is possible to combine the studies or contrast the findings in order to answer particular research questions. For example, this has been done with epidemiological data from the Isle of Wight and London studies in connection with the effects of multiple hospital admission (Quinton and Rutter 1976); the differentiation of varieties of reading disability (Rutter and Yule, 1973, 1975); and the effects of organic brain dysfunction (Rutter 1977b). The strategy is a strong one (Rutter 1970b), as replication is much the best test in science. It is hoped to use a similar approach with the longitudinal studies currently in progress which have been described in this chapter.

22. Epidemiological investigations of mental health, educational attainment, and social development of children and young people in Reykjavík, Iceland

SIGURJON BJÖRNSSON

The research reported in this chapter started as a cross-sectional investigation of representative samples of children and adolescents in Reykjavík, aged 5–15. Most of the data were collected during the years 1965 and 1966. This study has since been extended in various ways:

(1) By in-depth studies in specific areas;
(2) By follow-up studies in specific areas and on subsamples;
(3) By a general mental health follow-up study on the original sample.

In the following a summary of the cross-sectional investigation will be presented. Mention will be made of the in-depth studies and summary of the follow-up studies on subsamples. Lastly the main outlines of the general follow-up study, which is now in its beginning phase, will be described.

Cross-sectional investigation of mental health of children

The aims of this investigation were threefold:

(1) To study the validity of the American norms of the Rorschach test for Icelandic children;
(2) To standardize the Wechsler Intelligence Scale for Children;
(3) To investigate the incidence of mental disorders of children and relate them to various cognitive, educational, and socio-economic variables.

Materials and methods

The sample size and the sampling procedures were selected for the purpose of meeting the requirements of the WISC standardization, as well as by practical limitations. The size of the sample was 1100 children, aged 5–15 years, 50 children in each age/sex group. The children were examined as close to their birthday as possible. Each month, 50 children could be tested and their mothers interviewed.

The subjects were selected from the Reykjavík census of 1963. The investigation started in January 1965 with the 15-year age group and continued in descending age until December 1966 when it finished with the 5-year-old group. Thus the sample consisted of children born between 1950 and 1961.

First, we picked out from the census for investigation all those children in the respective age groups who had birthdays within a two-month period. This gave us 2330 children, theoretically one-sixth of all children in Reykjavík within these age groups. A number of children had then to be excluded on various grounds, e.g.:

(1) All children who had attended the Municipal Child Guidance Clinic for assessment or therapy as well as their siblings, as information already obtained about them and previous contact with the parents would have biased the outcome of the investigations. (The investigation was conducted by the staff of the Municipal Child Guidance Clinic of Reykjavík.)
(2) All families who were personally related to or acquainted with the investigators.

A total of 150 children were excluded for reasons (1) and (2). The remaining 2180 children were then listed in alphabetical order within each age/sex group.

(3) By descending age, all children on the list who had a sibling in an older age group on the list were excluded, i.e., an additional 219 children.
(4) By a random rule, 348 children were dropped from the list, leaving a pool of 1613 children, 75–80 children in each age/sex group. This constituted the pool of children which should provide a sample of 1100.
(5) Of this pool, 221 children had moved from the Reykjavík area permanently or temporarily, or could not be traced.
(6) Of those remaining, 201 children or their parents refused participation for some reason, and 91 were not needed, as the sample was complete before their turn came.

This sample of 1100 children represents 6·31 per cent of the population of children aged 5–15 years in Reykjavík.

The representativeness of this sample can of course be questioned. The exclusion of groups (1) and (6) is especially critical. It is reasonable to believe that they contain a higher proportion of mentally disturbed children, so that the percentage of mentally disturbed children arrived at in this study is likely to be somewhat low. Nevertheless the representativeness of the sample can to some extent be estimated by the fact that it proved to be entirely satisfactory for the standardization of the WISC test. IQs were evenly distributed for all age groups and no corrective measures had to be taken to obtain a normal distribution.

As regards the investigation of mental disorders and their correlates, variables are divided into two sets:

1. Five mental health variables;
2. Twenty-nine cognitive, educational, socio-economic, and demographic variables.

These variables will now be summarily described.

Three out of five mental health variables were based on observation, that is of the WISC-tester, the Rorschach-tester, and the interviewer of the mother. These workers were required to group the children into three categories:

1. Well-balanced children in good mental health;
2. Fairly well-balanced children, considered to be able to cope with their difficulties without expert help;
3. Emotionally disturbed children in poor mental health. These children were expected to need expert help.

The fourth mental health variable was constructed in view of the outcome of the Rorschach test. The variable was divided in three categories as before. Selection criteria for the categories were as follows:

To be selected into the first group the child should meet all the following criteria:

(1) R 10–15;
(2) W above the 25th percentile;
(3) D below the 75th percentile;
(4) F per cent below 100;
(5) All other determinants should be between the 10th and the 90th percentile except M, and FC could go above the 90th percentile;
(6) $F+$ per cent above the 50th percentile;
(7) A per cent lower than the 75th percentile;
(8) H per cent higher than the 25th percentile;
(9) t below the 90th percentile;
(10) No cards rejected.

To be selected for the third group the child should meet one or more of the following criteria:

(1) $F+$ per cent below the 10th percentile (below the 25th percentile if W per cent was above the 75th percentile);
(2) R 8 or below;
(3) C 2 or more;
(4) Rejected 3 or more.

The remaining children fell into the second group.

The fifth and the last mental health variable consisted of an assessment of mental health by means of clinical evaluation of symptom-loading in the child, as described by the mother in an interview with her. The interviewer had in hand a list of about 50 types of symptoms which were intended to cover the main bulk of symptomatological varieties of psychosomatic, behavioural, neurotic, and psychotic problems. In the construction of this list several textbooks and other sources on child psychiatry or psychopathology in childhood had been consulted. The mother was asked to report on all the symptoms with which her child had been afflicted since birth (the symptom list serving as a mnemonic aid to the mother). She was asked to describe each symptom, the age of the child at its onset, and its date of cessation, when this was the case. The interviewer evaluated the degree of severity of each symptom on the basis of the mother's information, on a three-point scale ranging from very slight symptoms to very severe ones. These data were then used by an independent worker for the definition of three categories of symptom-loading. These categories were defined in the same manner as for the other four mental health variables. For the classification of the children into these three categories the following six items were taken into account:

(a) The number of symptoms;
(b) The type of symptom;
(c) The degree of severity;
(d) The duration of symptoms;
(e) The constellation of symptoms;
(f) The age of the child.

Of the 29 cognitive, educational, socio-economic, and demographic variables three were derived from WISC scores: IQ verbal, IQ performance, and IQ full scale. The fourth variable was a Grade Point Average (GPA) from the final examination at the end of 6th grade, which marks the transition at 12 years into the lower secondary school. When computations were made for the initial investigation, only the 600 oldest subjects of the sample had passed this age. Grades have been collected later for the remaining subjects for use in continued studies.

The remaining 25 variables were all constructed from interview data (interview with mothers). These are:

(1) Family constellation. This variable was grouped into the following four categories:

(i)   Intact families. Both biological parents present in a common home;
(ii) Broken families, first category. One biological parent present and a parent substitute;
(iii) Broken families, second category. One biological parent present and no parent substitute;
(iv) Broken families, third category. No biological parent present.

(2) Change of residence. Reykjavík is a fast-growing city. During recent decades the geographical mobility of its inhabitants has been of two kinds: People move to the city from the country and the smaller towns, and families frequently change their domicile within the city. Although the interview contained very detailed information on residential change, a very simple scale was used where only the number of changes was taken into account, without regard to the nature of mobility. This scale consisted of five categories from no change to four or more changes (i–v).

(3) The number of children in the subject's family. This variable pertains to the total number of children which have been brought up together with the subject under study, the subject himself being included in the number. Included are half-siblings, adoptive, and foster children, whereas stillborn siblings, siblings who have died in their first or second year, and siblings who have been brought up elsewhere are excluded.

(4–5) The number of children in the parents' families. Two variables have been defined for the number of children in the mothers' and the fathers' families respectively. Here, nine categories were used, the ninth category including 9 children and more.

(6) The occupational status of the father. As no classification system of occupational groups that could be used in a socio-psychological study such as the present one had previously been constructed in Iceland, a classification for the present sample was wrought with many difficulties. As the problems in question and the

reasons for the construction of the present scale are the subject matter of a separate paper they will not be discussed here. The occupational scale contains the following six categories:

(i) Non-skilled manual work. Daily labourers, sailors, farmers, taxi chauffeurs, unskilled foremen, pensioners, persons on social welfare;
(ii) Skilled manual workers and artisans;
(iii) Non-skilled clerical work;
(iv) Technical work, lower managerial, artistic, teaching professions (elementary and secondary level);
(v) Independent businessmen, directorial and managerial occupations in business and industry;
(vi) Specialists with academic education, teachers at grammar school and university level. Higher officials in central and local government.

(7–8) The occupational status of maternal and paternal grandfathers. The same scale as for the foregoing variable.

(9) Working schedule of the father. A scale of four categories was constructed:

(i) Regular daytime working hours;
(ii) Irregular working hours;
(iii) Working in shifts;
(iv) Frequent absence from home for reasons of work.

(10) The mother's out-of-home employment. Three categories were used:

(i) Full-time out-of-home employment;
(ii) Half-time out-of-home employment;
(iii) No out-of-home employment (or less than half-time).

(11) Number of rooms in the subject's home. This variable is divided into nine categories, from one room to nine rooms per family.

(12–13) Community origin of the parents. Two variables give a measure of the parents' origin with respect to the degree of urbanization of the community in which they were brought up, one for the mother and one for the father. Both variables are classified into three categories:

(i) Rural communities;
(ii) Villages and small towns;
(iii) Reykjavík (and foreign countries).

Community origin is defined as the socio-geographical region among the three above-mentioned ones in which the parent had been brought up and spent all his childhood and youth. The denotation rural community covers only isolated farms, as other kinds of rural communities do not exist in Iceland. The maximum number of inhabitants in a village is usually 1000–500. The greatest towns outside Reykjavík comprise about 10 000 inhabitants, but most of them are much smaller. As parents brought up in foreign countries were very few, it was not considered necessary to put them in a separate category.

(14–15) Educational level of the parents. Two separate variables were intended to yield a measure of the parents' educational level. They were divided into four educational categories or levels, ranging from elementary to academic level:

(i) Elementary school (or less);
(ii) Secondary school. Vocational school (lower technical education);
(iii) Grammar school. Teachers' training seminary. Higher technical education;
(iv) University.

(16) The mother's attitude toward her own rearing. Clinical child guidance work often indicates that there is a relationship between the mother's attitude toward her own parents, especially her mother, and the presence or absence of emotional problems in her child. With the inclusion of this variable it was intended to put this hypothesis to a preliminary test. On the basis of indirect questioning and spontaneous material the interviewer formed an opinion as to whether the relationship between the mother and her parents had been a harmonious one, with warm and positive feelings, or whether her looking back on her own childhood was characterized by an upsurge of feelings of frustrations, bitterness, and sadness. This variable was divided into two categories: (i) positive attitudes versus (ii) negative. Obviously such a dichotomous distinction provides only a very crude measure, although it was not considered as practicable to operate with a more refined scaling in this context.

(17–21) The mother's child-rearing practices. During the interview the interviewer tried to evaluate the mother's educational attitudes toward her child. Sh had as a guideline a list with about 20 attitudinal items, which were assessed by indirect questioning, spontaneous information, and observational data. From these data five attitudinal variables were constructed:

(17) Warm/coldness. Three categories: cold, neutral, warm. The warm end was defined as accepting, understanding, child-centred attitude and infrequent use of physical punishment. The cold end was defined by the opposite characteristics. A neutral attitude meant that the interviewer was not able to infer either cold or warm child-rearing attitudes in the mother;
(18) Permissiveness/control. Again a three-category scale was used, ranging from a controlling attitude through neutrality to permissiveness. High control is characterized by restrictive practices, demands for obedience, and abstention from aggression toward peers and parents; stress on neatness and orderliness;
(19) Detachment/involvement. The three-category scale runs from anxious emotional involvement to calm detachment, with neutral attitude defined as before. Anxious emotional involvement was characterized by high emotionality in relation to the child, babying, protectiveness, and solicitousness for the child's welfare. Calm detachment meant the opposite of this attitude: lack of emotional contact with the child, a nonchalant and 'laissez-faire' attitude;
(20) Consistency/inconsistency. This is a dichotomous variable. Consistent attitudes were those where the mother seemed to have a reasonably well developed set of educational rules and principles and was able to put them into practice. Inconsistency meant the absence of such principles or a frequent transgressing of them;
(21) Aspiration. This variable was also dichotomous. The distinction was made between low to average level of aspiration and high level of aspiration. High level was characterized mainly by ambitious attitudes especially with regard to cognitive and learning achievement.

(22) The father's abuse of alcohol. The procedure consisted in asking the mother during the interview if she thought that her husband abused alcohol. Only two categories were coded: (i) no abuse, and (ii) abuse. No coding was made of the frequency or amount of drinking, drinking habits, or behaviour, or how long the problem had been going on. This variable is therefore a measure of the mother's estimate of the father's drinking as a marital and family problem, but does not necessarily reflect the frequency of male alcoholism as a medico-social problem.

(23) Marital adjustment. This variable was in many instances coded on the basis of the interviewer's evaluation, as direct questioning would often have been considered as inopportune. Two categories were used:

(i) Good or fair adjustment. Relatively stable and harmonious marriage;

(ii) Faulty adjustment. Frequent disputes, lack of co-operation between partners. Mother unhappy. Often question of divorce.

(24) Diseases during pregnancy of mother and birth of child. This variable is dichotomous: (i) no disease, (ii) disease(s).

(25) Physical diseases, accidents, and injuries to the child after birth. This variable takes into consideration the total number of diseases and/or injuries with which the child has been afflicted since birth. Only those diseases are included which were evaluated as being of a serious nature. This variable is divided into 10 categories, ranging from no disease to 9 diseases, which was the maximum reported for any one child.

Results

Table 22.1 shows the frequency distribution of children into the three categories of mental health according to the five methods of assessment. The group of mentally disordered children is of primary interest in the present context. The percentage of children in this group varies from 11·8 to 30·8 per cent. The mean for all five variables is 21·85 per cent (23·05 per cent for boys and 20·65 per cent for girls). No significant difference has been found in the mental health of older (10–15) and younger (5–9) children.

It is obvious that these variables are rather different as instruments of assessment (see Table 22.2 for coefficients of correlation, r, for the five mental health variables). The reader is referred to Björnsson (1974) for further discussion.

Table 22.3 shows the frequency of symptoms in children. Only active cases at the time of investigation were counted, without regard to severity or duration. By far the most frequent group of

TABLE 22.1

Evaluations of mental health of children. Frequency distributions (per cent)

	Variable value			
	No information	1 Good mental health	2 Fair mental health	3 Bad mental health
Evaluation by WISC-tester	1·9	24·3	53·3	20·5
Evaluation by Rorschach-tester	0	23·9	45·3	30·8
Evaluation by interview (mother)	0·4	34·0	53·8	11·8
Evaluation by Rorsch. method	0	34·4	38·5	27·2
Clinical evaluation symptom-loading	0·5	61·9	18·8	18·8

TABLE 22.2

Coefficients of correlations for five types of evaluation of mental health in children

Variables	Clinical evaluation	WISC-tester	Rorschach-tester	Interviewer
WISC-tester	0·17	—	—	—
Rorschach-tester	0·11	0·28	—	—
Interviewer	0·52	0·28	0·18	—
Rorschach method	0·06	0·17	0·65	0·14

TABLE 22.3

Psychological symptoms in children. Active cases at the time of the investigation. Frequency (per cent)

Type of symptoms	Boys	Girls	Total
Sleep disturbances	3·6	3·4	3·4
Eating problems	3·5	5·7	4·6
Stomach disorders	3·6	6·2	4·9
Headache	3·5	5·5	4·5
Allergies	3·6	3·6	3·6
Enuresis	8·4	6·6	7·5
Encopresis	2·2	2·6	2·4
Hyperactivity	0·6	0·4	0·5
Passivity	3·6	1·2	2·4
Stereotypy, tics, etc.	4·2	3·0	3·6
Nailbiting	7·3	8·1	7·7
Thumbsucking	0·7	0·7	0·7
Speech problems	7·8	2·6	5·2
Contact difficulties	9·6	8·6	9·1
Sensitivity, shyness, anxiety	30·4	30·2	30·3
Phobic reactions	2·4	3·0	2·7
Aggressive-destructive behaviour, Temper tantrum	5·5	2·5	4·0
Undisciplined behaviour, negativism	8·9	5·1	7·0
Truancy†	0·2	0·2	0·2
Vagabondage, running away	0·8	0·6	0·7
Lying, fabulation	0·8	0·0	0·4
Stealing	0·8	0·2	0·5
Inhibition, concentration difficulties†	3·8	2·2	3·0
Reading and writing problems†	11·5	4·3	7·9
Adjustment in school†	6·3	3·7	5·5
Behaviour problems in school†	0·8	0·2	0·5

† $N = 800$ (children of school age).

symptoms is 'sensitivity, shyness, and anxiety', 30·4 per cent for boys and 30·2 per cent for girls. 'Contact difficulties', which in many cases are just a different wording for 'shyness' are also frequent (9·6 per cent in boys, 8·6 per cent in girls). 'Reading and writing problems' are fairly frequent in boys (11·5 per cent), as also are 'undisciplined behaviour and negativism', 'enuresis', and 'speech problems'. Other behavioural problems such as 'lying' and 'stealing' are conspiciously low, so there is reason to believe that the mothers have been reluctant to report on these symptoms.

Table 22.4 shows the correlations of the different mental health variables with socio-economic, educational, demographic, and cognitive variables. The interpretation of Table 22.4 leads to the following main conclusions: Good mental health in the children is most clearly associated with good education of both parents, high occupational status of the father (and his father), the maternal attitudes of warmth and emotional involvement, high IQ of the children, and high school notes at 12 year's examination in elementary school. The following variables were found not to be associated with mental health in the children: working schedule of the father, mother's out-of-home employment, mother's level of aspiration, mother's community origin, the number of children in both parental families, and physical diseases in the child.

In-depth studies in specific areas

The following in-depth studies have either been finished or are in preparation:

Enuresis in childhood (Björnsson 1973);

Explorations in social inequality. Stratification dynamics in Iceland (Björnsson et al. 1977);

Constellations of psychological symptoms in childhood (Björnsson in preparation).

These studies are all further elaborations of specific aspects of the above-mentioned cross-sectional sample.

TABLE 22.4

Variables of mental health evaluation correlated with socio-economic, demographic, educational, and cognitive variables. Coefficients significant at the 0·01 level are in bold face

Evaluation of mental health in children	Clinical evaluation	WISC-tester	Rorschach-tester	Interviewer	Rorschach method
Family constellation	0·05	0·04	0·01	**0·08**	0·01
Change of residence	**0·09**	0·02	0·05	0·05	0·03
Number of children	0·05	0·06	0·10	0·06	0·04
Occupation of father	**0·11**	0·05	**0·12**	**0·17**	**0·11**
Working times of father	0·01	0·07	0·05	0·07	0·07
Mother's out-of-home work	0·01	0·05	0·03	0·01	0·01
Number of rooms	**0·10**	0·06	0·02	**0·14**	0·03
Marital adjustment	**0·17**	**0·09**	0·06	**0·25**	0·04
Mother's child-rearing practices					
Warmth	**0·23**	**0·19**	**0·15**	**0·34**	**0·10**
Permissiveness	**0·10**	**0·10**	0·03	**0·16**	0·02
Detachment	0·05	**0·15**	**0·11**	**0·14**	**0·11**
Inconsistency	**0·19**	**0·09**	0·05	**0·27**	0·04
Aspiration	0·03	0·03	0·06	0·07	0·07
Mother's origin	0·01	0·00	0·05	0·03	0·05
Number of children in mother's family	0·03	0·03	0·01	0·00	0·00
Occupation maternal grandfather	0·05	0·04	**0·10**	**0·12**	**0·09**
Mother's education	**0·09**	**0·09**	**0·10**	**0·15**	**0·08**
Mother's attitude toward own rearing	**0·17**	0·03	0·02	**0·18**	0·01
Father's origin	0·01	0·03	**0·09**	0·02	0·03
Number of children father's family	0·04	0·07	0·07	0·03	0·06
Occupation paternal grandfather	**0·08**	**0·09**	**0·12**	**0·12**	**0·11**
Father's education	**0·15**	**0·12**	**0·17**	**0·23**	**0·15**
Alcoholism in father	0·06	0·02	0·03	**0·17**	0·01
Diseases during pregnancy	0·06	0·05	0·01	**0·10**	0·01
Physical diseases in the child	0·06	0·02	0·05	0·05	0·05
IQ WISC full scale	**0·18**	**0·22**	**0·17**	**0·09**	**0·10**
GPA sixth grade	**0·32**	**0·25**	**0·24**	**0·44**	**0·21**
Age of children	**0·10**	0·01	0·03	0·06	0·06

Longitudinal studies in specific areas and on subsamples

At the present date three such longitudinal studies have been conducted:

Educational attainments of youth in Reykjavík (Guðmundsdóttir *et al.* 1975). In this study the final educational attainment of the oldest 400 individuals in the original sample was assessed and correlated with variables from the original study. Table 22.5 shows

TABLE 22.5

Final educational attainment of children correlated with cognitive, parental, and mental health variables

Variables	Contingency coefficient	$p \geqslant$
School marks (GPA)		
at 12 years	0·57	0·001
IQ WISC	0·53	0·001
Educational level		
of father	0·42	0·001
Educational level		
of mother	0·34	0·001
Occupational status		
of father	0·39	0·001
Mental health of		
child	0·29	0·001

the variables which were most highly and significantly related to educational level. The WISC variable used here is IQ full scale and the mental health variable is that of 'clinical evaluation of symptoms'. Table 22.6 shows the frequency distribution for the educational attainment of the subsample.

TABLE 22.6

Final educational attainment of 400 individuals age 19–25 years. Frequency distribution in percentages

Educational levels			
i lowest	ii	iii	iv highest
per cent 6·5	53·39	20·05	20·05

School dropout (Sigurðsson and Óskarsson 1976). The same sample as in the foregoing study (400 oldest of the original sample) was studied. A school drop-out index in three categories was constructed:

(1) Drop-out from school before 16 years of age;
(2) Drop-out from school after secondary school (12 years of schooling with no vocational schooling;
(3) No premature drop-out from school. The student has finished vocational or academic schooling.

Table 22.7 shows the frequency distribution for the three categories of school drop-out. The drop-out index was related to variables in the original study as shown in Table 22.8.

Juvenile delinquency in Reykjavík (Steindórsson *et al.* 1975). This is a follow-up study of the oldest 600 individuals in the original sample (aged 19 to 25 years) with regard to recorded law infractions. The sample was divided into three groups with regard to recorded (police records) infractions of law:

(1) No recorded infractions;
(2) Minor infractions;
(3) Either of two:
    (a) two infractions of the penal code, or
    (b) three or more infractions, whereof one is of the penal code.

TABLE 22.7

School drop-out of young people. Frequency distribution in percentages

| | Drop-out index | | | | |
	(i)	(ii)	(iii)	No information	Total
N	44	143	196	17	400
per cent	11·0	35·75	49·0	4·25	100

TABLE 22.8

School drop-out of young people correlated with cognitive, demographic, educational, and socio-economic variables

Variables	Cont. coeff.	$p \geqslant$
School marks (GPA) at 12 years	0·54	0·001
IQ WISC (full scale)	0·48	0·001
Language marks at 12 years	0·46	0·001
Reading marks at 7 years (1st grade)	0·41	0·001
Mental health of child (evaluation of symptoms)	0·26	0·001
Sex of child	0·17	0·01
Alcohol abuse of father	0·17	0·01
Community origin of father	0·20	0·01
Community origin of mother	0·10	N.S.
Infractions of law (according to juvenile delinquency study below)	0·10	N.S.
Family constellation	0·14	N.S.
Number of siblings	0·30	0·001
Occupational status of father	0·33	0·001
Marital adjustment of parents	0·24	0·001
Cold/warmth in mother	0·24	0·001
Permissiveness/control in mother	0·14	N.S.
Detachment/involvement in mother	0·22	0·001
Consistency/inconsistency in mother	0·14	N.S.
Aspiration of mother	0·18	N.S.
Education of mother	0·33	0·001
Education of father	0·33	0·001

N.S. = non-significant.

As can be seen in Table 22.9, 18 per cent of the sample had some recorded delinquency, although only 3 per cent had committed serious or repeated delinquent acts. Group (iii) differed significantly from groups (i) and (ii) on 8 variables out of 20 tested for. The variables were taken from the initial cross-sectional investigation:

Their (group iii) family constellation was more often broken;
Their fathers had lower occupational status;
Their fathers had lesser education;

The child-rearing practices of their mothers had been less consistent;
The outcome of final examination from elementary school was worse (lower mean grade point average at 12 years examination);
The outcome of final examination of compulsory schooling (15 years examination) was worse;
Many fewer girls were in group iii. (Out of 108 individuals in the sample who had a criminal record there were only 20 girls and 19 of them were in group ii.)
The individuals in group iii were significantly younger when first infraction was committed than those in group ii (15·3 years as compared to 18·98 years for group iii).

TABLE 22.9

Recorded delinquency in young people (19 to 25 years of age) in Reykjavík. Frequency distribution

Categories of delinquency		
i No infractions	ii Minor infractions	iii Serious or repeated infractions
N 492	90	18
per cent 82·0	15·0	3·0

A general mental health follow-up study on the initial sample

A general mental health follow-up study has recently been started and is expected to take several years. The intention is to interview as many as possible of the initial sample when they have passed their 25th birthday and before they are 30 years old. In this interview information will be gathered on various topics, including: Occupational status and occupational history; educational attainment and educational history; marital status, marital adjustment, and information on marital partner; recreational activities and interests; delinquency, latent and recorded; use of alcohol.

In addition to the interview a short personality inventory will be used (Life-satisfaction, job-satisfaction, by Gardell-Westlander). The main purposes of the follow-up study are:

(a) To assess clinically the mental health and general adjustment of the subjects;
(b) To compare their mental health status with previous assessment of the same subjects when they were children (initial study);
(c) To estimate the prognostic value of the first mental health assessment;
(d) To trace the most relevant socio-economic and educational variables conducive either to good or bad mental health at an adult age;
(e) To collect information on intergenerational change with regard to (i) educational attainment, and (ii) occupational status.

23. The Cambridge study in delinquent development (United Kingdom)

D. P. FARRINGTON and D. J. WEST

Introduction

The Cambridge Study in Delinquent Development is a prospective longitudinal survey of a sample of 411 males. It began in 1961 and is continuing until 1979. It has been directed throughout by Dr D. J. West, a psychiatrist, Professor of Clinical Criminology at Cambridge University. During the major period of analysis and reporting, Dr D. P. Farrington, a psychologist, now a Lecturer in the Cambridge University Institute of Criminology and Director of the Postgraduate Course in Criminology, was equally responsible with Dr West for the conduct of the research. The names of other persons who have worked on the Study can be found in the three books which have been published (West 1969; West and Farrington 1973, 1977). These books, together with other publications emerging from the Cambridge Study in Delinquent Development are contained in a list which can be obtained from the authors.

The sample

The 411 males in the study were first contacted in 1961 and 1962 when they were aged 8 and 9. At that time, they were all living in a working class area of London. The vast majority of the sample was chosen by taking all the boys whose names were on the registers of fourth-year classes in six state primary schools within a one-mile radius of a research office which had been established. In addition, 12 boys were included from a local school for the educationally subnormal, in an attempt to make the sample more representative of the population of boys living in the area. The intention was to include about 400 boys in the study. The sample size, while limited by staffing and budgetary considerations, was intended to be large enough to permit statistical comparisons (bearing in mind the likely proportion of official delinquents) yet small enough to permit individual interviews and detailed case studies.

The sample largely consisted of two cohorts of boys: 231 born between 1 September 1952 and 31 August 1953, who were recruited during the academic year beginning September 1961; and 157 born between 1 September 1953 and 31 August 1954, who were recruited during the academic year beginning September 1962. The younger age cohort was smaller because in two of the schools no more boys were included after the first year of intake. In addition, there were 23 boys born between 1 September 1951 and 31 August 1952, comprising all the boys in one class in one of the schools, who were first contacted towards the end of the academic year beginning September 1960. These boys, originally a pilot group, have been the first to be contacted each time the sample has been surveyed. Since the sample consists of complete age groups of boys, it is thought to be fairly representative of the urban working class population in the area at the time. It would perhaps have been better to deliberately select a random sample, but this was not possible in practice.

The boys were almost all Caucasian in appearance, and only 12, most of whom had at least one parent of West Indian origin, were negroid in appearance. In addition, the vast majority (371) were being brought up by parents who had themselves been reared in the United Kingdom or Eire. On the basis of their fathers' occupations, 93·7 per cent could be described as working class (categories III, IV, or V on the Registrar General's scale), in comparison with the national figure of 78·3 per cent, at that time. This was, therefore, overwhelmingly a traditional British white working class sample.

Procedure

Tests and interviews

The boys were given psychological tests in their schools when they were aged 8, 10, and 14, and they were interviewed in the research office at ages 16, 18, and 21. All these ages are approximate; for example, the tests at age 8 were actually completed at age 8 to 9. The psychological testing was carried out by male or female psychologists in the study team, while the interviews were carried out by young male social science graduates. All 411 boys were tested at age 8, while the numbers tested at ages 10 and 14 were 408 and 406 respectively. At age 16, 398 (96·8 per cent) were successfully traced and interviewed, while the figure at age 18 was 389 (94·6 per cent). Of the 22 youths who were missing at age 18, one had died, one could not be traced, 6 were abroad, 10 refused to be interviewed, and in the other 4 cases the parent refused on behalf of the youth. At age 21, the aim was to interview only the official delinquents and a random sample of non-delinquents, rather than the whole sample. At this age, 218 of the target group of 241 were interviewed (90·5 per cent).

In addition to the interviews and tests with the boys, their parents were interviewed in their homes by female social workers in the study team, about once a year from when the boy was aged 8 until when he was aged 14, in his last year of compulsory schooling. At age 8, the parents of 22 boys (5·4 per cent) were rated uncooperative by the social workers. Since the sample contained 14 pairs of brothers, the total number of separate families was 397. All figures here are based on boys rather than families. At the time of the final interview with the parents, when the boys were aged 14, it was possible to interview a parent of 399 (97·1 per cent). The boys' teachers also filled in questionnaires about their behaviour in school when they were aged 8, 10, 12, and 14. The numbers of completed questionnaires received at these four ages were 404, 389, 404, and 384, respectively.

Records of convictions

It was also possible to make repeated searches in the central Criminal Record Office in London to try to locate findings of guilt sustained by the boys, by their parents, and by their siblings. In order to obtain identifying particulars which would enable these searches to be carried out, the full name and date of birth of each family member, including the mother's maiden name, was sought during interviews. These data were checked against, and frequently supplemented by, information from medical and social service records and from birth certificates and marriage certificates obtained from the General Register Office in London. In theory, the Criminal Record Office contains details of all convictions for indictable and akin-to-indictable offences sustained in England and Wales by persons aged 17 or over at the time. In addition, it contains details of all findings of guilt for these offences sustained by persons under 17 in the London area, and it also contains details of many findings of guilt sustained by juveniles outside the London area.

Repeated searches were necessary, because convictions were sometimes located in one search but not in another. Occasionally, searching was hampered by an individual's use of several names, or by his possession of a very common name that was difficult to locate, or by files being temporarily misplaced or on loan to a police force. Convictions for comparatively minor indictable offences occurring in the North of England were not invariably reported to the CRO. In a few cases where information from the boy or elsewhere did not agree with that in the CRO, the discrepancies were resolved by reference to local police or court records. Since the CRO information was supplemented by extensive interviews and other enquiries, it is unlikely that any convicted boys in the sample escaped identification. Coverage of the parents' generation was less accurate, partly because findings of guilt, especially involving juveniles, were less likely to be reported to the CRO in former years, and partly because of the difficulty of securing accurate dates of birth of parents and maiden names of mothers. When offenders are known to have died, their names are deleted from the CRO, and there is also a tendency to 'weed out' records of minor offences after a certain number of years.

Access to the Criminal Record Office is controlled by the Home Office and, for purposes of research, it is very restricted, increasingly so since personal privacy has become a political issue. We were exceptionally fortunate. One member of the study team was allowed to visit the CRO on a number of occasions and was supplied with files for direct inspection and identification, and we were permitted to ask for the names of all the sample and their immediate relatives to be searched regardless of whether or not a conviction record was thought to exist.

Difficulties in securing co-operation

The initial contacts with the 411 boys depended upon the co-operation of the education department, the schools, and the parents. At first, the education department made a ruling that group tests could be given provided only that teachers were agreeable, but that any individual testing of children could not be done without the written consent of parents given on a prescribed form. During the second year of the research this rule was relaxed and a limited range of tests, which had to be approved by a psychologist representing the local authority, was permitted to be given to all the children. This involved re-visiting the schools to test children who had previously been missed, and meant that the children were not all the same age at the time they were first tested. Incompleteness in some of the measures was caused by the persistent absence of some boys from school and by their illiteracy and lack of verbal comprehension.

Because the study depended in large part on the access to school boys provided by the Education Authority, we were compelled in the early stages to limit the inquiry in the schools to matters which that Authority saw fit to allow. Since some of the topics in which we were interested, such as educational standards and the prevalence of delinquency, were sensitive areas politically, we were obliged to tread warily. There were many anxious moments, especially when journalists discovered the telephone number of the research office and kept demanding information. The worst crisis of this sort arose when a journalist, by devious means, managed to secure some of our data about the schools and printed them in garbled form, thereby providing material for a highly publicized but quite unfounded political squabble about standards of literacy in the schools.

The original names and addresses of the boys were supplied by the Education Authority, but we were not allowed to call on their parents to request their co-operation. Instead, an official letter, partly composed by the Education Authority and signed by headmasters, was sent to the parents with a request that they sign and post an enclosed form signifying their consent to a visit by someone from the study. Predictably, in an area where standards of literacy were not high, and reluctance to sign puzzling letters from headmasters was understandable, the response was poor (about 60 per cent). Various attempts were made to improve the situation, including reminders from headmasters, calls by co-operative parents on their less co-operative neighbours, and the use of local welfare agencies to secure introductions. However, none of these methods proved really effective. In 1963 it was decided that the research team had been long enough in the neighbourhood, and had established sufficient contacts of their own, for the psychiatric social workers to call on the parents directly, without involving the education department. Because of the long delay in contacting a small number of parents, a few homes were not visited until the boy had reached the age of 10.

In order that the psychiatric social workers might work in the way in which they were accustomed, and elicit the maximum co-operation, they were given a list of topics to be covered, but no fixed rules were laid down about the manner in which the information was to be sought. Interviews were completely free and unstructured. Although a few written notes were sometimes taken during interviews, the psychiatric social workers relied on dictating their impressions on to a portable tape recorder as soon as possible after a visit. The boy's mother was the primary informant, although the father was also interviewed in 70·8 per cent of the cases. Three or four interviews, each lasting about an hour, were usually needed to complete the case record forms, but the number and duration varied according to the intelligence and co-operativeness of the parents. Appointments were generally made in advance, but were often cancelled or not kept, and in some cases a great many abortive calls had to be made before a satisfactory interview could be obtained.

Problems with the early data

In retrospect, the earliest investigation into family background was too ambitious and insufficiently precise. Much of the data was too subjective and too much influenced by halo effects to be of use for research purposes. The early interview data might have proved more valuable if it had been possible to carry out more extensive pilot work, but the then Director of the Institute of Criminology did not agree to this in view of the uncertain duration of the research. In a longitudinal survey, the earliest measurements are particularly valuable, making pilot work even more important than in cross-sectional surveys.

The parents were told that this was a study of child upbringing and development, and that anonymous information was being sought which could be of help to children and parents in the future. In explaining the purposes of the research, the psychiatric social workers went into more detail with some parents than with others, depending on the interest shown or the questions asked. No special emphasis was placed upon delinquency problems, and the name of the Cambridge Institute of Criminology was never mentioned. Except for a few cases in which rather poor parents received small sums in cash to compensate them for giving up time for interviews, no rewards were given for co-operation.

The high response rate obtained in the later interviews with the youths was achieved at the cost of a great deal of interviewer effort and time, as was true of the earlier interviews with the parents. The interviewers would go to great lengths to track down a youth's address, using a variety of methods. Some were traced through the local housing department, some were located by probation officers, some were provided by neighbours, relatives, or the present occupants of old addresses, some were derived from marriage certificates or telephone directories, and letters were forwarded to some youths by the Department of Health and Social Security, the Post Office, or by employers. The interviewers would make repeated calls at an address in an attempt to find someone in, and would go back to try to secure an interview even if a youth refused on the first occasion. The youths were paid a small fee (about £1 an hour) for their co-operation.

Interviews at age 18

The interviews at age 18 were the most ambitious and extensive carried out with the youths themselves, and lasted two hours on the average. The vast majority were carried out in the research office and were tape recorded. What the youths said was then transcribed from the tape and typed directly on to interview schedules, so that it was possible for us to quote the youths verbatim. Since much of the interview concerned sensitive topics, it was essential to put the youths at their ease so that they would talk freely. They were assured from the start that the interview would be kept completely confidential, and that no one outside the research team would hear the tapes. In view of the questions about delinquent behaviour and delinquency convictions included in the interviews, many of the youths may have realized the interviewers' particular interest in these matters, but this did not reduce co-operation. For most of the youths, delinquency was a less sensitive topic than others such as sexual habits.

In retrospect, the interviews at age 18 were too ambitious, striving to obtain information on too many topics. The length and complexity of the interview schedule, and of the instruction manual, presented the interviewers with an exhausting list of points to be kept in mind. This opened the way for occasional lapses, in the shape of mistaken codings or questions not put exactly in the manner specified. In a few places the interviewers found it necessary to modify the instruction manual after the interviews had begun. All this required a great deal of labour at a later stage in rectifying faulty or inconsistent coding of responses.

The high response rate from members of the sample and their parents owed very little to the help of official agencies. A great deal of time and effort could have been saved, and more data could have been obtained, if it had been possible to obtain full and continuous collaboration from services and departments such as education, health, social services, employment, housing, taxation, penal, police, probation, and voluntary organizations. Our experience suggests that some departments jealously tend to guard their information from each other and from outside researchers. No doubt this policy is sometimes necessary and desirable. Confidential information, especially if detrimental to individuals, has often to be withheld from authorities with the power to take punitive action. From the point of view of research, however, the obstacles in the way of information gathering seem arbitrary and excessive.

The research called for passive observation without intervention. On occasion, however, the social workers could not refrain from advising troubled parents where to go for help with their financial, housing, or health problems. We do not know the effect on the boys and their families of being studied over such a long period. In retrospect, what we should have done at the beginning was to establish a control group of other boys from the original six schools, who could have been followed up in records but never contacted personally. We doubt if our occasional intrusions into their lives had much effect on the youths, but we cannot be certain about this. Contact with the mass media was studiously avoided until reports were published and it could not be prevented. At that point and ever since, care has been taken not to specify the area of the study or to release any information which might lead to the identification of individuals.

Some of the social workers were troubled by ethical considerations about carrying out record searches and inquiries about families without explaining to them the full extent and purpose of the research and, in some cases, in spite of the parents' express wish to take no part in the study. Unfortunately, in delinquency research the information needed is not always of a kind likely to be given voluntarily, certainly not by the more evasive and unco-operative families. We have justified our enquiries on the grounds of the advancement of knowledge, taking stringent precautions to preserve the anonymity of the families and the privacy of the case records, so that no individual could be harmed by the leakage of personal information.

Financial support of the study

Up to and including the interviews at age 21, the research was financed entirely by annually reviewed grants from the Home Office. Since then, when the Home Office discontinued their support, the research has been financed by a grant from the Social Science Research Council and Department of Health and Social Security acting jointly. The fact that there was no guarantee of renewal of the grant from one year to the next hampered planning, especially in the early stages. The Home Office exercised some control by vetting research plans before consenting to grant renewals, by demanding progress reports, and by insisting that any report for publication or any talk about the study should be submitted to them for prior approval. In practice, these conditions did not seriously limit our freedom, and they sometimes proved helpful as a check on the quality of the published research.

The organization of a long project is far from simple. A stable research team is essential for the continuity of assessments and for maintaining the co-operation of the subjects under investigation. This is not so easy to achieve when the staff are on annually renewable research grants and when they feel that they must move on or lose their place on some academic career ladder. Uncertainty about the length of contracts of employment was a continual source of anxiety and a hindrance to the recruitment and maintenance of research staff. Fortunately, there were minimal changes in the first few years when interviews with parents were at their most intensive stage.

The data

The family background data relating to the boys' development up to 10 years of age, together with the data collected from the schools at the same time, were coded and transferred to punched cards by 1964. Later data has been coded and transferred to punched cards as it has been obtained. In general, raw data from questionnaires and psychological tests (i.e. responses to each item) has been punched in addition to derived scores. All of this data is now stored on magnetic tape in the Cambridge University Computer Laboratory. We do not think that this information could be used as a data base except under the supervision of one of us. Despite our extensive coding manuals, there are many pitfalls in the data in which someone who was not thoroughly familiar with the project could fall.

The major aim of the project was to explore the antecedents and concomitants of delinquency in males. The officially delinquent minority was identified from findings of guilt recorded in the Criminal Record Office. Up to January 1977, 132 of the original 411 (32·1 per cent) have been convicted. Since the minimum age for findings of guilt in court is 10, as much of the early data as possible was collected and coded ready for future analysis at or before age 10, before it was known which members of the sample would obtain an official delinquency record. Ideally, a longitudinal survey should begin at or just before birth, but practical considerations meant that our survey was designed to begin just before the minimum age for conviction. It was fortunate for us that this minimum age was raised from 8 to 10 soon after the study had begun. We discounted three convictions which actually occurred under age 10, because only the older boys in the sample were exposed to the risk of sustaining such convictions. In addition to the official measure of delinquency, we also have self-reports of delinquent acts derived from the youths at ages 14, 16, 18, and 21.

Many different factors have been measured in this study, derived from many different sources. The aim in measuring so many factors was not only to test the myriad of hypotheses about the origins of delinquency but also to compare the relative importance of different factors (e.g. individual versus social) and to see whether some factors still remained important after controlling for other, more basic, factors. The longitudinal design meant that it was possible to trace the course of events, and to investigate the effects of specific events on the development of an individual.

Data collected in a longitudinal survey are intended to throw light on events in the distant future. If there is an intervening gap of several years, as in this study, ideas and theories are apt to change in the meantime. When the results are finally available, an investigator may feel that the factors which were thought to be most relevant when the project began are not the ones he would choose in the light of the most recent research. This is another reason for casting the net widely in the early stages of a longitudinal survey, in order not to leave out those factors which future researchers may want to know about. Even so, no one can foresee everything that will become of interest, and we have been repeatedly frustrated in having to tell subsequent enquirers that the particular points in which they were interested were not measured in our research. Moreover, as the work progresses, and it becomes evident that certain factors are of unexpected importance, there is inevitably regret that they were not investigated in greater detail. In a longitudinal survey, decisions taken at the start affect the research for years to come, for better or worse.

Results

'Official' juvenile delinquents

About one-fifth of the boys (84, or 20·4 per cent) were defined as official juvenile delinquents, because they were found guilty in court of an offence normally recorded in the Criminal Record Office and committed between their tenth and seventeenth birthdays. Six boys spent over a year of their juvenile life span outside England and Wales. In their cases, approaches were made to the appropriate authorities, as a result of which one was counted as a juvenile delinquent. The official conviction records were thus effectively complete for the whole sample. The majority of the offences were thefts, burglaries, and unauthorized takings of motor vehicles, and most were committed with one or two other persons, usually boys of the same age. Judging by the boys' descriptions of their offences leading to court appearances, their misbehaviour was often less serious than the ponderous legal terminology suggested. The juvenile delinquents were subdivided into 37 recidivists and 47 who were convicted only once as juveniles.

The official juvenile delinquents differed in many respects from their unconvicted peers on the predictive factors measured before age 10. On any particular factor, it was almost invariably the category which, on common sense grounds, would be defined as the most adverse that included the highest percentage of delinquents. For example, more delinquents were drawn from the poorest families, from those with low IQs, and from those with cruel, passive, or neglecting parents. In terms of significant relationships, we had an embarrassment of riches. The problem was to reduce the very large number of measured variables (about 200) to a more manageable number.

We were guided by certain principles. In particular, we thought that, from the point of view of theoretical or causal analysis, it was

desirable to have a number of variables which were each operational definitions and measures of only one theoretical concept. We tried to achieve this by identifying clusters of variables which were related empirically and theoretically, and then either choosing one variable as the best representative of this cluster or combining a number of the variables in the cluster into a single composite variable. As an example of the former method, all the measures of intelligence and attainment taken in the primary schools were closely correlated. We thought that, whatever else they were measuring, each of these variables measured intelligence, and so we chose non-verbal IQ as the purest measure of this theoretical construct, to represent this cluster.

As an example of the second method, the psychiatric social workers' ratings of maternal attitude, maternal discipline, paternal attitude, paternal discipline, marital disharmony, and parental inconsistency were all closely related. Parents tended to be seen as bad in many respects, or good in many respects, but rarely bad in some respects and good in others. It is probable that the psychiatric social workers had found difficulty in rating one aspect of parental behaviour independently of another, and this is one manifestation of the halo effect mentioned above. In view of these relationships, it was decided to combine all the variables into one global rating called parental behaviour. The rules of combination were very simple, both in this example and in others. Each boy was given 1, 2, or 3 points on each variable, and his scores were simply added over all the variables. The features contributing to the rating of poor parental behaviour were parents with cruel, passive, or neglecting attitudes, very strict, harsh, or erratic discipline, and parents who were in conflict with each other.

There were other reasons for combining variables. For example, the non-verbal IQ scores at ages 8 and 10 were combined (by averaging), on the grounds that the combined score would have less variability than either individual score. Measures of the same theoretical concept obtained from different sources were combined in the expectation that the biases present in the sources might cancel out to some extent. For example, the measures of troublesomeness obtained from teachers and peers were combined, as were the measures of daring obtained from parents and peers.

Another way in which the number of variables in the analysis was reduced was by eliminating those which were very subjective or not well defined. For example, the rating of mother's past health was eliminated because it depended on mothers' recollections and admissions of past events. The rating of present health of mothers, which in some cases was supplemented by hospital records, varied markedly with socio-economic status, as expected, with the lower status mothers having poorer health. However, poor past health was not related to socio-economic status, suggesting that the lower status families were underreporting. The rating of sibling disturbance was eliminated because there were marked differences between the psychiatric social workers in the proportion of boys said to have disturbed siblings, and these differences could only be explained by interviewer bias. The rating of unstable personality of mothers, which was intended to identify behaviour-disordered individuals who did not necessarily have anxiety symptoms, was eliminated because it was not defined very explicitly. In choosing between variables, those which were more objectively measured, those which were more sensitively measured (i.e. using a scale rather than a small number of rough categories), and those which were alleged to be important in the criminological literature were preferred.

By these various methods, the approximately 200 measured variables were reduced to about 20 key variables without, it was hoped, losing too much essential information. In order to compare each of these key variables with each other, the scores on all variables were divided approximately into quarters. This, of course, did involve a considerable loss of information, especially in the case of the more sensitively measured variables. However, it was justified in the interests of comparability, and produced some interesting results. For example, the average non-verbal IQs of the delinquent and non-delinquent groups were 95 and 101 respectively. In previous investigations of the IQs of delinquents, a difference of up to 8 points has sometimes been regarded as unimportant. However, when non-verbal IQ was scored on a comparable scale to poverty, large families and criminal parents, it was found that low IQ was a significant precursor of delinquency to much the same extent as the other major factors.

The final stage in the analysis was to investigate whether each key factor was significantly related to delinquency independently of each other key factor. This was studied by means of matching analyses. For example, low family income and large family size were both significantly related to each other and to delinquency. It might be argued, for example, that poverty is the real cause of delinquency and that delinquents only appear to come from larger families because they come from poorer families which happen to also be larger. If this were so, delinquents and non-delinquents would not differ significantly in family size when matched for family income. However, they did. Furthermore, delinquents and non-delinquents differed significantly in family income when matched for family size. These results show that family size and family income were independently related to delinquency.

On the other hand, separations of a boy from his parents for reasons other than death or hospitalization seemed to be significantly related to delinquency only because they were also associated with criminal parents. It could not be shown that delinquents and non-delinquents differed in separation experiences after matching for criminal parents, whereas they did differ in criminal parents after matching for separations. This suggests that parental criminality was the primary causal factor. These matching analyses were also used to investigate the masking of relationships. For example, the rating of a boy as 'nervous–withdrawn' was not significantly related to delinquency, but was significantly related to poor parental behaviour, which in turn was significantly related to delinquency. After matching for parental behaviour, it emerged that delinquents were significantly less nervous–withdrawn than non-delinquents. This suggests that the real negative relationship between a nervous–withdrawn temperament and delinquency was being masked by the positive relationship between nervous–withdrawn boys and poor parental behaviour, and between poor parental behaviour and delinquency. In turn, this suggests that delinquency and a nervous–withdrawn temperament were two alternative effects of poor parental behaviour.

These kinds of matching analyses do not allow for the possibility of non-linear interactions in the data, for example where a factor is positively related to delinquency at some levels of another factor and negatively related at other levels. However, significant interactions of this kind were very rare in our data. The matching analyses do allow us to satisfy Hirschi and Selvin's criteria of causality, namely that A causes B if A and B are associated, if A is prior to B, and if the association between A and B does not disappear when the effects of other variables related to A and B are taken into account. However, we have tended not to talk in terms of causes of delinquency because of the deterministic connotations of the word 'cause'.

Only two behavioural measures and five background measures survived these analyses, and were shown to be independently predictive of official juvenile delinquency. The delinquents were drawn from those who were rated troublesome and daring at their primary schools. They also tended to come from the poorer families, the larger-sized families, those with criminal parents, those suffering poor parental behaviour, and those with low IQs.

The five background factors were retrospectively combined to see if an improved prediction would result. However, the pro-

portion in the vulnerable group who became delinquents was only about 50 per cent, which was little improvement on troublesomeness alone. The use of more sophisticated methods of selecting and combining predictor variables also indicated that the limit of predictability with these data was reached in identifying a vulnerable group of which half become delinquents, in turn containing half of the delinquents. This limit probably reflects the importance of later factors in causing delinquency, the extent to which findings of guilt in court depend on essentially random or unpredictable events, and the impossibility of accurately measuring the predictive factors.

For completeness, we will mention some of the other factors which predicted delinquency, while realizing that these factors were of subsidiary importance to the ones mentioned above. The delinquents tended to come from families living in poor houses with neglected interiors, supported by social agencies, physically neglecting their children, and unco-operative towards the research. They tended to come from those born illegitimate, and from those who had experienced broken homes or separations from their parents for reasons other than death or hospitalization. They tended to be drawn from those with parents who were Roman Catholic, uninterested in education, who were lax in enforcing rules or under-vigilant, or who tended to endorse authoritarian child-rearing attitudes on questionnaires. Their mothers tended to be nervous and in poor physical health, while their fathers tended to have erratic job histories. In addition to their low intelligence and attainment, the boys tended to be clumsy on psychomotor tests and relatively small.

Some of the negative results were also of interest. Delinquents did not tend, to any significant extent, to come from low socio-economic status families or to have working mothers. Analysis of medical records of their births revealed no undue incidence of obstetric abnormalities. They did not tend to have a mesomorphic physique, they were not unpopular with their peers, they did not tend to be neurotic extroverts on personality questionnaires, and they were not in poor health.

'Self-reported' juvenile delinquents

All the preceding results, of course, apply to the official juvenile delinquents. Self-report and victim surveys indicate that the official records are very much the tip of the iceberg of offending. As an alternative measure of juvenile delinquency, we gave the boys a self-reported delinquency questionnaire at ages 14 and 16. This consisted of 38 delinquent or fringe-delinquent acts, and the boys were asked to say whether or not they had committed each one. As a measure of self-reported juvenile delinquency, each boy was scored according to the total number of different acts he admitted at either or both ages. The validity of these scores was confirmed by the fact that they significantly predicted future convictions for delinquency among unconvicted boys.

For ease of comparison with the 84 official juvenile delinquents, the 80 boys with the highest self-report scores, all of whom admitted at least 21 acts, were grouped together and called the self-reported juvenile delinquents. The overlap between the two groups was very marked, amounting to about 50 per cent. This suggests that, to a large extent, the boys who sustain findings of guilt as juveniles tend to be those who commit the most offences. While the official records are a poor measure of the incidence of offending, they are useful in separating out the more and less frequent (and serious) offenders.

No doubt at least partly because of the overlap between the two groups, our results in relation to self-reported delinquency were not markedly different from those obtained with official delinquency. The self-reported delinquents tended to be rated troublesome and daring at their primary schools, tended to come from poor, large-sized families, suffered poor parental behaviour, had criminal parents, and low IQs. This last result is interesting, as some researchers have suggested that delinquents have low IQs only because the less intelligent boys are more likely to get caught.

Criminal parents as a factor in delinquency

This survey has demonstrated, therefore, that five background factors are independently predictive of delinquency. However, we have not gotten very far in explaining the precise nature of the processes linking each factor with delinquency. As an example, consider the finding that criminal parents tend to have delinquent children. There are many possible explanations for this. One that we were not able to investigate is the hypothesis that some characteristic which bears on the likelihood of becoming a delinquent is genetically transmitted. We did try to investigate the hypothesis that criminal parents do not transmit delinquent behaviour, but merely transmit the likelihood of being convicted. In other words, it is suggested that boys who commit offences and have a known criminal father are more likely to be convicted than boys who commit offences and do not. We matched boys who had a criminal father with boys who did not, on self-reported delinquency. We found that, at all levels of self-reported delinquency, a criminal father greatly increased the likelihood of being convicted. This result could perhaps be explained if it was suggested that the sons of criminal fathers were more likely to conceal their offences, but the same result was obtained when the teacher–peer rating of troublesomeness was used as an index of bad behaviour, rather than self-reports.

Even though the sons of the criminal fathers were more likely to be convicted, this was not the sole explanation of the association between criminal fathers and delinquent sons, because self-reported delinquency was much greater for the sons of criminal fathers. Another explanation which was tested was that criminal fathers directly encouraged their sons to commit crimes or taught them criminal techniques. However, only four of the fathers were convicted of an offence with one or more of their children as accomplices, and the criminal fathers were generally critical of their sons' delinquency.

It may be that criminal parents produced delinquent sons because of some peculiarity in their child-rearing methods, and indeed they were said to exercise significantly poor supervision over their children. In this result, and in the demonstration that criminal fathers increased the risk of conviction, we could go some way towards explaining the link between criminal parents and delinquent sons, but this was not very far.

The school as a factor in delinquency

As mentioned earlier, it is possible in a longitudinal survey to trace the course of events and to investigate the effects of specific events on the development of an individual. As an example of a longitudinal analysis, we tried to investigate the effects on delinquency of going to different secondary schools. Almost all the boys were in six neighbouring primary schools at age 8. At age 11, they scattered to a much larger number of secondary schools, although the majority (335) went to one of 13 schools. From information given to us by the local Education Authority, we knew that these 13 schools differed dramatically in their delinquency rates, from one which had more than 20 court appearances per year per 100 boys aged 11 to 14, to another where the corresponding figure was only 0·3.

We were interested in investigating whether these large differences in delinquency rates were caused by some features of the schools themselves, or whether they merely reflected intake differences. We had ratings of troublesomeness in the primary schools made by teachers and peers, and we knew the extent to which these predicted official juvenile delinquency. We then found that there was a very marked tendency for the boys who were badly behaved in their primary schools to go to the high delinquency rate secondary schools. We also found that, on the basis of the known rela-

tionship between troublesomeness and delinquency, and the known troublesomeness ratings of the boys entering each group of secondary schools, we could predict the delinquency rates of these boys quite accurately. This suggests that the secondary schools themselves had very little effect on delinquency, and that the differences in delinquency rates between these schools were largely caused by intake differences.

Effect of criminal conviction on delinquency

Another example of a longitudinal analysis, this time more explicitly quasiexperimental, was a study of the effects on delinquent behaviour of being found guilty in court. If official processing in the criminal justice system had a deterrent or reformative effect, then it would be expected that a person's delinquent behaviour would decrease after he was convicted. On the other hand, it is possible that the stigmatizing and contaminating effects of convictions actually propel people into more delinquent behaviour than before. As a measure of delinquent behaviour, we used our self-reported delinquency scores at ages 14 and 18. Fifty-three youths were first found guilty in court between ages 14 and 18, and we found that, in relation to all the others, these convicted youths had significantly increased self-reported delinquency scores by the later age. This is in agreement with the idea that convictions produce a worsening of delinquent behaviour.

It could be argued that the convicted youths became worse because of some pre-existing differences between them and the remainder, rather than because of the effects of being convicted. In testing this, we matched the 53 convicted youths with 53 others not convicted up to age 18, on self-reported delinquency at age 14, on troublesomeness, and on the combination of 5 background factors mentioned earlier. Despite this rigorous matching procedure, the convicted group still worsened relative to the unconvicted group. We also tried to investigate whether the conviction was followed by a worsening of the delinquent behaviour, or whether the deterioration in behaviour came first and led to the conviction. We used our self-reported delinquency scores at age 16, and studied only the youths first convicted between ages 16 and 18. If the youths got worse before being convicted, it might be expected that those first convicted between 16 and 18 would already have deteriorated in behaviour between 14 and 16. However, this was not true. The significant difference in self-reported delinquency scores only appeared at age 18, after the youths had been convicted, suggesting that official convictions preceded increases in delinquents behaviour.

Differences between 'official' and 'self-reported' juvenile delinquents

At age 14, when the boys were in their last year of compulsory schooling, the differences between official juvenile delinquents and non-delinquents were similar in many respects to those found at age 8. For example, the delinquents were still said to have cruel, passive, and neglecting parents who were in conflict, although it must be remembered that the later social workers who made these ratings had access to the earlier social workers' ratings and to the delinquency records. A much more systematic attempt was made at age 13 to 14 to investigate parental discipline and boys' reaction to it, using a structured questionnaire given to the mothers. The results were rather disappointing, as significant relationships were conspicuous by their absence. It may be that parental discipline at age 14 is less important than at age 8. However, we are inclined to believe that our closely structured interview using set questions was a less effective method of obtaining information about parent–child relationships than the more free-ranging and unstructured approach employed by the psychiatric social workers in their earlier interviews.

At age 14, the official juvenile delinquents were still significantly lower on our measures of intelligence and attainment. At this age, we made a special effort to measure aggressiveness, a factor which had not been investigated earlier to any extent, largely because of the limitations imposed by the schools. The delinquents were much more aggressive than the non-delinquents, both in their self-reports of fighting and carrying weapons, and in the teachers' ratings of aggressiveness and disobedience in school. The delinquents also revealed more aggressive self-concepts in a semantic differential test, but they were not more aggressive in a projective technique (a picture frustration test). This unusual result probably reflects the inadequacy of this particular projective technique. Both at ages 14 and 16, the delinquents showed extremely critical attitudes to the police on a questionnaire, and said that their friends and acquaintances had committed many delinquent acts.

At age 18, the major comparison was between the 101 youths who had been convicted for an offence committed before the interview, and the remaining 288 youths interviewed. The pattern of offences leading to convictions changed somewhat as the youths progressed from the juvenile to the young adult age range. Thefts from employers, violence, fraud, damaging property, and possession of drugs became more common, while thefts from shops, vehicles, cycles, and automatic machines all decreased. There was little evidence of specialization in criminal careers, since the vast majority of offenders had been convicted of at least one crime of dishonesty. The small group of 18 youths who were found guilty between ages 10 and 12 proved to be unusually persistent offenders, averaging more than 5 convictions each by age 18. Taking into account later information, it seems that the peak age for conviction in this sample was 18.

During the interview, the youths were asked whether they had ever had to appear before a court. With the exception of seven who were interviewed in penal institutions, they had no reason to suspect that the interviewers knew about their conviction histories. Nevertheless, 95 of the 101 official delinquents admitted that they had been convicted, and two others admitted that they had been involved in the offences for which they had been convicted, although they denied being convicted. Conversely, only seven of the 288 non-delinquents claimed one or more convictions which could not be found in the Criminal Record Office. At least two of these youths were probably telling the truth, since they said that they had been convicted in provincial cities for comparatively minor offences, and it was possible to locate a record for one of these offences. The low incidence of concealment and exaggeration of convictions gave us some confidence that the majority of youths were trying to be truthful during the interview.

As a measure of self-reported delinquency at age 18, the youths were asked how often they had committed each of seven specified delinquent activities in the previous three years, namely damaging property, taking and driving away motor vehicles, receiving, burglary, shoplifting, stealing from slot machines, and stealing from parked cars. It was then possible to investigate how many of these delinquent acts led to findings of guilt in court. Burglary and taking and driving away motor vehicles were much more likely to be detected than the other offences. Roughly one in eight of the burglaries led to convictions, and one in 16 of the taking and driving away offences. These figures are very much lower than police clear-up rates, of course, largely because crimes known to the police represent only a minority of those actually committed. Because most offenders committed several offences, the likelihood of each offender being convicted at some stage was much higher than the likelihood of each offence resulting in a conviction. For example, nearly two-thirds of those who had committed at least one burglary had been convicted of burglary, and nearly two-fifths of those who had taken motor vehicles had been convicted of this offence.

The youths were also asked to give their usual motives for committing offences. Much the most common category of reasons given

(60 per cent) were rational ones. By and large, it seemed that the youths stole and burgled purposefully, for the material gains involved. The next most common category (20 per cent) were motives of excitement or enjoyment. Offences of damaging property and taking motor vehicles were particularly likely to be done for enjoyment, whereas rational motives predominated in all other cases.

The official delinquents at age 18 were very different from the remainder on almost every factor that we investigated, and were almost invariably at the socially deviant end of the spectrum. They drank more beer, they got drunk more often, they were more likely to say that drink made them violent, and they were more likely to get into trouble with the police after drinking. They smoked more cigarettes, and had started smoking at an earlier age. They were more likely to be heavy gamblers. They were more likely to have been found guilty of minor motoring offences, to have driven after drinking at least five pints of beer, and to have been injured in road accidents. They were more likely to have taken prohibited drugs such as cannabis or LSD, even though very few of them had been convicted of possessing these drugs.

The official delinquents were more likely to have had sexual intercourse, especially with a variety of different girls, and especially beginning at an early age, but they were less likely to use contraceptives. They were more likely to be living away from home, and did not get on well with their parents. They changed jobs more frequently, and tended to hold relatively well paid but low status jobs. They were more likely to be tattooed. They were more likely to go out in the evenings, and were especially likely to spend time hanging about on the street. They were more likely to go around in groups of four or more, and were more likely to be involved in group violence and vandalism. They were much more likely to have been involved in fights, to have started fights, to have carried weapons, and to have used weapons in fights. They were also more likely to agree with aggressive and anti-establishment attitude statements in a questionnaire.

Development of a scale for measuring antisocial tendencies

All these deviant characteristics tended to cluster together, so that the typical delinquent was socially deviant in a wide variety of different ways. It was decided to combine some of these factors to produce a scale to measure the degree of antisocial tendency in each youth. Inevitably, such a scale would be strongly linked with delinquency, because each of the component features was characteristic of delinquents. At the same time, however, it would be a measure of antisocial behaviour different from the type which usually led to official delinquency (i.e. property offences).

As a first step, 24 factors were chosen as the most important and relevant of those measured at age 18. Each seemed to be measuring a distinct theoretical construct. Eleven of these factors were eventually selected to constitute the scale of antisocial tendency. These were heavy gambling, heavy smoking, driving after drinking, use of prohibited drugs, sexual promiscuity, unstable job record, spending time hanging about, involvement in antisocial groups, most aggressive in behaviour, anti-establishment attitudes, and tattooed. They were combined very simply, because we just gave each youth one point for each factor which he possessed. Each youth's score, between 0 and 11, was used as an index of his antisocial tendency.

The principles governing the choice of these 11 factors are worth mentioning. As it was hoped to produce a measure which would reflect a general trait of antisociality, several factors which were unrelated to most of the others were the first to be eliminated. For example, the variable unco-operativeness, which referred to the difficulty of securing an interview with the youth, and which was significantly related to delinquency, was not significantly related to most of the other variables. Other variables were eliminated because they were too closely connected and were not independently related to delinquency. For example, a favourable attitude to prohibited drugs was closely related to the admitted use of such drugs, and was not related to delinquency after controlling for admitted drug use. The 11 factors which were finally chosen were all significantly related to each other. Nevertheless, each factor was to some extent independently related to delinquency, as shown by the fact that youths who had adverse ratings on both of two factors were more often delinquents than those with adverse ratings on only one factor.

Only 110 youths had four or more antisocial characteristics, but the majority of the delinquents (67·3 per cent) belonged to this antisocial minority. At the other extreme, 72 youths had none of the antisocial characteristics, and only three of them were delinquents. This shows the close connection between convictions for delinquency and a socially deviant life style at age 18.

Up to the end of 1974, when the majority of youths were aged 21, 120 of the 389 who had been interviewed at 18 were found to have had one or more convictions at some time in their lives. Of these 120 delinquents, 50 had both juvenile and adult convictions, 32 had been convicted only as juveniles, and 38 only as adults. Our earlier work showed that certain background features were significantly more prevalent among those destined to become juvenile delinquents than among the remainder of the sample. It was of interest, therefore, to see whether these same early background features would prove to be equally characteristic of those who were first convicted as young adults.

Like the juvenile delinquents, those first convicted as young adults tended to come from large families, tended to have criminal parents, tended to have low IQs at age 14, and tended to be rated aggressive by teachers at age 14. They also tended to come from poor families, to have been rated troublesome, in their primary schools, to have low IQs at age 10, and to have critical attitudes to the police at age 14, but in these cases the differences did not reach statistical significance because of the small numbers involved. Unlike the juvenile delinquents, those first convicted as young adults were not more likely to have suffered poor parental behaviour. This was an interesting difference between those first found guilty as juveniles and those first convicted as young adults, coupled with the demonstration of the lasting predictive power of most of the factors.

A longitudinal analysis of aggression

We carried out a special longitudinal analysis of aggression, based on teachers' ratings of classroom behaviour at ages 8, 10, 12, and 14, and self-reports of fighting at ages 16 and 18. Each of these measures was significantly related to each of the other measures, showing that aggressive tendencies were to some extent stable over time. Even the teachers' ratings at age 8 and the self-reports at age 18 were significantly related. A group of 27 violent delinquents was also identified, using conviction records up to the end of 1974. A youth was only included in this group if he had been charged with an offence that must have involved violence, or if a police report said that he had used, or threatened to use, physical violence against another person during the commission of an offence. Each of our measures of aggressiveness was significantly related to violent delinquency.

Violent delinquency was significantly predicted by many of the factors measured up to age 10, notably low family income, large family size, criminal parents, low IQ, harsh parental attitude and discipline, separations, and daring. An analysis based on partial Ø correlations showed that all except the first two of these factors were independently predictive of violent delinquency. The only factor which discriminated significantly between violent and non-violent delinquents was harsh parental attitude and discipline, which was twice as common among the violent delinquents. Low IQ and separations nearly discriminated significantly, but criminal

parents and daring were equally characteristic of violent and non-violent delinquents.

Most of the background factors which were related to violent delinquency were also significantly related to aggressiveness at ages 8 to 10. This was true of harsh parental attitude and discipline, criminal parents, separations, low family income, and daring. It might be suggested that these factors had already exerted their aggression-producing effects by ages 8 to 10, and that they were only related to violent delinquency because, as boys matured, there was a natural progression from aggression in school to violent delinquency. It was also interesting to enquire which factors predicted the emergence of aggressiveness for the first time at later ages. When those who were rated aggressive at ages 8 to 10 or 12 to 14 were eliminated, the only early factors which significantly predicted self-reported aggressiveness at ages 16 to 18 were low family income and criminal parents. This again shows the lasting predictive power of these factors. In an analysis designed to investigate the factors which would predict those boys, out of those rated aggressive at ages 8 to 10, who would go on to be rated aggressive at 12 to 14 and at 16 to 18, the most significant factor was separations.

At age 21, an attempt was made to interview all the convicted men in the sample, together with a random sample of non-delinquents. Of the 124 convicted men, 113 (91 per cent) were actually seen, and of the 117 non-delinquents 105 (90 per cent) were seen. Most of the contrasts between official delinquents and non-delinquents at age 21 were similar to those existing at age 18. The delinquents had much higher self-reported delinquency scores, reported more aggressive behaviour, expressed more aggressive attitudes, were more often unemployed, spent more on drink, were heavier smokers, and were more likely to have taken prohibited drugs (in the previous two years). Although the delinquents at age 21 retained their relatively extreme position in these respects, the extent of social deviancy in the sample as a whole had decreased since age 18. For example, the incidence of self-reported offences and the frequency of reported involvement in fights had decreased considerably in both the delinquent and non-delinquent groups, but without affecting the contrast between the two groups.

Effect of marriage on delinquency

Being already married at the time of the interview had a considerable effect on some of the social habits associated with delinquency, notably in reducing the amount spent on drink, reducing non-marital sexual intercourse, reducing the amount of time spent in the company of groups of males, and increasing the amount of outstanding debts. There was no evidence that aggression, unstable employment history, self-reported delinquency, or actual convictions were reduced by being married, at least not in the short term. In investigating the effects of marriage, men who had married between the interviews at 18 and 21 were matched with single men on factors measured at 18. There was no general tendency for delinquents to marry under the age of 21 more often than non-delinquents, but cohabitation without marriage, and marriage to an already pregnant bride, were both more common among delinquents.

Prediction of criminal careers

While in earlier years the emphasis was on predicting the onset of delinquency careers, the emphasis now is on predicting their end. The recidivists, defined as those with two or more convictions before their nineteenth birthdays, were divided into those who continued their delinquency careers by sustaining a further conviction before their twenty-third birthdays, and those who did not. After controlling for the number of previous convictions, other factors which predicted the likelihood of continuing delinquency included having other convicted family members, coming from large, low income families, and scoring high on the antisocial tendency scale at age 18. Since the most seriously delinquent group were the 35 continuing recidivists, an attempt was also made to predict them out of the whole sample. Using only the factors of extreme troublesomeness and convictions of other family members, both assessed at age 10, it was possible to identify a vulnerable group of 35, of whom 18 became continuing recidivists. These results once again demonstrate the continuing predictive power of the early social background factors.

Conclusions

Summing up the major findings of the Cambridge Study in Delinquent Development, it shows how a constellation of adverse family background factors (including poverty, large families, marital disharmony, and ineffective child rearing methods), among which parental criminality is likely to be one element, leads to a constellation of socially deviant factors in late adolescence and early adulthood (including drinking, gambling, drug use, reckless driving, sexual promiscuity, and aggression), among which criminality is again likely to be one element. It seems very likely that the young adult delinquents studied by us will recreate for their own children the same undesirable family environments, thus perpetuating from one generation to the next a range of social problems of which delinquency is only one feature.

We have show that persistent delinquency among working class males is a serious problem with many ramifications. In large part it is attributable to a minority of vulnerable individuals whose potentiality for a chronically antisocial life style is often apparent from an early age. These individuals create endless difficulties for themselves and others. The acts of dishonesty that typically bring them before the courts represent a small and perhaps relatively unimportant facet of their problem behaviour. However, these conclusions are not easy to translate directly into recommendations for social action.

Advantages of longitudinal surveys

Our longitudinal survey has many advantages over the more usual cross-sectional surveys of delinquency. In the usual comparison between a group of delinquents, often drawn from an institution, and a control group of non-delinquents, it is difficult to know the extent to which the characteristics of official delinquents are consequences rather than causes of getting caught by the police. Because of the possibility of establishing temporal ordering of factors, it is easier in a longitudinal survey to move from correlation to causation. The longitudinal survey avoids the problem of retrospective bias, or the fact that ratings or memories may be affected by the knowledge that a person has been convicted. In addition, it is possible in a longitudinal survey to investigate the stability of behaviour, and the effects of particular events on the course of development.

In the usual cross-sectional survey, the delinquents and non-delinquents are extreme groups, and comparisons between them may produce misleading results. In our survey, the delinquent minority developed naturally out of a comparatively normal sample of children, and the whole range of variation was present. It was therefore possible to assess more realistically the relative importance of different factors, and indeed the relative incidence of different kinds of personal and social adversities associated with delinquency. By measuring a large number of factors, it was possible to investigate the extent to which each factor was related to delinquency independently of others.

Some proposals for social action

The translation of research findings into social action is a task that many researchers find repugnant, perhaps because of a deep-seated cynicism about the ability of researchers to influence government policy. It calls for decisions whose full consequences cannot be foreseen, because of the mass of uncontrolled and interacting variables involved in any change of social policy. It calls for difficult value judgements, especially when conflicting needs and competing demands on scanty resources have to be weighed against each other. It calls for an appreciation of what is administratively practicable and tolerable to public opinion, as well as what is theoretically desirable. It also requires the consideration of wider social issues than delinquency, since what is good for delinquency prevention is not necessarily good for society as a whole. We have put forward a number of proposals, but we do not claim that they can be justified scientifically. They are ideas suggested by our research findings, but influenced by other considerations as well.

Some of our proposals are as follows. Even at the cost of taking a little away from the more fortunate members of the community, scarce welfare resources should be concentrated on the most vulnerable, namely the educationally retarded children of large, poor, criminal families. Their predisposition toward a socially deviant life style is often apparent from an early age. Since court appearances seem to exacerbate the problem, social action should be concentrated as far as possible outside the criminal justice system. Help received voluntarily from educational, health, and welfare agencies might prove to be more effective in preventing delinquency than convictions and penal treatment. Unfortunately, the families who are most in need of such help are often the most resistant and unco-operative. In some way, help by social agencies needs to be made more attractive and acceptable. Juvenile delinquents tend to come from families characterized by parental disharmony, cold, harsh parental attitudes, and erratic discipline. It would be desirable to train adolescents of both sexes in the practical skills of parenthood, and this might best be done within the school curriculum.

Longitudinal surveys based on passive observation, with no attempt to manipulate situations experimentally, provide clues to probable chains of cause and effect, but they cannot decisively rule out alternative explanations of varying degrees of plausibility. Because of this, they are even less suitable for forecasting the outcome of social intervention than for deciding between rival criminological theories. What is needed is social experimentation, involving random allocation of persons to different conditions. As an example of the kind of experiment that might be tried, a sample of vulnerable young men, identified by some of the criteria used in this research, could be allocated randomly to several groups, one of which would serve as a control and be left to the usual resources of the existing welfare agencies. Each of the other groups would be provided with a different kind of special help, or with a different combination of several kinds of help. The groups would need to be followed up over a substantial time to discover whether one form of intervention or another proved to have a particularly beneficial effect upon the school performance and social behaviour of their children.

Our conclusion is that longitudinal surveys involving experimental manipulations are the most desirable form of social research. It has always been advisable to precede large-scale social or legislative changes by smaller scale experiments designed to establish their likely effects, but this has hardly ever happened in practice. Our longitudinal survey has been valuable in securing the basic information with which to begin to think about explanatory hypotheses and plans for social action, but it is only a starting point. We hope that it will lead to further longitudinal surveys based on different populations, using experimental interventions.

24. The Malmö study (Sweden)

INGEMAR FÄGERLIND

The Malmö data set is unusual in several respects. It is composed of longitudinal data originally gathered from all 1544 third graders (most were ten years of age) in the private and public schools of the city of Malmö in southern Sweden in 1938. The population represented the entire spectrum of income groups and ability levels in the city. Information about educational and occupational careers of the members of the group is available from age 10 to 44. Data have also been gathered on spouses' social and educational background. In the 1970 to 1974 follow-up the educational careers of all their children have been mapped out. School marks for children who are in school age and above have been gathered as well as mental ability data for all boys who at age 18 have been at military conscription. The various data gathering phases are summarized in Table 24.1. The data set is available in a well documented data bank. Professor Torsten Husén who is now the scientific leader of the project has been involved in the project since 1938 and Ingemar Fägerlind, the present co-ordinator, has worked with the project since 1963.

There are unique historical reasons accounting for the Swedish law making most demographic data open to public perusal. Also a long tradition of accuracy and efficiency in public record-keeping exists in Sweden. The recent computerization of public record-keeping has made it still easier to locate people's records. The tracing of a person's home address, formerly quite a time-consuming task, has also become easier since the population registers for the entire country were computerized and the use of birth numbers, unique to every person, started. According to legislation passed by the Parliament (*riksdag*) in 1973, certain regulations were issued related to data registers of identifiable individuals, with the purpose of protecting privacy. A central agency, the Data Inspectorate, was established and researchers have to apply for permission to set up registers for research purposes.

Perhaps the most remarkable feature of the data in the study is that since the first follow-up in 1948, the number of cases lost has actually decreased over time. Since Malmö group members reached their mid-career they are less mobile and easier to trace through the facilities of the public record system.

An account of the data collected in the Malmö study will be given below. More detailed information about the search strategies and data gathering procedures may be found in the Husén *et al.* (1969) monograph and in reports in the Swedish language by Emanuelsson and Fägerlind (1968) and by Emanuelsson *et al.* (1973). In the data bank manual detailed information about all variables collected is available.

TABLE 24.1

Phases in the collection of the Malmö data set 1938 to 1974

Date of collection	Type of data	Size of sample	Source of data	Mode of collection	Principal researchers
1938	Group intelligence test	1544 (835 boys, 709 girls)	All third grade children in Malmö public and private schools	Pencil and paper tests	Hallgren (1939)
1942	Types of school to which students transferred, and scholastic rating	440	All children transferred to junior, secondary, or higher school	Teacher ratings	Hallgren
1948	Social data, school marks, IQ test at maturity	613	All male respondents enrolled for military service	Military records, pencil and paper tests	Husén (1950) Husén and Henricson
1958–65	Criminality data, social assistance and education data	104 about 1500	Central criminal register Central welfare registers Malmö schools and National Central Bureau of Statistics	Public records	Husén, Emanuelsson, Fägerlind, and Liljefors (1969)
	Income data	1236	County tax departments	Public records	
	Social background data, adult education, and occupational career data	1116	Questionnaires	Mail	
1971–3	Adult education, data on occupations and working conditions	1077	Questionnaire	Mail	Emanuelsson, Fägerlind, and Hartman (1973)
	Social welfare and criminality data			Public records	Fägerlind (1975)
1974	Second generation data	2690	School records Males enrolled for military service	School records Military records	

Collection of data

The 1938 data

The data were originally gathered by Hallgren (1939) in order to study the relationships between different environment factors and cognitive ability among school children. The ability test, devised and standardized by Hallgren, was composed of four subtests labelled: (1) antonyms, (2) sentence completion, (3) identical figures, and (4) disarranged sentences. Test results were gathered during the spring semester of 1938 for 835 boys and 709 girls, all third graders.

In keeping with the purposes of the study the data on social background consisting largely of information obtained from the public records, were gathered especially carefully. Information on unemployment, illness in the home, and public assistance received by the family, was obtained from school welfare registers. Information on number of siblings under sixteen at home was taken from the population registers. These registers also provided the information on father's occupation. Income data from the tax assessment registers included earnings and income from investments of both parents. An almost complete set of social background data is available for 792 boys and 679 girls.

The 1948 data

Ten years after the first data collection the male respondents were required to appear before a military conscription board in order to be examined with regard to their fitness for military service. This provided an opportunity to gather additional information about the male members of the population, including formal educational attainments, occupation at age 20, and mental ability data. Complete test score data were obtained for 653 men. No data were obtained for over-age and under-age males as testing was restricted to the males in the population who were due for military service in 1947 or 1948. Husén (1950) used the data to study the stability of mental ability measures over time.

Data from 1958 to 1965

An extensive follow-up effort was launched at the beginning of the 1960s. Through a search of the Swedish population registers 1375 (89 per cent) of the 1544 Malmö respondents were identified. Registers were also used to gather data on education, social welfare, income and criminality. A questionnaire was used to gather supplementary data on adult education, vocational career, and spouses' educational and social background. Replies were received from 1116 (81 per cent) of the 1375 persons that had been identified. For a more detailed description of the procedures and type of data gathered see Husén et al. (1969, pp. 46–53).

Data from 1970 to 1974

The latest follow-up was conducted in the early 1970s. Experience from data collection in the 1960s was utilized and, by a very careful search both in county and parish population registers, 50 persons that had not been located in 1963 were found. Only 18 persons of the original 1544 were not located, in most cases because information given in 1938 was wrong or incomplete. In 1972 some information was available for more than 98 per cent of the original population.

Supplementary career and educational data, including adult education, have been obtained by mailed questionnaires. Replies were received from 1077 (77 per cent) of the 1397 with known addresses. Income data from 1948, 1953, 1958, 1963, 1968, 1969, and 1971 have been gathered from tax registers. Information about social welfare and criminality during the 1960s and early-1970s has also been collected. Data about all children raised by the families in the population have been collected as well as school records for these children and mental ability data from the compulsory induction test for all boys older than 18 years of age.

Advantages of the project

Data from the study have been used to study many problems that arose during the years. As can be understood from the description above the project is mainly concerned with educational problems. However, some health data are available from the questionnaires. The social registers also contain information about health problems in the family, and problems with alcohol are especially recorded. The family situation is very well recorded as well as the economic situation of these families through the years. Fägerlind (1975) made a study of the economic benefits of education where conclusions were different than they would have been in a cross-sectional study. Emanuelsson (1974) studied the mentally disadvantaged from school to adult life and also found these data much more useful than cross-sectional data. Liljefors (1967) studied the background of persons available in the criminal records, a study that could be continued into the 1970s as data are available. At present the vocational and economic situation of the females is being studied.

As data are available for three generations very interesting studies could be performed, such as the transmission of mental ability from generation to generation. The investigators have great interest in contact with other European longitudinal projects and within certain limits service can be given to researchers from other institutions. Additional information about the projects is available from the Institute of International Education, University of Stockholm, S-106 91 Sweden.

25. Personality development during the school years: a longitudinal study of children in Germany (F.R.G.)

HANS THOMAE

Sample and programme

This chapter reports on a longitudinal study started in 1952 by C. Coerper, W. Hagen, and myself. The study was conducted up to 1961. The subjects of this study were tested for the first time when they entered school (at between 6 and 7 years of age). Approximately 1500 children came to our centres for the last time when they were 15 to 16 years of age. A sample of 126 cases was interviewed and tested again in 1964 when they were 18–19 years old.

At the beginning the sample consisted of approximately 2800 cases from 6 different areas of Western Germany: 3 big cities (Frankfurt, Nuremberg, and Stuttgart); one city with little industrial population (Bonn); one typical industrial city in the Ruhr area (Remscheid); and one rural area (county of Grevenbroich, west of Cologne). The loss of almost half of the cases can be explained by the fact that the subjects participated in the study voluntarily and lost motivation when they grew older or left school. The loss of cases is further due to the loose contact between the parents and the staff members, at least at the beginning of the study. The size of the sample as well as the whole design were determined by the fact that the study was started as part of a public health survey on the initiative of Prof. Hagen, former president of the Federal Health Office of Western Germany. One of the aims of the survey was to give school physicians more recent information on children's physique and health. These data were published by Hagen (1954, 1964), Hagen and Paschlau (1961), Mansfeld (1958), Mansfeld and Lang (1962), Scholz (1963), and others.

The sociological data collected in our study refer to socioeconomic status, the number and kind of persons belonging to the child's family, the parents' educational and professional background, the integration of family, country of origin, and other variables. A review of the main sociological data of the study is given by Ronge (1962).

The psychological programme was limited due to the conditions offered. Intelligence tests (items from Binet–Bobertag for the first three years, items from WISC-scale, Raven, Hawie for the following years), free drawing, sentence completion tests, interviews, and a psychomotor test were administered within a one to two hour session during the annual test periods. The behaviour of the child during performance of tests and the interview was rated on a nine-point scale for eight dimensions (Thomae 1954, 1963a; Mathey 1956). The selection of these dimensions was influenced by a model of personality which has its roots in clinical experience, especially in child psychiatry. Degree, form, and direction of the individual's activity, kind of orienting, regulating, and stabilizing mechanisms, and 'differentiation', are the main categories. The extent of agreement between raters on these scales was notably high when the psychologists had learned to rate the behaviour observed and nothing else (concordance measures according to Kendall (1962) in the range 0·5–0·8; significant at the 1 per cent level).

As the members of the team had to keep notes on details of the behaviour observed within the case histories it was possible to a certain degree to check the validity of the ratings for uniform application. Another check of these ratings was made by receiving reports from the physicians and social workers who sometimes made different observations. In addition, records from school and partial information from interviews with the mother were also available for purposes of confirmation. In the evaluation of the data we regard all our rating measures as ordinal scales.

Within each of the six centres the team consisted of a paediatrician or public health officer with similar training, one psychologist, and a part time social worker. To ensure the comparability of the data, the six teams met twice a year for training and discussion.

Evaluation of the study

The writer had the privilege of studying some of the case histories collected within the Berkeley Growth Study (Bayley 1964), the Guidance Study, the Study of Denver (Colorado), and that at Fels (Antioch College, Yellow Springs, Ohio), when he visited some of the centres of longitudinal research in the United States in 1952, and he is well aware of some of the shortcomings of our study. We tried to follow 5 per cent of our cases with the same range of methods as applied in most of the American studies. However, these case histories can be used only for illustrative purposes.

On the other hand I feel that our findings on the whole group may be of some interest for several reasons. First, the size of the sample enabled us to give a more representative description of children, especially of the physique, health, and general adjustment, than was possible in the very limited number of cases followed in the

American studies mentioned. Further, the social strata were not limited to the upper-middle class, as is the case in many of the American studies, and we were able to study the impact of a larger number of objective socialization variables upon child development. For example, we were able to compare children born in the area where they were now going to school with other children who had been born in parts of the former German 'Reich' which became parts of Russia, Poland, or Czechoslovakia in 1945, and whose parents moved to West Germany shortly before or after our subjects were born. As the living conditions after displacement were often very difficult for these families, it was expected that detrimental effects would appear in these children. Another group which could be compared with the 'average' child consists of the 312 illegitimate children included in the original sample. A third 'objective' socialization variable, the effect of which can be studied in a representative way with this large number of cases, is the question of working versus non-working mothers.

On the other hand the nature of our study did not permit any applications of scales for measuring attitudinal variables in the parents or teachers. It did, however, permit the study of some major socialization variables which sometimes are at least partially neglected in contemporary developmental psychology.

Statistical procedures

Hawell, who analysed our data of behaviour ratings by factor analysis, found that there is a very high degree of correlation between the scores for the different dimensions. We might say therefore that the raters judged one personality factor from different points of view. This factor can be interpreted as 'achievement-related activity' or 'adjustment to an achievement situation'. The dominance of this factor shows that the short testing situation did not allow us to assess the more expressive and emotional aspects of behaviour in many of the cases. The application of the same rating scale within another study which offered an observation period of three to five hours and which included achievement tests as well as personality tests, yielded two factors, one of which was called 'task-related activity' and one 'ego-control' (Essing 1966).

Comparison of extreme groups. One of the approaches to the analysis of our longitudinal data consists of the comparison of extreme groups. 'Extreme' in this connection refers to behaviours or performances which are rated high or low over the greater part of the observation period. Comparisons of this kind were given a preliminary testing in a series of studies by Kern (1959), Schadendorf (1958), Lietz (1960), Distler (1959), and Tägert (1962) for different aspects. The significant differences between the extreme longitudinal groups on one of the aspects relate to most of the other aspects of our rating scales. While this could be expected from the results of factor analysis (Essing 1964; Hawell 1963), other differences are to be explained in relation to theories of social-personality relationships. This is demonstrated by comparisons of subjects with consistently high or low scores in school achievement (Rank 1962; Knöpfler 1964; Klein 1965) and by comparisons of individuals with consistently high or low scores within all of the aspects rated by psychologists during the eight years (van Lieshout 1965).

Objective tests, too, offer a chance of systematic comparisons of consistency over a period of time. The one test which we had to change, in detail only, over the eight years was our psychomotor task (eye–hand co-ordination). The systematic comparison of cases with high and low scores in this task points to a number of social and personality conditions for 'accurate performance' (Steege 1966).

Another very important area for the longitudinal comparison of extreme cases relates to biological data. Hagen (1954), Mansfeld

(1958), Oster (1963), and others developed a measure for biological maturation which used most of the criteria elaborated in relevant literature (excluding bone age; X-ray of hand could be taken at only one research centre). Using these criteria it was possible to differentiate early- from late-maturing subjects on a great variety of other data. Within the first year of observation we could not find any significant psychological differences between early- and late-maturing groups. During the following years it was, however, possible to trace a number of significant differences in intelligence tests and in the behaviour ratings (Strickmann 1957; Thomae 1957; Schmidt 1965; Mansfeld and Strickmann 1965).

Use of external criteria. As mentioned above, we collected data on achievement in school, as given by teachers. In addition the teachers were asked to rate the behaviour of the children in school on dimensions similar to those described in our psychological rating scales. As the teachers' ratings arrived at our research centres several months after the testing time, these two sets of ratings can be regarded as independent of each other. Rank (1962), Knöpfler (1964), and Klein (1965) used these external criteria for systematic evaluations of the relationships between social conditions, personality, and adjustment in school.

We were also able to use data on adjustment to occupational training in small sections of our population. The first of these sections does not belong to the longitudinal sample which is the topic of this report. From 1952–4 we tried to follow a second population born between 1937–9 and leaving school in 1952 (*N* at beginning 1200). Between 1954–6 we gathered data on the occupational career of about 300 of them (Hagen *et al.* 1958). Some of our findings of social impacts on general adjustment will be reported here, although we want to report in particular on the sample born at the end of the war.

Of this sample a group of 70 cases from two centres was followed by Knöpfler (1964) through the time of their occupational training, using reports and questionnaire data from business and workshop owners and training specialists from large companies. The two groups of 'good' and 'poor' adjustment were compared with regard to the many variables mentioned above.

Review of main results

Socio-economic background and personality

According to the findings of Hetzer (1937), Hotyat (1956), Blomquist (1957), Himmelweit (1955), and others, we can expect better adjustment scores in children of high socio-economic status than in children of low socio-economic status. Within our study 'socio-economic status' is defined by the following data:

(a) Income of family;
(b) Father's occupation;
(c) Mother's occupation;
(d) Number of rooms in the home in relation to the number of persons living in this home;
(e) Rating of socio-economic conditions in the family by the social worker.

An analysis of the data from 1952–61 pointed to two larger groups which showed respectively high and low scores in at least four of the five scales related to achievement activity. These two groups were compared with children from more socio-economically favourable homes always scoring higher. In children from homes with lower socio-economic status we found a second trend defined by continuously rising scores, whereas in the high socio-economic status group there were three patterns of consistency and change, namely consistent high scores during the ten-year follow-up, fluctuating scores, and falling scores.

Although certain changes are explained by regression effects, the main finding refers to the stable high and low scores and the relationship between socio-economic status (SES) and consistency in rising and falling scores (Uhr *et al.* 1969). This finding points to an aspect of socialization which very often has been overlooked: Growing up in families with different socio-economic backgrounds is related to differences in the variety of developmental trends. Whereas children from families of higher SES show a high degree of variability, children from lower SES have only one choice: to stay on a low level of achievement-related activity or to try to increase this activity. This increase very often is related to an improvement of socio-economic conditions at home (Thomae 1968a).

SES was also related to school career. Rank (1962) found that pupils who got good grades in elementary school (up to age 13 years) consistently, and significantly more often came from families with satisfactory or good socio-economic background. While these data refer to our Nuremberg sample, Knöpfler's (1964) analysis of the data of 345 cases from Bonn and Remscheid found the reverse. Here especially, boys coming from favourable homes consistently more often got lower grades than those coming from poor socio-economic background. The differences are significant at the 1 per cent level in both studies. These divergent findings might be explained by differences in composition of samples and in parental attitudes toward children. It should be mentioned, too, that 'poor socio-economic background' in the Bonn and Ruhr area would be classified in the United States as 'lower-middle class'.

Very distinct differences between children from high and low socio-economic status appeared when we used the speed of somatic development as a dependent variable. Strickmann and Mansfeld compared a group of 276 boys and girls rated as 'early-maturing' during 4 years of observation with 212 children rated 'late-maturing'. Children from families with high incomes (DM 600 and more) were significantly more often 'early-maturers'; the children from families with low income more often 'late maturers' ($\chi^2 = 11\cdot4$; $p < 1$ per cent).

In addition early-maturers came significantly more often from higher occupational groups, from homes which offered more room for each member, from families whose socio-economic situation was rated as favourable by social workers, and from cities as compared with rural areas. These findings are in agreement with the theory of Bennholdt-Thomsen (1942), who regards this acceleration as an effect of interaction between a more stimulating enviroment and a more 'irritable' (activated) group of the population (see Lehr 1959, 1960).

Integration of family

R. B. Cattell (1950) introduced the term 'syntality' as a measure for the degree of 'togetherness', of 'intimacy' within a group. We prefer the term 'integration'. Within our study it was possible to record only major disturbances of the social structure of a family. Thus in 1955, 82·4 per cent of the families covered by the study were rated as 'integrated', 'socially intact', 7 per cent showed major disturbances, and 2.2 per cent were broken homes. The remaining cases refer to unknown conditions in the family. This rating of integration was done without regard to the completeness of the family. Even if one of the parents had died it could still be rated for the remaining members as 'fully integrated'.

On account of this lack of differentiation of our measure, any comparison between children from integrated and disturbed or broken homes has its problems. We must be aware that within the group of integrated families there is a wide variation of this integration. This may be one of the reasons why van Lieshout (1965) could find consistent trends towards only a small majority of children from disturbed homes within his group of 'low scorers'. On the other hand Uhr (1965) found that children who were rated consistently high in these aspects came more often from integrated homes than all the other types of development she had differentiated. If we turn to an external variable like 'achievement in school' we consistently find that 'poor achievers' come a little more often from disturbed homes than 'high achievers'. This is especially true for the ages 12–15 where the differences are significant at the 1 per cent level (Knöpfler 1964).

An objective criterion for an '0'-degree of integration of family is (at least in this country) divorce. Horn (1959) compared 100 school children of divorced parents within our population with the normal population of the study. The most distinct difference of these two groups is to be found in the rating of socio-economic situation, and throughout the years of observation it was rated consistently worse for children of divorced parents. Within the different behavioural aspects, the number of cases available for analysis dropped between 40 and 50. Sons of divorced parents are significantly more often rated high in activity, responsiveness, and emotional responsiveness for the ages 7–10. Daughters do not differ in these aspects from the normal sample. Within the aspects of adjustment, ego control, and security, sons and daughters of divorced parents significantly more often get low scores than those from 'normal' homes ($p < 1$ per cent). Intelligence scores and school achievement do not differentiate in a consistent and significant way between children and adolescents of divorced and non-divorced parents.

As in many other areas our findings did not confirm extreme opinions on the detrimental effects of the relevant socialization variable. However, they do give evidence of the impact of family integration in a more differentiated way. We might hypothesize from our data that an 'irritation' effect of divorce (high activation, high degree of responsiveness, low degree of adjustment and ego control) does exist, especially in the case of boys.

Working mothers and child development

At the beginning of the study our sample included 29·2 per cent children whose mothers worked outside the home. This proportion increased to 47·71 per cent within the first four years. At first it was possible to complete a comparison of children of working mothers with those of non-working mothers only for the first four years of observation (Schreiner 1963). This comparison was made in two ways:

(1) Differences between children whose mothers did not work at all during the whole period of observation, and those whose mothers worked continuously during this period;
(2) Differences between children whose mothers worked only at the beginning of the observation period, with those who worked only at the end of this period.

From statements and studies such as those by Speck (1956), Nye (1959), Rouman (1956), and Renier (1957) one could expect that children of working mothers would get lower scores in adjustment, ego control, and security. Our data do not confirm any of these statements. In boys there were no significant differences between the groups compared. If there are any trends toward differences they show better adjustment and achievement scores for sons of working mothers. However, none of these differences remains consistent throughout the period. In girls with working mothers we find better grades in school, a higher degree of differentiation and higher scores on ego control at a significant level during part of the observation period. However, none of these differences remains consistent throughout the period. We do not thus find significant differences in the proportion of children of working and non-working mothers within the groups of children with high and low scores. This is shown, too, by Ahrlé (1965) who analysed our data for the second period of observation (1955–9).

Legal status of child and development

More than 10 per cent of our sample consisted of illegitimate children ($N=312$). Of these only 2·3 per cent lived in foster homes, 37·7 per cent lived alone with their mothers, 42 per cent with their mother and a stepfather or with their mother and father (who had married after the child had been born: 4·2 per cent). The remaining children lived with relatives of the mother or foster families. As is shown by Schadendorf (1964) the socio-economic background of illegitimate children is worse than that of the control group. This statement refers to parent's occupation, family income, rating of social situation, and room–person ratio. However, these differences are significant only at the 5 per cent level during the first four years of observation. A consistent trend in differences between illegitimate and legitimate children relates to the number of persons in the family. The illegitimate child lives in a small family much more often than the legitimate child.

As far as personality variables are concerned there are significant differences in general activity within two years of observation (ages 9–10), the illegitimate children belonging to the more inactive group. For the last four years of observation there is a consistent (but not significant) difference for girls. Illegitimate girls are rated less often as very active when compared to daughters of married mothers. In boys these differences approach statistical significance for the ages 11–12 and 13–14. There are also consistent trends in degree of responsiveness. Illegitimate children more often get low scores and less often high ones than legitimate children. In boys this difference disappears at the age of 13–14.

The general adjustment score was lower for illegitimate children during the first four years of observation ($P<0\cdot01–0\cdot05$). These differences could still be observed in the last four years but were not significant. Ratings for ego control (as defined by our criteria) pointed to some very distinct differences between the two groups of children. During the first years of observation the illegitimate children got low scores for this significantly more often than legitimate children ($p < 1$–2 per cent). However, the percentages of children with low scores drop during these years in both groups. Between the ages 11 to 15 these differences become even less evident. Illegitimate girls still more often get low scores ($p < 5$ per cent) for ages 14–15; a similar relationship is also true for boys aged 11–15.

Comparing the general developmental tendencies as defined by Uhr and the writer, illegitimate children significantly more often show a rising tendency within most of the rated aspects than the control group. This points to the fact that there are several reaction patterns toward possible social impairment. One of the compensatory reactions is shown by this tendency of illegitimate children.

As the socio-economic background of illegitimate children generally is more unfavourable than that of legitimate children, Schadendorf (1964) compared illegitimate children with a group of legitimate children from the same socio-economic level. By this comparison many of the differences mentioned so far disappear. However, for the ages 6–10 Schadendorf postulates a 'primary syndrome' for illegitimate children. The first trait of the syndrome is called 'retardation of personality development' (as defined by low scores in adjustment, ego control, differentiation, and security). The impact of the socialization variable generally seems to be more consistent in girls.

Number of siblings and order of birth

The effects of size of family on child development have been studied by several writers (e.g. Blomquist 1957). Usually, children from small families show better adjustment and achievement scores than those from large families.

A preliminary evaluation of relevant data on 639 children made by H. Graumann (1966, unpublished) demonstrated that the items of the Binet–Bobertag intelligence test were passed more often by single children than by those from large families. Similar differences could be observed between children from families with 1 to 3 children on the one hand and children from families with 4 and more children on the other hand, when the ISC items were administered at the age of 9–10. The teachers' ratings showed consistent differences between children from small and large families with regard to dependency–independency. Children from large families are significantly more often rated as dependent by the teacher than single children. On the other hand, single children were significantly more often rated as unsociable by the teacher than those with siblings ($p < 0.05$). The behaviour ratings during the test situations show a significantly higher proportion of children of small families within the group of consistent high scorers, whereas children from families with 3 and more children belong more often to the low score group (van Lieshout 1965).

It would be premature to explain these data by any theory. The same is true for some of the findings of Mansfeld and Strickmann (1965), who compared 'early'- and 'late'-maturing children. The former came significantly more often from small families (1–2 children) ($\chi^2 = 22.48$, $p < 1$ per cent). It seems likely that this difference should be evaluated together with the socio-economic differences between these two groups of children.

As far as the position in the family is concerned, oldest children are rated by the teacher significantly less often as dependent than youngest children. In the categories sociability and dominating versus liking-to-be-dominated there is no difference between the oldest and youngest children. These findings can be evaluated by some kind of learning theory for the development of independence, adjustment, and ego control in older children; however, it is not easy to understand why oldest children belong significantly more often to the 'early-maturers', whereas the second, third, and fourth children significantly more often are rated as 'late-maturers' ($n = 1255$; $\chi^2 = 20.38$; $p < 1$ per cent) (Mansfeld and Strickmann 1965).

If these findings could be confirmed by further investigations they might contribute to some new ideas in the treatment of the nature–nurture problem.

Effects of displacement of family during or after the war

Around 9 per cent of our sample came from families which had to leave their homes in the eastern areas of Germany, Czechoslovakia, Poland, etc. The mothers of these children had especially stressful experiences during pregnancy (immediate war experience, occupation by foreign troops or transportation over 1000 miles under catastrophic conditions). After arrival in Western Germany many were brought to camps where they lived for years under very unsatisfactory conditions. Many of the fathers could not find work for which they were trained. Very often this group of displaced persons was regarded as 'alien' and 'marginal' by the citizens of the communities they had joined.

Generally it could be expected that children from these families should suffer from the after-effects of the stressful experiences of mothers around time of birth, of social and economic deprivation, and of failure in adjustment to new living conditions by the parents. Many essays and educational observations have stressed the possibilities of these impairments whereas other writers have found a general 'prematureness' in these children (for references see Brandt 1964).

A comparison of the socio-economic conditions of the 'native' and the 'displaced' families within the 6 regions of our survey showed that they differed especially with regard to living space. Only 15·2 per cent of the displaced families had at least one room per person; in native families the percentage was 29·2 at the beginning of our study. This difference remained at least unchanged until 1955 (the last year when we asked systematically for sociological data). The income level between the native and displaced groups differed at the 5 per cent level in 1952. By 1955 this difference had become less evident.

The ratings of the socio-economic conditions by social workers did not yield any differences between the groups compared here. This cannot be explained by errors of sampling, but reflects the effects of a state (federal) policy which tried to compensate the losses of the displaced groups by public assistance (and other socio-political actions). The data on adjustment and achievement within school, on intelligence scores, and on area of scores within each of the years of observation in behaviour rating do not point to any significant differences between children from native and displaced families (see Brandt 1964, pp. 31–47).

If the prevalence in developmental trends between the two groups are compared (Brandt 1964, pp. 74–84), the children from displaced families get more consistent scores in the psychological ratings than those from native families. This is not true for ego control. In this dimension the boys from displaced families often get high scores at the time of beginning school. In the following years the boys from displaced families more often get medium scores in ego control than the boys from the native families. Girls from displaced families most often get consistent medium or high scores for the aspects which are related to adjustment, ego control, security, and differentiation. Girls from native families more often get higher scores in activity, responsiveness, and emotional responsiveness. On the other hand, girls from displaced families most often get low scores on security. These findings might point to different attitudes of parents in displaced families compared to those in native ones. During the first years especially they stress adjustment and control of behaviour, whereas children from domestic families can experience a greater range of possible behaviours. With increasing age the demands in both groups become more and more similar. Hence the relevant differences disappear.

This is one of the examples which show that a longitudinal study of human development must try to keep up with the social-political history of the time covered by the study. If it had been possible to follow at least part of our sample from early childhood we would also have found considerable differences by cross-sectional comparison. On the other hand our findings show that those environmental stresses which are of a transient nature can be compensated for or regulated by social change and parental guidance.

Breastfeeding and personality

As we started to follow our children only from when they first went to school the psychoanalytical theories concerning childhood experience and personality development cannot be tested by our findings. However, for the problem of orality they may be of similar value as those of Sewell and Mussen (1952) or of Sears et al. (1957), who interviewed the mothers of their subjects at about the same age as the mothers of our subjects. As our children were 6–7 years old at this interview they were considerably younger even than the subjects in the studies of Blum and Miller (1952), Goldman (1950), and Thurston and Mussen (1951).

In our study this interview was conducted after the first medical examination. It covered the main medical dimensions of physical and mental development in infancy. It brought fairly reliable data on the kind of feeding, and in some cases the age of weaning, etc. Other data such as that on bladder and bowel training, educational problems, etc. we did not consider reliable enough. The data for kind of nutrition in infancy were complete for 2699 children. The data on time of breastfeeding is shown in Table 25.1; no sex differences were observed in this instance. The difference between this data and that of Sears et al. (1957) should not be regarded as a cross-national difference. Whereas these authors state that 60 per cent of their subjects did not breastfeed their children, in our sample only 13·8 per cent gave that answer.

The correctness of this answer cannot be doubted as there was no policy or public campaign favouring breastfeeding at the time when

TABLE 25.1

Duration of breastfeeding (in weeks), N = 2699

Group	A (No breastfeeding)	B	C	D	E
Duration (weeks)	0	1–12	13–20	21–52	52 and more
Number of cases	375	802	623	807	98

the interviews took place. Actually the high prevalence of breast-feeding can be explained by the fact that food was rationed at the time of the birth and infancy of our subjects, and breastfeeding was awarded higher ration tickets (coupons). The usual difference in feeding habits between the different social strata appeared only in the Ruhr district. It was not observable within the samples from Frankfurt, Stuttgart, or Nuremberg.

For the evaluation of possible effects of breastfeeding we compared only the data for the year 1955, when our subjects were 9–10 years old. The children from group A (no breastfeeding) did not differ from the remaining sample in intelligence, adjustment to school, activity, mood, responsiveness, general adjustment, and ego control. The same was true when we compared the children from group B (short period of breastfeeding) with those of group D (long period) or E (extremely long period). If we accept Erikson's revision of the psychoanalytical theory of the effects of oral gratification in infancy, we should expect differences between the groups A/B and D/E with regard to security. Actually these groups of children did differ significantly in the percentage of low scores within this dimension.

The higher proportion of children with low scores for security within the group of subjects with short experience of breastfeeding is especially remarkable. This finding may be related to the assignment of the polarity 'basic trust vs. basic mistrust' as a main theme for development in the oral stage (Erikson 1951). On the other hand, the majority of children with no or very short experience of breastfeeding got medium scores for security. A quarter of those with long experience of this kind got low scores. This shows that breastfeeding *per se* is only one variable among many influences effective during and after the oral stage.

Conclusions

If we compare the findings on the impact of seven groups of socialization variables, the most important dimension appears to be the socio-economic. The lack of evidence of the impact of integration of family in the dimensions of behaviour where it could be expected may be explained by the inadequacy of information available to us. This is not true for the other variables. Comparing the data on the legitimate and illegitimate children, i.e., two groups most clearly differentiated from each other in sociological terms, socio-economic status again proved to have a greater effect than legal status.

The fact that we did not find differences between children of working and non-working mothers, of children of native or alien status, or resulting from order of birth, may be explained by the more fundamental role of the variable socio-economic situation. Whereas the effect of the other variables can very often be compensated for by other factors (for instance the absence of the mother by the increased role of grandmother or increased intimacy between mother and child in families with working mothers), this is apparently possible, however, only to a minor degree, for the adverse effects of low socio-economic status.

Unfortunately we can evaluate the effects of parental attitudes on child development only by case histories (Hagen 1964; Thomae 1963*b*). Although no direct correlation can be stated, a close relationship between favourable socio-economic situation and favourable attitudes seems to be more likely than the reverse. This is shown by Ronge (1962) who pointed to the dominance of unfavourable socio-economic conditions within the non-integrated families of our study population. Experiences from clinical practice and from biographies of eminent men which seem to demonstrate reserved relationships of this kind, should not be used as a basis for general conclusions.

In this instance the results of Pattie and Cornett (1952) and Lehr (1965) who analysed early childhood memories, should be recalled. These were less favourable in subjects from low socio-economic backgrounds. No difference was observed in this respect between subjects from integrated or non-integrated homes (Lehr 1965).

We should not regard the differences between children from low and high socio-economic status as indications of direct relationships between these variables. Other factors, however, do have an effect within the range determined by low socio-economic status. This constitutes a barrier which apparently cannot be overcome so easily as other adverse factors. This statement does not at all call into question the value of the studies on the effects of those socialization variables which primarily attract the attention of contemporary students of child development. In particular it does not reduce the importance of studies on parent–child relationships. We hope that further analysis of our data will provide at least some information on these questions.

As this analysis is continuing, this report should not be regarded as a summary of all the findings of our study. As is the case with most other longitudinal studies, the analyses have not yet been completed. In particular, we have not been able to complete the analysis of the data on leisure time activities and personality. A preliminary study showed that concentration (rated by the school teacher) and ego control (rated by psychologists) were less favourably developed in the subjects who went most frequently to the cinema or watched television than in the control group (Thomae 1960*b*). Although this finding is contradictory to that of Himmelweit and Oppenheim (1958) it cannot be attributed to mere chance. As the raters had no knowledge about the leisure time of the respondents it cannot be explained by bias either. However, this will have to be tested by further longitudinal analysis.

On the other hand, we do not overestimate the impact of mass media and technological change. A series of cross-generational comparisons started by the author and his co-workers in 1949 show a great tendency toward very similar reactions in the generations born between 1910 and 1920 and those born twenty to thirty years later (Engels and Thomae 1950; Thomae 1962, 1969; Glöckel 1960). This similarity may suggest that the family background of the individual is more important than social or political change. The data available for the years 1949 to 1960, which brought a great deal of economic recovery and of consolidation of attitudes, also show that socio-economic conditions form an important frame of reference. They may be of less value than many of the emotional contacts which are usually stressed in socialization theory. However, they do exist.

Summary

This report describes the design, subjects, and methods of a

German longitudinal study on children and adolescents. It reviews the main trends of the evaluation of the data and the main results in relation to the possible effects of seven groups of socialization variables: socio-economic status, integration of family, work of mother, legal status, number of siblings and order of birth, displacement of family, breastfeeding. It also presents a preliminary discussion of the differences in evidence of these effects.

c. Prospective adult cohort studies

26. The longitudinal study of women in Göteborg, Sweden

TORE HÄLLSTRÖM and SVERKER SAMUELSSON

History

In the last two decades the biological aspect of the climacteric has received increased attention, partly because of the new interest in the changes in lipid and calcium metabolism and the associated increase in incidence of coronary heart disease and osteoporosis in the post-menopausal period. For psychiatrists the phases of endocrine changes in women have long been a focus of interest. The psychic changes associated with puberty, pregnancy, the postpartum period, and phases of the menstrual cycle have been the subject of intensive study. In the last few decades, however, there have been few advanced psychiatric studies on the climacteric.

It was felt that this situation called for a multidisciplinary approach designed to throw some light upon the climacteric from a number of different aspects: somatic, psychiatric, and social. With this aim, an investigation was undertaken in Göteborg during 1968 and 1969 on 1622 women selected so as to constitute a representative proportion of women in that town in the age strata 38, 46, 50, 54, and 60 years. The study was carried out by a number of research teams from several medical departments at the University of Göteborg. The project included psychiatric studies of a subsample of 899 women in the age strata 38, 46, 50, and 54 years. The sample was re-studied during 1974–5. One of the authors (Hällström) had the responsibility for the first psychiatric study while the responsibility for the prospective longitudinal psychiatric project now is shared by the authors. Associate Professor Calle Bengtsson is coordinator of the total project.

Rationale

Epidemiological investigations in psychiatry have mostly aimed at establishing the prevalence or incidence of various types of mental disorder in the general population or in selected portions of it. In these investigations, morbidity has usually been related to broad demographic factors such as sex, age, ethnicity, civil state, migration, and socio-economic status. In contrast to this, the present investigation was designed to apply epidemiological methods for the more detailed study of a series of specifically defined questions within a limited field.

The objective, defined at the beginning of the study, was to demonstrate any possible effect of the climacteric on mental health and sexual behaviour. A further aim was to undertake a comprehensive survey of the relations between biological, psychological, and social factors on the one hand, and, on the other hand, mental health and sexual behaviour in middle-aged women. With few exceptions, earlier psychiatric studies on the climacteric are performed on clinical samples and the generalizability of earlier findings are therefore questionable. It was thought that the epidemiological approach would allow more far-reaching con-

clusions to be drawn regarding the interplay between different kinds of factors in the causation of disturbances in mental health and sexual behaviour than previously had been possible.

Population

The selection of women for the psychiatric project was made by taking all those in the population register of the county authority who were recorded as resident in Göteborg on 1 January 1968 and who were born in the years 1914, 1918, 1922, and 1930. The subjects were examined six to eight months after they reached 38, 46, 50 and 54 years of age respectively. The menopause occurs on the average at the age of 50 years, and it therefore appeared natural to choose a group of 50-year-old women to represent this phase of the climacteric. The 46-year-olds consist in the main of pre-menopausal women and the 54-year-old women are mainly post-menopausal. The 38-year-olds form a pre-climacteric control group. It was thought advisable to include in the two middle groups a considerably larger number of subjects than in the youngest and oldest age strata. As far as the climacteric and its hormonal aspects are concerned, the two latter age groups are more homogeneous than the former and therefore do not have to be divided for analysis into different subgroups to the same extent as the two middle age groups.

To obtain a representative selection of suitable size and with the required age distribution, it was decided to extract from the women born in 1914 those born on the 12th of each month, from the women born in 1918 and 1922 those born on the 12th, 18th, 24th, and 30th of each month, and from the women born in 1930 those born on the 12th of each month and on the 18th of each odd month. This produced an original sample comprising 956 women. Of these 57 were selected for a pilot study, which was not included in the main psychiatric series, so this was finally composed of 899 women. During the interval between the selection procedure and the planned examination, seven women died and eight moved away from Göteborg. Eight hundred of the remaining 884 subjects agreed to take part in the study.

Method

The subjects were invited to a general health examination by means of an introductory letter sent out two months before the planned day of examination. About a week later a secretary made telephone contact with the subject and arranged a convenient day for the examination. A question form was then sent covering previous and current physical illness. This was intended to be filled out at home and brought to the examination.

The complete series of physical health tests occupied two to three days and took place at the Sahlgren hospital. The psychiatric examination took place within one to four weeks after the first series of physical examinations. The psychiatric interview was conducted by one of the authors (Hällström). The interview was structured in part with fixed questions and restricted alternative answers; in part it can be described as an orientated conversation on predetermined subjects in regular order. An 88-page question form was used to aid the interview. Answers to questions were coded as they were given, and in the informal part of the interview all answers were written down as accurately as possible. The psychiatric interview usually took one to two hours. During its course, observations were made on the subject's behaviour and these were coded immediately after the interview was concluded.

The interview consisted of questions covering certain personality traits, current psychic disturbance, leisure interests, circumstances of early life, psychiatric family history, schooling, employment, marital situation, other social circumstances, previous nervous disorder, sexual history, and it concluded with questions on menstrual history. The sections of the interview which had a free clinical character were regarded as the most important ones. During or after the interview, global ratings were made for a series of variables such as current disability grade, disability grade one year earlier, and mental health deterioration during the one-year period immediately predecing the examination. These ratings formed the basis for determination of prevalence and incidence rates of various kinds (See Tables 26.1–26.3).

Supplementary examination instruments were the Eysenck Personality Inventory (EPI), the Cesarec–Marke Personality Schedule (CMPS), and a phobia checklist. Data from record sources were

TABLE 26.1

Mental impairment (disability grade). Point prevalence rates (per cent) in different age strata

Disability grade	Age strata (years)					
	38 $N=111$	46 $N=309$	50 $N=290$	54 $N=90$	Totals N	per cent
0	63·1	61·5	61·0	48·9	481	60·1
1	23·4	24·6	28·3	33·3	214	26·8
2	10·8	10·4	6·6	11·1	73	9·1
3	2·7	3·6	3·4	4·4	28	3·5
4	0·0	0·0	0·7	2·2	4	0·5
Totals	100	100	100	100	800	100

Disability grades: 0 = Complete or almost complete freedom of symptoms; 1 = Mild symptoms and very little or no functional impairment; 2 = Moderate symptoms and clear functional impairment; 3 = Pronounced symptoms and work capacity greatly reduced; 4 = Severe symptoms and complete incapacity for work.

TABLE 26.2

Maximum disability grade during life: Reports from women in different age strata (per cent)

Maximum disability grade	Age strata (years)					
	38 $N=111$	46 $N=309$	50 $N=290$	54 $N=90$	Totals N	per cent
0	22·5	18·4	21·0	15·6	157	19·6
1	20·7	32·7	32·8	27·8	244	30·5
2	38·7	33·3	31·7	37·8	272	34·0
3	15·3	14·2	13·4	14·4	113	14·1
4	2·7	1·3	1·0	4·4	14	1·8
Totals	100	100	100	100	800	100

TABLE 26.3

One year incidences of different grades of mental illness in different age strata, including those with disability grade 0 one year before examination, and excluding those who had undergone oophorectomy or hysterectomy and those in the age strata 46, 50, and 54 years who were taking contraceptive pills

Age strata (years)	Remained well N	Maximal disability grade during the one year period			Totals N	Total incidence rate (disability grade 1+2+3) per cent
		1	2	3		
38	62	5	9	2	78	21
46	160	19	12	0	191	16
50	153	22	7	1	183	16
54	34	8	8	0	50	32
Totals	409	54	36	3	502	19

collected for the whole of the population selected for examination. Clinical records were examined at all treatment centres for out- and in-patient psychiatric care in Göteborg. Among other things, the number of treatment periods and age at each admission were coded. In addition to this, information was obtained from insurance records about periods of medically certified illness with psychiatric diagnosis for all the subjects selected for examination. Women with symptoms or signs of diseases were offered further control and treatment by members of the research staff or referred to specialists or general practitioners. Every participant also received a sheet with some laboratory data and a short clinical comment.

To get some idea of the reliability and validity of the mental health ratings, control studies of various kinds were made. Statements made by subjects during the interview about contact with psychiatrists and psychiatric treatment were compared with the information obtained from record sources and agreement was found to be good. To obtain some measure of inter-rater reliability in the assessment of the current grade of mental illness, tape recordings were made of 100 consecutive interviews. On the basis of these recordings, new ratings of disability grade were made by another assessor. The intraclass correlation coefficient was 0·77 (ratings on a five-degree scale). The corresponding rating for maximal grade of mental illness during the last 10-year period was compared with the records of certified illness with psychiatric diagnosis during the same period. Those rated as mentally well were found to have been certified sick in 8·6 per cent of the cases. With rising grade of mental impairment the frequency of certification gradually rose, reaching 100 per cent in disability grade 4.

Among the population who were invited to take part in the investigation, 11·0 per cent failed to attend. Of these, 0·9 per cent had moved away, 0·8 per cent had died, 0·3 per cent were not reached, and 9·0 per cent refused co-operation. In order to determine whether the drop-out group differed in any material respect from the investigated population, certain data were extracted from record sources for the two groups. Single women, widows, and those not employed are overrepresented in the drop-out group. No differences were found as regards migration, social group, occurrence of psychiatric hospital treatment, and medically certified illness with psychiatric diagnosis.

Results

As the investigation was concerned with the normal climacteric, women who had undergone bilateral oophorectomy, X-ray castration, or hysterectomy were excluded from the analyses, as were the small number in the age groups 46–54 years who were taking contraceptive pills. The climacteric was divided into four phases: (1) pre-menopause, with menstruation still regular, (2) peri-menopause, with irregular menstruation, (3) early post-menopause, when less than three years had elapsed since the last menstruation, and (4) late post-menopause, when three years or more had elapsed since the menopause.

The comparisons between different climacteric groups (see Table 26.4) showed no significant differences in the one-year incidence rates of mental illness (all diagnoses together), depressive

TABLE 26.4

One-year incidences of different grades of mental illness in different climacteric phases. Age strata 46, 50, and 54 years combined, including those with disability grade 0 one year before examination

Climacteric phase	Remained well	Maximal disability grade during the one-year period			Totals	Total incidence rate
	N	1	2	3	N	per cent
Pre-menopause	160	17	13	0	190	16
Peri-menopause	100	18	7	1	126	21
Early post-menopause	45	8	1	0	54	17
Late post-menopause	42	6	6	0	54	22
Totals	347	49	27	1	424	18

states, or in psychiatric morbidity as determined by an operationally defined scale which recorded different levels of symptomatic affliction. However, two single symptoms did occur significantly more frequently in certain climacteric phases: anxiety in peri-menopause and irritability in pre- and peri-menopause. A comprehensive analysis was undertaken to see whether various possible causal factors of mental illness were unequally distributed among the climacteric groups under comparison. This was found not to be the case. In view of these findings, the most probable explanation for the negative outcome of the testing of these hypotheses would appear to be that there are in fact no causal relations between any particular climacteric phase and the development of mental illness.

Sexual interest was significantly weaker among the post-menopausal women than among those in pre- and peri-menopause. In fact, sexual interest appeared to decline gradually as the climacteric advanced. This tendency is independent of age (see Table 26.5). The results show that there is also a tendency for sexual interest to decline with increasing age, irrespective of whether the climacteric is advancing or not. In a group of ageing women, these two trends operate together. As an example of their pressure it may be mentioned that 20 per cent of the married 38-year-olds reported weak or absent sexual interest. Among the 54-year-olds this figure had risen to 52 per cent. The same trends were found for most of the variables used as measures of different types of sexual functional capacity or changes in these.

An analysis was made of the relation between mental illness at the climacteric and a series of background factors. Those women who became ill during the climacteric (after 40 years of age) reported mental illness in their parents and strict upbringing in significantly larger numbers than did those who remained well. However, those who became ill for the first time at the climacteric differed only in minor degree from those remaining well as far as mental illness in the parents and unfavourable early environmental factors were concerned. The earlier in life the onset of the illness, the more prominently these negative background factors featured in the history.

Mental illness earlier in life was found significantly more often among those who had become ill during the climacteric than among those who had remained well throughout this time. However, it could not be shown that mental illness during puberty, pregnancy, or post-partum in a specific way increased the risk of recurrent illness at the climacteric.

Examination of current social circumstances brought out the following factors which showed significant relations with mental illness occurring during the year preceding examination: marriage disrupted by reason of separation, divorce, or death of the husband; serious problems with the children; unhappiness at work; and a large number of psychosocial stress factors in general. Among social variables which did not show any significant relation of this kind were social group, family income, civil state, amount of employment, childlessness, and the last child having left home.

Twenty-one per cent of women in the age group 46–54 years

TABLE 26.5

Proportion of women (per cent) who reported different types of changes in sexual interest in different age strata and climacteric phases

Age strata (years)	Climacteric phase	Changes in sexual interest				Total N	Total per cent
		Increase	No change	Some decrease	Great decrease		
38	Pre-climacteric	16	53	23	9	93	100
46	Pre-menopause	12	46	29	14	157	100
	Peri-menopause	16	33	29	20	54	100
	Early post-menopause					10	
	Late post-menopause					4	
	Totals	12	42	29	16	225	100
50	Pre-menopause	5	48	34	12	58	100
	Peri-menopause	4	32	43	21	75	100
	Early post-menopause	0	43	31	26	42	100
	Late post-menopause	7	21	48	24	29	100
	Totals	4	37	39	20	204	100
54	Pre-menopause					1	
	Peri-menopause					7	
	Early post-menopause	6	31	31	31	16	100
	Late post-menopause	0	24	39	37	38	100
	Totals	2	27	35	35	62	100

reported that they previously had had a mainly negative attitude about menopause; the remainder had either a neutral or a mainly positive attitude. In the peri- and post-menopausal women, no significant relation was found between previous attitude about menopause and the onset of mental illness during the year preceding examination.

To analyse the associations between different background factors and the declining sexual interest the women in peri- and post-menopause were divided into two groups, one consisting of those who had noted decrease or complete loss of sexual interest during the last five years, and the other those whose sexual interest had remained constant or had increased during the same period. Several variables indicated that the former group had a generally low sexual functional capacity. Those with declining sexual interest reported a low desired frequency of coitus, a low and decreasing capacity for orgasm, a low and decreasing actual frequency of coitus, and also a poor capacity for orgasm earlier in life. In comparison with the other group, these differences were all statistically significant.

Several other factors also showed differences between these two groups. These differences could in large measure be attributed to two main variables: social group and grade of mental illness. Women with declining sexual interest were overrepresented in lower social groups, they had lower grade school education, inferior vocational training, lower family income, smaller homes, and fewer artistic interests. The differences in respect of these factors were significant when the subjects were matched both for age and for grade of mental illness. However, when the matching was according to social group the differences were no longer significant.

The proportion of women with declining sexual interest increased in parallel with rising grade of mental disability. This trend was significant with matching both for age and for social group. A series of scales indicating the number of psychic symptoms of various types present also showed corresponding significant differences between the groups. Certain factors showed significant correlation with declining sexual interest, irrespective of age, social group, or grade of mental illness; these were physical illness of the husband, unhappiness at work, and external dyspareunia.

The cross-sectional character of the first investigation has made it necessary to work largely with retrospective data. Interpretation of some of the findings will be facilitated when results from the prospective study are available. The first study can thus be regarded as an initial contribution which will acquire its full value only after a follow-up study.

The test sample taken for examination has in most aspects been shown to be adequately representative of the normal population of Göteborg women in the relevant age strata. Probably most of the findings apply to middle-aged Göteborg women in general. On the other hand, it is uncertain how far the findings can be generalized to apply to women in other Swedish towns, in rural areas, in other countries of Europe, or in other cultures. To learn something of this it is advisable for similar studies to be made elsewhere. The authors thus would welcome contacts with other longitudinal projects for purposes of establishing cross-national or cross-cultural reliability of the findings. The relations found to exist between social factors, mental health, and sexuality presumably apply only in limited degree to societies very different in character from a European industrial city such as Göteborg. However, the relations between biological factors such as age and climacteric on the one hand, and mental health and sexuality on the other are probably more independent of the character of the society.

The follow-up study

The follow-up study was designed to give answers to the following questions:

(1) Which are the point prevalence, one- and six-year incidence rates of different disability grades, point prevalence rates of psychiatric symptoms and syndromes, and incidence rates of changes in sexual behaviour in the material?

(2) What is the outcome of those cases of mental illness found in the first study? Which are the indicators of good and bad prognosis?

(3) Which are the associations between biological, psychiatric, psychological, and social background variables and incidence of mental illness?

(4) To what extent do certain life changes influence the risk of developing mental illness? Do any of the background variables make the women more vulnerable or resistant to that risk?

Of those 1462 women who attended the initial study (total project), 1302 participated in the follow-up study (89·1 per cent), which means 80·3 per cent of those initially sampled. Twenty-six women had died during the interval between the two examinations. If these subjects are excluded, the participation rate was 90·7 per cent, and also if those women among the non-participants who had moved from the city during the period are excluded, the participation rate was 94·4 per cent. In the subsample attending the psychiatric project the participation rate is 84·6 per cent.

In the follow-up study the interviews were semistructured and were aided by a 26-page questionnaire. Current psychiatric symptoms were rated on a seven-degree scale (Comprehensive Psychopathological Rating Scale). Reported symptoms were: worrying over trifles, inner tension, autonomic disturbances, muscular tension, phobias, hostile feelings, derealization/depersonalization, hypochondriasis, sadness, pessimistic thoughts, inertia, fatiguability, concentration difficulties, failing memory, inability to feel, indecision, compulsive thoughts, rituals, reduced sleep, suicidal thoughts, delusional ideas, hallucinations. Observed symptoms were: apparent sadness, elated mood, hostility, labile emotional responses, lack of appropriate emotion, autonomic disturbances, sleepiness, distractability, withdrawal, perplexity, blank spells, disorientation, pressure of speech, reduced speech, specific speech defects, flight of ideas, incoherent speech, perseveration, overactivity, slowness of movement, agitation, involuntary movements, muscular tension, mannerisms and postures, hallucinatory behaviour.

The occurrence of 53 psychosocial stressors during one year was assessed. During and immediately after the interview various components of the mental health status and changes in this during the last six years were rated.

The psychiatric interviews are finished and the data are coded and transmitted to OCR sheets. No results are available yet. The data from the investigation of 1968 and 1969 are on tape and further analyses are under way. As regards the future, we hope to be able to study the sample a third time after another six-year interval (1980 to 1981). The subjects' anonymity is protected and the project is approved by the ethical committee of the Faculty of Medicine at the University of Göteborg.

The project has received financial support by grants from the Medical Faculty of the University of Göteborg, the Göteborg Medical Society, Transatlantic's Foundation, the Psychiatric Resarch Fund at the Department of Psychiatry of the Sahlgren Hospital, the Royal Society of Science and Art in Göteborg, and the Swedish Medical Research Council. Yearly grants are received from the Swedish Medical Research Council with termination date in June every year (Project No. B75-27X-4578-01 to B80-27X-4578-06B).

27. A prospective epidemiological study of depressive, psychosomatic and neurotic disturbances (Switzerland)

J. BINDER and J. ANGST

Research questions

The project is concerned with minor psychiatric disturbances. By this we mean disturbances with psychosomatic, depressive, and neurotic symptoms. Because of the use of standardized interviews as the main research technique, subjects can not be examined somatically nor be investigated in a detailed anamnestic inquiry. Thus diagnoses are possible only at the level of psychiatric syndromes. The following disturbances are excluded from our definition of minor psychiatric disturbances: antisocial behaviour, psychoses, and drug addiction.

Although it is generally accepted that the problem of minor psychiatric disturbances is very important, we do not know enough about the prevalence and the course of these disorders. Because most studies have been based on samples of psychiatric patients or of general practice patients they show a bias towards more serious disorders. Remarkably little is known about the normal course and outcome of less serious psychiatric disorders.

The minor psychiatric disturbances are of great practical and sociomedical importance because of:

1. Their high prevalence in the general population;
2. Their high social costs in terms of consumption of medical services, absenteeism, etc.;
3. Their not being recognized as such, so that many patients find themselves in continuous medical treatment;
4. They are, for the individual concerned, a burden and an impediment.

The research project envisages investigating the following areas:

1. Prevalence of psychosomatic, depressive, and other neurotic symptoms and interdependence of these symptoms;
2. How the symptoms change in the course of time (change of symptoms, spontaneous development of untreated minor psychiatric disturbances);
3. Course and outcome of disturbances as a function of psychological and social variables as well as of the individual 'illness behaviour';
4. Social impairment resulting from these disturbances (frequent consultation of doctors, impairment in working capability, absenteeism, social marginality, etc.);
5. Psychological and social conditions linked with the occurrence of minor psychiatric disturbances.

The main purpose of this investigation is a descriptive analysis of the course of minor psychiatric disturbances and their consequences for the social life of the subjects. Aetiological aspects of these disturbances are of minor relevance because the research design doesn't allow the collection of data about constitutional disposition and about the early stages of the socialization process.

Methods

A panel of 600 subjects will be interviewed several times during a first period of four years with a standardized psychiatric–sociologi-cal interview. The sample consists of 600 subjects of the age of nineteen or twenty years stratified according to the degree of psychiatric impairment. The central methodological concern will therefore be the definition of the universe, the selection of the subjects who will be included in the panel (psychiatric screening), and the psychiatric–sociological interview.

Universe

The universe consists of the whole Swiss population of the canton Zurich born in 1958 (females) or 1959 (males). The canton of Zurich is mostly an urban area with an occupational structure that offers employment in the sectors of industry and services, but it also includes rural areas at its periphery. For practical reasons the foreign population cannot be included in the study. This is regrettable not only because of the numerical importance of this population segment (about 10 per cent), but also because the foreigners in Switzerland, coming to a large extent from southern Europe, mostly occupy the lowest positions in the social stratification system.

This sample will be subjected to a psychiatric screening device—the questionnaire SCL-90-R that has been developed by Derogatis (1974). The SCL-90-R is a self-rating questionnaire with nine scales of clinical significance. It will make it possible to identify subjects with different patterns of minor psychiatric disturbances in order to get a sample that includes subjects with psychosomatic, depressive, neurotic, and diffuse disturbances. From the approximately 16 000 persons exposed to the psychiatric screening, 300 males and 300 females will be selected for this prospective investigation. The universe that has been screened may be useful for other epidemiological projects in the future.

The psychiatric screening procedure

Males. All Swiss men of the age of nineteen have to show up for the military conscription. The military authorities let us carry out the screening during the conscription. Thus, it is possible to have a complete screening of the entire population of males of the age of nineteen. The psychiatric screening is accomplished by the personnel of the Research Direction and the subjects are informed that it has nothing to do with the military authorities. Different pretests have been carried out to insure that the situation of conscription has no influence on the psychiatric screening.

Females. In Switzerland it is not possible to reach the complete population of females in a similar way. Because females are very important in a project dealing with minor psychiatric disturbances we have to accept a screening procedure for females with certain imperfections.

In Switzerland young people become of age when they are twenty. For administrative reasons, all communities establish registers of their twenty-year-old inhabitants. Nearly all communities of the canton of Zurich are offering us these registers for the purpose of our research. It is planned to carry out the psychiatric screening for females by postal enquiry with the same questionnaires as those used for the males. On the basis of a pretest we expect a return rate of 70 per cent. Thus it is possible that the sample of female subjects will not be completely representative. We expect an overrepresentation of women with higher education.

Contact with subjects and protection of their anonymity

The 600 subjects selected for the panel will be contacted by interviewers (students of medicine and psychology that are specially trained for the project) after receiving a written announcement. Our project will be presented as 'a sociomedical investigation into the prevalence of physical and mental disturbances'. Because the project is of strictly scientific character it is not possible to use public agencies or mass media to inform the sample.

The repeated interviewing of the same subjects doesn't allow an anonymous interview. The subjects will be assured that all their answers are under strict medical secrecy. All the information will be stored on a computer without personal identification and will not be available for public use.

Drop-outs

The problem of drop-outs in the prospective study has not yet been solved. The main difficulty will be those subjects who are unwilling to collaborate. The tracing of subjects who changed their addresses won't be of great practical difficulty in a country as small as Switzerland. A similar study that has been carried out at our research department led to a drop-out rate of 43 per cent when the subjects were reinterviewed by a mailed questionnaire after three years. However, an analysis of these data permitted us to analyse the non-respondents.

Psychiatric–sociological interview

The core of the research project consists of repeated interviews. It is planned to accomplish an intensive psychiatric interview soon after the psychiatric screening as well as two interviews during the course of the project, each after a time of about two years. All the three interviews of the prospective study are compatible in their methodology and investigated topics, so that they will be comparable with each other.

Because of the large number of interviews it is impossible to have them carried out by trained psychiatrists. Relying on existing psychiatric interviews our interviews shall however be standardized so that they can be accomplished by advanced students of medicine and psychology after special training. Recent investigations by Wing (1976) show indeed that an abbreviated version of the present State Examination (9th version) can be used for epidemiological field research by lay interviewers. The psychiatric–sociological interview includes the following topics:

Somatic ailments and mental disturbances;
Consultation of doctors, attitudes concerning illness and the use of medical services (illness behaviour);
Personality;
Attitudes, values;
Interactions in family, work, leisure;
Life Change Questionnaire, and long-lasting stress in social interactions;
Socio-economic background variables.

During the first interview anamnestic indications will also be collected. A pretest of the reliability of anamnestic indications shows that they have to be gathered with great care.

Data analysis

Data will be stored on electronic media in order to carry out statistical analyses with computer programs. It is planned to use the SPSS Program Package (Nie *et al.* 1975), which integrates data management with various statistical procedures. The use of multivariate statistical techniques will also be of great importance.

Administrative considerations

The project has been initiated by the Research Department of the Psychiatric University Clinic in Zurich with strictly scientific aims. Grants for the project have been available through the Schweizerischer Nationalfonds zur Förderung der wissenschaftlichen Forschung. This organization, primarily financed by the Swiss Confederation, gives grants for fundamental research for a period of three years. A continuation of later funding is possible.

Appendix: results of different pre-test investigations Bias of psychiatric self-rating through openness and situational influences

In a series of preliminary investigations it had to be decided if the situation of military conscription is suitable for the collection of such personal information as are topics of psychosomatic and neurotic disturbances. It may be expected that several subjects dissimulate their disturbances whereas others malinger, depending on whether they are motivated or not to do military service.

To control the influence resulting from the subject's perception of some interrelation between the psychiatric screening and the military authorities, we devised the following experimental design: The instructions that subjects were given before completing the questionnaire were modified from day to day, in such a manner that the subjects had to presume different interrelationships between our research project and the military authorities. There were three types of instructions:

1. In the instructions the medical secrecy as well as the independence of the military authorities were stressed, and a written declaration of this, signed by the Research Director, was given to every subject. The subjects were asked to put their names on the questionnaires for practical reasons (confidential/not anonymous).
2. In the instructions the medical secrecy as well as the independence of the military authorities were stressed, but there was no written declaration. Subjects were asked not to put their names on the questionnaires (confidential/anonymous).
3. In the instructions there was no statement about medical secrecy or independence of military authorities. Subjects remained thus unsure about the relation between the psychiatric screening and the military authorities. Subjects were asked to put their name on the questionnaires (not confidential/not anonymous).

To measure the influence of the situation of conscription, the mean scores of the SCL-90 scales in the three experimental groups were compared. Table 27.1 shows consistently that the scores of psychiatric disturbances are highest for all scales in the condition 'written declaration of confidentiality' and lowest in the condition 'not confidential/not anonymous'. In the anonymous condition the scores of psychiatric disturbances are between the two extremes with only one exception. On the other hand an analysis of variance shows that there is no significant difference between the mean values of the scales in the three different experimental groups. This result may be summarized as follows: the more the subjects perceive a relationship between the psychiatric screening and the military authorities, the less they indicate complaints. The correlation is extremely weak so that it may be neglected for the practical purposes of our research.

Comparing the 'illness dissimulation' scores between the different experimental groups we got a similar result. The scale 'illness dissimulation' has been constructed in the line of a lie scale (Baumann *et al.* 1974). Least dissimulation was found when confidential treatment of the answers was assured, most dissimulation

TABLE 27.1

Analysis of variance with different instructions (A: written declaration of confidentiality; B: confidential/anonymous; C: not confidential, not anonymous) and Pearson correlations (r) with dissimulation of illness

SCL-90 subscales (N=1122)	Mean scores			Level of significance	eta²†	r
	A	B	C			
Somatization	1·53	1·48	1·48	N.S.	0·0028	0·26
Obsessive–compulsive	1·71	1·67	1·64	N.S.	0·0030	0·29
Interpersonal sensitivity	1·63	1·63	1·55	N.S.	0·0041	0·28
Depression	1·60	1·58	1·56	N.S.	0·0008	0·29
Anxiety	1·64	1·64	1·60	N.S.	0·0011	0·33
Anger–hostility	1·58	1·62	1·56	N.S.	0·0018	0·26
Phobic anxiety	1·29	1·28	1·24	N.S.	0·0045	0·22
Paranoid ideation	1·71	1·70	1·65	N.S.	0·0019	0·20
Psychoticism	1·48	1·46	1·46	N.S.	0·0005	0·27
Total SCL-90 distress level	1·58	1·57	1·53	N.S.	0·0025	0·32
PND scale (N = 808)						
Dissimulation of illness	9·50	9·51	9·73	N.S.	0·0042	

† eta² = correlation ratio = explained variance
N.S. = not significant

when confidential management was not mentioned. The difference is not statistically significant either, and the different experimental conditions explain less than 0·5 per cent of the variance in the scale scores.

An earlier investigation (Ruppen *et al.* 1973) showed that the situation of conscription doesn't involve serious response bias in answering very personal questions. Ruppen *et al.* compared questionnaires that had been filled out either anonymously or not anonymously and found no significant differences.

Another problem when using psychiatric self-rating questionnaires consists in conscious or unconscious tendencies of subjects to answer questions untruthfully. The reasons for such biases may be psychological factors (defences) or a conscious conformity with social norms and expectations. Table 27.1 shows correlations between the scale 'illness dissimulation' with the scales of the SCL-90. As expected, all subscales of the SCL-90 show significant negative correlations with these scales. The magnitude of the correlation coefficients between 'illness dissimulation' and psychological distress scales means that about four to ten per cent of the variance of the distress scales may be explained by the factor 'illness dissimulation'. These strong correlations make it necessary to control the factor of dissimulation in further studies. The size of the correlations between dissimulation scale and distress scales approaches very closely the values that were found in other studies (Phillips and Clancy 1970).

The reliability of previous histories

Another preliminary study was concerned with the issue of the reliability of questions about previous history that the subject has to answer about somatic and psychiatric symptoms during his youth and about social background variables. For a test of reliability we compared case records with the answers of mailed questionnaires, which were sent to the subjects.

All pupils in Zurich show up for routine medical inspections three times during school. Many of them contact the school doctor for individual consultations. Thus there is a case record for each pupil in Zurich. This allowed us to select 212 records of pupils born in 1956. The records have been analysed and coded with respect to different criteria of somatic, psychiatric, and social factors or disturbances. A mailed questionnaire was then sent to the 212 subjects of the age of twenty. In this questionnaire there were exactly the same items that we had coded when analysing the case records. We asked the subjects which of these disturbances they had suf-

fered from during school. The subjects were not informed that we were in possession of their case records from the school doctor.

In spite of two follow-up letters only 50 per cent of the subjects returned the questionnaires. There was a bias towards response from subjects with better education and less social and psychological disturbances during school time. We do not consider this bias as severe because we want to check the upper limit of reliability of our anamnestic questionnaire.

Table 27.2 shows the sensibility of the questions in the anamnestic questionnaires. Sensibility of a screening instrument means the capacity to identify a case correctly, and is defined as the ratio of correctly identified cases, over all cases according to medical records of the school doctor. Symptoms with a prevalence of less

TABLE 27.2

Sensibility of the questions in the anamnestic questionnaires

Symptoms	Sensibility per cent
Repetition of one school year	83·3
Deferred entrance into school	81·8
Subjects wearing glasses	76·2
Choleric	70·0
Special courses in logopaedics	69·2
Bad posture	66·7
Inhibited character	62·1
Attending special type school (for mental deficiency)	60·0
Gymnastics for better posture	57·1
Stay at a sanatorium	50·0
Brain concussion	47·1
Skin disease	46·2
Special training for dyslexia	42·9
Middle ear infection	41·7
Severe illness	41·2
Stay at hospital	40·0
Severe headaches	38·5
Enuresis	38·5
Heavy nervousness	38·5
Depression	36·8
Attending special type school (for behaviour disorder)	17·6
Frequent bronchitis	16·7
Frequent sleeping disturbances	5·3

than 10 per cent were excluded from the table. In general Table 27.2 shows a low sensibility, e.g. a poor correspondence between disturbances as identified by the school doctor and the answers to the anamnestic questionnaire. Table 27.2 doesn't allow us to conclude that questions about a special topic (e.g. about somatic disturbances, about neurotic disturbances, or about social behaviour) are answered more or less reliably. But there is some tendency for the more reliable items to consist to a higher degree of questions about achievement in school, physical impairment, and behaviour disorders; whereas the less reliable items consist of questions about illnesses and neurotic symptoms.

The most important conclusion resulting from this preliminary investigation is that previous history indications collected with a questionnaire have a very poor reliability. It may be that the reliability can be improved by shortening the time period for which anamnestic data are collected, e.g., only the last five years and not the whole school period as we did in our questionnaires.

An analysis of non-responders to a mailed questionnaire

In a follow-up study about drug consumption 1413 males aged 22 received a mailed questionnaire. In a previous project (on military conscription three years beforehand) all these subjects had been asked about their drug consumption, personality characteristics, and social background. Questionnaires were returned by 56·6 per cent of the sample. In another preliminary investigation we tried to find out what bias results from the fact that a large part of the sample did not respond.

The groups of responders and non-responders, respectively, were compared on the basis of the data collected in the first questionnaire. This analysis showed correlations between response tendency and social status of the parents, as well as with indicators of social marginality. A high educational and occupational status were the most important determinants for responding to the questionnaires. Social background, for example place of residence or social status of the parents, has an influence on the response tendency only via a complicated interactive relationship.

Two other factors that have a relevant influence on willingness to fill out the questionnaire are living with the parents at the age of twenty, and not smoking cigarettes. If we control for these two variables, several other correlations with indicators of social marginality (drug consumption, psychiatric treatment) and response tendency are revealed as spurious correlations.

Considering in addition the results of the personality test (Freiburger Persönlichkeits-Inventar FPI, Fahrenberg and Selg 1970) we can draw the following picture of the non-responders: they are sociable, dominant, and uninhibited, but they are less willing to answer the questions openly; according to their occupation, education, and regional origin they more often come from lower social strata; they enter into the adult world at an earlier age, which results in an earlier separation from the parents, in higher income, but also in taking over adult behaviour (e.g. smoking).

We can summarize the results of this analysis as follows: the bias that results in a prospective epidemiological investigation is not directly related to the symptoms of interest (for example drug consumption, psychiatric treatment); however, there is such a social selection among the respondents and the drop-outs, that in the long run the number of subjects with symptoms of interest decreases (Binder et al. 1979).

Summary

In this research project the occurrence and the course of minor psychiatric disturbances shall be investigated in a general population sample of 300 young men and 300 young women who will be contacted by interviewers during a period of at least four years. The project actually is in the stage of planning and pretesting. The most important research questions concern symptom change of minor psychiatric disturbances, the influence of social and psychological factors on the course of the illness, and the impairment in social functioning as a consequence of those disturbances. The results of three preliminary investigations are reported.

28. Health in progressive old age (The Netherlands)

R. J. VAN ZONNEVELD

Introduction

In 1954 the Advisory Committee on Gerontological Research of the Organization for Health Research TNO (Toegepast Natuurwetenschappelijk Onderzoek, Applied Scientific Research) in The Hague, The Netherlands, decided to organize a nation-wide study among the aged to acquire a better insight into their health status, their health problems, and a number of psychosocial variables considered relevant to the health of old people.

Prior to this, a health survey undertaken by van Zonneveld in 1954 (with the help of about 70 nearly-graduating medical students) had brought forward a number of data on the health status of the aged and the resulting needs for various types of care. This earlier survey was mainly conducted using oral answers to a structured, partly pre-coded questionnaire; in part, the results were also obtained from simple functional tests, including a memory test. The random sample was stratified according to sex and age and was comprised of 3000 people of age 65 and over in the city of Groningen, The Netherlands; this made up approximately one-

fourth of the aged population in that city. This report does not deal further with the Groningen survey (1954); details can be found in van Zonneveld (1954).

The motivation for conducting a larger nation-wide study was to get more detailed data on the health status and symptoms of disorders of old people than had been obtained in the Groningen study, in order to allow the committee a better judgement as to what kind of gerontological research, and which fields, should be encouraged and supported.

Another objective of conducting a nation-wide study was based on the hope that the results would provide a certain insight into the question of periodic physical examination of this older age group by general practitioners. The inclusion of general practitioners in scientific research was in itself considered to be of great importance: among other factors, participation in such a gerontological study might, for many of these physicians, lead to a greater interest in medical research in general and in particular in the health of the aged.

The beginning: a cross-sectional survey

In order to place the nation-wide project in the context of the longitudinal study that originated from it, a description of the cross-sectional survey is presented here. The actual investigations consisted of an extensive medical history, a physical examination of the sort that can be performed in a general practitioner's office (including some measurements and laboratory investigations), and an extensive structured interview (partly with a set of pre-defined answers) on psychological, sociological, and social issues, including a memory test. These were carried out by the general practitioner of the sample person. (In The Netherlands almost all people have a general practitioner; only those who are permanently in a hospital or a nursing home no longer have one.) The survey was conducted by R. J. van Zonneveld, M.D., Ph.D., who had experience in conducting extensive health surveys of the aged and who was the co-ordinator of gerontological research of the Organization for Health Research TNO. All the statistical problems (e.g., the questionnaire, sampling, processing, calculations, etc.) were continuously discussed with or solved both prior to and during the survey by the Statistical Department TNO.

Although the survey was not particularly geared to the mental health of the aged, a great many data were collected on this point, as can be seen from the questionnaire in the book: *The health of the aged* (1961), by R. J. van Zonneveld, which is the full report on the plan, organization, methods, results, discussion, and conclusions of the survey.

Investigators

For various reasons it was decided to commit the investigation to the aged individuals' own physicians. These physicians would inherently have a better idea of the general health of the subjects and of other circumstances involved than would any other medical investigator. The choice also fell particularly on the general practitioner because as a whole he was the most likely to have the subject's confidence. This consideration weighed heavily in relation to certain of the questions because of their confidential nature. The physicians who participated in the preparatory phase of the investigation were confirmed in this conclusion by their own experience. Further, on the basis of experience gained in other studies of the health of aged individuals, the physicians were of the opinion that superficial investigation, consisting of only a few questions and a limited physical examination, would not supply the desired data. For many reasons which will not be gone into here, they also considered unsatisfactory an arrangement by which each physician would carry out only a part of the investigation, the rest being done by special investigators, or one by which the whole study would be done by a small mobile team of physician–investigators. As previously mentioned, it was also hoped that the inclusion of the general practitioner in this study of the aged would have the effect of giving a number of them an increased interest in geriatric problems.

The aged subjects

It is self-evident that the willingness of the subjects of the investigation to let themselves be studied was essential. Various studies in this and other countries had shown that in general the reaction of this population group to being investigated was not so adverse as had sometimes been expected, but in the present case, among other factors, an actual physical examination was involved which might indeed cause some people to object. It was for this reason that it was considered so important that the individual's own physician do the examination. It was also left to the investigating physicians themselves to decide how they would approach the people who were designated as subjects. In many cases this came about on the occasion of a visit during which the doctor told his candidate something about the survey. A few investigators did this by means of a short letter. In many cases it was possible to bring up the subject during an ordinary house or office visit. Most of the aged patients were quite ready to take part, indeed they were sometimes even very anxious to do so. It was not unusual for persons who were not considered for the investigation themselves to wish to be one of the 'lucky ones'. There were, of course, aged individuals who did not wish to participate.

Since it seemed useful to inform the aged not only personally through their physicians but also more generally, the investigation was made the subject of several articles on old-age problems in publications read by many of them, as well as of a radio talk on the medical aspects of the old-age problem. In this connection it should be added that on its own initiative one of the big morning newspapers wrote about (not entirely accurately) the survey, which was by then in progress, and short pieces on it appeared in some other newspapers with large circulation.

From the above it may be clear that no special approval for this survey was obtained, but that a lot of co-operation was received from a large research organization, many officials, general practitioners, and the aged themselves. Since the general practitioner did the actual investigation, the old person benefited immediately when some abnormality was found which had to be investigated or treated further.

The subject's anonymity was protected by putting only a code number on his or her form. The code numbers were stored in such a way that no one other than the project leader, the subject's own doctor, and a few administrative personnel, who had to stick to professional secrecy, would know the names. In the report only general findings were presented, never personal details. Included in the information collected were some data on the parents of the subject (age and cause of death, state of health during life).

The longitudinal study

When the survey, which actually took place in the years 1955 through 1957, was finished, a great number of doctors who had participated in the survey, as well as Dr R. J. van Zonneveld, expressed the wish for a follow-up. The main rationale was to detect, if possible, symptoms or other variables in the beginning of the study, which could predict in a manner the quantity and quality of life after the first (or early) examinations. Another rationale was partly to find out what the reasons for certain changes were: e.g., would the decrease in height or memory test results with advancing age found in the cross-sectional study also be found in the longitudinal study? In other words, was the decrease due to selective death, to a general ageing process, or to secular changes? This new (longitudinal) study was funded by the Organization for Health Research TNO.

The same old people as in the survey, as far as they were still alive, were again interviewed and examined by the same doctors, as long as they were still in practice. Otherwise their successors, who were sometimes medical doctors of a hospital or nursing home (both for physical or mental patients), undertook the investigation.

Determination of the sample

It would have been ideal if it could have been so arranged that the investigators (the general practitioners) as well as the persons to be investigated, satisfied the requirements of a statistically reliable sample. In practice, however, this was impossible with regard to the former because participation was on a voluntary basis; this undoubtedly led to a certain amount of selection of the investigators. A connection between this selection and the actual health of the aged subjects is, however, most unlikely. Since they assumed this work voluntarily, many of the doctors could be supposed to be among the most conscientious investigators, and, should this supposition be accurate, it could only be counted to the advantage of the survey. The representativeness of the sample of the investigators can also be in part determined by analysing such factors as geographical distribution over the country, etc.

For the sake of clarity, it should be repeated that in principle the same subjects were re-examined and re-interviewed along exactly the same lines as during the first round, by the same physician–investigator. Of course, it could not be the same general practitioner in many instances, due to various reasons such as death or moving away of the doctor, or moving away of the old person to another place, etc. Thus, at the beginning 374 doctors participated; by the fifth round (until February 1970) more than 920 doctors (among them 40 specialists) were involved in this longitudinal project.

Representativeness of the subjects in the sample. On the basis of a number of calculations an attempt was made to find out whether the investigated individuals were more or less representative of the entire group of aged in The Netherlands. For each age group and sex, the distribution by provinces, the socio-economic standing, the religious affiliation, and the marital status in the sample and in the total population (the latter obtained from the Central Bureau of Statistics) were compared.

It can be said that the sample in general did indeed contain a reasonable cross-section of the aged in the population in the whole of The Netherlands for the period 1955–7. The general validity of the data is limited only by the fact that the aged in institutions, no longer treated by their own general practitioners, were not included in the survey. The percentage of aged which, according to the Central Bureau of Statistics data, lived in non-profit homes and institutions in 1956 comprised about 6 per cent of all aged persons of 65 and over. Some of these, however, were undoubtedly still treated by their own doctors, as the investigation also indicated. For the sake of completeness, it should also be said that old people are sometimes admitted to mental institutions and treated there by staff members although they remain on the lists of their own physicians. It may thus safely be assumed that at least 95 per cent of all the aged belonged to the total collective group from which the sample was chosen.

In evaluating the results it must be continually kept in mind that the age composition of the sample did not agree with that of the same group in the actual population since in the sample an attempt was made to have approximately equal age groups. The total percentages for men, for women, and for both sexes together thus apply only to the frequency in the sample. It is for this reason that as an aid to further orientation, figures are given by van Zonneveld (1961) for the lowest and highest frequency of a given factor in the various subgroups. When the percentages for a given datum in the successive age groups consistently show little mutual difference it can be assumed that in the total aged population such percentages will in all probability also be found. The percentages in each separate age group in the sample of course hold for the whole age group concerned, within the previously noted limitations.

Selection of the sample. Date and year of birth, and address were provided by municipal population registers and registers of the sick funds. There was no geographical delimitation. The subjects had ages between 65 and about 100. The delimitation of the sample subjects was determined by lot through the Statistics Department TNO. The investigator was notified by this department which numbers had been chosen by their lot. Each number represented the name of an aged individual on the doctor's list or card system. When one of the indicated subjects could not be examined for some reason, the investigator was to take the number preceding the original subject's number (where this was 1, then the last of that group). If this subject was also unavailable, the next preceding

person was to be taken. Once chosen, a subject was to be examined if at all possible. Those who had died or no longer belonged to the doctor's practice, for example because they had moved away, were self-evidently eliminated. Within reasonable limits as much persuasion as possible was to be used on those who were hesitant. In some cases the physician could drop some parts of the examination if necessary. If that was insufficient, then he was, if at all possible, to find out the reason for the refusal. It need hardly be said that the seriously ill were not to be disturbed by the examination, as well as anyone in whom the smallest unfavourable effect might be anticipated. The investigator was to wait in such cases until reasonable recovery had taken place, or try on the basis of his notes from previous contact with the patient to fill out the questionnaire as far as possible. It was expressly intended that any deaf, blind, or demented persons should be included.

After an investigator had concluded his work, he was always asked whether the subject was the originally indicated subject or whether changes had been made and, if so, what the reasons for these had been.

Loss of subjects. Of the 243 changes which became known, 38 per cent of these changes were caused by refusals, 30 per cent by death of the subject before he could be examined, 18 per cent by change of physician (e.g., through change of residence, admission to a hospital or nursing home, etc.), and 14 per cent for other causes. Only for the refusals is there a definite difference between the sexes to be found: women refused twice as often as men. It is almost self-evident that the number of changes due to death was highest for the older groups. The relatively large number of changes in the older groups due to changing physicians can be explained in terms of the more frequent necessity at that age for admission to an institution where the individual's own physician cannot continue his treatment. For the rest, the number of changes due to changing physicians was limited to ± 1·5 per cent of the subjects examined.

Because of insufficient administrative staff, particularly at the first re-examination, many old people appeared to have dropped out, as too little attention could be given to tracing subjects when they had moved. Since every person in The Netherlands has to be registered in the municipality where he lives and to give notice of his migration, had there been adequate staffing it would have been relatively easy to follow them throughout the country.

The number of refusals by the aged was very small. Most of them appreciated the continuing extra attention paid to them. Although the actual number of refusers was probably somewhat larger than appears (a few doctors reported that they had given up participating in the study after having from the very beginning failed to interest subjects), the number of known refusers was limited to 3 per cent of the sample, which can be called encouragingly small.

In general it can be said that the subjects remained very co-operative, as only a few per cent were lost through refusal at each assessment. The low refusal rate can largely be explained by the fact that the subjects were contacted and informed personally by their own family doctor, and the extra interview and examination by him provided more information on the physical, mental, and social conditions of the old person, thus often leading to better treatment and a better patient–doctor relationship. As in the great majority of cases the doctors preferred to examine the subjects in their own offices, free transportation between home and office was offered to those old people who were in need of this.

The loss of subjects by death was far greater: of the original 3174 subjects, during the first five years 1005 died, between five and eight years 406 had died, and between eight and eleven years 279, totalling 1690 in the first eleven years. Through various calculations it became known that 152 deaths were not reported, so that after eleven years no more than 1307 subjects, at most, could participate. Because of obvious reasons (the aim being to follow up only those who had been investigated in the initial round) there was no replacement of the drop-outs.

In longitudinal studies of particularly old people there exists, of course, a strong bias, as the remaining persons (those who did not die in the meantime) become more and more a selected group (in a way: survival of the fittest). There is no reason why those old people investigated after 11 years should be different from old people of the same ages in the total population, unless one assumes that the first group had a more thorough medical follow-up. From other data of this longitudinal study, however, it appears that in general in The Netherlands very many old people are seen rather often by their general practitioners.

A total of about 2·5 per cent of the original subjects dropped out because of death even before they could be examined for the first time, since there could be an interval of up to $2\frac{1}{2}$ years between the ascertainment of the original sample and the actual investigation. In The Netherlands about 55 000 people over 65 died annually around 1956, i.e., ± 6 per cent of all the aged. The reported percentage, which indicates mortality in a period of more than two years and pertains to a sample which is older than the average for the actual population of the aged, is thus appreciably lower than that for the population at large. This can probably be ascribed largely to the selective effect already remarked on of excluding aged people no longer treated by their own general practitioners (patients in many types of institutions).

At the time (the 1950s) there did not exist registers on physical and mental health (or morbidity), criminality, and suicide among the aged in The Netherlands. However, general data on mortality causes were obtainable because death certificates with the cause indication legally have to be sent by the medical doctor who confirms death to the medical doctor of the Central Bureau of Statistics (CBS). In case the latter has doubts about the death cause he checks it with the doctor who filled in the certificate. It is stated that the accuracy of this system is very good. In principle it is impossible for an outsider to get information on the death cause of a certain person from the CBS. Rarely such data are given in case of a scientific study, but then the Chief Inspector of Public Health (the Chief Medical Officer) has to ask permission from each medical practitioner for each given case.

An attempt was also made in the beginning to match the causes of death of persons deceased between two successive rounds of re-examination. Although the assistance of the Central Bureau of Statistics, which collects the death certificates, the Medical Chief Inspectorate of Public Health, and the approval of most doctors to disclose the cause of death, were obtained, the work was so elaborate and complicated that the lack of sufficient administrative staff again forced us, after several hundreds of death certificates had been collected, to stop this part of the suvey. The rationale had been to see whether and which of the diseases at later age finally led to death. (Of course it is often very difficult to assess the actual cause of death in very old people.)

Although a great many persons were 'lost' particularly in the first five years, it appeared after a statistical evaluation that drop-outs (not those because of death) did not differ significantly in various respects from those who were still in the survey. So it was possible to follow up a rather great deal of the orginal sample, although sometimes subjects dropped out during one or two rounds but could later be picked up again.

From the above it may become clear that this longitudinal survey met with an enormous amount of difficulties, but as far as is known to me, it is still the only nation-wide longitudinal survey on health and psychosocial variables in people of 65 and over.

Information on mental state

Concerning the mental state, attention was given to the way time was spent, the degree of adjustment to old age, to feelings about being old, the place of the old person in society, and to a memory test. Since it did not seem proper here to use the choice of one of several indicated answers, in relevant instances the answer as given by the subject was to be noted. The questions concerning how time was spent had to do with the reading of newspapers, magazines, and books, listening to the radio, attending various sorts of performances, how Sundays were spent as well as vacations, holidays, and 'free time', whether the individual was still busy with a profession or hobby, his contact with family, friends, and acquaintances, and feelings of boredom and loneliness. In the section concerned with adjustment, the physician attempted to find out a little more about how the subject reacted to circumstances arising from old age, such as the death of the spouse, the childrens' leaving home, deterioration of health, and retirement. By means of a few questions, an attempt was also made to perceive the feelings harboured by the subject in relation to his advanced age, his idea of his place in society, and what expectations he had of the future.

The memory test. To get an insight into the memory function, as a part of intelligence, a number of questions from the Wechsler Memory Scale were used. Among them there are questions about personal orientation, general orientation, and orientation of time and place; there is a request to say the alphabet, to do a little arithmetic problem, and to do a simple financial problem; finally, there is a test for visual and auditory memory. The evaluation of the marks obtained had to be made differently from the one used by Wechsler.

Re-examinations. The re-examinations took place about 5, 8, 11, 14, 16, and 17 years later, after the period 1955 to 1957, thus in 1960–2, 1962–5, 1966–8, 1969–71, 1971–3, and in 1974. The re-examination in 1974 was the last one, but with a shortened questionnaire and procedure. When the doctors could not spend as much time as in the first examination, a short questionnaire and a small actual examination procedure were used.

Technical details

The data collected on structured and mostly pre-coded questionnaires were partly coded by the doctors themselves, and partly by administrative personnel; the coding was controlled by the two medical doctors (the project leader and a collaborator, Dr A. Beek). Afterwards they were put on punch cards, for storing later during a certain time on tape and then back on new punch cards. The subjects can always be identified for purposes of follow-up.

Several data analyses have been completed with the help of computers. Special attention was given to comparisons of data from the first and second rounds (interval of five years) and to a great many data from each of the first four rounds (intervals of 5, 3, and 3 years).

The data which were coded and put on punch cards were processed by computers according to the wishes of the original leader of the project, Dr R. J. van Zonneveld, and another medical doctor with experience in surveys, Dr A. Beek. In continuous co-operation with van Zonneveld, Dr Beek undertook the very laborious task of working further on the results produced by the computer and writing the concept of the report on the first eleven years, i.e., the results of four successive rounds of examinations. For some chapters the help of a statistician and another medical doctor could also be obtained. The whole concept was reviewed and complemented by Dr A. Beek and Dr R. J. van Zonneveld. The report of the longitudinal study of the first eleven years was published by Gezondheidsorganisatie TNO) in 1976 under the title: *De gezondheid in de voortschrijdende ouderdom* [*Health in progressive old age*]. It contains a rather extensive summary in English. (Copies are obtainable free of charge from Dr R. J. van Zonneveld, Director, Postbus 297, 2501 BD The Hague, The Netherlands.) Articles on partial findings of this longitudinal study have also been published in several Dutch and international journals or proceedings of international congresses.

The data on the fifth, sixth, and seventh rounds have been coded, punched, and for computing purposes, have been transferred to tape; at the moment, the data are in the process of being computerized, according to a number of wishes and to the possibilities of the material.

The writing of the report in which comparisons will be made, also with regard to the so-called longevity quotient, will start in the latter part of 1979. This report will then contain data on a small number of old people followed up (by interview and examination) over a period of about 17 years. These data, in part, will also give information on the mental condition of old people.

The longitudinal study was funded from 1954 through 1975 by the Organization for Health Research TNO, a semi-governmental research organization; for the statistical process now (1977) being undertaken, a grant has been obtained by the Prevention Fund, a fund which receives its income from health insurance sick funds and laws.

Special problems encountered

In the foregoing several difficulties have already been mentioned. A few may be repeated or added here, including both realized and potential ones:

1. *Funding* was in general not a great problem. The costs for direction, administration, statistical analysis, and publication, were paid out of a grant from the Netherlands Organization for Applied Scientific Research TNO, under whose auspices the study was performed. The actual investigators, the general practitioners, decided that in spite of the many hours (up to 40) they had to spend in examing the elderly, they would do this for free. There was the added advantage that population registers of municipalities and patient registers of sick funds provided names, birth dates, and addresses of subjects without costs. Only at the last stage, the statistical analysis of data from the seventh round, was the organization mentioned above unable to pay for the costs; then the Prevention Fund was willing to provide a grant. Moreover, during the last years of analysis and reporting the project leader did not receive any remuneration.

2. The *following of subjects* is, in principle, not difficult in The Netherlands as everybody has to be registered in the municipality where he lives, and can be traced each time he moves more permanently to another municipality. Yet a small number of subjects was lost, because sometimes after a few years the examining doctor no longer knew whom he had examined, or the subject had another doctor (in consequence of removal or for other reasons) who was not willing to co-operate in this study. Also, inaccurate information caused some losses.

3. *Staffing.* A major lesson to be learned from this longitudinal study was the underestimation of administrative staff needed for good administration. Particularly in the beginning it gradually appeared that much more time was needed for this work, and thus many subjects were not examined in time or at all. The situation could partly be improved later by having additional competent personnel, and by examining drop-outs in a later round.

4. Another problem was the fact that the collaborating *doctors had less time available* in later rounds, so that some of them could only fill out small forms. Loss of subjects and the frequent unavailability of the doctors (who were also getting older!) resulted in only 108 subjects, of various ages, being followed up in the very extensive way over the course of 17 years.

5. *Data analysis.* Particularly in the beginning, the analysis of complex data obtained at successive times (longitudinally) appeared to be very difficult, since at that time sophisticated methods were not yet developed. To some extent this is still the case.

6. The *co-operation of the subjects* themselves was in general quite good, as has already been stated. (Some of them did drop out, out of their own free will.)

7. Co-operation with *national or local administrative units* was in general very good.

A short review of changes in psychosocial variables in progressing age

In the following a number of results with respect to psychological variables and mental status from the longitudinal study of old people will be briefly mentioned. However, in general this study was not set up to contribute to the early detection of mental health problems.

Most of the following data are given with regard to the so-called longevity quotient (LQ), which is the ratio (formulated on statistical grounds) between the expected lifespan on a certain date and the actual age reached (Palmore 1969). The influence of the factors investigated could in this way be approached in a more refined manner.

Living independently. Although this situation is influenced by a host of factors, the mental condition of the person is also involved. In the first investigation it appeared that after the 74th year, more than half of the aged no longer live independently. Women gave up their independence sooner than men did, but in many cases they changed their minds.

Opinion on health. From the relation to lifespan it appeared that the opinion of the general practitioners concerning the health of the aged person was better founded than that of the aged person him/herself.

Activities of daily life. As expected, disturbances in the ADL (activities of daily life)-functions had a strongly unfavourable influence on the LQ, and this was also the case with disturbances in domestic management and in management of money.

Memory test. The results of the memory test showed cross-sectionally as well as longitudinally a steady decrease of scores with increases in age. This deterioration of the memory was significantly greater when the life duration of the testees appeared to be shorter. Almost none of the physical characteristics investigated by us showed such a clear connection with longevity as the here-mentioned component of psychical life (memory).

Other factors. In agreement with expectations, the aged who were still, more or less, working reached a higher mean age than those who were not.

Interest in newspapers appeared to have, as contrary to interest in the radio, a favourable correlation with the LQ. The percentages of women reading the newspaper regularly were lower and dropped more rapidly than those of the men; the cause of this difference probably is of a secular nature.

Although feelings of loneliness and/or withdrawal had the expected unfavourable correlation with the lifespan, a non-optimal contact with children appeared to be of no great importance. One would expect that the women who in the fourth round were still doing some (usually domestic) chores were less bored than the men who did not; however, the reverse proved to be true.

An overview of the relation between a number of psychosocial variables and the longevity quotient is given in Table 28.1.

Provisions for health care

The opinion of practitioners about the needed facilities for the aged appears to have changed considerably in the course of the last decades, due to increasing interest in the aged. In the period from 1960 to 1964 twice as many practitioners have insisted on more

TABLE 28.1

Relation between a number of variables of a psychosocial nature and the Longevity Quotient (LQ)

Variable	LQ for sex and age groups							
	M 65–74 years		M ≥ 75 years		F 65–74 years		F ≥ 75 years	
Still working	*0·98*		*1·09*		*0·93*		*1·00*	
No longer working		*0·77*		*0·86*		*0·67*		*0·79*
Being bored never or sometimes	*0·92*		*0·98*		*0·91*		0·93	
Being bored often		*0·59*		*0·67*		*0·56*		0·81
Reading newspaper daily	*0·92*		*0·98*		0·91		*0·97*	
Reading newspaper never or occasionally		*0·71*		*0·84*		0·83		*0·79*
Listening to radio often	0·89		*0·98*		0·90		0·93	
Listening to radio never or occasionally		1·00		0·83		0·80		0·84
Not being withdrawn, not lonely	*0·92*		*1·00*		*0·92*		*0·96*	
Being withdrawn, lonely		*0·78*		*0·79*		*0·79*		*0·79*
Contacts with children good	0·92		0·97		0·89		0·92	
Contacts with children not very good or non-existing		0·92		0·89		0·79		0·89

Significant results ($P < 0.05$) are in italics.

facilities for intramural assistance than practitioners who did so for extramural help; in the period 1968 to 1972 the proportion was the same. In the first-mentioned period there was a greater demand for nursing homes than for residential homes; in the second period the reverse was the case. There was a demand for more facilities for acutely decompensated aged persons living independently.

The many wished-for improvements mentioned by the practitioners include: more possibilities for convalescence, social stimulation, job provision, periodic check-ups, and more trained auxiliary staff.

Advantages of longitudinal research

Many physiological or pathological processes of ageing can only be analysed and understood through very complicated and time-consuming longitudinal studies. The study described here was able to contribute somewhat to alleviating the problem of how to predict certain diseases, abnormalities, and death at later ages. A striking example is that the results of the memory test were the best predictors of longevity.

From the original survey population a select group of 'long-living' persons was selected. This group was comprised of those persons from the original age group of 65 to 75 who were still alive after eleven years, and with whom the survey could be repeated three times using the full questionnaire. There were 56 men and 52 women in this group. This subsample came closest to the ideal of a longitudinal survey; the changes over the years of a great number of variables could be followed up.

As has been stated before, the purpose of this research is partly to predict aspects of physical, mental, and social well-being in very old age. The aim is also to follow up the changes (or non-changes) of a number of measurable variables, including a memory test. There is no doubt that only longitudinal studies can help in providing certain data on changes during the *process* of ageing.

Conclusions

At present Dr R. J. van Zonneveld, as an individual, is responsible for the project. Data from the study are being used in postgraduate and undergraduate teaching of gerontology. Whether or not there is an impact on public health is difficult to say; certainly the effect is not a direct one.

Data from other European studies show that it would be very useful to have groups working to establish cross-national reliability of future findings and maximum exploitation of already available data.

29. The Bonn longitudinal study of ageing—an approach to differential gerontology (F.R.G.)

HANS THOMAE

Introduction

The planning and design of the Bonn Longitudinal Study on Ageing (BLSA) was determined to a great degree by findings which pointed to the increasing interindividual variability of biological, social, and psychological processes in older age. Several outstanding approaches to the study of human development in late life pointed to 'very large individual differences in intellectual perfor-

mance among older persons' (Birren *et al.* 1972) and to different 'life styles' (Reichard *et al.* 1962; William and Wirths 1965; Maas and Kuypers 1974; Havighurst 1975). Cross-sectional studies like that of Birren and Morrison (1961), Granick and Friedman (1967), Green (1969), and Rudinger (1974) pointed to differences in mental consistency and decline between persons from different educational backgrounds. Due to the great impact of education many cross-sectional findings on mental decline are misleading as educational opportunities were worse for the cohort born between 1870 and 1900 than for those born in the period 1930–60.

Cross-sectional as well as longitudinal studies point to health as a determinant of differences in mental and personality development (Birren *et al.* 1963a; Spieth 1964; Lehr *et al.* 1972; Rudinger 1974). The assessment of this interindividual variation in biological and psychological findings became one of the main issues in longitudinal studies like the Duke Study (Beek *et al.* 1968; Palmore 1974a, b) and the Bonn Longitudinal Study of Ageing (Thomae 1976).

Longitudinal studies were criticized because of the increasingly selective and biased character of their samples. However, they can be defended against their critics if they are focused on differential aspects of ageing rather than on normative aspects. They can demonstrate interindividual variability in ageing and some of the conditions of this variability. From this point of view they are instruments of prediction as well as control of certain 'styles' or 'patterns' of ageing.

General hypothesis and strategy

The general hypothesis for the design of BLSA refers to the complex character of the conditons which determine this interindividual variability. Therefore the design was oriented more along the lines of 'global' longitudinal studies which require the inclusion of a great number of variables as opposed to studies which are focused on a limited number of hypotheses and can concentrate on one to three variables (e.g. Owens 1966). However, our preference for the more global type of longitudinal study is not only based on the expectation that ageing is an extremely complex process which differs under various biological, social, biographical, and person-specific conditions. The history of the great longitudinal studies on children, which were started in the United States in the late-1920s or early-1930s shows that some of the most valuable results of these studies emerged from hypotheses or theories which became relevant many years after the studies were started. When the Child Guidance Study (McFarlane 1938) began in 1928, nobody cared about 'coping styles' or 'central orientations'. However Bronson (1966) was able to analyse the data collected in that study from 1928 to 1942 in terms of these constructs, which had become important aspects of developmental theory since the late-1950s. She also could order early childhood data from 1928–36 along a dimension of 'expressive–outgoing versus reserved–withdrawn' defined by her in 1966, and correlate these data with interview data from the same subjects as adults (Bronson, 1967).

The very detailed analysis of the interviews with the mothers of the children of the Guidance Study provided by McFarlane (1938) enabled Honzik (1967) to interpret her findings on early childhood environmental correlates of mental growth until 30 years, in terms of constructs defined 35 years after the beginning of the Guidance Study.

The careful registration of observational data on the children of the Fels Longitudinal Study enabled Moss and Kagan (1964) to have these data rated approximately 30 years later and to correlate them with ratings of interviews with the same subjects when they were adults. In fact, the most important aspect of this study rests on the definition of these rating scales which reflect the status of psychological theory between 1945 and 1960 rather than that of 1928.

As we keep our records available for future analysis we expect that they too will provide material for testing hypotheses which today are unknown. In any case, we tried very hard to plan the study in a way which would offer data for different kinds of theories and approaches. On the other hand, the study had to have several restrictions in order to be practicable. As we included a fairly extensive psychological testing programme, we had to limit the medical programme owing to financial as well as psychological reasons. However, a general health rating of each subject was made at each measurement point (m.p.) by a specialist of internal medicine. Furthermore all survivors at the fifth m.p. (1972) had the most important tests in the University Hospital for internal medicine.

A second limitation refers to the assessment of learning and social conditions preceding transition into old age: they could be assessed only by interviewing the subjects themselves. Therefore, our findings are related to the reported socialization history rather than the 'real' one. Our findings will have to be checked by the few studies which exist so far related to longer age ranges (for instance Owens 1966; Maas and Kuypers 1974; Palmore 1974a, b).

It was decided to take time enough to assess the physical, psychological, economic, and social situation of the subjects as it was perceived at each of the measurement points. We tried to pay attention to the time perspective of this situation. Therefore, at each of the measurement points we devoted one 3-hour interview to the assessment of 'present situation', one interview (between 2–4 h) to that of the past, and a third one to the assessment of the future outlook. Each interview was tape-recorded and as the tapes are still available it will be possible to use our data for future evaluations and hypothesis testing in the same way as has been done with the very extensive records of the longitudinal studies of children and adolescents in Berkeley (Bronson 1967; Baumrind 1966) and in Yellow Springs (Kagan and Moss 1962).

The schedule of our procedures at each of the first four measurement points (see below) demonstrates that we assigned the major part of the week during which our subjects were available to interviews. This decision can be explained firstly by methodological preferences which can be traced in the Berkeley studies (Jones 1958) in the same way as in ours. In our case this decision can be further supported by theoretical considerations which were formulated in terms of a cognitive theory of personality (Thomae 1968a), or of ageing (Thomae 1970) which places special emphasis on the nature of behaviour as a dependent variable of the situation as perceived by the individual. As our subjects were well motivated to co-operate in our study their responses in the interviews can be regarded as rather valid ones to their perceptions of present, past, and future life situation. On the other hand, we applied intelligence and personality tests to get information as objective as possible on their psychological situation. As cognitive and motivational aspects of behaviour are interrelated to each other in a very complex manner, it was decided to introduce as many variables as possible in order to be able to identify different patterns of ageing and the cognitive, motivational, social, and biological correlates of these patterns.

The design of the study was influenced by the author's experience gathered as psychological director of the German Longitudinal Study on children (Coerper *et al.* 1954; Hagen and Thomae 1962) and by longitudinal studies on middle-aged white collar employees (Lehr and Thomae 1958) as well as on a sample of men and women born 1885–1930 (Lehr and Thomae 1965; Lehr 1969). The final design was discussed with many colleagues from Bonn and other universities.

Master plan and measurement points

The planning of the study goes back to the years 1962–3. The pretests and the sampling started in 1964. So far we have been able to test and interview our subjects at six measurement points (m.p.):

m.p. (I): 1 April 1965 – 31 March 1966
m.p. (II): 1 April 1967 – 31 March 1968

m.p. (III): 1 April 1968 – 31 March 1969
m.p. (IV): 1 April 1969 – 31 March 1970
m.p. (V): 1 September 1972 – 31 July 1973
m.p. (VI): 1 September 1976 – 15 July 1977

In twelve years the sample was reduced by about 58 per cent of the original number of 220 subjects.

Sample and sampling procedures

Most longitudinal studies on aged persons use volunteers who are motivated by organizations or agencies (Birren *et al.* 1963b; p. 7) or by their co-operative attitude toward friends, colleagues, or relatives who ask them to participate (snowball technique, Palmore 1970; p. 4; see also Stone and Norris 1966; p. 575).

We tried very hard to draw a random sample of the western part of Western Germany (Ruhr area, Cologne, Bonn and suburbs, Frankfurt, Mannheim, Heidelberg) for our study. However, in the same way as many previous researchers we faced many difficulties in doing so. Sampling procedures for a two-hour interview are a completely different matter compared to a complex psychological and medical examination which requires travel to and attendance at a university institute for a whole week.

Therefore we completed our random sample with referrals from welfare organizations and industrial plants to whom we explained our aims and plans. We required that persons participating should be in good health and live in their own household. The subjects we included had to be able to travel to Bonn by train and stay in a small hotel near the institute, or, for those in the Bonn area, reach the institute every day using public transportation. At the last measurement point some subjects were brought by taxi. Another selection requirement was lower middle class or (to a small percentage) middle middle class status. We tried also to control the sample for religious background and place of birth (Western Germany versus former German provinces which belong now to Russia, Poland, and Czechoslavakia).

The original sample consisted of 118 men and 104 women which is not representative for our population. The smaller number of women included is to be explained by the greater anxiety of elderly women at undergoing psychological or medical testing. At the fifth measurement point there were 64 men and 56 women left. Most of the women were housewives; some of them had never worked outside their own household. White collar employees of the medium and lower ranks, civil servants, and skilled workers were the occupations of the majority of the original as well as the longitudinal sample. The marital status distribution is typical for the older generation. Most participants were married, especially the men. A greater number of women were single or widowed.

A major decision had to be made regarding the age cohort. In order to analyse possible effects of retirement one-half (approximately 110) of our subjects (59 men, 51 women) were looking forward to retirement or had retired no more than 2 years before the first point of measurement. A second cohort consisted mainly of persons who had retired 3 to 12 years before our study started.

This resulted in a design which included 4 groups of men and women of lower middle class status:

(1) Men born 1900–5;
(2) Women born 1900–5;
(3) Men born 1890–5;
(4) Women born 1890–5.

This design made it possible to combine longitudinal and cross-sectional comparisons. The two cohorts did not differ regarding socio-economic status, and health differences were confined to the group of older women at the beginning of the study. However, the biography of the older cohort during childhood and adolescence was characterized by the experience of peace and security, although they very often reported great economic need and few opportunities for better education or occupational training. The adulthood of the older men was influenced by military service during the First World War whereas the older women very often either had lost their first husband or fiancé in this war or were separated from their husbands for years. Very often they reported great economic difficulties and even starvation at this time.

Only very few of the 'younger' men were soldiers in the First World War (for the last year). Most of them were adolescents during this war and had to work quite hard to help support their families. A time remembered by both groups in the same intense and negative manner was around 1930 when there was widespread unemployment in Germany.

During the time between 1933 and 1945 most of our older subjects did not favour the Hitler regime. One survived many years in a concentration camp, others belonged to Christian groups in the silent opposition, and only a few apparently were supporters of the regime. On the other hand, the group born 1900–5 included at least one member of the SS-troop and several active party members as well as quite a few supporters of the regime. Most of the younger groups were in the German Army in the Second World War and most of them reported their experiences as prisoners of war. From these data a cross-sectional comparison of our cohorts is reasonable, although the main emphasis of our study was on the longitudinal analysis.

Overview of measured variables

One set of variables which was assessed was related to social conditions existing immediately before the interview. Aside from careful assessment of the socio-economic situation we used the interview schedules of the cross-national study on adjustment to retirement (Havighurst and DeVries 1969) to assess the degree and quality of social participation of our subjects. This schedule was supplemented by inventories related to leisure time activities, etc.

A second set of information to be gathered was related to the past. We collected data on the life history from childhood up to the time of marriage and/or end of training for a job and inquired systematically about the time during and after the Second World War in which most of the 'younger' men (born 1900–5) had to participate as soldiers. Using the time of the West German currency reform in 1948 as a reference point made it very easy to elicit quite detailed reports on the situation as it existed at the time regarding income, job, housing conditions, health, and family. The interviewers tried not only to cover the situation as it was experienced. They asked in a detailed way for descriptions of how our subjects coped with different aspects of the situation.

The same procedure was followed for the reference times 1955 (i.e. 10 years before the first interview), 1965, 1966, 1968, 1970, and 1972. These reference points in time made it possible for most subjects to remember a very stressful situation and the ways they coped with it. Our data on perceived stress during these years from 1948–72 point to a continuous decrease which resulted in a decrease of information regarding the ways to cope with problems. However this whole section will receive special attention in the future evaluation of our data.

A third set of data was related to plans for the year following the interview and in the more distant future. From a complex set of items we tried to rate extension and quality of future time perspective, attitudes toward health and death, etc.

Our test data included the HAWIE (German standardization of WAIS) in the 1·, 3·, 4·, and 5· m.p.s; the Raven Progressive Matrices in the second and fifth years. These tests are used in most studies on ageing, but tests for checking psychomotor performance at high speed are less frequently used. We applied the Mierke apparatus (or Kieler Determinationsgerät) in which subjects have to react to irregular patterns of coloured flashes and of sounds with increasing speed (see Mathey 1968). Two other tests to measure psychomotor adjustment were used only in the first and last years of the study: A Pursuit Rotor learning task and the Beck apparatus. Projective techniques, used especially during the first years, were the Rorschach and Behn–Rorschach, Wunsch-Probe ('Wishtest' according to Wilde).

Since questionnaires adapted for aged persons from the lower middle class were not available at the time of the beginning of our study we used the Riegel Inventories (Riegel and Riegel 1960) which had been developed with an aged population in Northern Germany in the late 1950s. They try to assess several aspects of attitudinal rigidity, dogmatism, and attitudes toward present and future time. Data on health and standard medical data (blood pressure, vital capacity, reflexes, etc.) were recorded at each m.p. in a standardized situation. In the last year, a half-day clinical check-up was added.

Selective findings

Cognitive functioning

The performance scores of the Wechsler Intelligence Tests pointed to improvement until m.p. (IV) in the 'younger' cohort and to a continuous decline until m.p. (V) in the older group. For the whole sample, therefore, the time effect shows no significance in the analysis of variance done by Rudinger (1976). In verbal scores there was a two-point decline from m.p. (I)(51·5) to m.p. (IV) (49·6). However this time effect explained only 1 per cent of the total variance, whereas education accounted for 20 per cent of the variance in the Wechsler results. The cognitive performances of persons in better SES conditions remained better than that of persons with lower SES throughout the time.

Whereas the intelligence measures of men were clearly superior to those of women at the beginning of the study the scores of men decreased whereas those of women held or even improved. This may be explained by the stimulating effect of our study programme especially for many of the single or widowed women.

Psychomotor performance and reaction speed

Psychomotor or sensor motor performance of our subjects was measured by the Kieler Determinationsgerät at all m.p.s by Mathey (1976). The experimental task required an immediate reaction to various optical and auditory stimuli presented at varying speeds. The analysis of the data from the years 1965–72 pointed to significant differences in the performance on this task between the cohorts and sexes. It demonstrated, too, an increase in the number of trials necessary to reach the criterion from the first to the fifth m.p. However, even more striking was the increase in the interindividual variability from the younger to the older cohorts. From m.p. (I) to m.p. (V) the level of performance in the multiple reaction task was significantly correlated with health as assessed by the clinician. While this was true for m.p. (I–V), correlations between psychomotor performance and SES were significant only at the beginning of the study.

Summarizing his analysis Mathey concluded that psychomotor or sensory motor age, 'largely a matter of vitally important flexibility, activity, and general performance tendencies, is different from chronological age' (Mathey 1976; p. 49).

Formal aspects of behaviour

Computing approximating 38 variables measured from m.p. (I)–m.p. (V) related to personality, SES, health, intelligence, etc. Grombach (1976) found that time (7 years) could account for about 1 per cent of the total variance in the behavioral ratings

whereas education and SES proved to be the more relevant variables. Better health and education were correlated with higher activity and adjustment.

Focusing on questionnaire data regarding rigidity, attitude toward others and toward the future, Angleitner (1976) found that rigidity scores were decreasing rather than increasing from m.p. (I) to m.p. (V). Only in the scale of personality rigidity was there an increase during this time, which suggests that items stated in the first person and relating to concrete situations (by asking what actions the subject would take personally) are more endorsed over a 7-year period (Angleitner 1976; p. 78). As many of the items for personal rigidity refer to attitudes, e.g. toward skyscrapers as compared to homes with gardens, or to an unfamiliar dish, it would be wrong to over-emphasize this finding. In any case, it was shown that different aspects of rigidity may change in a different way.

Perceived life space

According to cognitive theories of personality, the situation as perceived rather than the situation itself will control human behaviour. From the many measures we took to assess the perceived life space of our subjects, Fisseni (1976) analysed patterns of consistency and change of extension of life space (especially future time perspective), perceived stress and conflict, and life satisfaction.

Good health was associated with a pattern of consistent high scores of extended life space; poor health was related to restricted life space. Similar relationships existed regarding SES. Regarding perceived stress there was a striking sex difference. One group of men showed declining scores for stress perception from m.p. (I)–(II) and from (IV)–(V), but consistently increasing scores from (II)–(III) and (III)–(IV). On the other hand a group of women reported consistently low scores for perceived stress. Generally in the women's group there was a tendency towards steadying the pattern of not complaining, whereas among men on the whole this pattern fades away. The differences between objective and perceived stress as predicted by a cognitive theory of ageing can be observed especially regarding health, which was one of the areas for possible stress perceptions. One group of our subjects was in poor health at most of the m.p.s, but did not perceive stress in health, family, or housing situation. Another group was of poor health, but was worried only about housing problems, not about health. A third group described as being in good health, was yet worried about health and family life.

Patterns of coping

Within the interview on the life history and on the economic, housing, family, and health problems as existing at each of the m.p.s we also tried to get reports on how our subjects tried to cope with these situations. From our pretests we developed a list of 15 reaction patterns. The staff members rated the information on the reactions to reported problem situations on a 7-point scale. Conference ratings as well as control ratings by two to five raters were made resulting in an 85 per cent rater agreement.

At the first m.p. we asked our subjects not only about problems existing at the present situation but also about the way they experienced the end of the Second World War, and especially the currency reform in 1948, by which almost everybody lost his savings. As this time was recalled in a very detailed way we could use this situation as a source for the classification of the adjustment patterns.

The rank order correlation between the adjustment patterns reported for 1948 and 1965 is not significant. The difference in the structure of overall adjustment to the situation is explained especially by differences in the rating scores for four adjustment patterns. Adjustment to the institutional aspects of the situation, i.e. adjustment by applying to the employment office, the former employer, the trade union, or local authorities, was most important for getting or keeping a job in 1948. It was not so important in 1965 when half of these men were retired, and problems in this area usually had to do with getting the highest possible pension or finding a post-retirement job.

Another major technique or adjustment pattern to a situation with very poor occupational opportunities (and a high degree of economic disorder) is using whatever chance is offered to get a job (i.e., using chance opportunities). This involves looking around for jobs, keeping good contacts with people who know something, and motivation as well as flexibility to accept whatever is offered. It can be understood very easily that this adjustment pattern was not relevant in the occupational situation for men around or past retirement age in an affluent society with (relatively) high pensions. On the other hand, in 1948 these men (about 45 years of age) did not react in an evasive manner to the occupational situation, and they could not solve the problem by identifying with the aims and successes of their children or grandchildren.

During the years in which we observed our subjects their economic situation as well as housing conditions improved. Also the problems related to family generally were not as serious as in the years after the war when the old parents waited for their sons to return from prisoner of war camps in Russia or elsewhere. Therefore the opportunity to gather information on reactions to problem situations decreased. One of the most important forms in which our aged persons reacted to failure or shortcomings in the economic or housing situation was some kind of 'identification with the achievements and aims of children'.

Many of our low-income subjects told us, after they reported their economic situation: 'Well, I myself had poor luck, but my son (grandson, daughter, etc.) made it'. Their offsprings' success was experienced as their own success. Even if the situation of the children or grandchildren was not extremely good, it could be perceived in a manner which provided satisfaction or helped in coping with feelings of dissatisfaction regarding the economic and/or occupational situation. Some of these reactions may be combined with cognitive distortions, but for many of our subjects the economic and occupational status of their offspring was not only a monetary asset but even more an aid in the cognitive restructuring of their own situation, especially regarding economic aspects.

This process of restoring the emotional or cognitive balance, e.g. in light of discrepancies between desires and achieved goals, by identification with the status of offspring, is one example of a group of techniques which can be defined as techniques of 'cognitive restructuring'. This cognitive restructuring of the situation is one of the main instruments for restoring an internal balance in aged persons who very often are faced with situations which can be changed in the way they are perceived, but not in reality. Besides identification with offsprings' status we could observe three other forms in our subjects:

(a) Positive interpretation of events (e.g. 'I am quite fine, if you compare my lot with that of poor Mr X'.);
(b) Revision of own expectations (e.g., 'Well, as long as you are young you believe you must get everything, but when you get older you learn to enjoy whatever you have.');
(c) Acceptance of the situation as it is (e.g., 'Well, it could have been worse'. or 'Who knows what this will be good for?').

It is quite evident that this type of problem-solving differs entirely from achievement-oriented behaviour, which always involves some change in the external world.

There are some similarities between cognitive restructuring and adjustment to the needs and habits of others (e.g., paying compliments, not talking too loud at home because of conflict with some neighbours). However, adjustment always remains an active effort which maintains a given goal whereas cognitive restructuring more often is related to situations which require resignation or insight into the unchangeable character of the situation. On the other hand, cognitive restructuring is not identical with passive reaction, mood of general resignation, depressive reaction, or evasive behaviour. Whereas these reactions preserve the unbalanced situation, cognitive restructuring has the aim of restoring balance. This group of techniques or problem-solving devices certainly differs from a fifth group which includes different forms of assertive behaviour like resistance to socially required demands or appealing to the next higher authority (e.g., regarding pension).

Preliminary data available so far concerning consistency and change of these five strategies for problem-solving of the economic and occupational situation, point to decreasing scores for achievement-orientated behaviour are at the mean point of the rating tency in scores from the first to the fifth measurement point. Whereas these trends were similar in all groups, mean scores for men are always higher by 1–1·5 points.

This finding has to be interpreted with reference to the decrease in economic problems from 1948–65 and the consolidation of this situation during the following years. Whereas mean scores for achievement-oriented behaviour are at the mean point of the rating scales, they drop to 3–3·8 in men and to 1–2 in women. This finding means that achievement-orientated behaviour can still contribute very much to economic balance in old age but far less than before. However, this kind of strategy is consistently more observed than all of the remaining strategies combined. This identifies our sample as a group of aged men and women who react to their problems in a rather active way. This statement is supported by the variability of scores for adjustment in its different forms. Mean scores centre around 2·5 in the four age/sex groups in 1948 and around 1·0 between m.p. (I) and m.p. (V).

The trends for cognitive restructuring of the situation differ in the sex groups: In both men's groups there is an increase from 1948–72 (from 0·9–1·6). This would confirm our expectation that cognitive restructuring of the situation will become a major strategy for problem-solving in situations which cannot be changed by one's own effort. However, we have to mention a sex difference: In women scores are rather consistent from 1948 to 1965 (0·8–1·0 in the older and 1·7–1·9 in the younger age group) and decreased from m.p. (I) to m.p. (V).

On the other hand we observed an increase in assertive behaviour from 1965–73 in both women's groups. This rising trend for assertive behaviour can be observed even more in both men's groups (from 1·1–2·5 in the younger, 0·4–1·25 in the older group). Passive reactions got consistently low scores in the older age groups and the younger women's group (2–4) at all measurement points. Men of the cohort 1900–5 who scored low in 1948 and 1965, gave reports on their situation from 1965–73 resulting in a score for passive reactions ranging from 1·0 to 1·8. Generally we might state that the amount of strategies reported was rather low in the years of observation. We might predict a decisive increase in times of economic depression. Generally more active strategies are prevailing with active opposition scoring higher with increasing age than before, and achievement-orientated behaviour scoring lower.

Whereas there are some indications that cognitive restructuring as a strategy of solving problems which cannot be solved by changes in the social (or biological, etc.) reality, will become more relevant with increasing age, we could not confirm this for the women's groups. This may be explained by reference to the situation as perceived by them: Apparently it was more often perceived as something which can be changed than by men who 'knew about the realities of life'. This opinion would be supported by the increase of scores for assertive behaviour. Generally we may state that the role of cognitive restructuring of the situation for adjustment to ageing could not be adequately assessed in our study. We might find it represented more often in samples of impaired aged for which this strategy might serve as the only successful one. Furthermore, this way of problem-solving may be utilized more often in samples representing normal ageing in which distortion of the balance between self and social system may be reported more frequently. In any case, we expect from our findings that the ways of restoring balance between the aged and the biological–social systems cannot be reduced to one dimension like autonomy–dependency (William and Wirths 1965). As there are different ways of maintaining and restoring this balance there might be more patterns of ageing or life style in terms of this focal development task in old age.

Objective health, subjective measures of health, and behaviour

Health as assessed by the clinician, and health as perceived by our respondents differed in about 75 per cent of our cases. Men especially perceived their health as better than it was rated after the medical assessment, whereas in women there was a tendency to perceive oneself as less healthy than the medical tests indicated.

On the other hand more behavioural correlates of subjectively perceived health attained a satisfactory level of significance (Olbrich 1977). Activity related to control and improvement of health was dependent on perceived stress in the area of health. Correlations between activity and indicators of sclerosis of heart insufficiency were rather low. On the other hand, performance on a perceptual-motor task (Mathey 1976) was influenced by sclerosis rather than by perceived stress on health. From data like this we may conclude that neither the environment nor the objective health is 'isomorphically perceived.' This confirms the view which holds that cognitive representations are a function of factors which go beyond those of the present stimulus situation (Olbrich 1977).

Survivors and non-survivors as assessed at the beginning of the study

As in most longitudinal studies on aged subjects the comparison of those subjects who survived until the end of the study and those who died was part of our research programme (Lehr and Schmitz-Scherzer 1976). Of the 222 men and women of the BLSA sample tested in 1965, 45 had died in the seven years up to 1972. As expected, the older cohort had a higher percentage of death (28 per cent) than the younger one (13·5 per cent).

The comparative analysis of the data on survivors and non-survivors at the first measurement point showed that non-survivors had more sclerotic symptoms. There was no difference, however, in respect to physicians' ratings of general health, cardiovascular insufficiency, etc. The most striking difference pointed to measures of intelligence. In agreement with several other longitudinal studies the survivors had higher scores (95·8 compared to 84·2 of the non-survivors). In the psychomotor performance task the survivors reached the 50 per cent correct response criterion faster than the non-survivors. Survivors and non-survivors differed also regarding their personalities at the first measurement point: the survivors were rated as more active, better adjusted, and of higher mood or morale during the interview and testing session. Concerning SES the survivors were of a slightly higher status.

Lehr (1977) believes that these findings on survivor versus non-survivor differences point to a system of interactions. Aged persons who are most active show more initiative and are more interested in their physical surroundings. Cognitive functioning is influenced in a favourable way from this stimulation. Finally it can be hypothesized that higher degree of activity in survivors facilitates coping with crises situations such as illness, physical stress, or emotional stress.

Conclusions

Longitudinal samples of aged persons—'normative' or 'elite' groups?

Considering the many deprivations, stresses, and personal losses reported by most of our subjects, all of them could be regarded as 'survivors' of serious strains even at the first point of measurement. The men in particular were survivors in the true sense of the word. According to census data of the FRG (1961), 1890–5 cohorts consisted of approximately one million men and 1·658 million women; the 1900–5 cohorts included 2·076 million men and about 2·5 million women. These sex differences in survivorship are only partially explained by the two World Wars. More recent calculations point to the decreasing life expectancy for men in the next ten years (Schwarz 1974) compared to a slowly increasing life expectancy of women. This difference is explained by some writers with reference to the occupational situation of men as entailing more severe stress and other conditions conducive to coronary vascular disease in middle age.

Against this background our subjects might be defined as a biological 'elite' even if they have by no means attained the status of centenarians. Those especially who were able to come to us at all points of measurement from 1965–77 may be regarded as examples of 'successful' ageing. This is also true if we consider the high degree of 'normality' and of continuously well-adjusted behaviour in the survivors of our study.

By defining the ageing pattern of our survivors as examples of successful ageing we would avoid the problem of delineating the degree of normality in terms of 'averageness' of this group. Perhaps this normal or average process of ageing can be found in an area between the elite life of our survivors on the one hand and that of less successful, ill, and/or disabled persons living in institutions on the other hand. It will not be easy to rate the distance between this successful group and the area of normal ageing. However, this normal area is to be located closer to the successful pattern than to the patterns defined by increase of dependency, helplessness, or social isolation.

According to findings from a random cross-sectional sample covering the age range 65–90 we can locate the normal group rather close to the elite group of the BLSA survivors (Schmitz-Scherzer et al. 1974). This sample (415 men and women, aged 65–80) was studied from a medical, sociological, and psychological point of view at Muenster, Westphalia. It will be referred to, therefore as the Muenster sample.

The Muenster sample medians for cognitive functioning, psychomotor performance, and personality variables such as activity were only 0·2 to 1·5 points below those of our longitudinal sample. Another difference between this cross-sectional sample and the BLSA sample refers to social isolation. Whereas most of our subjects reported a high degree of social participation (see Olbrich and Lehr 1976) there was a greater percentage of perceived isolation in the Muenster sample (Schmitz-Scherzer et al. 1974): 18·8 per cent of the men and 29 per cent of the women said that isolation was the greatest problem in their lives. Another area of concern was income: 15·1 per cent of the men and 11·8 per cent of the women reported serious problems in this area compared to 5–7 per cent who did so in the BLSA. Finally there was a difference regarding health: while this was rated as 'average' to 'good' in BLSA by the physician, 50 per cent of the Muenster sample suffered from at least two health problems (especially coronary and respiratory diseases, and orthopaedic problems).

As the social stratification of the BLSA and the Muenster sample were identical, we might hypothesize that the differences in cognitive functioning, social participation, and perceived economic situation are to be explained primarily by different coping techniques. Perhaps the better health of the BLSA sample enabled our subjects to respond to their problems in the active manner which according to Lehr and Schmitz-Scherzer is a main correlate of survivorship.

Generally, however, a cross-sectional sample of non-institutionalized aged persons is very similar to our longitudinal sample and very much unlike a sample of institutionalized and mentally or physically disabled persons. Therefore, successful ageing defined by survivorship in our sample comes rather close to 'normal ageing' and if there exists something like 'elite' ageing (like that of centenarian or professional persons) it will be still a different pattern of ageing, not that of the BLSA subjects.

Unfortunately, the image of the deteriorated, helpless, or at least dependent old person has been reinforced by many clinical experts generalizing unduly from their experiences with physically or mentally impaired patients. Even if samples like ours here are to be defined as an elite group (although they belong mainly to lower SES), studying them can help in revising stereotypes that have emerged from experiences with physically and/or economically highly dependent persons. The reports on our findings published so far have been evaluated by many clinicians, social workers, and the general public as a much needed counterbalance to negative stereotypes of aged persons. The image of ageing we should like to reinforce is neither optimistic nor pessimistic. It is realistic, i.e. adapted to the highly complex and variable process of ageing. Therefore, our approach emphasizes the study of different patterns of ageing, the control of conditions for a well-balanced process of ageing, and the prevention of developments which may result in impairment and disability.

In agreement with many other findings we recommend an active orientation toward and within old age and an integration of the aged into society based on solid knowledge of their capacities rather than on stereotypes.

30. A prospective follow-up study on the epidemiology of drug, tobacco, and alcohol consumption (Switzerland)

MARTIN SIEBER and JULES ANGST

Introduction

Because the drug consumption of young people can change very quickly, one single study on a sample gives an incomplete picture of the habits of drug consumption. In 1971 and 1974, two surveys were made for 19-year-old males in order to establish possible changes relating to the consumption of drugs, alcohol, and tobacco. The population groups investigated ($N=2785$ in 1971, $N=1617$ in 1974) came from three different geographical areas of the canton of Zurich.

A longitudinal study gives us a better impression because we can see the individual pattern of drug consumption during an observed period. Follow-up studies are also important because we can separate out groups with a special pattern of drug consumption (high risk groups). The correlation of these high risk groups with different variables can show us where prophylactic or therapeutic intervention could be effective.

In 1971 we started with a three-year prospective follow-up study on 19-year-old males. We were especially interested in knowing something about the percentage of drug users and about the change in their pattern of consumption. We were also interested in their personal and social development and in the correlation of a special pattern of consumption with some variables of the personal and social situation. In this study we also make similar and comparative analyses with the users of cigarettes and alcohol. Thus, we do not think of drug consumption as an isolated phenomenon.

Research questions
The object of this study was:

(1) To group subjects with different developmental patterns of consumption (increase, decrease, permanent heavy consumption, and no consumption), and to find the percentage of these groups with different risk of drug dependence;
(2) To relate social, economic, and personal characteristics with these groups. The results relative to drug consumption will be compared with those relative to alcohol and tobacco consumption. Therefore it will be possible to identify the characteristics which are specifically typical of drug consumption.

Methods

The follow-up sample consists of 841 men of the canton of Zurich, Switzerland. They are selected from a survey we made in 1971, where we investigated all 19-year-old men in the canton of Zurich born in 1952 ($N=6325$ men). They were questioned about their consumption of drugs, alcohol, and tobacco. We got the social characteristics of the proband and his parents as well as information about personality (Personality Inventory FPI) and social attitudes. The 841 selected subjects were re-examined three years later in 1974. We mailed every subject a questionnaire about his present situation and drug consumption, and we also again used the personality inventory FPI. In addition we made personal interviews with 178 subjects.

The 841 subjects were divided into different groups with typical developments of drug consumption. In this classification we took into consideration the different drugs, the degree and duration of consumption. Drugs are here operationally defined as cannabis, hallucinogens, stimulants, and opiates. Clinical and statistical considerations lead to the following groups with a different development in drug consumption:

Group A: non-consumers ($N=387$);
Group B: young consumers, first consumption after age 19 ($N=31$);
Group C: subjects with terminated consumption ($N=252$);
Group D: subjects with continual, moderate consumption ($N=121$);
Group E: subjects with increased consumption ($N=50$).

All information was first punched and then put onto a magnetic tape for electronic data analysis. In three different methodological studies we were concerned with the following problems:

(1) Methods to raise the quota of responders in surveys with mailed questionnaires;
(2) Analysis of the non-responders in regard to social, economic, and personal characteristics;
(3) Study of the reliability of surveys made with mailed questionnaires.

Preliminary results

The development of drug and cigarette consumption in men between the ages of 19 and 22 years shows that there are two different patterns of development (Table 30.1).

TABLE 30.1

Patterns of development of drug and cigarette consumption in men aged 19–22 years

Percentage of	Development of consumption	
	Drugs	Cigarettes
Non-consumers	high	low
New-consumers (first consumption after the age of 19)	low	high
Subject with terminated consumption	high	low
Risk to social disintegration when heavy consumption is continued	high	low

We could not make an accurate comparison with the consumption of alcohol but the present results show that the development of alcohol consumption is similar to that of cigarette consumption.

The results indicate that prophylactic measures against the abuse of tobacco and alcohol consumption after the age of 19 should reach the whole population, whereas the prevention of drug dependence is more efficient when concentrated on groups with a high risk of drug dependence. The prevention of drug dependence is very important because a high degree of consumption leads very quickly to social disintegration. It seems that problems of young people and of puberty are more connected with drug consumption than with the consumption of alcohol or tobacco.

The analyses in regard to socio-economic characteristics, social attitudes, and personality show that there are differences between the four groups A, C, D, and E which have a different pattern in the development of drug consumption. Especially the difference between the groups D and E is remarkable; the subjects of group D came more often from upper class families and had a better education than the subjects of group E.

Most personality traits and attitudes did not change in the observed interval. This shows that many personality traits and attitudes are formed before the age of 19 and before the 'drug career' and social disintegration begin. The results show that there is no correlation between the degree of drug consumption and a change of personality. This means that the pharmacological effect of the drug could not be proven in the form of a change in some personality traits, because the personality did not change very much in all four groups.

The preliminary results show that the heavy and constant consumers are confronted with several problems and that the drug dependence is only one problem among several. Some of these problems or characteristics are the following:

(a) Non-conventional, non-conforming lifestyle;
(b) A different system of norms and values in regard to social performance;
(c) Weak social integration, tendency to be in marginal social groups;
(d) Low or moderate attainment in school or professional education;
(e) Little professional success, unfavourable professional and financial situation;
(f) Socio-economic status of parents: lower class;
(g) Restricted relations with other persons;
(h) Frequent physical and psychic complaints;
(i) Emotional lability, depressive symptoms, low self-confidence.

Therefore drug prevention must not only be concentrated on the undesired behaviour of drug consumption itself, but should also include all areas connected with the development of a low self-esteem, and feelings of helplessness and inferiority.

31. Occupation and alcoholism: cause or effect? A controlled study of recruits to the drink trade (Scotland)†

MARTIN A. PLANT

Introduction

Alcoholism rates vary very greatly between different social groups, including occupations (Plant 1975a, 1978, 1979). The exact prevalence of alcoholism in the community remains unknown because many alcoholics do not seek treatment from medical and other agencies, and many of those who do often fail to be recognized as problem drinkers (Wilkins 1974). Probably the most reliable indicator of the prevalence of alcoholism is mortality due to liver cirrhosis (WHO 1951). Even so, this indicator is far from perfect since most alcoholics do not die from liver cirrhosis, and not all of those who die from this disease are alcoholics.

Some occupations carry a far greater risk of alcoholism than others. Table 31.1 shows the 24 occupational groups in England and Wales (males) which had the highest liver cirrhosis mortality ratios in 1961. Each of these occupational groups had at least twice the average rate of mortality due to liver cirrhosis. (Standardized mortality ratios are calculated taking into account the age composi-

tion of an occupational group. The average standardized mortality ratio is 100.)

Three main factors have been advanced to explain these differences. First, work situations where alcohol is readily available to be consumed during working hours, have been cited as conducive to high rates of alcoholism (Glatt 1967; Wilson 1940). This factor may be relevant to alcohol production and distribution jobs, and to jobs which require social drinking as part of role performance. Second, strong social pressure to drink is suggested as an influential factor relevant to occupational groups such as seamen, servicemen, and commercial travellers (Amark 1970; Brun-Gulbrandsen and Irgens-Jensen 1967; Carney and Lawes 1967; Clarke 1949; J.I.F. 1947; Rose and Glatt 1961; Wallinga 1956). The third factor associated with high occupational levels of alcoholism is separation from normal sexual or social relationships, when the work situation creates an isolated occupational group with restricted social outlets, such as domestic servants, seamen, or oil rig workers (J.I.F. 1947; Strauss and Winterbottom 1949; Department of Trade 1975a, b).

† Reprinted (with modifications) from Plant (1978), by courtesy of Marcel Dekker Inc.

Workers engaged in alcohol production are traditionally purported to be particularly vulnerable to becoming alcoholic (Wilson 1940). The most reliable evidence for this is the incidence of mortality due to liver cirrhosis which is much higher among workers (and their spouses) producing and distributing alcohol than in the general population (Mellor 1967; Kessel and Walton 1971; Glatt 1972; Hitz 1973). The Registrar General's decennial supplement on occupation in England and Wales (Office of Population Censuses and Surveys 1978) showed that amongst drink trade workers such as publicans and bar staff mortality due to liver cirrhosis was exceptionally high. Table 31.1 shows the twenty occupational groups which had the highest liver cirrhosis mortality rates 1970–2:

TABLE 31.1

Male liver cirrhosis mortality (England and Wales 1970–2)

Occupational group	Standardized Mortality Ratio
Average occupation	100
Publicans, innkeepers	1576
Deck, engineering officers and pilots, ship	781
Barmen, barmaids	633
Deck and engine room ratings, barge and boatmen	628
Fishermen	595
Proprietors and managers, boarding houses and hotels	506
Finance, insurance brokers, financial agents	392
Restaurateurs	385
Lorry drivers' mates, van guards	377
Cooks	354
Shunters, pointsmen	323
Winders, reelers	319
Electrical engineers	319
Authors, journalists and related workers	314
Medical practitioners	311
Garage proprietors	294
Signalmen and crossing keepers, railways	290
Maids, valets and related service workers	281
Tobacco preparers and product makers	269
Metallurgists	266

Undoubtedly, people engaged in alcohol production are particularly likely to receive medical treatment for alcoholism and alcoholic psychoses. Between 1970 and 1973, 2·8 per cent of males treated for those conditions at the Royal Edinburgh Hospital were brewers, distillers, and allied workers, while, according to the 1966 sample census these groups comprised only 0·4 per cent of Edinburgh's labour force. The Registrar General (Scotland) provided information indicating that alcohol production workers have particularly high mortality due to suicide and motor accidents. Amongst comparable workers in England and Wales (1961) the suicide rate was low, but motor accidents were 57 per cent higher than amongst the general population.

The only detailed post-war study of drink producers (Frank *et al.* 1967) examined 450 Austrian workers, 200 of whom worked in a brewery. This investigation showed that the proportion of heavy drinkers in the brewery was double that amongst the other workers. Physical examination revealed liver damage in more than a quarter of the brewers, a significantly higher rate than amongst all other workers. The researchers suggested that these differences may have been due to the greater availability of alcohol for the brewery workers. Table 31.2 presents the major research on occupational factors in alcoholism.

While there is general agreement upon the high prevalence of

drink-related problems amongst those engaged in drink production, little has been done to investigate what factors lead to these industrial hazards. Two alternatives merit attention and provide the main objectives of this study:

(1) To ascertain whether alcohol production attracts workers who are already heavy drinkers or alcoholics, or who appear likely to become such;

(2) To examine how workers' drinking habits change over time after recruitment to the alcohol production industry.

Method

In order to assess possible selection factors influencing levels of industrial alcoholism new recruits to the drink trade were compared with new recruits in other industries. This was made possible by the help of five companies: three alcohol producers—brewers and distillers, and two other firms. All were situated in the Edinburgh area and recruited male manual workers from a broadly similar catchment area. All the firms operated similar shift systems and provided comparable conditions of work. These companies were chosen in order to obtain interviews from a total of 300 newly recruited workers: 150 brewers and distillers and 150 controls. New recruits were interviewed consecutively until the two study groups had been completed. None of the respondents had been in his current employment for longer than 3 months.

Data were collected using a standardized interview schedule which included questions on the following topics:

(1) Description of current job;
(2) Employment history;
(3) Education;
(4) Smoking habits;
(5) Drinking habits;
(6) Assessment of light/heavy drinking;
(7) Experience of drink-related problems;
(8) Drinking at work;
(9) Perception of workmates' drinking habits;
(10) Parental drinking habits;
(11) Drinking habits of wife, girl friend, etc.;
(12) General biographical data—age, marital status, criminal record, recent bereavements, income.

The interview schedule, containing 129 separate questions, was constructed by the author. Altogether 102 of these items had previously been used in three earlier studies (Edwards *et al.* 1972; Plant 1975b; Dight 1976). The other 27 questions were introduced for this investigation. The schedule was pretested firstly amongst 6 members of the University Department of Psychiatry at Edinburgh University, and then amongst 6 male manual workers in Edinburgh. No major problems being evident, the fieldwork procedure was piloted amongst 20 male manual workers in a Stirlingshire distillery. Each of these men was interviewed with the schedule and also in a semi-structured manner in order to check the reliability of the main items relating to alcohol consumption, drink-related problems, and employment histories. Pretesting and piloting revealed no evidence of unreliability, but the likely validity of data collected with this schedule is less dependable. Interview surveys of drinking behaviour are widely reported to produce a distorted pattern of alcohol consumption, invariably an underestimate (Summers 1970; Pernanen 1974). It is likely that respondents, especially if they are in fact heavy drinkers or alcoholics, will significantly underreport their real alcohol consumption (Schmidt 1972). Conversations with people in the liquor industry indicated that at least some

TABLE 31.2

Research on occupational factors in alcoholism

Author	Year	Method	Type of subjects	Number of subjects	Main findings	Study limitations
Wilson, G.B.	1940	Review of mortality data published by Registrar General (U.K.)	British brewing workers	—	Between 1860 and 1932 there was an excess mortality amongst British male drink trade workers of 80 000–90 000	Does not include all involved in alcohol and distribution
J.I.F.	1947	Participant observation	Merchant seamen	Unspecified	Suggests that seamen are highly vulnerable to alcoholism due to job situation and peer pressure to drink heavily	Impressionistic
Clarke, R.E.	1949	Review of hospital admissions	Hospitalized white male alcoholics	1695	Alcoholism most prevalent amongst low status individuals	Not based upon representative occupational groups
Strauss, R. and Winterbottom, M.T.	1949	Interview with subjects and their employers	Female domestic servants and their employers	216	Domestic servants significantly heavier drinkers than general community. Excessive drinkers in this group soon detected and dismissed	Little evidence about occupational groups
Wallinga, J.V.	1956	Observation of hospitalized patients	Hospitalized U.S. Navy and Marine alcoholics	94	Peer pressure to drink with armed forces milieu led to alcoholism	
Rose, H.K. and Glatt, M.M.	1961	Interview survey	British seamen	1000	Heavy drinking commonplace, high risk of alcoholism. Suggested prone personality type likely reason for high incidence of alcoholism	No data on personality of subjects *before* becoming seamen
Mellor, C.S	1967	Literature review	Varied	—	Alcoholism especially commonplace in alcohol production and distribution trade and amongst merchant seamen	Cites previous research General
Glatt, M.M.	1967	Clinical records	Private alcoholic patients	50	High proportion of high status professionals	Private patients are unrepresentative of hospital population
Brun-Gulbrandsen, S. and Irgens-Jensen, O.	1967	Sample survey interview assessment	Norwegian naval conscripts	3447	Alcohol abuse a major problem amongst seamen. Suggested that people prone to abuse alcohol entered the merchant navy	No control group
Carney, M.W.P. and Lawes, T.G.C.	1967	Review of hospital records	Male alcoholic patients and non-alcoholic patient controls	40	No clear association between alcoholism and occupation, though alcoholics were more likely to have attained senior military ranks	Numbers too small a basis for generalization
Kessel, N. and Walton, H.	1967	Review of British mortality data	Occupational groups (males)	—	Publicans have liver cirrhosis mortality rate nine times the expected level	
Amark, C.	1970	Review of hospital records	Hospitalized male alcoholic patients	199	Commercial travellers, seamen, those in literary and artistic occupations were overrepresented	Numbers small
Glatt, M.M.	1972	General literature review including references to British occupational mortality data			Liver cirrhosis mortality rate high amongst occupations with easy access to alcohol	
Hitz, D.	1973	Sample interview survey	White males aged 21–59 resident in San Francisco	786	Some occupations are especially tolerant of heavy drinking, and amongst such groups drink-related problems are greater than elsewhere	Findings do not include whether men in 'high risk' occupations were heavy drinkers prior to current employment
Department of Trade (U.K.)	1975a	Discussions with key people in British fishing industry	British fishermen	—	About 15 per cent of fishermen are thought to be excessive drinkers. The 'hard core' are young men aged 18–35	Impressionistic
Department of Trade (U.K.)	1975b	Discussion with key people in British merchant navy	British Merchant Seamen	—	Alcohol abuse widely considered the main cause of indiscipline amongst seamen	Impressionistic

respondents had underreported their alcohol consumption, and in some instances interviewers concluded that they were given 'socially acceptable', untruthful replies to questions about drinking behaviour. Even so there is no particular reason to suppose that the alcohol producers were markedly different from the control group in this respect.

Fieldwork was carried out between March and December 1975 by six males. Three of the interviewers were behavioural scientists and two were nurses in the Alcohol Problems Clinic at Edinburgh. Three of the interviewers had previous interviewing experience and all six were thoroughly trained in the use of the interview schedule before commencing fieldwork. Interviews averaged 20 min in duration and no tangible problems were encountered. The success of fieldwork is largely attributable to the help and co-operation throughout of both managements and trade unions.

Results and discussion

Response rate

Three hundred interviews were completed. In addition there were 8 refusals, 6 of which were from alcohol production workers. The net response rate was high: 97·3 per cent. Workmates of some of those who refused commented that these individuals were not co-operating because they wished to conceal their heavy drinking. This, if true, is consistent with evidence that heavy drinkers are especially unlikely to co-operate with surveys of drinking habits (Schmidt 1972). This high response rate is probably attributable to the fact that interviewing was conducted during working hours.

Background characteristics of the study group

One hundred and fifty male manual workers were interviewed in each of the two subgroups. Their distribution according to age is shown in Table 31.3. A significantly higher proportion of the alcohol producers than the controls were under 25 years of age ($\chi^2 = 7.9371$; $df = 1$; $p < 0.01$).

TABLE 31.3

Number of alcohol producers and controls according to age

Age	Alcohol producers	Controls
Under 25	74	49
26–35	50	59
36–45	24	31
46 and above	2	11
Total	150	150

Country of birth. There were 135 alcohol producers and 122 controls who had been born in Scotland ($\chi^2 = 3.9091$; $df = 1$; $p < 0.05$). Only 3 alcohol producers and 12 controls had been born outside the United Kingdom.

Marital status. Consistent with the greater youthfulness of the alcohol producers, a significantly higher proportion of these men were still unmarried than amongst the controls: 58 compared with only 37 ($\chi^2 = 6.1617$; $df = 1$; $p < 0.02$). Only 9 of the alcohol producers were separated or divorced compared with 21 of the controls ($\chi^2 = 4.1642$; $df = 1$; $p < 0.05$). This discrepancy is *not* explained by the higher proportion of older men amongst the controls. There were no significant differences in divorce or separation rates between alcohol producers and controls of the same ages.

Fathers' occupation. Of the 300 respondents, 264 reported that their fathers were, or had been, manual workers: 134 of the alcohol producers and 130 of the controls. This difference was not significant.

Education. Of the 300 respondents, 245 had no educational qualifications. Only 23 of the alcohol producers and 32 controls reported that they had some form of qualification ($\chi^2 = 1.4248$; $df = 1$; N.S.). Most of those in both subgroups were unskilled workers without either academic or occupational qualifications, however lowly. Their chances of attaining clerical or other non-manual jobs were thereby severely limited.

Previous employment. There was no significant difference between the alcohol producers' and the controls' previous experience of working in alcohol-related occupations. Fifty-one of the alcohol producers and 53 controls had formerly worked in alcohol production or distribution. There were no significant differences in the levels of previous alcohol-related employment of the different age groups. The alcohol producers were significantly more likely to have poor employment records than the controls, reporting having had more than 5 jobs in the previous 5 years, or that they had previously been in non-manual jobs, and were thereby downwardly mobile; 31 compared with only 12 ($\chi^2 = 8.7955$; $df = 1$; $p < 0.01$).

Hours of work. The alcohol producers were significantly less likely than the controls to be working on a shift rota: 80 compared with 112 ($\chi^2 = 13.9033$; $df = 1$; $p < 0.001$).

Wage levels. There were no significant differences between the reported weekly earnings of the two subgroups. The average of the alcohol producers was £38.20 compared with £36.40 for the controls ($t = 1.4486$; $df = 298$; N.S.; two-tailed). In addition there were no significant differences between the alcohol producers and the controls when age was taken into account.

Reasons for applying for present job. In view of the absence of differences in wage levels between the subgroups, it is interesting that the alcohol producers were significantly more likely than the controls to report that they had been attracted to their new job by good wage levels: 45 compared with 26 ($\chi^2 = 4.0434$; $df = 1$; $p < 0.05$). In addition, the alcohol producers were significantly more likely than the controls to state that 'security' had been their primary attraction: 19 compared with only 5 ($\chi^2 = 6.5967$; $df = 1$; $p < 0.05$).

Drinking patterns. The main indication of alcohol consumption used in this investigation is total drinking during the week preceding the interview. This is calculated on the basis of units of alcohol each equivalent to either half a pint of beer/lager/cider/stout, etc., or to a single glass of wine or spirits, roughly one centilitre of absolute alcohol. The average amount consumed during the previous week by the alcohol producers was 33·13 units, compared with only 21·40 units for the controls ($t = 3.8204$; $df = 298$; $p < 0.001$). (Since the distribution of alcohol consumption approximates to a Log Normal Curve, t-tests relating to consumption have been log-converted.)

In addition to the overall higher level of consumption amongst the alcohol producers (Fig. 31.1) they also consumed more amongst each of the three age groups (Fig. 31.2). Amongst those age 35 and under, this difference was statistically significant but was not significant amongst the older men (Table 31.4). In addition to their generally lower level of alcohol consumption, the controls were significantly more likely than the alcohol producers to report that they had not drunk any alcoholic beverages during the preceding week: 29 compared with 11 ($\chi^2 = 8.3365$; $df = 1$; $p < 0.01$).

The heaviest drinkers. Seven individuals—6 alcohol producers and one control—reported that they had drunk more than 100 units (equivalent to 50 pints of beer or 100 glasses of spirits) during the

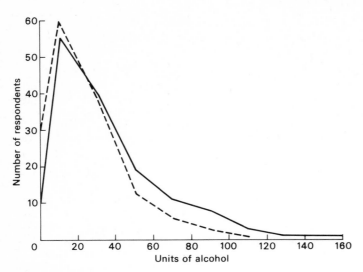

FIG. 31.1. Previous week's alcohol consumption: (——) alcohol producers; (– – – –) controls.

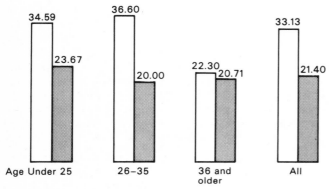

FIG. 31.2. Average previous week's alcohol consumption: (□) alcohol producers; (▉) controls.

TABLE 31.4

Average previous week's alcohol consumption

Age	Alcohol producers	Controls	Level of significance (two-tailed)		
Under 25	34·59	23·67	$t = 2\cdot0864$;	$df = 121$;	$p<0\cdot05$
26–35	36·60	20·00	$t = 2\cdot8371$;	$df = 107$;	$p<0\cdot01$
36 and above	22·30	20·71	$t = 1\cdot8682$;	$df = 66$;	N.S.
Total	33·13	21·40	$t = 3\cdot8204$;	$df = 298$	$p<0\cdot001$

week preceding the interview. These individuals represent 4·0 per cent of the alcohol producers and 0·7 per cent of the controls. Together these 7 respondents consumed 11·0 per cent of the total alcohol reportedly consumed by the 300 respondents during the previous week. This result is broadly consistent with Dight's finding in her *Survey of Scottish drinking habits* (1976) that 3·0 per cent of males consumed 30·0 per cent of the total alcohol drunk by the population. Also consistent with Dight's study was the fact that all the 7 heaviest drinkers were aged 35 or less.

Existing research (Schmidt 1972) suggests that heavy drinkers often underreport their real drinking habits. It is accordingly very likely that these findings underrepresent the actual level of drinking within the study group.

Assessment of heavy drinking. Respondents were asked to state

their assessments of the quantities of beer and whisky a man would need to consume in a week to be counted as a heavy drinker. There was no significant difference between the alcohol producers' and the controls' average estimate of what amount constitutes a heavy whisky consumption: 3·85 bottles and 3·67 bottles respectively.

The alcohol producers produced a higher average estimate of heavy beer consumption than the controls, 61·75 pints compared with 55·69 pints. Like the discrepancy for whisky drinking, this overall difference was not significant ($t = 1\cdot5147$; $df = 285$; N.S. two-tailed). Even so, the alcohol producers were significantly more likely than the controls to state that a heavy beer drinker would consume at least 80 pints in a week: 36 compared with only 18 ($\chi^2 = 6\cdot739$; $df = 1$; $p<0\cdot01$).

Effects of work situation on drinking behaviour. The alcohol producers were significantly more likely than the controls to state that they had begun to drink more since starting their new jobs: 32 compared with only 6 ($\chi^2 = 18\cdot8328$; $df = 1$; $p<0\cdot001$). There were 81 alcohol producers and only one control who admitted that they drank illegally while at work. These findings appear to substantiate the view that some individuals do drink more in job situations where alcohol is freely available than they would otherwise have done.

Perceived drinking habits of fellow employees. Significant differences were evident between the two subgroups' reported perceptions of the drinking habits of those they worked with in their new jobs. This topic aroused more reticence or reluctance to reply than any other item in the interview. Altogether 166 of the 300 interviewed failed to comment upon their workmates' drinking habits. Many had not been in their new jobs long enough to evaluate their colleagues' drinking habits. Others clearly believed they would have been disloyal to comment, regarded the question as an intrusion into their friends' privacy, and declined to reply for that reason.

The alcohol producers were significantly more likely than the controls to supply information on this topic: 95 compared with only 39 ($\chi^2 = 40\cdot7975$; $df = 1$; $p<0\cdot001$). This difference is striking, since the alcohol producers appeared generally more likely than the controls to regard drinking at work as something tangible they could discuss, whereas the controls clearly regarded it as either none of their business, or as an area of essentially secret behaviour. Respondents were asked what percentage of their workmates they regarded as heavy drinkers. The 95 alcohol producers who replied to this question produced a significantly higher average estimate than the 39 controls: 37·2 per cent compared with 29·3 per cent ($t = 23\cdot9311$; $df = 132$; $p<0\cdot001$; two-tailed).

Smoking. There was no significant difference between the ratios of smokers to non-smokers amongst the alcohol producers and the controls. One hundred and nine of the former and 120 of the latter reported that they sometimes smoked tobacco ($\chi^2 = 1\cdot8545$; $df = 1$; N.S.). These ratios did not vary significantly with age, although only 4 of the 42 controls aged 36 and over were non-smokers.

There were no significant differences between the proportion of alcohol producers and controls classified as heavy smokers (smoking either at least 20 cigarettes daily or 3 ounces of tobacco weekly). Forty-seven of the alcohol producers and 56 controls were heavy smokers ($\chi^2 = 0\cdot9462$; $df = 1$; N.S.). The prevalence of heavy smoking does not significantly relate to age.

Alcohol-related problems

Physical damage. Respondents were asked if they had ever suffered from the following physical conditions associated with alcohol abuse: stomach ulcers. tuberculosis of chest, and liver cirrhosis.

Stomach ulcers. The alcohol producers were significantly *less* likely than the controls to report that they had had a stomach ulcer: 10 compared with 23 ($\chi^2 = 4\cdot9029$; $df = 1$; $p<0\cdot05$).

Tuberculosis of chest. Four of the alcohol producers had had tuberculosis compared with only one of the controls. These numbers are too small to justify a statistical comparison.

Liver cirrhosis. Three of the alcohol producers stated that they had had liver cirrhosis compared with only one of the controls. Again, these numbers are too small to warrant statistical comparison.

Altogether, 17 of the alcohol producers and 16 of the controls reported having at least one of these physical symptoms; of these 3 individuals, one alcohol producer and two controls had suffered from two of the three symptoms. These differences are non-significant. Physical damage was *not* significantly associated with age.

Other problems. Respondents were asked whether or not they had experienced any of 18 listed problems connected with heavy drinking. Altogether 227 of the 300 respondents reported that they had experienced at least one of these difficulties. The alcohol producers reported an average of 2·8 problems, compared with 3·5 for the controls. Both in terms of individual problems, and the overall number of problems reported, there was no significant difference between the two subgroups.

Amongst the alcohol producers aged 35 or less, 13 individuals reported having experienced 8 or more problems. None of the older alcohol producers had experienced this number. This difference is consistent with the higher average alcohol consumption reported by the younger alcohol producers. Even so, there was no significant difference between the proportions of younger and older alcohol producers who had experienced 4 or more problems ($\chi^2 = 2·0994$; $df = 1$; N.S.).

Taking the physical symptoms and the 18 other problems associated with alcoholism together, these findings do not lend support to the conclusion that the alcohol producers had experienced more difficulties associated with alcohol than the controls. Even so, a minority in both subgroups, 4·0 per cent, reported that they had experienced at least 10 of the 18 problems, and clearly constitute an 'at risk' group.

Family drinking problems. There were no significant differences between the proportions of alcohol producers and controls reporting that either of their parents had experienced drinking problems, or had been alcoholics. Fourteen of the alcohol producers and 20 controls reported that their mothers had experienced drinking problems ($\chi^2 = 0·8292$; $df = 1$; N.S.). Thirty-two of the alcohol producers and 37 controls stated that their fathers had experienced drinking problems ($\chi^2 = 0·5000$; $df = 1$; N.S.). Five of the alcohol producers and 13 of the controls reported that their wives, fiancées, or girlfriends had experienced some form of drinking problem ($\chi^2 = 2·8959$; $df = 1$; N.S.).

Age of spouse/partner. It has been frequently asserted that alcoholic males marry markedly older women (Kessel and Walton 1971; p. 107). This study revealed no significant differences between the two subgroups in relation to the relative ages of their wives, fiancées, or girlfriends. Eleven alcohol producers and 13 controls reported that they had older partners, while 11 alcohol producers and 16 controls had younger ones.

Criminal records. Fifty-seven of the alcohol producers and 61 controls had been convicted of at least one offence (excluding minor motoring infringements). This difference was not significant; neither was there a significant difference between the numbers of alcohol producers and controls who had been given a custodial or suspended sentence (indicating a more serious offence) ($\chi^2 = 3·6684$; $df = 1$; N.S.). Even so, the alcohol producers were significantly less likely than the controls to report that they had been convicted of an offence related to alcohol abuse: 8 compared with 28 ($\chi^2 = 11·3952$; $df = 1$; $p < 0·001$). This difference may be due to the effects of screening out alcohol offenders during selection for employment in the drink trade. Alternatively, respondents engaged in brewing and distilling may have been more likely than controls to deny or conceal their alcohol-related convictions.

Parasuicide (attempted suicide). Twelve respondents, 3 alcohol producers and 9 controls, reported that they had at some time taken an overdose. While these numbers are too small to justify a statistical comparison, they do indicate that the alcohol producers were certainly no more likely than the controls to have made a parasuicidal gesture. All twelve of these respondents were aged 35 or younger, which is consistent with evidence that parasuicide in the Edinburgh area is most prevalent amongst younger people (Kennedy *et al.* 1974).

Psychiatric illness. There was no significant difference between the proportion of alcohol producers and controls who reported that they had at some time had trouble with their nerves: 17 and 23 respectively ($\chi^2 = 0·7211$; $df = 1$; N.S.). Reported experience of psychiatric illness was not related to age.

Conclusions

The findings of the initial phase of this study indicate that there were some important differences between new recruits to the drink trade and recruits to other industries. The main distinctive characteristics of the alcohol producers upon recruitment were their significantly higher level of alcohol consumption and their poorer employment records. Together, these factors suggest both a degree of self-selection and a higher level of disturbance amongst the alcohol producers. It would appear that the alcohol producers were more likely than the controls to be sliding down the social scale. This is consistent with the view that the drink trade *attracts* at least some individuals who are predisposed by their life experiences to become alcoholics.

In addition, it appears clear that once in their new jobs, the alcohol producers in general, were more likely than the controls to perceive their working environment as conducive to illicit drinking, and to regard those with whom they worked as people who drank heavily. The fact that such illicit drinking is widespread is clearly shown by these findings. In addition during fieldwork a great deal of anecdotal information was collected from people at all levels in brewing and distilling firms indicating that illegal drinking during working hours is widespread. Discussions with those encountered during data collection also suggested that newly recruited workers are subject to strong social pressures by established employees to drink during working hours. This situation is certainly not confined either to male or to manual workers in the drink production trade. It is likely that these results are attributable at least in part to the screening process involved in appointment to the drink trade. Some of the most disturbed drinkers may have been excluded. It is notable that in spite of their heavier drinking habits, the alcohol producers did not *appear* to have experienced more alcohol-related problems than the controls.

It is also a clear possibility that the alcohol producers were more likely to deny such problems than the controls. Surveys of drinking habits certainly provide only an indication of the real situation. Even so, these findings lend support to the view that the drink trade does recruit more than its fair share of heavy drinkers and individuals likely to become alcoholics. In addition, the evidence further supports the view that once in the drink trade strong social pressures encourage workers to use the available alcohol. Illicit drinking appears to be the norm rather than the exception. Many of those interviewed volunteered that they drank because their jobs were hot and dusty. Several suggested that they would prefer to use soft drinks, but that these were not freely available. Beyond doubt, some workers have more chance to drink than others. For example, drivers, coopers, and tun-room workers, seem to have great freedom to drink regularly.

These results are preliminary ones. It is proposed to re-interview the study groups one year and two years after the initial interview. These results will be published in due course. It would be even more interesting to examine new recruits to occupational groups with even higher alcoholism rates, such as publications and innkeepers.

One possible way of reducing the harm caused by alcohol abuse in the drink trade is to move vulnerable or potentially vulnerable workers, when identified as such, into jobs with minimal opportunity to drink. Screening by interview is unlikely to be effective, since workers can easily give misleading information about their drinking habits. Some respondents *certainly* provided inaccurate information during this survey.

While questioning employees about their drinking habits is likely to be unfruitful, it would be possible to examine periodically the physical health including liver function, of workers as was done by Frank *et al.* (1967). Few companies require such regular medical examinations, yet these could be especially valuable in the context of the liquor industry.

Discussions with people at all levels in the industry revealed a general awareness that alcohol abuse is a widespread occupational hazard. The drink trade clearly has a particularly pressing need to control such abuse. Many problem drinkers can be identified in their work setting and the industry as a whole would benefit from adopting proper policies on alcoholism: encouraging or even coercing those employees who require it, to take paid leave for treatment, and guaranteeing the jobs of those who do take advantage of such schemes. At present few British firms have initiated such policies, even though these appear highly successful (Gordon 1976) and problem drinkers seldom seek treatment until a major social disaster, such as dismissal from their job, befalls them. The cost to the liquor industry due to alcohol abuse is beyond doubt enormous, if incalculable. Both employees and management would benefit if a concerted policy was undertaken to identify and to help problem drinkers while they are still useful, productive employees.

A complete account of this follow-up study is available in Plant (1979a). A summary of the whole study is also available (Plant, 1979b).

d. Prospective community cohort studies

32. Shetland: the effects of rapid social change on mental health (Scotland)

DEBORAH J. VOORHEES-ROSEN and DAVID H. ROSEN

Overview

Until 1972 the Shetland Islands were known primarily for their ponies and woolen sweaters. Few people, even in Great Britain, knew the remote location of these windswept islands in the North Sea, 250 miles from Aberdeen, Scotland. The veil of anonymity was lifted when oil was discovered off Shetland's shores and plans were made to transform this sleepy group of islands into the home of Europe's largest oil port. In the near future, where once only small fishing boats bobbed up and down in the waters around Shetland, giant super-tankers will appear.

The metamorphosis of Shetland from a rural, seafaring community to an industrial one presents a rare opportunity to study the effects this change will have upon the people and their way of life. Taking advantage of this unique situation, we traveled to Shetland in March 1975 to begin a longitudinal study designed to measure the impact of changes associated with the oil developments on the health and the way of life of the islanders.

The overall objective of our Shetland Health Study is to try to determine whether or not the change from an isolated, rural community to a more industrialized one, over a relatively short period of time, will adversely affect the health, particularly the mental health, of the islanders and precipitate an increase in certain indices of social disorder (crime, divorce, and suicide). It is our hypothesis that industrialization and the expected subsequent changes will have a deleterious effect upon the islanders' way of life (social disorganization) and on their physical and mental health, an effect that can be measured over time.

To test this hypothesis, we have initiated a longitudinal and prospective study that contains two major substudies. One of these, the General Survey, examines the prevalence of treated psychiatric morbidity and the prevalence of certain indices of social disorder. The other, the Individual Survey, involves the study of two populations: one a target population living in direct proximity to the planned oil industrial complex; and the second a control population living in an area of the island designated as a conservation region and less likely to be directly affected by the developments. A stratified random sample from each population was interviewed during the base-line phase of the study (July 1975 to Jan 1976) and the same subjects will be interviewed again at intervals following the opening of the oil port and construction of the oil complex. The first of these follow-up studies was conducted in the summer and fall of 1978. The General Survey is designed to give a broad picture of certain social and physical changes that are expected to occur on the islands and in its population over time, whereas the Individual Survey will examine the reactions of individuals to change and factors that might be important in the aetiology of those reactions.

Rationale

For more than a century there has been controversy about whether or not industrialization and modern civilization cause increases in social problems and mental illnesses. In the nineteenth century, Esquirol (1830) attributed increases in rates of mental disorders to the progress of industry, commerce, and civilization in general. Kraepelin (1909) also suggested that the stresses of civilization have led to an increase in psychiatric disorders.

These contentions were supported by Mead (1947a) who maintained that urbanization and subsequent cultural changes pose a serious threat to both personality and social integration, and that changes that increase the heterogeneity and complexity of a society give rise to 'more and more special forms of psychosomatic expressions' (Mead 1947b). Mead's assumption that 'primitive' and non-industrialized societies are actually less complex and less stressful than modern complex societies has been called into question (Beagelehole 1949). According to Wallace (1961), heterogeneity and cultural change *per se* do not lead to increases in neurotic and psychosomatic complaints but, rather, these are the responses of individuals to the more complex society's failure to meet their needs and wants.

Sorokin (1957) suggested that in periods of transition from one fundamental form of culture to another the society becomes so complex and the individual so strained that an increase in social disintegration and individual nervous breakdowns is an inevitable result. Slotkin (1960) held that forced rapid industrialization leads to severe cultural disorganization and its attendant social and personal maladjustment.

An increase in psychiatric disorder in Africa has been linked to industrialization in Ghana (Field 1960) and culture change in Nigeria (Leighton et al. 1963). In an address to an international meeting on *Industrialization and mental health* in 1964, Lambo (1965) said that 'industrialization in its present form and speed contributes to social dis-integration and conflict'. In studies carried out in Africa of communities that had experienced rapid industrialization, Lambo found higher prevalence rates (when compared to control populations) of the following: delinquency, drug addiction, alcoholism, prostitution, venereal disease, crime, and sociopathic behaviour. It was felt that these problems were caused by the erosion of traditional ways, with changes in attitudes and values and a decreased sense of belonging, and the dissolution of primary familial bonds, leading to the social isolation of individuals.

Other studies have attempted to measure the mental health of a population living in an industrial and urban environment. Most of these present the 'after' pictures, in that they have taken place in urban centres after a significant degree of industrialization has occurred. These studies present a fairly consistent pattern of higher rates of mental disorder (except for manic-depressive illnesses) in the economically poorer sections of the city and among the poor. These results are significant in that future research can be designed to determine whether people who become mentally disturbed and are unable to obtain gainful employment 'drift' eventually into these poorer sections of the city, or whether living in these areas of the city plays a part in causing mental disturbance. Faris and Dunham (1939), in one of the first ecological studies of mental disorder in an urban environment, found that higher rates of poverty, unemployment, crime, and suicide were also present. In later work, Faris (1947) further developed the theory from his and Dunham's 1939 work, that the central city is an area of high mobility and social disorganization, populated mainly by the poor, and that this mobility acts as a form of isolation that might tend to precipitate the isolation behaviour of the schizophrenic.

A more recent examination of the mental health of an urban population can be found in the Midtown Manhattan Study (Srole et al. 1962; Langner and Michael 1963), a study of the prevalence of psychiatric disorder in an urban setting. Interviews were carried out by trained personnel, and then psychiatrists, on the basis of the interview material, determined the gross typology of mental disturbance and the degree of impairment. The results indicated that 25 per cent of the individuals interviewed were psychiatrically impaired and that no fewer than 81·5 per cent had symptoms of some sort. Using a similar methodology, the Stirling County Survey, a major epidemiological study in a rural setting (Nova Scotia), found that 24 to 42 per cent of the persons interviewed were psychiatrically impaired and that 57 to 69 per cent were considered 'psychiatric cases' (Leighton 1959; Hughes et al. 1960; Leighton et al. 1963). However, as Goldberg (1972) pointed out, neither study (Midtown Manhattan or Stirling County) validated its interview guide by having psychiatrists clinically assess a subsample of the group to determine if mental health ratings made from the interview data were corroborated by direct psychiatric examination. The theory developed in the Stirling County Survey is similar to Faris and Dunham's theory of social disorganization. Leighton and co-workers found 'a much higher prevalence of psychiatric disorders in the disintegrated groups than in others'. Social disintegration, according to these investigators, can occur in all communities, rural and urban. It is relevant to our Shetland study that at least two indicators of social disintegration (cultural confusion and rapid change) as defined by Leighton will occur in our target population, and the opportunity therefore exists to test the validity of this theory in Shetland.

Selye (1956) has pointed out that the failure to adapt to the stresses of 'the ever-changing conditions on this globe' has given rise to many common diseases such as nervous and emotional disturbances, high blood pressure, gastric and duodenal ulcers, and certain types of rheumatic, allergic, and cardiovascular diseases. However, as has been noted by several researchers, reaction to stress must be examined in light of the individual's attitudes to stressors, because change or stress that the individual perceives as threatening to him (whether others do or not) poses a greater problem to the individual's ability to adapt to that change (Wolff 1950; Hinkle 1974; Mechanic 1974; Brown 1974). Therefore, as a community changes from a rural to a more industrialized setting, a mere examination of the physical and psychological changes that occur would mean little without an examination of the attitudes the people in that community have toward the change.

Attempts to quantify change in an individual's life were initiated in the work of Holmes and Rahe (1967), who showed a positive relationship between the number of life change units experienced over a given time period and the onset of illnesses. There has been increasing interest in measuring life events and determining how these interrelate with medical and psychological symptoms and illnesses (Gunderson and Rahe 1974; Dohrenwend and Dohrenwend 1974a). Rahe has demonstrated that the degree of life change has pathogenic significance, and this is important since the greater the number of life changes, the greater the risk of subsequent morbidity (Rahe 1969). Horowitz and co-workers (1974) have shown that recent events are rated as more stressful than remote events. Both Rahe's and Horowitz's work seem pertinent to our Shetland research in that we postulate that the change to a more industrial society could be reflected in an increase in life changes for the individuals in that society. Inclusion of a life events scale would allow quantification of these events and their recency.

Both Levi and Cobb have outlined models for understanding the impact of the industrialization process and stressful life events, respectively, and how these lead to the onset of medical and psychiatric symptoms and illnesses (Carlestam and Levi 1971; Levi 1974; Cobb 1974). Both emphasized the interacting variables of the psychosocial stimuli, past experience, genetic predisposition, social situation, psychological defences and coping mechanisms, and disease. During stressful periods of rapid social change due to industrialization and urbanization it has been suggested that some people are more vulnerable to environmental influences than others. Levi (Carlestam and Levi 1971) has shown that this is particularly true for the young, the elderly, and the handicapped.

Some investigators do not link an industrial and urban environment with an increase in psychological disturbance. Inkeles and Smith (1974) carried out a large scale, cross-cultural, six-nation study involving nearly 6000 men. They found no significant difference in the levels of psychiatric symptomatology in men living in urban and in rural settings. In fact, they found that 'the more modern the individual the better his psychic adjustment as measured by the Psychosomatic Symptoms Test'. However, because the study was carried out with only working men between the ages of 18 and 32 years, generalizations from this work must be limited, and there is a need for a thorough test of the hypothesis involving a population with more diverse demographic characteristics.

To our knowledge, aside from our Shetland Health Study, there have been no planned, prospective, longitudinal investigations into the effects of rapid social change associated with industrialization on the physical and mental health of the people who inhabit that changing environment. This might be because of the many uncontrollable variables involved in such research and because industrialization tends to occur in areas of great heterogeneity and highly mobile populations that would be difficult to study over a long period of time.

We are aware of only one study, by Sasaki (1960), that touches on this problem, and it examines changes in indices of social order without discussing changes in mental health. He found that the discovery of oil near a Navajo reservation in New Mexico and the subsequent change from a poor, non-industrialized environment to a relatively affluent and industrialized one, correlated positively with an increase in broken families, divorces, neglected children, alcoholism and lawlessness. Sasaki originally was collecting baseline social data to study the effect of the introduction of new agricultural techniques upon the community, but he changed his focus when oil was unexpectedly discovered in the vicinity. It is uncommon that an investigator can anticipate such rapid industrialization and change and carry out the necessary base-line studies from which change can be measured. Had Sasaki not been in the area collecting base-line data before oil was discovered, perhaps there would not have been enough time for investigators to collect such data before environmental and mental health changes began to occur.

Many investigators concerned with psychiatric epidemiology have suggested studies which support the research design we are using in our Shetland study. In the summary of the Stirling County Study, D. C. Leighton *et al.* (1963) discussed the most desirable form of research needed:

Incidence is, by its nature, a more sensitive indicator than prevalence for detecting response to variations in circumstances. If large probability samples are drawn and the same individuals re-examined at intervals, the results would have the advantage of incidence, plus a general increase in our appreciation of variation through time.

Lin and Standley (1962) agreed, adding that:

prospective longitudinal studies of a general population may be regarded as an ideal method of obtaining epidemiological data on mental disorder, provided the sample remains reasonably stable and the research design constant throughout the whole period. One great advantage of prospective studies is that they permit the collection of accurate and objective information on uniform materials, independent of histories based on personal recollection. Moreover, they diminish the risk that the observer may interpret past histories in the light of the hypothesis the study is designed to test. Prospective studies of this type can provide accurate information not only on the onset and evolution of mental illness, but also on the little-explored question of spontaneous recovery. In other words, this type of study may clarify the natural history of mental disorder. . . . Since the sample is under observation over a period, a better understanding is possible of the roles of predisposition and environmental factors in determining the onset of mental disorder. The time-lag between the onset of the illness and the discovery by the community can also be observed more accurately. A greater awareness of social changes and attitudes in relation to mental disorder becomes possible.

Mechanic (1974) has stated, 'In the near future we have most to learn from field studies of adaptation to particular stress events over time. Such involvement requires greater emphasis on prospective and processual studies'. Dohrenwend and Dohrenwend (1974b), Cooper (1973), Kiev (1972), Reid (1960), and Opler (1956) have also supported the need for prospective longitudinal epidemiological studies in psychiatry.

Even though prospective studies generally are recognized as a most desirable form of research, they can have certain drawbacks. Among potential problems is migration of the population. Fremming's (1947) success in tracing 92 per cent of his original cohort after 50 years was attributed to the fact that he selected a small Danish island as the site for his longitudinal study. This is clearly one of Shetland's assets.

The setting

There are some intrinsic qualities of the Shetland Islands that are quite desirable for a prospective and longitudinal study. First, Shetland is geographically isolated, which tends to prevent migration. A lack of housing presently limits in-migration and the local government plans to control the rate at which new houses are built. A factor currently controlling out-migration is the present economic prosperity. There has been virtually no unemployment in the islands since the mid-1960s; at first this resulted from the success of the fishing and knitting businesses, but now it is because of oil-related work. Thus, at present the endogenous population is a relatively stable one, which is necessary in a long-term follow-up study.

The homogeneity of the population also makes Shetland attractive for a study of this kind. The way of life and livelihood is similar for the majority of islanders. Most people are born and raised on the islands and as a result there is a 'collective Shetland identity'. There is a strong feeling of community and a sense of belonging, exemplified by the native dialect, music, dances, customs, and folklore (Nicolson 1972; Zetland County Council 1973; Marwick 1975).

Shetland's greatest asset for a prospective longitudinal study is the unique phenomenon that is taking place there. By 1980, Shetland will be a major receiving and processing site for North Sea oil, and the character of the islands will change from a basically rural and seafaring existence to a more industrialized one. The magnitude of the change is apparent when one considers that if Shetland were an independent country, it would be the sixth largest oil-producing nation in the world (Clark 1975). Since the oil fields are all more than 60 miles offshore, a great deal of time is required to plan and lay oil pipelines to Shetland. This, plus delays resulting from adverse weather conditions (with waves over 75 feet high and gales with winds over 116 m.p.h.) and technological problems (such as a section of laid pipeline floating to the surface), have provided adequate time and opportunity for us to collect base-line data of a medical, psychological, social, and ecological nature from which change can be measured after the oil industry is established in Shetland.

There are other valuable aspects of Shetland's unusual experiment in nature. The local government's success in getting a bill through parliament enables them to contain and control the oil developments, and by law all major oil-related industrial developments must be built in the Sullom Voe region. The Delting district, where the planned industrial complex will be located, became our target area. The Walls–Sandness and Sandsting districts in a remote are of Shetland that will not be directly affected by the developments were selected as the control area.

Because of the significant amount of oil discovered, the oil industry will be in Shetland for at least 25 to 30 years and some of the oil companies predict a much longer period. Therefore, the effects on people over a long period of time can be studied, an important factor, since Krapf (1964) proposed a time span of three generations as a reasonable 'incubation period' for socio-pathological effects of rapid social change.

Theoretical framework

Some operational definitions should precede the description of our theoretical model.

1. *Industrialization*: The use of technology and science in the production of goods and involving 'the use of complex technological equipment which can neither be owned nor operated by a single worker, extensive division of labour, formal industrial

organization, and interdependence between the industrial organization and the wider society' (Slotkin 1960). In Shetland the following aspects of urbanization will be associated with industrialization: the depopulation of rural areas, and an increased population density in settlements that provide a wider, more specialized range of goods and services, such as communication and transportation technology, energy supply and its side-effects–noise, air and water pollution (Carlestam and Levi 1971).

2. *Stressors*: Stimuli or situations thought to play a role in the aetiology of various somatic and psychiatric disorders (Dohrenwend and Dohrenwend 1974c).

3. *Organismic variables*: Those personal qualities, physiological, psychological, and demographic, that characterize the individual and that may affect the individual's response to stressors (Abdellah and Levine 1970).

4. *Environmental variables*: Those external factors, both physical and social, that can impinge on the individual and affect his or her reactions to stressors (Abdellah and Levine 1970).

5. *Modernity*: A 'syndrome' of attitudes, values, and behaviour that have emerged to reflect 'up-to-date', rather than old or traditional, views as measured by the O.M. Scale (Inkeles and Smith 1974).

The model of our *theoretical framework* (Fig. 32.1) was constructed to aid in the explanation of the effects of the industrialization process and other stressors on the health, specifically the mental health, of individuals.

Components 1, 2, and 3 in the model represent some classes of variables that could act independently or with each other as stressors for individuals in our study. For example, industrialization could produce a life change event (major change in work, e.g., leaving fishing for employment on an oil rig) which could lead, in turn, to problems in the individual's work life (role ambiguity), and act as a stressor impinging upon the individual. Each of the variables in these boxes also could act independently to produce stressors that affect the individual directly, i.e., a life event (death of a parent) need not be directly linked to the variables in component 1 or 3.

Components 4 and 5 outline the intervening organismic and environmental variables that might interact with the stressors to influence a person's response to them. For example, we hypothe-

size that positive attitudes to the oil developments will correlate negatively with symptom formation.

The relationship between the different components can be complex, with many variables interacting to influence a response. However, we believe it is necessary to attempt to measure certain of these complicated associations between variables in order to gain a better understanding of the relationship between rapid social change and mental health. The discussion that follows includes a more detailed description of some of the items used to measure the variables we are studying and the rationale for their inclusion in the interviews done in the Individual Survey.

The Recent Life Events Questionnaire and items regarding stressors in an individual's work, economic, community, and family life were included in an attempt to understand how these variables affect the relationship, if any, between rapid social change and symptom and disease formation. It has been reported that there is a significant overall correlation between increased life events and physical and psychological symptoms (Rahe 1974; Markush and Favero 1974). We are interested in examining whether the industrialization process is associated with an increase in life events and if an increase in life events also correlates positively with increased medical and psychosomatic symptoms.

The questions concerning stresses in one's work, economic, community, and family life (Component 3) were drawn from the 'Problems of everyday life' questionnaire developed by Dr L. I. Pearlin at N.I.M.H. in the United States. These items were included to try to ascertain what relationship they might have with the industrialization process, and to determine if these stressors were acting independently to influence symptom or disease formation. For example, if people living in the target area reported a significantly higher number of these problems on follow-up than those living in the control region, a case could be made that the changes associated with industrialization included a higher incidence of these stresses in their lives. However, if there is no significant difference between the rates of symptom or disease formation in the two populations, we will determine whether reports of increased physical and mental symptoms correlate with increased reports of stress in the subjects' family, work, and community life. Of course, these are merely a few examples of the numerous possible interactions that are being examined.

Also drawn from the 'Problems of everyday life' questionnaire

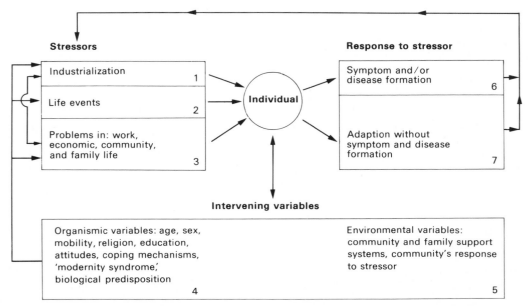

Fig. 32.1 The effects of the industrial process and other stressors on the health and mental health of individuals.

are certain items designed to measure coping mechanisms. We believe, as do many investigators (e.g. Coelho *et al.* 1974), that basic styles of coping (e.g., denial) act as intervening variables and can significantly affect an individual's response to stressors, and that it is important to attempt to measure what influence various coping mechanisms have on the formation of symptoms and diseases.

Another intervening variable to be examined is degree of 'modernity' as measured in the O.M. Scale developed by Inkeles and co-workers (1974). Data from the O.M. Scale also might help to describe the process of a change to a more industrialized community. For example, is the industrialization process associated with a shift from traditional attitudes to more 'modern' ones? If so, according to Inkeles and Smith's findings one would expect fewer psychosomatic symptoms in individuals with high modernity scores.

Another variable thought to be important in an individual's response to stressors is the person's attitudes toward the stressors (Wolff 1950; Hinkle 1974; Mechanic 1974; Brown 1974). Therefore, a ten-item scale designed to measure attitudes toward the oil developments and their effects on Shetland was developed and included in the study's interview guide.

We chose to study symptoms of psychiatric disturbance rather than to attempt to diagnose 'psychiatric cases'. We did this because we concur with Kiev (1972) that

symptoms are not only medically important; they are perhaps the phenomenon *par excellence* to be investigated cross-culturally, since many symptoms are learned, in much the same way that behavioural patterns, attitudes, and beliefs are. Many symptoms occur in individuals who are not suffering from illness and it may be possible to compare their experiences with those of others who develop specific illnesses, by clarifying in only one group the mechanism involved in the development of the disorder.

We considered several methods of assessing psychiatric symptoms, such as interviews by trained personnel as done in the Midtown Manhattan Survey (Srole *et al.* 1962; Langner and Michael 1963), and the Stirling County Survey (Leighton 1959; Hughes *et al.* 1960; Leighton *et al.* 1963), and clinical interviews by psychiatrists as done by Essen-Moller (1956) and Hagnell (1959) in their Swedish studies. We chose the General Health Questionnaire (G.H.Q.) for measuring psychiatric symptomatology, not only because it is a reliable and objective method, but also because it is economical, simple to administer, and would be easy to replicate in other studies. The General Health Questionnaire is a 60-item, self-administered questionnaire that takes only 10–15 min to complete. This questionnaire has been found to be a reliable and valid screening device to determine current symptoms of psychiatric disturbance (Goldberg 1972). Because the G.H.Q. is designed to detect symptoms only present in the past three to four weeks, we also included questions in our interview guide regarding psychosomatic symptoms experienced in the past year. This was done to try to make our measurement of symptoms more comprehensive.

Research plan

In 1973, when we first learned of the unique opportunity that existed in Shetland to conduct a longitudinal study, we went to the islands to discuss the possibility of doing such a study with local officials. We met with the directors of the health and social services and the chief executive of the local county government, as well as with general practitioners in the regions where we proposed to carry out our interviews. We discussed the objectives of the study and involved them in the initial planning. By including these individuals early in the planning phase, we formed a strong foundation of local interest and support that was invaluable when we returned to Shetland in 1975 to collect data for the base-line phase of the study.

The final research design was formulated after several meetings with Shetland representatives. That design includes two substudies, the General Survey and the Individual Survey. The General Survey involves monitoring reported data on ecological, epidemiological, and sociological change and is designed to give an overview of the general impact of the oil developments. The Individual Survey involves interviewing two populations (the target and control) in Shetland and is designed to examine individuals' reactions to change and variables associated with these reactions.

The general survey

We obtained base-line data for a 12-year period (1963–75) before the major oil developments on the following: reported psychiatric morbidity, figures on crime, suicide, and divorce, and air, water, and noise pollution levels.

Five times a year, the Kingseat Hospital (affiliated with the University of Aberdeen) holds a psychiatric clinic in Shetland. At those times, psychiatrists see individuals who have been referred to them by the local general practitioners. This is primarily an out-patient clinic but they do refer people to their in-patient service. Shetland general practitioners also send patients directly to Kingseat Hospital when the psychiatric clinic is not on the island. Thus, the psychiatric services are uniform for the entire population. When Shetland clinics are held, each person is interviewed prior to psychiatric examination, to gather demographic data and information about psychiatric and medical history. Place of birth and place of residence (one and five years previously) is also obtained, so it is possible to examine reported psychiatric morbidity for those who have always lived in Shetland, those who were not born in Shetland, but lived there more than five years, and those who have recently migrated there. Information pertaining to psychiatric treatment (both for in- and out-patient therapy) is available, including admission and discharge diagnoses and modes of treatment. An up-to-date file is kept, and each time an individual is seen a report is placed in his or her file. Records are discarded when subjects die or move out of the northeast region of Scotland, a task easily accomplished because of the centralized record keeping of the British National Health Service. These reports form part of the North East Scottish Psychiatric Case Register that dates back to 1963 and represents an accurate data base that is accessible to mental health researchers through the Research Unit of the Department of Mental Health, University of Aberdeen (Baldwin and Evans 1971). We obtained permission to utilize data from this Register and we have worked closely with the past (Dr David J. Hall) and present (Dr Peter C. Olley) Directors of the Research Unit.

Data on crime were obtained from the local and district police departments (Zetland Constabulary Chief Constable's Annual Report, 1963–1968; and Northern Constabulary Chief Constable's Annual Report, 1969–1974). Data on suicide figures came from the Scottish Registrar General's annual reports (1963–1975). Data on divorces were gathered from census reports (Annual Reports Registrar General Scotland 1963–1975). Base-line data on various forms of environmental pollution were obtained for eventual possible correlation with mental and physical symptoms and illnesses. Water and noise pollution data were provided by Douglas Smith, the Director of Shetland government's Department of Environmental Health. Air pollution data were collected from the British government's Department of Industry Warren Springs Laboratory reports (Department of Industry 1975).

The individual survey

In order to obtain base-line data of a more specific and personal nature, we conducted structured interviews and administered questionnaires to individuals living in the target and control populations. The target region was geographically delineated as the area surrounding the future oil port and industrial complex. This area also corresponded to a local political district as well as a medical region served by one general practitioner.

We selected a stratified random sample in the target region of persons between the ages of 15 and 60 years. This was done by first compiling a list of all persons on the local general practitioner's National Health Service rolls. (The Shetland County Health Board reports that at least 95 per cent, and probably more, of the county's population is registered with the National Health Service.) The total number for the 15–60 age range was 445. We reviewed the list with the doctor and excluded 47 individuals who had died, moved, or who were unable to be interviewed for medical reasons (e.g. severe mental retardation). We divided the remaining 398 into the following sex–age groups: males and females, ages 15–19, 20–29, 30–39, 40–49, and 50–59. Our initial sampling goal was 300 people from the target population. Therefore, we selected randomly from each age group the number that would be equivalent proportionally for a total population of 300. We continued selecting subjects past the needed number until they were exhausted, in order to create a random list of alternates. For example, in the 15–19 age group there were 29 males in the doctor's population of 398. We randomly selected 22 males for this age group (the equivalent number for a population of 300). The remaining 7 subjects were selected randomly and placed on an alternate list.

The control area was geographically defined as the Walls–Sandness district. This area on the west side of the mainland was chosen because in the past the way of life has been similar to that in the Delting district and its population's sex and age characteristics were similar to those in the target area. The control area has been designated as a conservation area and there are no oil developments planned for this region. There will be some indirect effects from the oil developments on this and other districts, but these will be of a very different nature from the effects on those actually living near or next to a rapidly developing industrial complex and port, with hundreds of incomers moving into the district. After compiling a list of all subjects on the local general practitioner's National Health Service rolls and excluding certain subjects as we did in the target area, we had a population of 305 individuals. We used the entire population of 305 as our sample for the control area. In order to form an alternate list, we randomly selected 131 subjects from a bordering region of the Sandsting district. The same methodology was used in excluding subjects and in randomly selecting alternates to represent an age and sex distribution proportioned to that of the entire Sandsting district.

Individuals to be sampled were then sent a letter from their general practitioner introducing the co-investigators and the other physician and nurse who assisted with the interviewing. The letter explained that we were conducting a General Health Survey that involved the subject answering some questions regarding his or her health and way of life. If possible, the study's secretary telephoned the subject and tried to arrange an interview appointment. An unforeseen difficulty in scheduling was that only 40 per cent of all possible contacts had telephones. This delayed our interviewing efforts considerably, since many hours were spent locating isolated homes to schedule interviews. It was not unusual to make several trips to contact individuals, since a substantial number were home at unpredictable times (this was especially true for working males).

Subjects who were 'too busy' working or 'not keen' to participate or who refused to participate when our secretary contacted them by telephone were put into a follow-up group for personal contact later. All these individuals eventually were contacted personally, at least once, by an interviewer who further explained the study and the importance of their participation.

Most interviews were carried out in the subject's home, to minimize inconvenience to him/her. Before each interview, the subject was given a consent form to sign. This informed consent is a requirement of the United States government to protect subjects who participate in research studies. The form explained generally what their involvement in the study would entail (i.e., being interviewed and filling out three questionnaires). It also informed the subject that all the information obtained from the interview and questionnaires was completely confidential and that all subjects would remain anonymous. Each subject received a number and his or her name never appeared on the interview or questionnaire forms.

From the structured interviews data were collected on the following subjects:

a. Demographic;
b. Mobility (number of residences in and out of Shetland);
c. Medical history (check list of illnesses);
d. Psychiatric symptoms (check list of symptoms);
e. Family medical history (check list of illnesses for subject's mother and father);
f. Use of tobacco and alcohol (quantity and frequency);
g. Social class and occupational background (including questions concerning stressors of work situation);
h. Economic status (average monthly income and questions concerning financial stresses the subject might be experiencing);
i. Educational level;
j. Religious background;
k. Community life (including involvement in community clubs and organisations, ratings of community, and changes in activity patterns over the past two years);
l. Methods of handling personal problems (support systems and coping styles);
m. Rating of family life (questions regarding stressors in marriage and of being a parent);
n. O.M. (modernity) scale (questions designed to measure traditional and modern opinions).

Questions concerning all the above were to be included in the interview, and the following three forms were given to the subject to complete at the end of the interview:

a. Recent Life Events Questionnaire (as developed by M. Horowitz et al. 1974);
b. General Health Questionnaire (developed by D. Goldberg 1972);
c. Attitude Scale (designed to measure general favourable versus unfavourable attitudes to the oil developments).

All information concerning the subjects' report of illnesses, treatment for illness or symptoms, and use of medication, was cross-checked with their general practitioner for validation (prior to signing the consent form the subject was told we would check with his or her doctor regarding only the medical questions to assure that that information was as accurate as possible).

All interviews were completed by the end of January 1976, and, with a few exceptions, each interview was conducted with just the interviewer and subject present. The total number of people interviewed was 263 in the target area and 270 in the control region. The refusal rates were 22·65 and 21·05 per cent, respectively, for the target and control areas.

People who refused did so for various reasons. The village 'grapevine' spread several erroneous rumours about our study that seemed to make some people resistant to participating in it. Most of the rumours developed from certain individual's reactions to specific parts of the interview. For example, from questions concerning an individual's financial situation, a rumour developed that we were undercover agents for the tax collectors. Another rumour was circulated that we asked detailed questions about the sexual life of the subjects. Initially we did not utilize the mass media to inform the community of our study, and retrospectively feel that was a mistake. When these rumours were at their peak, we did have an article in the local paper explaining our project and subsequently there was less resistance to participating in our study.

Others refused because they felt the interviews were too long. It took a minimum of 50 min to complete the entire interview and questionnaires; however, the average interview session was one hour and 30 min and occasionally an interview would last two or two and a half hours. These longer interviews occurred when the subject was interested in talking longer about something in the interview or discussing something totally unrelated. However, when some prospective subjects heard about these longer interviews, they were not anxious to participate and some refused because of the time requirement. Retrospectively, had the interview been shorter and taken an average of one hour, we feel that our refusal rate would have been lower. The interviews done during the first follow-up were designed to meet this shorter time requirement.

Follow-up studies

The first follow-up study took place during the summer and fall of 1978. At that time the coinvestigators returned to Shetland and collected follow-up data for both the General and Individual Surveys.

The difficulty of population migration in a prospective longitudinal study is always a potential problem, but for reasons discussed above, we believe out-migration of the Shetland population will be minimal. If, however, out-migration does take place, it will have a greater effect on the General Survey than on the Individual Survey. If an interviewed subject moves we will be able to trace him or her because we have the name of a friend or relative we can contact who will know the new address. We plan to interview as many of these subjects as possible, to determine if their move was in any way linked to the oil developments, and to ascertain their current physical and mental health status. To determine how migration will affect the General Survey, we will monitor the data published on migration from Shetland by the British Census Office.

We realize that an increase in the provision of medical and psychiatric services to the islands might improve the detection and reporting of psychiatric disorder. An increase in reported psychiatric morbidity might reflect improved detection rather than a real increase in mental disturbances. If additional physicians begin practising on the islands, there would be one way to examine the extent their practices might alter the reporting of psychiatric morbidity. The referring physician of an individual sent to the psychiatric clinic or hospital is recorded in the case registry data and, therefore, rates of referrals from Shetland physicians can be examined. We shall also carefully monitor changes in the health and social services of the island to examine how these changes might affect reported psychiatric morbidity.

The follow-up interviews will concern changes that have occurred in the individual's health and way of life since the first interview was done. The tools for assessing illnesses and symptoms will remain the same, and as in the first survey, we will validate responses with the subjects' general practitioners. We will also reassess their attitudes toward the oil developments, level of 'modernity', number of life events, and changes that have occurred in their community, family, work, economic, and social life. As a service to the participants, we plan to offer them a brief summary report of changes in their health that have developed since they were first interviewed.

Preliminary results

The following is a summary of the findings from the General Survey, and some of the findings from the Individual Survey with a focus on the prevalence of psychiatric symptoms and 'cases' in the interviewed population.

The general survey

Population. During the past century, the population of Shetland gradually decreased from 31 670 in 1861 to a low of 17 245 in 1966. With the economic prosperity of the late 1960s and the discovery of oil, the population increased to 17 327 in 1971 and to an estimated 19 069 in 1975. The female-to-male ratio has begun to equalize in recent years. The 1951 ratio of females to males was 115 to 100, in 1961 it was 109·3 to 100, and in 1971 it was 107·7 females to 100 males. This increase in the number of males in Shetland is due, in part, to better economic conditions that have allowed working-age men to stay in Shetland. The trend of out-migration was reversed in the period from 1966 to 1971 and a population increase was documented as a result of both natural increase and in-migration.

Reported psychiatric morbidity. Currently data are only available for the years 1963 through 1971 from the North East Scottish Psychiatric Case Register. Examination of Table 32.1 reveals that the total number of psychiatric patients has increased from 162 in 1963 to 219 in 1971 with a peak of 232 in 1968. One-year prevalence rates parallel these figures with a rise from 9·3/1000 in 1963 to 13·4/1000 in 1968 and then a drop to 12·6 per 1000 in 1971. On average 1·2 per cent of the total Shetland population were in psychiatric treatment during the years 1963–71. This is lower than the 2 per cent that Mazer (1976) reports in his study of psychiatric disorders on the island of Martha's Vineyard. The fact that Martha's Vineyard had a year round mental health clinic probably accounts for this difference. In Shetland, as elsewhere, women tend to utilize psychiatric services more than men.

TABLE 32.1

Total number of psychiatric patients per year and one-year prevalence rates

Years	Males	Females	Total	Prevalence rates per 1000 population
1963	77	85	162	9·3
1964	84	89	173	9·9
1965	91	96	187	10·8
1966	95	100	195	11·3
1967	101	115	216	12·5
1968	112	120	232	13·4
1969	105	114	219	12·7
1970	99	120	219	12·7
1971	92	127	219	12·6

The varieties of psychiatric disorders are evident in Table 32.2. The percentage of psychotic disorders has decreased from 35 per cent in 1963 to 25 per cent in 1971. The main decrease in the psychoses has been from the group of affective psychoses. There has been little fluctuation in the overall percent of neurotic cases, but this is a function of an increase in depressive neuroses coupled with a decrease in other neuroses. Alcoholism and the personality disorders remained relatively steady.

The proportions of men and women in the prevalence data are very similar to those found in the incidence data (Tables 32.3 and 32.4). Register data in Table 32.3 reveals that for the entire Shetland population, the number of new cases per year decreased from 71 (38 males and 33 females) in 1963 to 36 (14 males and 22 females) in 1971. There was no significant difference in the total number of first referrals for males as compared to females for the 9 years 1963–71. Among the new cases of men, more than half (57 per cent) were single and 29 per cent were married. For women, the

TABLE 32.2

Percentage of total cases by diagnosis per year

Diagnosis	1963 (N=162)	1964 (N=173)	1965 (N=187)	1966 (N=195)	1967 (N=216)	1968 (N=232)	1969 (N=219)	1970 (N=219)	1971 (N=219)
Psychoses	35	34	28	26	25	22	20	23	25
Schizophrenia*	13·5	12	13	11	13	14	12	12	14
Affective	18·5	18	11	12	10	6	6	8	7
Other**	3	4	4	3	2	2	2·	3	4
Neuroses	39	36	40	39	40	38	44	41	40
Depressive	27	23	29	28	31	34	37	36	35
Other	12	13	11	11	9	4	7	5	5
Alcoholism	5	6	5	6	4	8	6	5	4
Personality disorders†	5	7	7	4	3	3	4	6	6
Other††	11·5	13	15	17	20	23	19	19	21
Nil psychiatric†††	5·5	4	5	8	8	6	7	6	4
Total	100	100	100	100	100	100	100	100	100

   * Includes paranoid states.
  ** Includes organic psychoses.
   † Includes sexual deviation and transient situational disorders.
 †† Includes psychophysiologic disorders, special symptoms, childhood disorders, and ageing.
††† Includes not known and not applicable.

TABLE 32.3

Total number of new psychiatric cases per year

Years	Males	Females	Total
1963	35	36	71
1964	29	37	66
1965	34	28	62
1966	31	34	65
1967	27	35	62
1968	38	33	71
1969	25	29	54
1970	12	26	38
1971	14	22	36
Total	245	280	525

TABLE 32.4

Percentage of new cases by diagnosis and sex for the period 1963–71

Diagnosis	Males (N=245)	Females (N=280)
Psychoses	13	18
Schizophrenia*	7	3
Affective	5	11
Other**	1	4
Neuroses	38	57
Depressive	27	46
Other	11	11
Alcoholism	13	1
Personality disorders†	9	5
Other††	25	18
Nil psychiatric†††	2	1
Total	100	100

   * Includes paranoid states.
  ** Includes organic psychoses.
   † Includes sexual deviation and transient situational disorders.
 †† Includes psychophysiologic disorders, special symptoms, childhood disorders, and ageing.
††† Includes not known and not applicable.

opposite was true, 46 per cent were married and only 35 per cent were single. A significant sex difference was noted for referrals of widowed men and women, with almost four times as many widowed women as men being referred for treatment (11 per cent women and 3 per cent men). This is partially related to age, because women in Shetland outlive males. Table 32.4 presents a listing of the diagnostic categories by percentage of new cases (male and female) referred for psychiatric treatment during the 1963–71 period. Neurotic depression was the most common form of mental disorder among the new cases for both males (27 per cent) and females (46 per cent). Alcoholism was 13 times more frequent among males than females. Affective psychosis was twice as common among women as men, whereas schizophrenia was twice as frequent in males than females. There were no diagnoses of drug dependence made during the study period.

Suicide. There were 14 suicides (ten males and four females) in the period 1963–73, or a mean of 1·27 suicides per year. It is noteworthy that all of the female suicides occurred in the period 1970–3. The overall suicide rate equals 7·5/100 000 which is considerably lower than the rates for Scotland (9/100 000) and for England and Wales (11·5/100 000) (Kreitman 1972).

Divorce. The number of divorced people in the Shetland population increased steadily from 1951 through 1971. In the 20-year period, 1951–71, the small percentage of divorces in the population more than doubled, rising from 0·17 per cent in 1951 to 0·43 per cent in 1971. The per cent of divorced people in Shetland is lower than that of Scotland as a whole for the same period, with 0·30 per cent of the Scottish population divorced in 1951 and 0·70 per cent in 1971 (Census 1961, 1966, 1971).

Crime. Through 1975 there has been no homicide in Shetland for more than a century, and serious crimes had been absent from the Shetland society for the same period. Table 32.5 summarizes the crime reports for 1963–75 and shows a trend of increase in most forms of crime through 1973 and a marked jump in 1974 and 1975. The number of people detained in the Lerwick jail has increased from 61 in 1970, to 128 in 1973, and 313 in 1975. It also must be noted that during this 13-year period the number of law enforcement personnel also increased from 17 in 1963, to 24 in 1972, and 27 in 1974. However, the increase in crimes

TABLE 32.5

*Shetland crime statistics**

Year	Police Personnel	Class I against person	Class II against property w/violence	Class III against property w/o violence	Class IV malicious injury to property	Misc. offences	Total crimes or offences	Total juvenile offenders	Drunk driving	Road accidents fatal or non-fatal	Aliens registered
1963	17	9	11	64	1	339	426	14	6	2/56	2
1964	19	9	11	52	1	345	420	13	2	2/57	2
1965	20	16	19	53	2	350	440	10	2	1/63	3
1966	20	10	12	50	1	371	449	6	6	1/86	8
†1967	19	11	27	64	—	284	306	1	1	2/65	5
1968	19	5	23	70	3	312	413	6	6	0/62	7
1969	19	4	15	33	3	266	321	8	7	0/90	6
1970	21	22	18	94	2	316	453	3	8	4/95	6
1971	22	13	23	81	6	306	430	20	16	1/91	7
1972	24	17	25	97	3	432	578	23	16	2/117	6
1973	23	15	22	96	4	644	788	23	58	1/104	11
1974	27	13	28	206	13	1030	1303	65	67	2/105	20
1975	—	17	45	196	3	1174	1444	49	52	0/72	146

* Yearly reports from Zetland Constabulary (1963–8); Northern Constabulary (Caithness, Orkney, and Zetland) Headquarters–Wick (1969–74); and Expanded Northern Constabulary, Headquarters–Inverness (1975).
† Breath testing for alcohol started in compliance with the Road Safety Act 1967.

was proportionally higher than the increase in law enforcement personnel.

It is noteworthy that the dramatic rise in miscellaneous crimes and crimes against property parallels the period of the oil developments in Shetland. The number of aliens (mostly male construction workers) registered in Shetland also increased from 2 in 1963 to 146 in 1975 when the oil-related work was underway.

The individual survey

Generally, the preliminary results from the Individual Survey confirmed our assumption that during the base-line period both the target and control populations would not differ significantly on most of the major variables tested. The general demographic make-up was similar for both populations, with no appreciable differences in age and sex. There were few differences in the sociological profile of the two populations. The control population reflected ties to the more traditional Shetland way of life in that 50·9 per cent were still involved in crofting (small, subsistence-level family farms) compared to only 33·3 per cent of the target population and 10 per cent more control individuals (13·4 versus 3·4 per cent in the target area) had the lowest monthly family income of £50 (=$100) or less. However, the control region had fewer native Shetlanders (81 versus 88·6 per cent in the target area) and more people with education beyond secondary school (36·5 versus 22·2 per cent in the target area).

There was no statistically significant difference between the target and control population report of medical and psychiatric disorders except for those listed in Table 32.6. There was no statistically significant difference between reports of symptoms in the target and control populations except for the symptom 'feeling tired and rundown'. Here, the difference between the target population (27·7 per cent) and the control population (36·8 per cent) was significant ($p = 0·01$). The reports of the use of psychoactive and analgesic medication did not differ appreciably except for the use of tranquilizers; 6·7 per cent of the control population reported taking tranquilizers compared with 3·8 per cent of the target population, and again this was statistically significant ($p = 0·01$).

Psychiatric disturbances. Of the entire population, 64·3 per cent indicated on the General Health Questionnaire that they were experiencing no psychiatric symptoms. This accounts for the overall low mean GHQ symptom score of 2 ($\bar{x} = 1·9$ target and $\bar{x} = 2·07$

control). Women in both populations had higher mean scores than men ($\bar{x} = 2·7$ for women versus $\bar{x} = 1·3$ for men). Non-Shetlanders had higher mean GHQ scores than Shetlanders, in general, and when controlled for residence (target versus control) and sex. Further demographic analysis reveals that the mean GHQ scores were higher for divorced ($\bar{x} = 3$) and widowed ($\bar{x} = 3·6$) than for the married ($\bar{x} = 2·2$) single ($\bar{x} = 1·9$) or separated ($\bar{x} = 0·5$).

TABLE 32.6

Illnesses with a statistically significant difference in prevalence between the target and control populations

Illness	Target population		Control population	
	Occurred past year†	Occurred before 1 year ago†	Occurred past year†	Occurred before 1 year ago†
High blood pressure	5 (1·9)	4 (1·5)	15 (5·6)	15 (5·6)
Anaemia	3 (1·1)	14 (5·3)	10 (3·7)	29 (10·7)
Asthma	10 (3·8)	15 (5·7)*	5 (1·8)	10 (3·7)*

† Per cent in parentheses.
* $p = 0·05$; all other differences in Table 32.6 between the target and control region were statistically significant at $p = <0·01$ using a hypergeometric test for comparing two proportions when sampling without replacement.

Our study corroborates the findings of most psychiatric epidemiological studies (Dohrenwend and Dohrenwend 1974d, e) that higher rates of mental disturbance are associated with the lowest social class. As Table 32.7 shows, Shetland subjects in the lowest social class have the highest mean GHQ score. However, this is not an inverse relationship because those in the highest social class do not have the lowest mean GHQ scores. In addition, people with educations at the college and university level as a group have a higher mean score on the GHQ ($\bar{x} = 2·81$). However, those with less than a college education make up 88 per cent of the target and control population. Thus, while those in the lowest extreme of the socio-economic spectrum indicate the highest psychiatric symptom level, individuals in the upper extreme also report relatively high symptom levels.

From clinical studies during the development of the GHQ, it was determined that an individual who checked 12 or more symptoms

TABLE 32.7

Mean GHQ score by social class of entire (target and control) population

Social class**	Mean GHQ score	N
I Profession	4·00	2
II Skilled	1·95	150
III Intermediate	1·40	250
IV Semi-skilled	2·73	66
V Unskilled	1·50	4
**VI Unemployed, Retired,	5·04	25
Students	2·96	24
Entire population	1·99	521*

* 521 represents the number of subjects out of the 533 total who completed the entire GHQ.
** We use the British system of assigning social class, which groups the unemployed, retired, and students together; however, in our analysis we separated the students from the unemployed and retired.

could be considered a possible psychiatric case (Goldberg 1972). Table 32.8 presents the prevalence of such GHQ 'cases' as well as the prevalence of 'depression' and 'trouble with nerves' found in the illness and symptom section of the interview. The per cent of GHQ cases in the target area was 4·6 and in the control area it was 3·4 per cent; this difference in per cent of cases in the two areas is not statistically significant at the $p = 0.05$ level. When we examined other self-reports of treated psychiatric symptoms from our interview, such as: 'feeling depressed' or having 'trouble with your nerves', the psychiatric symptom level increased slightly. This increase can generally be attributed to the longer time period which the subject could report having had a symptom or illness.

Although direct comparison of these prevalence rates with those of other studies is difficult due to methodological differences, as a general reference, it seems useful to place our Shetland results in a context of those from other community surveys. Our prevalence rates are within the low range of those found in seven general practice surveys in Great Britain where one-year prevalence rates ranged from 4 to 13 per cent of the population at risk (Shepherd *et al.* 1966). Our results are lower than those found in a survey of a rural North Carolina Community where 10 per cent of the population had some 'psychiatric disorder' (Cassel and Tyroler 1961). And they are significantly lower than the 31 per cent 'impaired' found in a rural Florida county being affected by urbanization (Schwab *et al.* 1973), or the 37 per cent 'probable cases' found in the Stirling County Survey (Leighton *et al.* 1963).

TABLE 32.8

Prevalence of psychiatric symptoms and disorder in the target and control populations

Symptom or disorder	Target†	Control†	Total†
General Health Questionnaire—			
12 or more symptoms (past month)	12 (4·6)	9 (3·4)	21 (4·0)
Depression—			
symptom (past year) total	54 (20·5)	51 (18·9)	105 (19·7)
symptom (past year) treatment	11 (4·2)	16 (5·9)	27 (5·1)
Trouble with nerves—			
symptom (past year) total	21 (8·0)	27 (10·0)	48 (9·0)
symptom (past year) treatment	10 (3·8)	19 (7·0)	29 (5·4)
Trouble with nerves—			
disorder (entire life) total	38 (14·5)	38 (14·1)	76 (14·3)
disorder (entire life) treatment	22 (8·4)	28 (10·4)	50 (9·4)
disorder (past year) treatment	7 (2·7)	10 (3·7)	17 (3·2)

† Percentages in parentheses.

Summary

We have described the general methodology of a longitudinal, prospective epidemiological study designed to examine the impact that oil-related developments will have on the mental health and social order of the Shetland islanders. Preliminary findings from the first survey, carried out during the early construction phase of the introduction of oil to Shetland, have been presented. These results focus on the official reports of treated psychiatric disorders, suicide, divorce, and crime (The General Survey) as well as examining the prevalence of psychiatric symptoms and possible 'cases' in the two interviewed populations (the Individual Survey). Data from the General Survey covers the pre-oil period 1963–73, except for crime reports where data were available through 1975. The crime reports show a marked increase in total crimes during the same period the oil-related construction work began in Shetland.

Results from interviews with 533 Shetlanders indicate that during the early transition of Shetland becoming more industrialized there was no statistically significant difference in psychiatric disturbance between the target and control populations. The prevalence of possible psychiatric cases (defined as 12 or more symptoms checked on the General Health Questionnaire) was 4 per cent for the entire Individual Survey population. Some variables associated with a higher mean GHQ score are: being female, not born in Shetland, coming from the lowest social class, and having academic education beyond secondary school.

Significance

This longitudinal prospective study in the Shetland Islands can potentially furnish knowledge not previously available concerning the effects that major social change might have on the aetiology of mental disturbances. Because the social changes will be those associated with the industrialization of a previously rural community, information from the study could lead to a refinement of theories that link industrialized environments with increased mental and social disorder. Assuming a strong correlation exists between rapid industrialization and increased psychiatric morbidity, the study could provide information concerning the characteristics of individuals 'at risk' in a situation of social change. If the results indicate there are no significant correlations between industrialization and mental and social disorders, an examination of the actions taken by the Shetland government to avert such problems may yield information which could be utilized by other communities facing similar situations.

The Shetland Health Study also will add to the body of knowledge concerning the incidence and prevalence of psychiatric symptoms and illnesses. Such information would establish a broader data base which could aid in the prediction of disease development. This in turn could help in planning and providing for medical and social services.

Acknowledgements

The base-line phase of the Shetland Health Study was conducted from March 1975 to May 1976, in Shetland, and funded by grant MH26997 from the National Institute of Mental Health (NIMH) in the United States. NIMH also awarded an additional three year grant (June 1976 to June 1979) to analyse data from the base-line study and to plan, complete and analyse the results of the first follow-up study (planned for June–October 1978).

When working in Shetland, the co-investigators are attached workers to the MRC Unit for Epidemiological Studies in Psychiatry, University of Edinburgh, Edinburgh, Scotland. Norman Kreitman, the director of this unit, and his staff, particularly Jack Ingham and John Duffy, have provided valuable consultation and assistance since the inception of the Shetland project. We would also like to express our appreciation to the following individuals for their help: Albert J. Hunter, Robin and Janet Ditchburn, and Margaret Shimmin, general practitioners in Shetland, for assisting us in the Individual Survey; Peter Olley and David Hunter of the Research Unit, Department of Mental Health, University of Aberdeen for providing data for the General Survey; Gary Lapid and Barbara Weisstub-Lapid of Stanford University, for carrying out over half of the Individual Survey interviews; Rose Ray, University of California San Francisco for data analysis and statistical advice; Dorothea Leighton and Jurgen Ruesch for their encouragement and helpful comments.

33. The Berlevåg project on psychiatric morbidity (Norway)

CHRISTIAN ASTRUP

Introduction

During the years 1939–45 Bremer was the public health officer of Berlevåg. Using 31 March 1944 as a counting date, he studied the psychiatric as well as the somatic health of the population. Bremer found that 20 per cent had some kind of psychiatric disorder (Bremer 1951).

A follow-up and re-examination of the population was carried out during the years 1972–5. The project was organized by researchers from the University of Tromsø. The coastal express steamer takes 26 hours from Tromsø to Berlevåg (500 km). The plane is often unable to land during the winter storms, and one does not save much time by taking the plane (distance 700 km via Kirkenes).

The community of Berlevåg is a fishing village at 71 degrees north. During the 1944 German retreat the village was burned and the inhabitants evacuated, but after the war practically all returned. We had Bremer's 1944 list of 1325 persons, a list of persons living in Berlevåg on 31 December 1971 and on 31 March 1974. The population was stable between 1971 and 1974, and made up 1856 persons on the last list.

Methods of investigation

The project was introduced by discussions and meetings with key persons in the community. Letters were also sent to all adult persons on the 1971 list. The aim was to provide maximum psychiatric assistance. Between 1972 and 1974 three psychiatrists worked for 4 months in Berlevåg during the summers. In addition, one of them travelled monthly to Berlevåg through 1973–5. The team collaborated closely with the public health officer of the community. Altogether 13 per cent of the population consulted one of the psychiatrists.

Information about psychiatric morbidity was also collected through the Norwegian Central Register of Psychotics, registers from the psychiatric hospital in Tromsø, the public health officer, relatives of patients and key informants (Bjarnar et al. 1975a, b).

As one measure of psychiatric morbidity we have used a questionnaire—Harvard programme, 1969, health and family life survey. With minor modifications, this is the same questionnaire as described by Leighton et al. (1963). A sample of the population has also been studied with a psychophysiological test battery (Smith-Meyer et al. 1976).

Questionnaire study

During the summer of 1973 a team of students interviewed a sample of the population using the above-mentioned questionnaire. The interviewers were well received, and only 5 per cent of the sample refused to answer. The age distribution corresponded well to the population census of 1970, although men were underrepresented. The reason for this appeared to be that it was more difficult to meet with men in their homes.

Among 618 respondents above 18 years of age, 37·3 per cent complained about nervousness 'sometimes' or 'often'. Dividing the sample into those above and below 40 years of age, the latter had slightly more symptoms. Marital status, place of birth, and migrations before or after age 20, were rather independent of nervousness. Factors found to be strongly associated with nervousness were: not living with biological parents before 16 years of age, family problems, economic worries, poor health, and lack of self-confidence.

'Sometimes' or 'often' 39 per cent had to 'take it easy' on their job; 42·5 per cent had felt down or hopeless; 29·1 per cent experienced so much restlessness that they could not sit for a long time in a chair; and 30·4 per cent had used drugs to calm their nerves. Several other answers support an assumption that as many as 37·7 per cent subjectively felt nervousness.

Sleep disturbances were noted among 28·5 per cent. They were clearly associated with nervousness. Below 30 years of age 15 per cent had sleep disturbances as compared with 40 per cent in the 60–9 age group. Of the single persons, 22·2 per cent had sleep disturbances as compared with 42·7 per cent of the widows and widowers. This probably reflects the age differences. The permanently disabled showed 50·8 per cent with sleep disturbances which appears to be associated with effects of psychiatric and somatic illness. It also turned out that sleep disturbances were most pronounced during the winter. Compared with Stirling County (Leighton et al. 1963) the frequency of nervousness and sleep disturbances are rather similar.

Psychophysiological study

We studied 78 subjects using the Kenff–Rosanoff word association test, and 69 using a psychophysiological procedure. The physiological functions selected for registration were heart rate, skin conductance response, and thoracal and abdominal respiration. Seven groups of stimuli were used: conditioning, mental arithmetic, controlled respiration, habituation, a rhythm test, controlled respiration, and stress stimulation. A detailed description is given by Smith-Meyer et al. (1976). Clinically the persons were divided into four groups: normal controls, conduct disorders, neurotics, and psychotics.

An analysis of variance with groups, stimuli, and conditioning was carried out. Group differences were not significant. The conduct disorder group is rather heterogenous. Excluding it from the analysis, the group differences become significant at the 5 per cent level.

The interaction between groups and stimuli is found to be significant. With skin conductance responses, psychotics and neurotics showed signs of autonomic inhibition compared with conduct disorders and normal controls. All groups, except psychotics, showed cognitive effects in conditioning. No differences between the groups could be established for the stereotype indexes, but the Berlevåg sample appeared to have unusually high stereotype indexes. With word associations the patient groups were markedly different from controls, with most deviations in psychotics and least deviations in conduct disorders. The psychophysiological findings may be used in prophylactic psychiatry for early detection and treatment.

A comparison of word associations in samples of the Oslo and Berlevåg populations suggested that the associative network was very similar in the two populations. There are differences with regard to verbal fluency, response types and reaction times. It is unresolved whether these differences measure psychiatric morbidity or reflect a culture-dependent character of the word association test. However, the author will 'guess' that there is less morbidity in Berlevåg.

Clinical measures of psychiatric morbidity

All psychiatric patients were classified using the ninth revision of I.C.D. Before the onset of intensive field work during the summer of 1973, we registered 153 non-psychotics and 85 psychotics in Berlevåg (Bjarnar *et al.* 1975a). This count is based on Bremer's 1944 list of 1325 persons, as well as a list of persons living in Berlevåg in 1971 (1800 persons). The number of non-psychotics is obviously too small, comprising mainly the more severe states. In the 1971 population there were 41 psychotics, which gives life prevalence of 2·3 per cent compared with 2·9 per cent in Bremer's study.

Another survey of morbidity was made in the spring of 1974. This time we included all persons of the Central Register who had been born in Berlevåg, or who were resident there at the time of admission to psychiatric institutions. This increased the number of psychotics to 134. Altogether 80 per cent had been treated in psychiatric institutions, 10 per cent in other institutions, while 10 per cent were ambulant only. The number of non-psychotics was 336 in the spring of 1974. Among these, 20 per cent had been treated in psychiatric institutions, 6 per cent in other institutions, while 74 per cent were out-patients.

Among the 470 cases classified according to I.C.D., 300 persons were found in the population list of 1971. This makes up 19·5 per cent of the population, as compared with 9 per cent before the field study in the summer of 1973. The total psychiatric morbidity nearly reaches the 20 per cent found by Bremer (1951). During the field study in the summer of 1974, two psychiatrists spending one month each in Berlevåg, located only 8 new cases through their personal

interviews. This suggests that the psychiatric morbidity was already well known before field work this summer.

Our psychiatric field work has mainly been through offering maximum psychiatric assistance. Unlike other investigations such as Essen-Møller (1957) and Hagnell (1966b), we did not go from house to house to have psychiatric interviews with the whole population (although this was done with the questionnaire). In this respect our method of investigation is more like that of the Samsø study (Strømgren 1968; Nielsen 1976). An important weakness of our method is that personal interviews with psychiatrists are limited to those who are willing to consult the psychiatrists. Nevertheless, we have by now found 23·6 per cent, about the same as in the Samsø and Lundby (Hagnell 1966b) studies.

By now we have counted all persons with mental disorders on our 1974 list, exactly 30 years after the census date of Bremer. There are altogether 391 persons with mental disorders, or 21·5 per cent of the population. The population of the municipality of Berlevåg consists of 2 populations, one of 1647 persons in the proper Berlevåg fishing village and one of 209 persons living 15 km away in Kongsfjord fishing village. The latter population consists to a great extent of Finnish and other migratory factory workers who by and large were unknown to us.

The most correct method would be to measure separately the morbidity in the two communities. In Kongsfjord the morbidity was only 10 persons out of 209 in the population, or 4·8 per cent. This is obviously due to poor registration. In the Berlevåg fishing village the population is 1647 persons. They had 389 persons with mental disorders, and 47 of them were psychotics. Thus the total morbidity is 23·6 per cent and the morbidity of psychosis is 2·86 per cent. The total morbidity lies close to that of Bremer. It remains to be analysed to what extent the diagnostic distribution differs in order to see if the finer analysis suggests increases or decreases during the 30 years.

Conclusions

Preliminary findings from the Berlevåg project will be presented here. The total morbidity as well as the morbidity of psychoses is about the same in 1971 and 1974 as in 1944 and corresponds to the morbidity found in Danish and Swedish field studies. Using the questionnaire method, the morbidity rate lies close to that of Stirling County. Psychophysiological data may be used for prophylaxis and for comparisons of morbidity in different areas as in Oslo and Berlevåg. The author will guess that word associations indicate less psychiatric morbidity in Berlevåg than in Oslo.

34. The Lundby study on psychiatric morbidity (Sweden)

OLLE HAGNELL

Overview

The purpose of the Lundby study is to make a survey of the mental health of a 'normal population' during a 25-year period of life. In 1972, it had been 25 years since Essen-Möller *et al.* (1956) carried out the first population study at Lundby, which included 2550 persons. This total population was again investigated in 1957 by Hagnell (1966a, b) regardless of where the people lived. Hagnell also investigated the newcomers (1013 persons) in July 1957, and conducted both a cross-sectional and a longitudinal study. The Lundby study thus includes 3563 persons (Table 34.1).

With a cross-section date of 1 July, 1972, Hagnell and Öjesjö have again examined the persons who are included in the 1947 and 1957 Lundby studies. In all three investigations the drop-out rate has been retained at about 1 per cent. The population now consists of two main groups, one which was examined in 1947, 1957, and 1972 or up to their death, and one which was examined in 1957 and 1972 or up to their death. These two groups are analysed partly separately and partly together. In certain respects, it will also be of importance to be able to carry out comparisons between the two groups. The interviews have been carried out in the same way and under comparable circumstances in 1947, 1957, and 1972. Even

TABLE 34.1

Survey of all inhabitants in Lundby 1947 and/or 1957 (3563)

| | In Lundby 1947, (2550) | | | | | | In Lundby 1957 only, (1013) | | |
| | Men | | | Women | | | | | |
Age 1947	In Lundby 1957	Moved 1947–57	Dead 1947–57	In Lundby 1957	Moved 1947–57	Dead 1947–57	Age 1957	Men	Women
							80+	8	4
70+	39	6	57	28	5	77	70–79	7	8
60–69	63	16	33	74	13	32	60–69	11	10
50–59	88	14	14	113	11	10	50–59	43	32
40–49	158	32	10	140	34	5	40–49	55	52
30–39	138	50	4	137	40	1	30–39	84	75
20–29	86	87	7	75	53	0	20–29	65	80
10–19	105	106	2	69	113	0	10–19	69	70
0–9	147	49	1	139	69	0	0–9	169	171
Total	824	360	128	775	338	125	Total	511	502
		1312			1238				

though the investigations are fundamentally similar, the two latest were more detailed, and the investigators could profit from the experiences of the former studies. We have also had to adapt ourselves to the changes in the population over time.

One of the examiners, Hagnell, carried out most of the examinations himself in 1957, and has conducted a great part of the examinations in 1972. Essen-Möller made more than a quarter of the examinations in 1947, and a few per cent in 1957 but nevertheless, took part in the discussions concerning the cases. In 1972 Essen-Möller also participated in the discussion. In this way, the same manner of evaluation and the same psychiatric tradition has been maintained during the complete investigation sequence. Additional information from various sources has been collected all three times although the relative importance of these has changed in accordance with the changes in the population. Hospital records have been important all three times. Key informants were more useful in 1947 and 1957 than in 1972. Information from social insurance offices was more important in 1972, e.g. sick leaves, hospitalizations, pensions due to illness, economy, etc.

In the 1947 study the sample was defined such that each person was counted only once. It was a prevalence study carried out by Essen-Möller and three other psychiatrists from Lund. In 1957 Hagnell made a prevalence study of the people in the same geographical area (2563 persons), and a prospective longitudinal study that included all who had moved out of the Lundby area (698 persons). In the 1972 study only those who had been included in a previous study were included: 2828 persons were alive; 735 were dead; 1 per cent (31) had emigrated; 50 per cent still lived in Lundby; 10 per cent had moved to rural areas; 10 per cent had moved to cities with more than 100 000 inhabitants; 30 per cent had moved to other densely-populated areas.

The 1947 Lundby prevalence study

In the introduction to Essen-Möller's monograph (Essen-Möller *et al.*, 1956) he writes:

The psychiatric population study here presented is in some respects a pursuit of other aims than are usually to the fore in this field. A main principle was to attempt some sort of description of *all* inhabitants, beyond those exhibiting conspicuous mental disease and abnormality. Thus a number of minor and normal variants of personality are included into the registration, and physical ailment also is accounted for.

The idea was to study, in an unselected population, the frequency of these

mental variants, their interrelations, and their distribution by age-groups, groups of physical ailment, and, in a subsequent paper, groups of families. This type of an approach to the 'natural history' of personality was motivated by the conviction that mental differentiation is accomplished, not by the influence of human relations exclusively, but by an interaction of such influence with basic individual differences biologic in origin.

To diagnose the variants of personality in which we were interested we endeavoured to make a personal though brief interview with every person belonging to the population investigated, and succeeded in seeing 2520, or about 99 per cent, out of 2550 inhabitants.

To be sure, the task is anything but clearly limited, since the qualities offering themselves for registration are of course endless in number, and their definitions diffuse. It can hardly be expected that different investigators will attain in the matter of personality variation the same good consistency of results as is usual in works on psychosis and mental defect. And yet an attempt, at least, of this type of work would seem advisable in view of its possible usefulness to clinical psychiatry, genetics, and demography.

Essen-Möller and co-workers personally interviewed 98·8 per cent of the inhabitants of Lundby, and exhaustive information concerning some of the remainder enabled them to make an appraisal of the mental health condition of 99·3 per cent of the population. The aim of the investigators was not only to get to know whether there was or had been any mental disorder, but also to make an appraisal of the personality of each of the 2550 inhabitants. Because their interest was concentrated as much on the normal personality as on the mental deviations, we can be certain that all of the inhabitants were accorded equal interest and comparable appraisal.

In the 1947 prevalence investigation, Essen-Möller described the population from the aspects of mental disorders, normal and abnormal personality traits, somatic conditions and social characteristics.

In order to give a glimpse of what the first report contains Tables 34.2, 34.3, and 34.4 are presented.

Familial interrelatedness in the Lundby population. The total general consanguinity, up to and including degree 1/32 prevailing between any of the 2550 inhabitants living in Lundby 1 July 1947 has been studied by Essen-Möller.

Lundby 10 years later—The 1957 Lundby incidence study

In 1957, after a 10-year interval, I repeated the study. I sought out and interviewed all of those who on 1 July 1947, were registered in Lundby: 698 had moved, 1599 still lived there in 1957, and 253 had died during the decade. It was possible to interview 99 per cent of the survivors and to obtain information about all except one of those who had died.

The field studies of 1947 and 1957 were fundamentally similar, although the latter is more detailed, mine being based on the experiences of Essen-Möller in his investigation.

Lundby has a densely built-up area where 40 to 50 per cent of the population live; the rest live in the rural area. The population represents demographically that of the most southern province of Sweden concerning, for instance, sex, age, marital status, and income. Lundby has good communications; it is in no way isolated.

The data collection is based on personal investigation of the subjects and on information from other sources. Before the personal investigation, a letter was sent to each subject to explain the object of the investigation and to identify the investigator. Before the field study began, I took great pains to inform and confer with communal representatives, teachers, police, doctors, and clergymen. Through these, information was rapidly spread throughout the community concerning the aims and objects of the investigation; this helped me considerably. It was, for instance, very valuable to be able to refer to these persons should any subject want more infor-

mation about me or the investigation. Another point that I paid particular attention to at the first contact with the subject was to identify myself, whether or not this was asked for.

The object of the interview was to make a complete appraisal of the subject. The interview method largely agrees with that used in psychiatry, especially in out-patient work. However, it was somewhat more systematized and focused. Nonetheless, it was a free interview with free formulation of the questions, which were put in the order dictated by the individual case.

The interview was divided into two parts. The first followed a definite line with prearranged questions; then there ensued a period of free conversation. At the interviews, I took with me a predetermined questionnaire. This was solely to ensure that I would remember the points to cover and not to overlook anything. The questions were formulated to suit the subjects. I considered it necessary to proceed in this manner when investigating a whole population such as that of Lundby, which is rather heterogeneous. I frequently had to explain and reformulate a question. Sometimes,

TABLE 34.2

Survey of mental diagnoses, by sexes, age-groups, and investigators, 1947

Age-group	Oligo-phrenia	Pathol. dullness	Intellectual deterioration severe	mild	Personality deviation major	minor	Early asthenia severe	mild	Late asthenia severe	mild	Somatic-asth. complaints pres.	prev.	Chalarophrenia severe	mild	Asociality, alcoholic ab. pres.	prev.	Autonomic instability pres.	prev.	Psychosis pres.	prev.	Neurosis pres.	prev.	Previous asthenia
	a	b	c	d	e	f	g	h	i	k	l	m	n	o	p	q	r	s	t	u	w	x	y
Women																								
80+	—	1	5	8	4	1	1	—	6	7	12	1	—	—	2	—	—	—	—	—	—	—	2
70–9	—	—	4	9	5	13	4	3	17	10	34	5	1	3	1	1	5	—	1	1	—	3	6
60–9	—	3	—	—	10	28	13	9	34	11	47	10	3	6	2	1	18	5	4	3	3	12	10
50–9	—	3	—	—	6	33	15	4	37	21	58	18	5	11	3	1	22	6	5_2	3	3	11	19
40–9	—	—	—	—	9	41	16	6	46	24	55	12	27	11	4	—	15	10	2	2	7	15	14
30–9	4	4	—	—	7	34	15	9	25	31	46	18	36	19	3	1	26	8	—	2	6	18	23
20–9	2	—	—	—	1	24_1	12	5	16	10	26	7	24	25	—	—	8	6	—	—	3	4	12
15–19	—	1	—	—	2	10	13	5	4	1	10	2	14	25	5	1	7	2	—	—	—	1	6
10–14	2	1	—	—	1	9	11	5	—	—	10	4	23	11	—	—	—	2	—	—	1	—	1
5–9	1	2	—	—	—	2	11	3	—	—	4	5	13	10	—	—	1	—	—	—	—	—	4
0–4	1	1	—	—	—	1	—	4	—	—	—	2	2	5	—	—	—	1	—	—	—	—	—
60+	*—*	*1.7*	*3.9*	*7.4*	*8.3*	*18.3*	*7.9*	*5.2*	*24.9*	*12.2*	*40.6*	*7.0*	*1.7*	*3.9*	*2.2*	*0.4*	*10.0*	*2.2*	*2.2*	*1.7*	*1.3*	*6.6*	*7.9*
40–59	*—*	*1.0*	*—*	*—*	*4.8*	*23.6*	*9.9*	*3.2*	*26.5*	*14.4*	*36.1*	*9.6*	*10.2*	*7.0*	*2.2*	*0.3*	*11.8*	*5.1*	*2.2*	*1.3*	*3.2*	*8.3*	*10.5*
15–39	*1.5*	*1.3*	*—*	*—*	*2.5*	*17.1*	*10.1*	*4.8*	*11.3*	*10.6*	*20.7*	*6.8*	*18.6*	*17.4*	*2.0*	*0.5*	*10.3*	*4.0*	*—*	*0.5*	*2.3*	*5.8*	*10.3*
0–14	*1.3*	*1.3*	*—*	*—*	*0.3*	*4.0*	*7.4*	*4.0*	*—*	*—*	*4.7*	*3.7*	*12.7*	*8.7*	*—*	*—*	*0.3*	*1.0*	*—*	*—*	*1.9*	*5.2*	*7.8*
15+	6	12	9	17	44	184_1	89	41	185	115	288	73	110	100	20	4	101	37	12_2	10	9	17	92
	0.6	*1.3*	*1.0*	*1.8*	*4.7*	*19.6*	*9.5*	*4.4*	*19.7*	*12.2*	*30.7*	*7.8*	*11.7*	*10.6*	*2.1*	*0.4*	*10.8*	*3.9*	*1.3*	*1.1*	*9.6*	*1.8*	*9.8*
Total	10	16	9	17	45	196_1	111	53	185	115	302	84	148	126	20	4	102	40	12_2	10	23	64	97
	0.8	*1.3*	*0.7*	*1.4*	*3.6*	*15.8*	*9.0*	*4.3*	*14.9*	*9.3*	*24.4*	*6.8*	*12.0*	*10.2*	*1.6*	*0.3*	*8.2*	*3.2*	*1.0*	*0.8*	*1.9*	*5.2*	*7.8*
Investigator																								
A	3	4+1	—	2	18	42+1	27+1	12+1	48	38	77+1	32+3	26+3	14+4	7	1	38	13	2	3	10+1	24	38+2
B	—	2+1	6	5	6	62+2	26+3	7+2	46	24	76+4	18+2	32+5	19+3	2	2	21	8+3	8	3	4	19	14
C	1+2	1+1	2	8	7	43+5	22+17	17+8	59	22	87+6	16+4	45+28	62+17	3	—	29+1	12	—	1	—	17	37+2
D	2+2	5+1	1	2	13+1	36+4	14+1	5+1	32	31	48+3	7+2	7+2	5+2	8	1	13	4	—	3	8	4	3+1
Men																								
80+	—	—	7	6	1	4	—	—	1	1	3	1	—	—	3	2	1	—	1	—	—	—	—
70–9	—	—	4_2	17	9	21	1	3	4	10	26	9	—	—	3	10	3	—	—	2	2	—	3
60–9	—	—	2	8	18	25	2	1	8	17	37	10	—	2	21	18	1	5	—	3	1	8	6
50–9	2	—	—	2	10	41	4	1	10	13	24	18	5	1	23	4	9	3	1	3	2	6	11
40–9	1	1	1	1	17_1	62	3	2	8	12	33	22	2	9	19_1	12	8	4	1	4	3	8	13
30–9	2	2	—	—	15	57	4	3	7	14	31	16	5	12	17	6	12	3	—	4	4	6	12
20–9	1	—	—	—	13	40_1	6	—	4	4	19	16_1	10	27	21_1	8	5	2	—	4	2	2	8
15–19	4_1	1_1	—	—	8_1	13_1	2_1	3	—	—	12	2	16_1	17	6_3	2_1	3	2	—	—	—	1	6_1
10–14	2	3	—	—	5	6	5	1	—	—	9	5	10	11	3	2	—	2	—	—	—	—	8
5–9	2	2	—	—	3	6	4	5	—	—	9	3	10	12	4	—	—	2	—	—	—	—	8
0–4	1	1	—	—	—	1	1	5	—	—	4	—	3	2	—	—	1	1	—	—	—	—	—
60+	*—*	*—*	*6.1*	*14.5*	*13.1*	*23.4*	*1.4*	*1.9*	*6.1*	*13.1*	*30.8*	*9.3*	*—*	*0.9*	*12.6*	*14.0*	*2.3*	*2.3*	*0.5*	*2.3*	*1.4*	*3.7*	*4.2*
40–59	*0.9*	*0.3*	*0.3*	*0.9*	*8.5*	*32.6*	*2.2*	*0.9*	*6.0*	*7.9*	*18.0*	*12.7*	*2.2*	*3.2*	*13.3*	*5.1*	*5.4*	*2.2*	*0.6*	*2.2*	*1.6*	*4.4*	*7.6*
15–39	*1.4*	*0.6*	*—*	*—*	*7.4*	*22.5*	*2.5*	*1.2*	*2.2*	*3.7*	*12.7*	*7.0*	*6.3*	*11.5*	*9.0*	*3.3*	*4.1*	*1.4*	*—*	*1.4*	*1.2*	*1.8*	*5.3*
0–14	*1.7*	*2.0*	*—*	*—*	*2.7*	*4.4*	*3.4*	*3.8*	*—*	*—*	*7.5*	*2.7*	*7.8*	*8.5*	*2.4*	*0.7*	*1.7*	*1.7*	*—*	*—*	*—*	*—*	*5.5*
15+	10_1	4_1	14_2	34	91_2	263_2	22_1	13	42	71	185	94_1	38_1	68	113_5	62	42	19	3	19	14	31	59_1
	1.0	*0.4*	*1.4*	*3.3*	*9.2*	*25.8*	*2.2*	*1.3*	*4.1*	*7.0*	*18.2*	*9.2*	*3.7*	*6.7*	*11.1*	*6.1*	*4.1*	*1.9*	*0.3*	*1.9*	*1.4*	*3.0*	*5.8*
Total	15_1	10_1	14_2	34	99_2	276_2	32_1	24	42	71	207	102_1	61_1	93	120_5	64_1	47	24	3	19	14	31	75_1
	1.1	*0.8*	*1.1*	*2.6*	*7.5*	*21.0*	*2.4*	*1.8*	*3.2*	*5.4*	*15.8*	*7.8*	*4.6*	*7.1*	*9.1*	*4.9*	*3.6*	*1.8*	*0.2*	*1.5*	*1.1*	*2.4*	*5.7*
Investigator																								
A	3+1	0+1	1	9	34+1	73+4	6+2	3+2	15	17	66+6	28+3	7+3	7+3	29	17	16+1	6+1	—	8	5	15	10+3
B	2	1	9	11	21+3	81+2	3+1	5+3	12	18	46+2	27	9+2	11	34	12+1	7	8	1	2	3	9	13+1
C	2+3	1+1	2	13	20	69+4	9+3	5+4	8	23	56+7	25+1	19+10	42+18	23+1	22	12	2+2	—	4	6	3	24+9
D	2+1	1+4	—	1	14+4	39+3	3+4	0+2	7	13	17+7	13+4	2+8	8+4	22+6	10+1	7+4	3+2	2	5	—	4	10+3

Indexes denote inhabitants not personally interviewed. + = children.
Italicized numbers are percentages.

for instance, the subject replied 'No' to a question concerning whether he had ever been hospitalized. If I then had the feeling that the answer ought to have been 'Yes', I would later return to the topic and ask it in another way. The answer would often then be: 'Of course, I've been hospitalized. I was there at such-and-such a time for such-and-such a complaint.' Throughout, the subjects experienced the interview more in the light of a conversation than as a regular questioning. There are naturally disadvantages with this method. This mainly concerns the fact that the answers are interpreted by the interviewer before being written down.

Throughout the interview, the behaviour of the subjects was observed and was described with about 50 variables, for instance, the nature of the contact, the occurrence of tension, anxiety, defect, rigidity, and normal personality variants, according to Sjöbring (1973). These behaviour traits were graded. This more circumscribed description was always complemented with a free description of the subjects.

When discussing a study such as this, we must bear in mind that we are not dealing with a hospital or institution population. The contact problems of doctor and interviewer are altogether different in a field study such as this from what they are in the consultation

room of the doctor. It is most important for the investigator to be able to master his own anxiety.

The length of the personal investigation was ½ to ¾ hour. I got information about those who had died from those who knew them best and followed as far as possible the investigative method that I have just described. It is possible to obtain information about moves, cause of death, marital status, military service, number of children, and so on through the official census.

It is always hard to explain the process and quality of interviews in psychiatric epidemiological field work. At a meeting in ARNMD E. M. Gruenberg said:

I think that Dr. Hagnell has some problems in getting across to us. One is that Swedish is his native language which he overcomes pretty well. Another one is that Lund is a medical centre with a special psychiatric subculture that is highly developed. This has developed over a couple of generations so that even within Sweden some of the concepts that Dr. Hagnell uses, I gather, are not always read or grasped.

I would like to say something about his data-gathering methods. Eight years ago when Dr. Hagnell was starting his investigation I had the privilege of visiting the department in Lund and met him there for the first time. I was impressed by two things. When I asked whether I could go out on an interview with him, he was amazed that anybody would be interested

TABLE 34.3

Subjective complaints, by sexes, age-groups, and investigators, 1947

Age-group	Tics, enuresis t	Tics, enuresis pr	Sleep disturb. t	Sleep disturb. pr	Swooning t	Swooning pr	Vertigo, dizz. t	Vertigo, dizz. pr	Headaches t	Headaches pr	Migraine t	Migraine pr	Veg. reactions t	Veg. reactions pr	Spells, fits t	Spells, fits pr	Sensations t	Sensations pr	Fatigue pr	Nervousness pr	Huntedness pr	Susc. to adv. pr
Women																						
80+	1	—	5	5	1	1	7	7	4	4	1	—	—	—	—	—	—	—	15 } 34·5	1 } 6·4	4 } 11·6	2 } 9·1
70–9	—	—	14	14	7	3	26	24	11	7	1	—	3	2	1	1	1	1	23 }	6 }	9 }	8 }
60–9	1	1	19	16	7	—	33	28	27	18	6	—	9	7	2	—	16	15	40 33·6	26 21·8	33 27·7	37 31·1
50–9	—	—	33	27	5	2	33	25	31	20	5	2	14	8	6	5	10	10	46 34·3	39 29·1	44 32·8	30 22·4
40–9	—	—	30	23	5	2	26	21	34	26	16	10	16	7	4	1	8	6	47 26·3	40 22·3	86 48·0	48 26·8
30–9	—	—	16	9	10	4	19	12	36	13	17₁	11₁	26	22	7	3	6	5	30 16·9	43 24·2	77 43·3	55 30·9
20–9	—	—	1	1	8	6	7	6	23	17	9	8	14	10	3	3	—	—	24 18·8	23 18·0	35 27·3	17 13·3
15–19	—	—	2	2	5	2	2	2	8	7	3	2	7	7	2	—	—	—	11 12·1	14 15·4	14 15·4	11 12·1
10–14	4	3	—	—	4	1	4	3	7	6	1	1	—	—	2	—	—	—	3 3·3	13 14·3	—	1 1·1
5–9	4	3	4	—	—	—	—	—	1	1	1	1	1	1	—	—	—	—	—	16 15·8	—	—
0–4	—	—	1	—	1	—	—	—	—	—	—	—	—	—	1	1	—	—	—	2 1·9	—	—
60+	2	0·9	38	16·6	15	6·6	66	28·8	42	18·3	8	3·5	12	5·2	3	1·3	17	7·4	78 34·1	33 14·4	46 20·1	47 20·5
40–59	—	—	63	20·1	10	3·2	59	18·9	65	20·8	21	6·7	30	9·6	10	3·2	18	5·8	93 29·7	79 25·2	130 41·5	78 24·9
15–39	—	—	19	4·8	23	5·8	28	7·1	67	16·9	29₁	7·3	47	11·8	12	3·0	6	1·5	65 16·4	80 20·2	126 31·7	83 20·9
15+	2	0·2	120	12·8	48	5·1	153	16·3	174	18·5	58₁	6·2	89	9·5	25	2·7	41	4·4	236 25·1	192 20·4	302 32·2	208 22·2
0–14	8	2·7	5	1·7	5	1·7	4	1·3	8	2·7	2	0·7	1	0·3	3	1·0	—	—	3 1·0	31 10·4	—	1 0·3
Total	10	0·8	125	10·1	53	4·3	157	12·7	182	14·7	60	4·8	90	7·3	28	2·3	41	3·3				
Present	7	0·6	97	7·8	21	1·7	128	10·3	136	10·9	35	2·8	64	5·2	14	1·1	37	3·0	239 19·3	223 18·0	302 24·4	209 16·9
Investigators																						
A			39+2		18+1		46		46+1		13+1		32		11		16		73	44+ 2	75	42
B	+3		37		12+2		42+1		51		16+1		19		3+3		8		71+2	42+ 6	75	42+1
C	2+4		32+2		15+1		40+1		43+4		21		26+1		7		14		51	66+21	85	77
D	+1		12+1		3+1		25+2		34+3		7		12		4		3		41+1	40+ 2	67	47
Men																						
80+	—	—	—	—	1	—	1	1	3	3	—	—	—	—	—	—	1	1	1 } 17·6	—} 5·9	1 } 3·9	5 } 4·9
70–9	—	—	12	9	1	1	22	17	8	4	1	1	1	1	—	—	2	2	17 }	6 }	3 }	3 }
60–9	—	—	25	19	2	—	23	18	17	11	1	1	4	—	1	—	1	1	20 17·9	9 8·0	16 14·3	13 11·6
50–9	—	—	15	9	1	—	17	10	26	16	5	2	8	6	3	2	2	2	19 16·4	12 10·3	23 19·8	12 10·3
40–9	2	2	17	8	6	4	11	3	37	21	3	1	11	8	1	1	1	1	18 9·0	15 7·5	46 23·0	13 6·5
30–9	2	1	16	10	4	2	11	8	26	15	1	1	14	13	3	3	2	1	12 5·8	23 12·0	39 20·3	25 13·0
20–9	3	3	7	3	6	2	7	6	19₁	11	3	2	6	3	—	—	3	3	14 7·8	11 6·1	23 12·8	9₁ 5·0
15–19	1	1	2	1	4	2	2	2	7	6	1	1	3	—	2	—	—	—	3 2·6	3₂ 2·6	7₁ 6·0	1 0·9
10–14	4	4	6	5	2	—	1	1	4	2	2	2	1	1	—	—	2	1	2 2·1	6 6·3	—	—
5–9	2	1	2	1	1	—	3	2	6	6	—	—	2	—	4	2	—	—	1 1·2	5 6·0	—	—
0–4	1	1	3	3											2	1	—	—	4 3·5			
60+	—	—	37	17·3	4	1·9	46	22·4	28	13·1	3	1·4	5	2·3	1	0·5	4	1·9	38 17·8	15 7·0	20 9·3	18 8·4
40–59	2	0·6	32	10·1	7	2·2	28	8·9	63	19·9	7	2·2	19	6·0	4	1·3	3	0·9	37 11·7	27 8·5	69 21·8	25 7·9
15–39	6	1·2	25	5·1	14	2·9	20	4·1	52	10·6	9	1·8	23	10·7	6	1·2	5	1·0	29 5·9	37₂ 7·6	69₁ 14·1	35₁ 7·2
15+	8	0·8	94	9·2	25	2·5	94	9·2	143	14·0	19	1·9	47	4·6	11	1·1	12	1·2	104 10·2	79₂ 7·8	158₁ 15·5	78₁ 7·7
0–14	7	2·4	11	3·8	3	1·0	4	1·4	10	3·4	2	0·7	3	1·0	7	2·4	—	—	3 1·0	15 5·1	—	—
Total	15	1·1	105	8·0	28	2·1	98	7·5	153	11·7	21	2·8	50	3·8	18	1·4	12	0·9				
Present	13	1·0	68	5·2	11	0·8	68	5·2	95	7·2	12	0·9	33	2·5	9	0·7	11	0·8	107 8·2	94₂ 7·2	158₁ 12·0	78₁ 5·9
Investigators																						
A	4+2		44+7		8+1		31		44		6+1		17+2		5		—		36	22+ 3	29	16
B	1+1		23		11		22		40+1		9		13		2		—		28	15+ 2	47	14
C	3+2		21+3		5		31+1		44+4		2		10		4		—		30+1	24+ 6	52	30
D	0+2		6+1		1+2		10+3		14+5		2+1		7+1		0		—		10+2	16+ 4	29	17

t = total, pr = present, + = children, index = not personally interviewed. Italicized numbers are percentages.

TABLE 34.4

Other traits as observed at interviews, 1947

Age-group	Viscous, sticky W	M	Tense, restless W	M	Tired, lachrymous W	M	Hypo-, chalarophrenic W	M	Dry, brittle W	M	Torpid, indolent W	M	Primitive, rude W	M	Hypomanic, eretic W	M	Dysphoric W	M	Heavy, gloomy W	M	Less accessible W	M	Eccentric, paranoid W	M
80+	—	2	1	—	2	2	—	—	—	2	—	—	—	—	4	4	—	—	1	—	1	—	—	—
70–9	7	7	5	5	11	7	4	—	4	3	2	3	2	1	9	6	5	—	2	1	1	5	2	2
60–9	12	6	21	6	19	11	9	2	7	8	7	11	—	5	6	6	8	2	4	3	14	9	3	2
50–9	23	17	35	14	13	5	16	6	10	11	5	16	4	2	9	8	—	4	3	5	9	5	2	3
40–9	17	22	49	29	17	6	38	11	17	20	11	11	4	2	6	8	7	11	6	2	11	16	2	6
30–9	11	13	38	33	25	3	55	17	13	17	9	24	10	6	2	6	5	8	2	1	13	16	3	1
20–9	6	5	14	15	12	3	49	37	15	11	14	20	—	4	3	1	—	—	3	1	5	18	—	2
15–19	2	1	5	5	6	—	39	32	17	2	7	16	5	1	2	2	2	1	2	1	3	4	—	—
10–14	1	—	5	8	2	1	34	21	5	1	8	—	4	2	2	2	1	—	1	—	—	—	—	—
5–9	—	—	5	4	4	1	23	22	2	1	1	1	1	1	3	2	—	—	—	—	—	—	—	—
0–4	—	—	1	2	—	2	7	5	—	—	—	—	—	—	1	2	1	—	—	1	—	—	—	—
60+	19	15	27	11	32	20	13	2	11	13	9	14	2	6	19	16	13	2	7	4	16	14	5	4
40–59	40	39	84	43	30	11	54	17	27	31	16	27	8	4	15	16	7	15	9	7	20	21	4	9
15–39	19	19	57	53	43	6	143	86	45	30	30	60	15	11	7	9	7	13	9	3	21	38	3	3
15+	78	73	168	107	105	37	210	105	83	74	55	101	25	21	41	41	27	30	23	14	57	73	12	16
per cent	*8·4*	*7·3*	*18·0*	*10·7*	*11·2*	*3·7*	*22·5*	*10·5*	*8·9*	*7·4*	*5·9*	*10·1*	*2·7*	*2·1*	*4·4*	*4·1*	*2·9*	*3·0*	*2·5*	*1·4*	*6·1*	*7·3*	*1·3*	*1·6*
0–14	1	—	11	14	6	4	64	48	7	2	9	1	5	3	6	6	2	—	1	1	—	—	—	—
per cent	*0·3*		*3·7*	*4·8*	*2·0*	*1·4*	*21·5*	*16·6*	*2·4*	*0·7*	*3·0*	*0·3*	*1·7*	*1·0*	*2·0*	*2·1*	*0·7*		*0·3*	*0·3*				
Total	79	73	179	121	111	41	274	153	90	76	64	102	30	24	47	47	29	30	24	15	57	73	12	16
per cent	*6·4*	*5·7*	*14·5*	*9·4*	*9·0*	*3·2*	*22·3*	*11·9*	*7·3*	*5·9*	*5·2*	*7·9*	*2·4*	*1·9*	*3·8*	*3·6*	*2·4*	*2·3*	*1·9*	*1·2*	*4·6*	*5·7*	*1·0*	*1·2*
Age deviation	+39	+30	+14	−37	+23	+45	−224	−177	−58	−3	−33	−65	−15	−2	+46	+36	+20	−11	+6	+8	+11	−26	+11	+8
Investigator Adults																								
A	20	23	57	31	24	10	40	14	17	10	14	30	6	5	12	8	11	18	9	7	23	34	3	1
B	23	21	46	28	16	6	51	20	14	20	17	25	8	8	9	16	8	9	6	1	12	13	4	5
C	23	23	33	29	45	13	107	61	26	29	9	25	5	5	9	11	1	—	3	3	8	13	3	7
D	12	6	32	19	20	8	12	10	26	15	15	21	6	3	11	6	7	3	5	3	14	13	2	3
Children																								
A	—	—	1	1	—	2	7	6	—	1	2	—	—	1	—	1	—	—	1	—	—	—	—	—
B	—	—	—	2	1	1	8	2	—	—	1	—	2	—	1	—	1	—	—	—	—	—	—	—
C	1	—	9	6	5	1	45	28	6	1	3	—	1	1	2	3	—	—	—	—	1	—	—	—
D	—	—	1	5	—	—	14	12	1	—	3	1	2	1	3	2	1	—	—	—	—	—	—	—
Capacity																								
7	1	1	3	3	1	1	1	2	2	2	1	—	—	—	—	1	—	—	1	—	2	—	1	
6	18	21	40	39	13	11	45	33	12	25	5	9	5	6	10	9	6	18	4	1	5	10	3	7
5	47	45	101	54	84	23	139	55	57	40	29	55	10	12	17	21	16	8	17	7	37	42	6	7
4	8	4	18	10	6	—	22	10	11	5	16	30	7	2	9	5	3	2	2	4	11	12	3	—
3	—	1	5	—	—	2	2	1	—	1	4	2	3	1	5	3	—	—	—	1	2	—	—	
?	4	—	1	—	1	—	1	—	1	—	—	3	—	—	—	—	—	2	1	2	4	—	1	
Oligophrenia	—	1	0+2	1+1	—	—	—	4	—	1	0+1	2	—	—	0+1	2+2	2+1	—	—	—	1	1	—	—
Validity																								
8	—	—	—	—	—	—	1	—	—	—	—	—	—	—	1	—	—	—	—	—	—	—	—	—
7	4	7	4	5	1	4	7	1	4	1	1	2	1	4	4	5	—	2	1	1	—	3	—	—
6	23	25	21	20	22	4	55	24	15	15	5	24	6	7	14	16	4	9	7	—	8	12	5	3
5	29	24	45	29	36	16	71	41	26	22	33	49	10	8	19	11	13	13	—	6	25	35	5	8
4	16	9	58	42	25	9	52	35	25	32	11	19	5	1	1	7	6	5	7	4	11	15	1	3
3	2	8	33	9	20	4	22	3	11	3	5	3	3	1	3	1	3	—	8	2	9	5	1	1
2	—	—	6	—	—	—	1	—	—	—	—	—	—	—	—	—	—	—	—	1	1	—	—	—
?	4	—	1	1	1	—	1	1	2	1	—	4	—	—	—	—	1	1	1	3	3	—	1	
Solidity																								
7	2	2	1	1	1	—	1	—	1	—	2	—	—	—	—	—	—	—	1	—	1	—	—	
6	4	16	9	19	12	7	17	12	9	21	6	19	1	4	2	1	1	8	4	3	4	10	1	3
5	39	27	80	42	53	20	94	47	40	32	26	44	9	11	17	20	15	14	13	6	36	43	5	8
4	24	24	58	40	32	9	87	42	29	15	19	29	12	5	18	15	9	5	6	3	11	14	5	2
3	6	3	9	4	6	1	10	3	2	5	2	5	3	1	4	5	1	1	—	—	2	2	1	1
2	—	—	—	—	—	—	—	—	—	—	—	—	—	—	—	—	—	—	—	—	—	—	—	—
?	3	1	1	1	1	—	1	1	1	1	—	4	—	—	—	—	1	2	1	—	3	—	2	
Stability																								
8	—	—	—	—	—	—	—	—	—	—	—	—	—	—	—	—	—	—	1	—	—	—	—	—
7	—	6	4	11	2	—	4	8	3	20	—	7	1	1	1	3	1	3	2	—	3	7	—	5
6	9	27	36	44	18	9	50	57	31	33	17	39	3	8	5	6	2	12	4	2	11	29	4	5
5	18	19	59	32	24	9	58	24	22	11	16	29	7	6	7	11	12	9	8	3	21	23	4	3
4	31	17	44	16	39	13	71	15	19	9	15	21	9	4	13	17	9	5	5	7	14	10	2	3
3	16	4	24	3	21	6	26	—	6	—	7	2	5	2	14	4	2	—	4	1	5	1	2	—
2	1	—	—	—	—	—	—	—	—	—	—	—	—	—	1	—	—	—	—	—	1	—	—	—
?	3	—	1	1	1	—	1	1	2	1	—	3	—	—	—	—	1	1	—	—	3	2	—	—
Maj. pers. dev.	8	12	9	15	4	5+1	4+1	4+2	5	6	7	22	5	7	13	6	2	8	1	4	13	26	8	6
Sev. early asth.	10	1	21+7	4+4	19	2+1	35+18	6+6	14+3	2	4	1	4+1	—	1+2	1	3	—	6	2	3	—	—	—
Sev. late asth.	22	5	69	17	54+3	7	7	7	16	4	11	2	3	—	2	1	5	—	12+1	2	8	1	—	—
Sev. intell. det.	1	—	—	1	—	1	—	—	—	—	—	2	—	—	—	—	—	—	—	—	—	—	—	—

+ denotes children.

enough to take the trouble. He had absolutely no difficulty in having a stranger along, particularly, I suppose, because I did not understand Swedish. However, I could understand a great deal of the emotional communication that was going on between Dr. Hagnell and his subject; these were very real interviews with real interactions between two people, and if the person had anything to say he was obviously saying it. I cannot say anything about the content because I could not understand it.

The other thing that impressed me a great deal occurred when we came back to the Medical Centre that evening. Dr. Hagnell's seniors were very interested in listening to tape recordings of his interviews that I had made. They listened to them and, to my amazement, with no prior discussion, each pulled a piece of paper out of his pocket and wrote down the classification of how he interpreted that case before he would begin to discuss the interview in any way with his colleagues. The first question was: would we agree in the way we perceive this particular case? This has evidently been standard procedure in Lund for years. I mention this to you because it is hard to know the quality of an investigator's data-gathering mechanisms if one has not seen it on the ground and, having had that privilege, I thought that I would tell you that I was very deeply impressed by it.

[see Hagnell 1969].

Hospital records were used to a large extent. The entire population was compared with the record archives at the psychiatric hospitals within the region that Lundby belongs to. Practically all out-patient care in psychiatry was carried out at these hospitals. All subjects who had been admitted to Lund's Lasarett—the central hospital for Sweden's most southern province and a university hospital—were registered during the entire 10-year period irrespective of what clinic they had been admitted to. The records of these hospitalizations were investigated, mainly for the purpose of tracing mental disorders. Concerning those who had been to other hospitals, I corresponded with these hospitals and, when necessary, also with private practitioners and others who had treated the patient.

It is practical to use key informants because they can be expected to know almost every inhabitant in this relatively limited population. Doctors, police, and others who have lived in Lundby for a long time and who know the population well were used as key informants.

Non-responders have a strong tendency to distort the results in psychiatric population studies. They are selective. Persons with mental abnormalities and disorders, such as psychopaths and alcoholics, have a strong tendency to disappear in this sort of investigation. By utilizing the Swedish census, it was possible to trace the subjects; the non-responders could be kept at about 1 per cent in both the 1947 and 1957 investigations.

Problems of definition of mental disorder

Definition of what should be considered a 'case of sickness' is, according to the manual *Measurement of morbidity* (1954), not practicable because such a definition can never be appropriate to all diseases. The general intention is that it should cover the whole course of one disease in one person as far as that course is relevant to the particular enquiry concerned.

A demarcation line cannot always be sharply drawn between mental disorders and normal conditions. Practically all individuals have at one time or another felt symptoms that are 'psychiatric', such as feelings of anxiety or depression. If people are closely questioned, it is possible that 'psychiatric' symptomatology would be shown by almost 100 per cent of the population or some other percentage sufficiently high to justify doubt as to the usefulness of the definition.

A psychiatrist–examiner may be alert for psychiatric symptoms and may give such symptoms undue weight. On the other hand, he may be too aware of this possibility and attempt to neutralize the tendency, by underestimating the case.

It must be emphasized that a clinical judgement regarding the significance of certain symptoms as showing mental illness does not depend solely on the words of the interview. It is, rather, an evaluation of the totality, which includes also the proband's general behaviour and non-verbal communication, the interpersonal contact, and so on. In addition, information from other sources should be used for a final integrative adjudication. This should reduce underemphasis or overemphasis occasioned by the psychiatrist's bias.

Pugh and MacMahon (1960) state:

A common error is to overestimate the degree of certainty required in the descriptive phase of epidemiology. The aim in this phase is to make observations . . .

The existence of descriptive observations whose basis is uncertain ought not to be a deterrent in forming hypotheses if the uncertainty is known and kept in mind. If all descriptive observations capable of 'noncausal' interpretation were discarded, little raw material would be left for building any hypothesis.

Objective criteria are comparatively few. Usually it is easier to measure not the illness itself, but some incident associated with it. Such information is of a factual nature, of a 'historic character', e.g. medical treatment, consultation, report to Official Temperance Board, sick leave, absence from work, legal abortion, sick pension, EST, suicide, or divorce.

While objective and factual criteria have the advantage of being more easily defined, it goes without saying that operational definitions of mental illness based upon such factual criteria are not in every respect reliable. For example, Official Temperance Boards in some places or at certain times intervene more frequently than others do; some people seek psychiatric advice or care to a far greater extent than others do. Even here, a subjective evaluation of the cases brought to notice becomes necessary in order to justify approximate comparability.

The fact remains, as Blum (1962) and Gruenberg (1963) have stressed, that case finding methods must always be related to the objectives of the particular study. If we seek for treatable cases in a community, we should establish criteria quite different from those to be employed in a study that seeks to identify the persons in a community for whom, by virtue of their diagnosis, psychiatric services have traditionally assumed responsibility. Indeed, an epidemiological research aim that seeks to identify only poor treatment probability cases is conceivable: in order, for instance, to determine differential characteristics or to set up evaluation programmes using experimental therapies.

In this study different definitions are tried and compared in order to merge more subjective and more objective views and to be able to make comparisons with other studies.

The problem of how to arrange the collected data into categories permitting tabulation, statistical treatment, and epidemiological analysis has been so excellently discussed by Dorothea and Alexander Leighton with co-workers (D. Leighton *et al.* 1963; A. Leighton *et al.* 1963, 1964) that all work in this field must be influenced by their views.

Different aspects of the concept of mental disorder can be registered. The following description follows mainly that of the Leightons:

Symptom pattern. This is a purely phenomenological grouping of symptoms in different patterns and has no aetiological or causal significance.

Degree of impairment may vary according to:

a. The individual's conscious feeling of stress and insufficiency;
b. The observation powers of the relatives who live with the proband, or those of the doctor consulted;
c. The extent of incapacity—primarily work incapacity;
d. The ease with which the symptoms can be identified as psychiatric symptoms.

Degree of certainty of psychiatric symptomatology. This is based on the investigator's feeling of certainty that what he has registered is really a psychiatric case. Uncertainty as to whether it is psychiatric symptomatology may depend upon (*a*) vague symptomatology and (*b*) inadequate information. The degree of certainty was subdivided as follows:

A=Absolutely certain or almost certain psychiatric symptomatology.
B=Symptomatology may be of psychiatric origin.
C=Cannot be entirely excluded as psychiatric symptomatology.
D=No psychiatric symptomatology.

In the present study, however, the cases came almost exclusively under subdivisions A and D. The few that could be listed under B and C were therefore also referred to A or D. It was similar in the Leightons' own studies. They found that when more information was procured more cases could be listed under A or D.

Duration. The length of time the mental decompensation has lasted.

Mental morbidity during the decade 1947–57

The morbidity in the population during the 10-year period can be described in various ways. It is possible, as I have shown here, to calculate incidence of mental disorder during the 10-year period for those who have never before been mentally ill. This makes it possible to calculate the expected illness risk.

It is, of course, also possible to calculate the incidence of mental illness during the 10-year period irrespective of whether the subjects were ill or healthy before 1947. The annual incidence can be calculated and a measure of the average annual incidence during the 10-year period obtained. Various episodes of disorder can be used, and it is possible to show how the incidence varies for different disorders and for persons with different characteristics in the base-line period, 1947. This gives us a picture of the dynamics in the incidence of the disorders..

The meaning of a case of mental disorder in a population study such as this must depend upon the purpose of the study. To be able to compare one's own study with other morbidity studies and to get a better perspective of one's own study, it is of value to take into account the morbidity in the total population not merely through one index of mental disorder, but through a set of indices, each based on different definitions of what is meant by a 'case of mental illness'.

As indicators of a 'case of mental disorder', I have chosen:

(1) admittance to psychiatric hospital (psychiatric clinic or mental hospital);
(2) visit to psychiatrist;
(3) my diagnosis of mental illness (my diagnosis of mental illness is based on my interpretation of the case through information from various sources).

The incidence and expectancy of mental disease

In the calculation of risk, I have used as a basis the part of the population that was not then ill or had not been ill before 1 July, 1947. The figures are then corrected for the time that those who had died were not observed.

In Figure 34.1, the risk of falling ill is illustrated by three different indicators of mental disorder.

Concerning the definition 'admitted to mental hospital for the first time during the 10-year period', there is a peak in the age group of 30 to 39 years. Concerning the definition 'consulted a psych-

iatrist for the first time during the 10-year period', there is a peak in the earlier middle age.

How many cases of mental illness are found if a psychiatrist investigates an entire 'normal' population? Figure 34.1 shows that the incidence of mental disorder by this latter criterion far exceeds the two previous ones. It can be seen that the peak already there by the two previous definitions shows here also in somewhat earlier middle age. The figure shows that onset occurs in many in the 20- to 30-year ages. Most of the cases here are neuroses.

Figure 34.1 also shows that there is another peak; this is to be found in the older age groups and is mental disorder associated with ageing. Many old persons are ill, but few are admitted to mental hospitals or cared for by psychiatrists. Social criteria play a large role in the selection of those admitted to mental hospitals. In the mental hospital in the region, there is a preponderance of unmarried old people. In the corresponding normal population, this is not so.

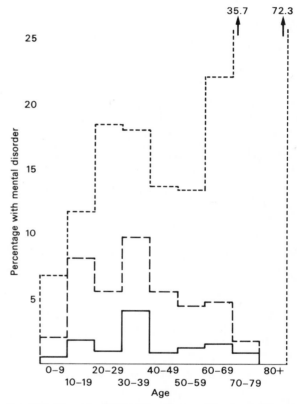

FIG. 34.1. The risk of falling ill as illustrated by three different indicators of mental disorder: (-----) the author's diagnosis of mental illness; (– – –) consulted a psychiatrist; (——) admitted to a psychiatric hospital.

With the aid of the incidence figures, a calculation of disease expectancy (Table 34.5) can be made. In that event, a fictive or artificial population must be created by combining all of the observed 10-year groups into one single generation. It must be assumed that a generation of newborns lives to an old age and that the fictive generation thus created is subject to the same influences, as far as variation of the disorders is concerned, as occur during the 10-year period observed here. The method that I employed to carry out this procedure can best be illustrated by Hardy–Weinberger morbidity tables.

Fuller explanations of the headings and procedures in Table 34.5 follow:

Column a. Age at cross-section date 00:00 hrs between 30 June and 1 July 1947.

TABLE 34.5

Method for calculation of disease expectancy

a Age (1947)	b Census population (1947)	c Persons who did not consult a psychiatrist before 1 July 1947	d Persons who did not consult a psychiatrist before 1 July 1947 × 10	e Obs. years lost through death (1947–57)	f Total exposure in person years	g No. of persons observed during 10-year period	h Consulted a psychiatrist (1947–57)	i Rate 10-year (observed incidence rates)	k Complement of 10-year rate	l The cumulated likelihood of remaining healthy Q	m Estimated cumulated risk of becoming ill
80+	20	20	200·0	−104·0	= 96·0	9·60	0	0·00000	1·00000	0·70403	0·29597
70–9	82	82	820·0	−180·5	= 639·5	63·95	2	0·03127 ± 0·02176	0·96873	0·70403	0·29597
60–9	112	107	1070·0	−141·5	= 928·5	92·85	3	0·03231 ± 0·01834	0·96769	0·72676	0·27324
50–9	116	108	1080·0	−56·5	= 1009·5	100·95	6	0·05944 ± 0·02352	0·94056	0·75103	0·24897
40–9	200	196	1960·0	−45·0	= 1915·0	191·50	8	0·04178 ± 0·01445	0·95822	0·79849	0·20151
30–9	192	184	1840·0	−9·5	= 1830·5	183·05	11	0·06009 ± 0·01756	0·93991	0·83331	0·16669
20–9	180	172	1720·0	−13·5	= 1706·5	170·65	6	0·03516 ± 0·01396	0·96484	0·88658	0·11342
10–19	213	212	2120·0	−22·5	= 2097·5	209·75	13	0·06198 ± 0·01665	0·93802	0·91889	0·08111
0–9	197	197	1970·0	−8·5	= 1961·5	196·15	4	0·02039 ± 0·01009	0·97961	0·97961	0·02039
Total	1312	1278	12 780·0	−589·0	= 12 191·0	1219·10	53	0·04347 ± 0·00584			

Column b. Census population, 1947. Number of inhabitants in the area at cross-section date, 1947.

Column c. Number of persons who have not consulted a psychiatrist before the cross-section date, 1947.

Columns d, e, and f. Correction for those who died and, therefore, were not observed for the entire 10-year period. The total number of years, reduced by the number of years lost through death. Years lost for other reasons (individuals not traced) were not subtracted; their number is very small.

Column g. The corrected number of observation years divided by 10, *i.e.*, the number of persons observed during one decade.

Column h. Number of individuals who consulted a psychiatrist during the time 1 July 1947, and 30 June 1957.

Column i. Refers to the risk an individual in a certain age group runs of becoming ill during a 10-year period.

Column k. The complement of the 10-year risk, one minus *i*; that is to say, the risk of not falling ill, in other words, of remaining mentally healthy.

Column l. Of the number in a given 10-year period, a certain proportion remains healthy after 10 years of observation (= *k*). This part, now 10 years older, is presumed to form the basis of the next age group and after a further 10-year observation to be reduced by the number observed to fall ill; that is to say, the *k*-value in that age group. Thus, a successive multiplication of the values in column l by the values in column k from the youngest to the oldest age group gives the number of completely healthy who remain of a thus 'created' generation of newborns.

Column m. Each of these successive products is again reduced from one: thus, we get the calculated cumulative risk of becoming ill; that is to say, the risk that is run up to a certain age or throughout life of falling ill.

Table 34.6 shows the risk during a 10-year period of being admitted for the first time to a psychiatric hospital. The observed incidence, all ages, during the 10 years is 1·4 per cent for men and 2·1 per cent for women. If the cumulative risk is calculated, it is found that throughout life it amounts to 10·8 per cent for men and 18·6 per cent for women.

Table 34.7 shows the risk during a 10-year period of consulting a psychiatrist for the first time. The 10-year incidence is 4·3 per cent for men and 7·1 per cent for women. If the cumulative risk is calculated, 29·6 per cent is obtained for men and 42·0 per cent for women.

If we include all who have had some kind of mental disorder for the first time during the 10-year period (a disorder diagnosed by me), the 10-year incidence is 11·4 per cent for men and 20·3 per cent for women. As mental illness I have only included conditions which are acute, defined, and pronounced as to symptoms and onset. They must also indicate a disease or a deviation from the patient's usual mental capability and capacity for work. They must affect him as real suffering and reduce his general psychophysical

TABLE 34.6

The rate during a 10-year period of admittance to psychiatric hospital for the first time

Age (1947)	Number of persons with no previous admittance to psychiatric hospital (1 July 1947)	N	First time in psychiatric hospital (1947–57) Mental hospital + psychiatric department	Rate 10-year	Estimated cumulated risk
Men					
80+	20 (9·60)	0	(0+0)	0·000	0·108 ± 0·027
70–9	82 (63·95)	1	(1+0)	0·016	0·108
60–9	108 (93·85)	1	(0+1)	0·011	0·093
50–9	111 (104·60)	2	(0+2)	0·019	0·084
40–9	197 (192·50)	2	(0+2)	0·010	0·066
30–9	187 (184·10)	6	(3+3)	0·033	0·056
20–9	175 (173·65)	0	(0+0)	0·000	0·024
10–19	212 (209·75)	4	(2+2)	0·019	0·024
0–9	197 (196·15)	1	(0+1)	0·005	0·005
Total	1289 (1229·15)	17	(6+11)	0·014	
Women					
80+	35 (16·05)	0	(0+0)	0·000	0·186 ± 0·027
70–9	73 (48·05)	0	(0+0)	0·000	0·186
60–9	110 (97·50)	2	(2+0)	0·021	0·186
50–9	128 (123·25)	1	(0+1)	0·008	0·168
40–9	171 (168·60)	5	(2+3)	0·031	0·161
30–9	172 (171·35)	9	(2+7)	0·055	0·135
20–9	125 (125·00)	3	(1+2)	0·025	0·084
10–19	181 (181·00)	3	(1+2)	0·017	0·061
0–9	208 (208·00)	1	(0+1)	0·005	0·045
Total	1203 (1139·80)	24	(8+16)	0·021	

well-being, which often forces him to consult a doctor. As to the dividing line between neurosis and psychosis, stress was laid essentially on the presence or absence of insight. Psychosomatic conditions, alcoholism, and mental retardation are not counted as mental decompensation states in this part of the analysis. The cumulative risk is 43 per cent for men up to 60 years of age, whereas it is 73 per cent for women.

In Tables 34·8 and 34·9, I have made a space between the age groups 50 to 59 and 60 to 69. The figures are uncertain for these higher age groups. There are mainly two reasons for this: partly, it

TABLE 34.7

The rate during a 10-year period of consulting a psychiatrist for the first time

Age (1947)	Persons who in 1947 had never consulted a psychiatrist		Consulted a psychiatrist (1947–57)		Rate 10-year	Estimated cumulated risk
			a	In-patient + out-patient		
Men						
80+	20	(9·60)	0	(0+0)	0·000	0·296 ±0·039
70–9	82	(63·95)	2	(1+1)	0·031	0·296
60–9	107	(92·85)	3	(1+2)	0·032	0·273
50–9	108	(101·60)	6	(2+4)	0·059	0·249
40–9	196	(191·50)	8	(2+6)	0·042	0·202
30–9	184	(183·05)	11	(6+5)	0·060	0·167
20–9	172	(170·65)	6	(0+6)	0·035	0·113
10–19	212	(209·75)	13	(4+9)	0·062	0·081
0–9	197	(196·15)	4	(1+3)	0·020	0·020
Total	1278	(1219·05)	53	(17+36)	0·043	
Women						
80+	35	(16·90)	0	(0+0)	0·000	0·420 ± 0·037
70–9	72	(47·05)	0	(0+0)	0·000	0·420
60–9	107	(94·50)	6	(2+4)	0·063	0·420
50–9	127	(122·25)	4	(1+3)	0·033	0·380
40–9	170	(167·60)	12	(5+7)	0·072	0·360
30–9	171	(170·35)	24	(9+15)	0·141	0·310
20–9	123	(123·00)	11	(3+8)	0·085	0·197
10–19	181	(181·00)	19	(3+16)	0·105	0·122
0–9	208	(208·00)	4	(1+3)	0·019	0·019
Total	1194	(1130·65)	80	(24+56)	0·071	

can be difficult to decide whether it is really a first time onset (a senile man can easily have forgotten a depression in his youth); partly, the large non-response occasioned by the death of observed subjects can to some extent distort the figures. If the highest age groups are included, a cumulative risk of more than 90 per cent is obtained for both men and women. The figures are high, but we must bear in mind two points: the possibility of a newborn remaining healthy throughout a long life and the inclusion of slight mental disorders.

We can restrict ourselves to the inclusion of ill persons who are moderately or severely impaired. If only severe mental disorders are included—severe depressions, psychosis, pronounced neuroses—which have been profoundly serious for the affected person, we get a 10-year incidence of 3·1 per cent for men and 4·0 per cent for women (Table 34.8 and 34.9). The cumulative risk up to 60 years of age is almost 8 per cent for men, somewhat more than 15 per cent for women.

Women have a greater morbidity than men by all of the criteria of mental disorder that I have employed in this study. With the criterion 'my diagnosis of mental illness', some of the differences are due to the fact that the definition chiefly contains so-called mental decompensation states and not those conditions such as alcoholism, psychosomatic illness (such as peptic ulcer, myocardial infarction), and certain forms of acting out which are more common in men than women. However, even if these are also included, there is still a greater morbidity for women than men.

Description of the diagnostic groups used in this study

Since the various types of mental illnesses merge into one another, only the most prominent symptoms will be described here.

1 and 2. Anxiety. The main symptom in this group is anxiety, a feeling of danger, disaster, dissolution, and the feeling of 'being blown to bits'. The cause of this anxiety is unknown to the patient, and he feels helpless against it.

In addition to more or less long-standing anxiety, the patient has anxiety attacks. They are often delimited, and a type of panic reaction in which the patient clings to a member of his family. The anxiety attacks are often accompanied by cardiac symptoms: tachycardia, nervous sensations around the heart, feelings of suffocation, sensations or pain in the chest, dizziness, feelings of fainting, anxiety often described by the patient as 'death anxiety', and fear of dying from heart trouble. The patient also suffers from anxiety feelings in the epigastrium, diarrhoea, frequent urination, fear of serious illness, e.g. malignant tumours and symptoms that usually come from organs from which there is normally a certain degree of sensation: heart, lungs, stomach; not from 'mute' organs. The patient may suffer from restlessness and sleep difficulties: may often wake up at night with anxiety, although the anxiety may come at any time.

1. Anxiety is a prominent symptom in the case history. More acute anxiety is episodically demarcated without any prominent

TABLE 34.8

Degree of impairment, men. Rate of contracting a mental illness for the first time during the 10-year period 1947 to 1957

Age (1947)	Persons at risk; without known mental illness before 1947		Mild + Medium + Severe			Medium + Severe			Severe		
	N	After correction for deaths	*N*	Persons without known mental illness before 1947	Estimated cumulated risk	*N*	Persons without known mental illness before 1947	Estimated cumulated risk	*N*	Persons without known mental illness before 1947	Estimated cumulated risk
80+	16	(8·40)	6	0·714	0·916 ± 0·047	6	0·714	0·869 ± 0·073	4	0·476	0·647 ± 0·119
70–9	74	(56·90)	21	0·369	0·707	17	0·299	0·538	12	0·211	0·326
60–9	96	(82·95)	15	0·181	0·536	13	0·157	0·342	6	0·072	0·146
50–9	98	(92·30)	10	0·108	0·434 ± 0·036	9	0·098	0·226 ± 0·035	3	0·013	0·079 ± 0·023
40–9	176	(172·25)	11	0·064	0·365	4	0·023	0·135	2	0·012	0·048
30–9	172	(171·05)	17	0·099	0·322	8	0·047	0·115	3	0·018	0·037
20–9	165	(163·70)	21	0·128	0·247	2	0·012	0·071	0	0·000	0·020
15–19	110	(108·70)	9			2			1		
10–14	96	(95·05)	0	0·074	0·136	4	0·029	0·060	2	0·015	0·020
0–9	193	(192·15)	13	0·068	0·068	6	0·031	0·031	1	0·005	0·005
Total	1196	(1143·45)	129	0·113		71	0·062		34	0·030	

TABLE 34.9

Degree of impairment, women. Rate of contracting a mental illness for the first time during the 10-year period 1947 to 1957

Age (1947)	Persons at risk; without known mental illness before 1947		Mild + Medium + Severe			Medium + Severe			Severe		
	N	After correction for deaths	N	Persons without known mental illness before 1947	Estimated cumulated risk	N	Persons without known mental illness before 1947	Estimated cumulated risk	N	Persons without known mental illness before 1947	Estimated cumulated risk
80+	30	(15·10)	11	0·728	0·964 ± 0·016	7	0·464	0·800 ± 0·054	4	0·265	0·524 ± 0·083
70–9	68	(43·80)	14	0·320	0·866	12	0·274	0·626	7	0·160	0·352
60–9	89	(78·65)	21	0·267	0·802	14	0·178	0·485	7	0·089	0·229
50–9	103	(99·25)	16	0·161	0·730 ± 0·026	5	0·054	0·374 ± 0·038	2	0·020	0·154 ± 0·030
40–9	147	(145·80)	33	0·226	0·679	15	0·103	0·341	8	0·055	0·136
30–9	148	(147·35)	40	0·271	0·585	18	0·122	0·265	8	0·054	0·086
20–9	117	(117·00)	31	0·265	0·430	11	0·094	0·163	2	0·017	0·034
15–19	89	(89·00)	19			6			2		
10–14	90	(90·00)	11	0·168	0·224	6	0·067	0·076	1	0·017	0·017
0–9	206	(206·00)	14	0·068	0·068	2	0·010	0·010	0	0·000	0·000
Total	1087	(1031·95)	210	0·204		96	0·093		41	0·040	

psychiatric symptomatology. Often attacks of cardiac anxiety, 'death anxiety', and feelings of suffocation. (*anxiety*)

2. Anxiety as a prominent symptom and in addition other psychiatric symptoms such as depressive. (*anxiety + other*)

3, 4, and 5. Tiredness. Nervous fatigue, low threshold for fatigue, wearies quickly, feels weak and worn out. Tendency for headaches 'like a pressure or band around the head and pain in the neck'. Subjective memory difficulties, owing to reduced ability to concentrate, but without such objective signs as found in organic syndromes. Hypochondriac sensations and imaginings. Insomnia is often prominent. Irritability and a certain degree of tearfulness, feelings of displeasure, vagueness, general feelings of disinclination, feelings of being stressed, of being overworked, lack of energy, feeling of tension, inadequate ability to relax, trembling, and shaking. The last-mentioned symptoms, of course, merge into those labelled 'anxiety', but there are no attacks, and tiredness is the dominant symptom. There is often a multitude of different symptoms, but many men complain about epigastric pain.

3. The nervous fatigue is by far the dominant symptom. (*tiredness*)

4. Nervous fatigue together with other psychiatric symptoms such as anxiety. (*tiredness + other*)

5. Nervous fatigue present with psychosomatic symptoms in the shape of epigastric pain. (*tiredness +stomach nerves*)

6 and 7. Depression. Lowered mood, depressive feelings, tendency to guilt feelings, gloomy outlook, reduced activity, reduced self-esteem, lowered enjoyment of life and feeling of low vitality, anxiety, fear, terror, lack of initiative. Has more difficulty than usual, and unable to carry out his daily responsibilities. Many patients continue their usual work; however, the symptoms become an increasing strain and the work suffers. Sometimes retardation is present. Pertaining to daily rhythm the patient is worse in the morning and better towards evening. Often he has sleep disturbances and wakes up early in the morning. Loss of appetite and weight.

6. This depressive syndrome is well demarcated without other more prominent psychiatric symptoms. (*depression*)

7. Depression occurs with other psychiatric symptoms. (*depression + other*)

8 and 9. Mixed neurotic symptoms. A number of cases fall under this heading that do not fit in with those described above.

8. Mixed neurotic symptoms. No symptom is especially dominant. (*mixed neurosis*).

9. Mixed neurotic symptoms that involve the personality to a deeper degree. (*mixed neurosis 'deeper'*)

10. Neurotic symptoms + somatic illness. Includes cases that are somatically and psychiatrically ill at the same time. The somatic illnesses are of a serious nature. (*neurosis + somatic illness*).

11. Child neurosis. Nervous symptoms in a patient under 15 years of age. They often have a history of behaviour disturbances. (*child neurosis*)

12. Schizophrenia. Follows Bleuler's concepts of schizophrenia. This classification is reserved for psychoses marked by a strong tendency to retreat from reality, by inappropriate emotional reactions, unpredictable disturbances in stream of thought, regressive behaviour, and often, by a tendency to 'deterioration'. These symptoms are present in the absence of confusion, depression, or mania and without distinct evidences of psychogenic or somatic origin. (*Schizophrenia*)

13. Other psychoses. These are not so frequent in this population and have therefore been collected in one group. Examples: confusions, paranoia, borderline psychosis, psychogenic psychosis. No manic states were diagnosed, otherwise they would have been included here. Depressive psychoses (three) are classified in groups 6 and 7, Depressions. (*other psychoses*)

14. Organic syndrome. Reduced comprehension and alertness, memory difficulties and slower reactions, rigidity in thinking, concentration difficulties, lowered ability to separate the important from the unimportant, tendency toward concrete behaviour, emotional and affective lability, irritability, and lack of emotional gradation. The patient may also suffer from headaches, vertigo, increased fatigueability, and hypersensitivity to light and warmth. (*organic syndrome*)

15 and 16. Pathological ageing. Includes all patients with psychiatric symptomatology who were 60 years of age 1 July, 1947.

15. Senile neuroses. Patients with psychiatric symptoms who

were over 60 years of age 1 July 1947, and where the patient had insight into his illness. (*senile neurosis*)

16. Senile psychoses. Patients with psychiatric symptoms who were over 60 years of age 1 July 1947, and who had no insight into their illness. (*senile psychosis*)

Groups 1–14 are patients who had not had their 60th birthday before 1 July 1947. Alcoholics have been grouped separately and are not included in the above-mentioned groups if the patient does not have a symptomatology of the above described kind at the same time as his alcoholism.

If the population is distributed into diagnostic groups, it is found that mental decompensation states with tiredness and anxiety are very common, particularly among women (Table 34.10).

TABLE 34.10

Cumulative risk up to 60 years of age for various diagnostic categories of mental illness

	Men	Women
Anxiety	0·058 ± 0·018	0·153 ± 0·028
Anxiety + other	0·022 ± 0·011	0·073 ± 0·022
Tiredness	0·042 ± 0·015	0·188 ± 0·025
Tiredness + other	0·006 ± 0·006	0·117 ± 0·021
Tiredness + 'nervous stomach'	0·071 ± 0·022	0·048 ± 0·020
Depression	0·050 ± 0·048	0·097 ± 0·036
Depression + other	0·028 ± 0·014	0·105 ± 0·025
Mixed neurosis	0·060 ± 0·020	0·118 ± 0·027
Mixed neurosis (severe)	0·011 ± 0·008	0·093 ± 0·079
Neurosis + somatic illness	0·039 ± 0·018	0·052 ± 0·019
Schizophrenia	0·021 ± 0·011	0·007 ± 0·002
Other psychoses	0·011 ± 0·011	0·028 ± 0·014
Organic syndrome	0·054 ± 0·021	0·014 ± 0·010

On the whole, there is a preponderance of women in the neurosis groups, conspicuously mixed neuroses, anxiety, tiredness, and depression. Schizophrenics, rather few for a study of this proportion, are around 1 per cent. Organic syndromes have a preponderance among men.

The frequency of strokes is about the same in both sexes. Of 26 men with strokes, 12 had pronounced mental symptoms, with confusion and delusion, whereas of 21 women, only four suffered in that respect. This was a significant difference between the two sexes ($p < 0·01$). These findings support Gruenberg's (1961) hypothesis that severe mental illnesses in men are often combined with arteriosclerosis. So far, I have reported about the risk of having an onset of mental illness for the population in its entirety.

A discussion of the extent to which mental diseases have developed in various subgroups in the part of the population that was judged healthy in 1947 follows. This concerns demographic groups, subjective complaints, observed personality traits, and somatic conditions.

Table 34.11 is one of the tables on which are based larger survey tables concerning predisposing factors. In this example from 1947, most of the women are housewives whose husbands are skilled industrial workers.

The headings on these tables refer to the following:

Age in 1947;
Persons at risk (number of persons observed for 10 complete years with the characteristic in question, e.g. skilled workers). Correction for mortality gives the figures with decimal point;
E = The number of expected cases of mental disease in this group if the frequency were the same as for the entire investigated population;

TABLE 34.11

Incidence rates of mental diseases in the group 'skilled worker, artisan, etc.'

Age (1947)	Men Persons at risk	E	O	Crude average annual incidence	Women Persons at risk	E	O	Crude average annual incidence
50–9	11·15	1·1	1	0·010	10·75	1·7	3	0·028
40–9	33·95	1·8	3	0·009	29·00	6·4	8	0·028
30–9	39·65	3·9	6	0·015	37·00	10·0	16	0·043
20–9	41·55	4·8	6	0·014	20·00	5·3	8	0·040
15–19	31·00	2·3	1	0·003	11·00	2·1	4	0·036
15–59	157.30	13·9	17	0·011	107·75	25·5	39	0·036
O/E		1·2				1·5		
CR		N.S.				3·42; $p < 0·001$		

O = The number actually observed who suffered an onset of mental disease during the 10-year period;
O/E = The quotient observed: expected;
Crude average annual incidence (number of persons observed to number of persons at risk divided by 10). Possible statistical differences, e.g. in the condition between skilled workers and unskilled workers, have been calculated with regard to age. It is expressed with a critical ratio CR: for example, for women skilled workers, the CR = 3·42 gives p < 0·001.

Table 34.12 shows the risks of falling ill in various demographic groups. In the upper part of the table, occupations are listed; there is a significant risk for skilled workers but not for any other occupational groups. The figure for farmers is possibly somewhat low. No differences can be found for economic groups, contrary to most other population studies.

The number who were married somewhat exceeds the unmarried, although it is more usual to find more unmarried among the mentally ill. It must be remembered, however, that this latter refers solely to severe conditions. Here, it also concerns a large group of slightly affected persons.

Women who still live in Lundby or who have moved to a rural district or to a town of less than 100 000 inhabitants are not subject to any increased risk, unlike those who have moved to a town of more than 100 000 inhabitants. Among the latter, there are 50 per cent more mentally ill than expected. Concerning men, the risk of falling ill is already manifest among those who have moved to a town of more than 10 000 inhabitants.

Those with certain forms of subjective complaints (Table 34.13), but not necessarily ill in 1947, have a worse prognosis. This is the case with somatic-asthenic complaints: that is to say, sleep disturbances, headaches, and vertigo. This also applies to headaches alone and migraine alone.

The lower part of Table 34.13 lists the mental complaints. Fatigue is found among both men and women, whereas nervousness and 'huntedness' (being compulsively driven, people who cannot relax) is found more in women than in men.

This is what the subjects reported in 1947. Table 34.14 shows traits that the investigators observed in 1947.

The absence of lesional traits, lesional in the sense of the Sjöbring (1973) psychology, has a good prognostic significance.

For those judged chalarophrenic—a subgroup of Sjöbring's lesions—the prognosis is unfavourable. Here, I wish to call to mind that Nyman (1952), as well as Nilsson and Smith (1962), have shown that the occurrence of chalarophrenia is related to a prolonged electroencephalogram rhythm.

Sjöbring's normal variances have in many instances proved to have significance for somatic and psychosomatic disorders (Table

TABLE 34.12

Incidence rates of mental diseases in various demographic groups

Demographic group	Men						Women					
	Person years observed 1947–57	Observed number with mental disease, O	Crude average annual incidence /100	Age specifically expected number with mental disease, E	O/E	p	Person years observed 1947–57	Observed number with mental disease, O	Crude average annual incidence /100	Age specifically expected number with mental disease, E	O/E	p
Total population (15–59 years)	7087·5	62	0·9				5984·0	136	2·3			
General and unskilled labourer, etc.	1926·5	17	0·9	17·0	1·0		1134·0	28	2·5	27·3	1·0	
Farm labourer etc.	621·5	5	0·8	6·1	0·8		240·5	7	2·9	6·9	1·0	
Minor farmer with additional occupation	442·5	4	0·9	3·5	1·1		400·0	11	2·8	8·9	1·2	
Farmer	1451·0	11	0·8	12·7	0·9		1198·0	17	1·4	26·3	0·6	0·10
Skilled worker, artisan, etc.	1573·0	17	1·1	13·9	1·2		1077·5	39	3·6	25·5	1·5	0·001
Light manual labour, white collar professions	1030·0	7	0·7	8·7	0·8		1841·5	34	1·8	40·3	0·8	
<6·000 Swedish crowns/year	4536·5	42	0·9	40·6	1·0		3568·0	85	2·3	80·5	1·0	
>6·000 Swedish crowns/year	2368·0	20	0·8	19·7	1·0		2243·5	50	2·2	51·5	1·0	
Married	3828·5	33	0·9	30·6	1·1		3877·0	98	2·5	90·4	1·1	0·10
Unmarried	3164·5	28	0·9	29·2	1·0		1970·0	35	1·8	42·4	0·8	0·10
Rural area	730·0	1	0·2	6·8	0·2		570·0	14	2·5	13·4	1·0	
Urban area <10 000 inhabitants	494·0	5	1·0	4·4	1·1		320·0	4	1·3	7·0	0·6	
Urban area 10 000–100 000 inhabitants	410·0	5	1·2	3·9	1·3		370·0	9	2·4	8·8	1·0	
Urban area >100 000 inhabitants	693·0	9	1·3	6·2	1·5		450·0	15	3·3	10·1	1·5	0·05
Abroad (2)												

TABLE 34.13

Incidence rates of mental diseases among persons with various kinds of subjective complaints

Item	Men						Women					
	Person years observed 1947–57	Observed number with mental disease, O	Crude average annual incidence /100	Age specifically expected number with mental disease, E	O/E	p	Person years observed 1947–57	Observed number with mental disease, O	Crude average annual incidence /100	Age specifically expected number with mental disease, E	O/E	p
Somatic asthenic complaints (present + history)	1545·5	20	1·4	13·2	1·5	0·05	2007·0	61	2·0	44·4	1·4	0·001
Somatic asthenic complaints (present only)	975·0	14	1·4	8·3	1·7	0·10	1594·5	51	3·2	35·0	1·5	0·001
Sleep disturbance	320·0	7	2·2	2·8	2·5	0·05	534·5	19	3·6	11·2	1·7	0·01
Swooning	190·0	3	1·6	1·7	1·8		260·0	6	2·3	6·0	1·0	
Vertigo and dizziness	355·5	5	1·6	3·1	1·4		682·5	16	2·3	14·5	1·1	
Headaches	918·5	13	1·0	7·7	1·7		1090·0	35	3·2	24·2	1·5	0·01
Autonomic instability	255·5	2	0·8	2·2	0·9		730·0	23	3·2	16·1	1·4	
Autonomic instability (present only)	145·5	2	1·4	1·3	1·5		560·0	18	3·2	12·2	1·5	0·10
Vasomotor lability etc.	235·5	2	0·9	1·9	1·1		520·0	16	3·1	12·0	1·3	
Spells and fits	60·0	1	1·7	0·6	1·7		70·5	1	1·3	1·4	0·7	
Sensations other than climacteric	10·0	0	0·0	0·1			147·5	5	2·2	3·1	1·6	
Migraine	150·0	3	2·0	1·4	2·1		373·5	15	4·0	8·9	1·7	0·01
Mental complaints												
Fatigue	500·0	7	1·4	4·6	1·5		1210·0	39	3·2	26·6	1·5	0·01
Nervousness	372·5	2	0·5	3·4	0·6		1086·5	42	3·9	24·1	1·7	0·00001
Huntedness	1088·5	9	0·8	9·1	1·0		2085·5	71	3·4	47·7	1·5	0·000001
Susceptibility to adversity	488·5	8	1·8	4·2	1·9	0·025	1242·0	36	2·9	28·2	1·3	0·10

TABLE 34.14

Incidence rates of mental diseases among persons with some personality and behaviour observations at interviews

	Men						Women					
Item	Person years observed 1947–57	Observed number with mental disease, O	Crude average annual incidence /100	Age specifically expected number with mental disease, E	O/E	p	Person years observed 1947–57	Observed number with mental disease, O	Crude average annual incidence /100	Age specifically expected number with mental disease, E	O/E	p
Pathological variation												
Evident	266·5	1	0·4	2·0	0·5		197·5	5	2·3	4·5	1·1	
Evident + probable	1263·5	12	0·9	10·5	1·1		1876·0	65	3·5	40·7	1·6	0·000001
Evident + probable + conceivable	3569·0	40	1·1	31·1	1·3		3716·0	110	3·0	83·0	1·3	0·00001
No	3511·0	22	0·6	30·6	0·7	0·05	2268·0	26	1·1	52·4	0·5	0·00001
Tense, restless	833·0	7	0·8	7·1	1·0		1180·5	35	3·2	26·4	1·3	0·05
Tired, lachrymose	477·5	3	0·7	3·9	0·8		590·5	18	3·0	13·8	1·3	
Chalarophrenia	948·5	14	1·5	8·7	1·6	0·01	1702·5	46	2·7	40·1	1·2	
Chalarophrenia severe	281·0	5	1·7	2·7	1·9	0·10	855·5	32	3·7	20·5	1·6	0·01
Dry, brittle	527·0	8	1·5	4·6	1·7	0·10	640·0	18	2·8	14·5	1·2	
Viscous, sticky	468·5	4	0·9	3·8	1·1		430·4	11	2·6	9·0	1·2	
Torpid, indolent	732·5	6	0·8	6·6	0·9		400·0	11	2·8	9·4	1·2	
Primitive, rude	150·0	1	0·7	1·4	0·7		140·0	1	0·7	3·2	0·3	0·08
Hypomanic, eretic	232·0	1	0·4	1·9	0·5		199·5	6	3·0	4·0	1·5	
Dysphoric	190·0	3	1·6	1·5	2·0		130·0	3	2·3	3·1	1·0	
Heavy, gloomy	52·5	0	0·0	0·4	0·0		110·0	3	2·7	2·5	1·2	
Less accessible	188·5	3	1·6	1·5	2·0		310·0	10	3·2	7·0	1·4	
Eccentric, paranoid	60·0	1	1·7	0·6	1·7		60·0	1	1·7	1·4	0·7	
Schizoid	358·5	4	1·1	3·0	1·3		80·0	2	2·5	1·9	1·1	
Ixoid	200·0	1	0·5	1·5	0·7		222·0	4	1·8	4·7	0·9	

34.15). Twenty men and 22 women had contracted a cancer during the decade. In women, a connection with substable personality was found, according to Sjöbring's model of normal personality dimensions. The incidence is comparatively higher among the more substable ($N = 156$; 5·5 expected versus 10 observed) than among the slightly substable ($N = 318$; 8·7 versus 10 observed). The observed number of cancer cases in substable women ($N = 474$) was 20 compared to 14·2 cases which would have been expected if the substable women had had the same age-specific cancer incidence rates as all women in the study. A trend of solidity is possibly found for mental disorders: more subsolid fell ill than did mediosolid and more mediosolid than supersolid.

Asocial men run less risk of contracting mental disorder; asocial women run more risk.

The tendency for infection shows, especially among women, a very unfavourable prognosis with strong statistical significance. Men with circulatory diseases or peptic ulcer, particularly those in the 40 to 59 age group, are more vulnerable (Table 34.16).

The incidence and duration of episodes of mental illness in a total population

I work here with the *pattern of mental illness episodes*. In my monograph of 1966, only the first incidences were considered. Here I am concerned with any episode observable during the ten years. All those registered and interviewed in the population in 1947 are included, irrespective of whether they consulted a doctor, treated as well as untreated. In this presentation, I deal primarily with: (1) ages at onset of mental illness, and (2) duration of neuroses.

For every episode of mental illness, data were obtained on diagnosis, degree of impairment, and date of onset and termination. Onset and termination were mostly recorded by month, although sometimes this was impossible and I then had to record the quarter and even in some instances the half-year.

The measurement of both relapses and remissions enables us to dispense with thinking of mental illness as a lifetime characteristic

TABLE 34.15

Persons who from July 1947 to June 1957 contracted cancer compared with persons of the same age who during the same period did not contract cancer

	Men		Women	
	Cancer (20)	Controls (160)	Cancer (22)	Controls (176)
Superstable	8	41	2	29
Mediostable	2	46	0	54
Substable	10	73	20	93
	$0·30 > p > 0·20$		$0·005 > p > 0·001$	

of an individual, and we do not miss—as is otherwise so easy—the acute brief conditions and the fluctuating patterns of such illness. The age of the proband is known at the onset of each episode of illness and so the age-specific incidence of the onset of episodes may be calculated.

The curves of the average annual incidence of onsets of episodes of mental illness (Figs. 34.2, 34.3, and 34.4) are bimodal in both sexes. The men's first mode is at 30–9 years; the women's is at 40–9 years. There are certain differences between the two sexes. For women, the curve rises strongly up to the 20–9 age; it then remains on the whole constant, except for a small maximum in the 40–9 age.

From and including the sixties, the average annual incidence falls markedly and then rises again in the highest ages– over 80 years. For men, the curve shows a decline from the thirties to the fifties; however this is by no means so obvious as for women. For women, the first mode is a decade later than for men. The second mode for both sexes is in the highest age-groups, and for 80 and over the ratio is higher still.

Thus it is reasonable to regard the bimodal curves as reflecting two groups of illness: the first group with its onset mostly before the age of 30, the second in the later decades of life. These groups may

TABLE 34.16

Incidence rates of mental diseases among persons with various physical ailments

Item	Person years observed (1947–57)	Observed number with mental disease, O	Crude average annual incidence /100	Age specifically expected number with mental disease, E	O/E	p
Men						
Proneness to infections	1818·0	20	1·1	16·5	1·2	
Orthopedics	1351·5	16	1·2	11·2	1·4	
Chronic polyarthritis	30·0	0	0·0	0·3		0·10
Rheumatic fever	280·0	2	0·7	2·6	0·8	
Encephalitis and meningitis[1]	182·0	2	1·1	1·7	1·2	
Endocrine disturbances[1]	48·5	0	0·0	0·4		
Circulative diseases[1]	303·5	8	2·6	2·8	2·9	0·001
Peptic ulcer	197·5	3	1·5	1·3	2·3	
Peptic ulcer 40–59 years[1]	187·5	3	1·6	1·2	2·5	0·05
Women						
Proneness to infections	1885·5	64	3·4	43·0	1·5	0·00001
Orthopedics	250·0	9	2·4	17·6	1·1	
Chronic polyarthritis	200·0	3	1·5	4·1	0·7	
Rheumatic fever	240·0	6	2·5	5·2	1·1	
Encephalitis and meningitis[1]	203·5	8	3·9	4·5	1·8	0·05
Endocrine disturbances[1]	350·0	13	3·7	7·9	1·7	0·025
Circulative diseases	500·0	14	2·8	10·3	1·4	
Peptic ulcer	120·0	3	2·5	2·5	1·2	
Peptic ulcer 40–59 years[1]	80·0	2	1·8	1·4	1·4	

[1] X^2 test used, age group 15–59 years.

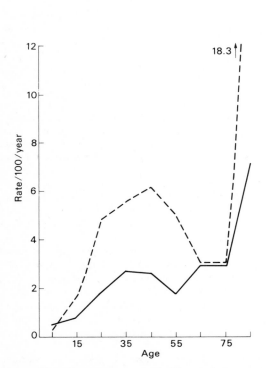

FIG. 34.2. The average annual incidence of all mental diseases: (——) men; (----) women.

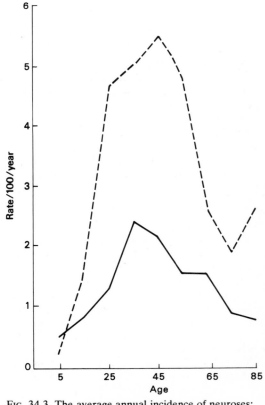

FIG. 34.3. The average annual incidence of neuroses: (——) men; (----) women.

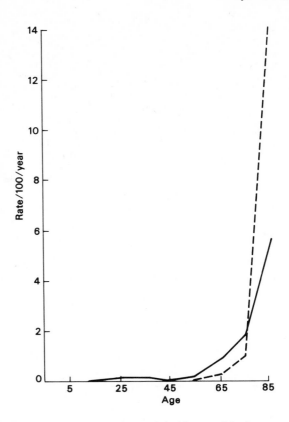

FIG. 34.4. The average annual incidence of brain syndromes: (——) men; (----) women.

be named the 'middle-years-maximum' (MYM) and the 'rise-with-age' (RWA).

The average duration of episodes of mental illness for psychoses and brain syndromes is about two years, for neurosis eight to nine months (Table 34.17).

Lifetime prevalence

In the present study, the lifetime prevalence per hundred is for:

Psychosis	1·7
Neurosis	13·1
Mental deficiency	1·2

If psychoses of the elderly are excluded, the percentage decreases from 1·7 to 0·96. By mental deficiency is meant an IQ below 70.

With Leighton's criteria of neurosis, the percentage in the present study increases to *circa* 35–40 per cent, psychosis remains at *circa* 1 per cent and mental deficiency increases to *circa* 10 per cent. This shows definitely that the criteria used in defining mental disorders are of great importance. An intelligible comparison between different studies cannot be made without keeping this in mind.

Point prevalence 1957

Point prevalence is calculated for mental disorders, subjective complaints, personality traits, psychophysiological symptoms (Tables 34.18–23).

Lundby 25 years later

In order to find out if the proband is living in Sweden and if so, his present address (on the cross-section date in 1972), all probands included in our sample, 3563, after special permission by the

TABLE 34.17

Number of episodes of mental illness, and mean duration, by sex and diagnosis (the figures in brackets include all those ill at cross-section day, 1 July 1947)

Diagnosis	Episodes		Persons	
	Number of episodes	Mean duration (months)	Number of persons	Mean duration (months)
Men				
Neurosis	188 (198)	8·0 (8·3)	134 (140)	11·2 (11·7)
Psychosis	20 (27)	22·7 (47·9)	17 (24)	26·6 (53·9)
Brain syndrome	46 (54)	28·3 (33·2)	46 (54)	28·3 (33·2)
Women				
Neurosis	407 (430)	8·9 (10·2)	282 (298)	12·8 (14·6)
Psychosis	21 (34)	15·5 (47·4)	19 (32)	17·1 (50·4)
Brain syndrome	33 (43)	31·7 (32·7)	33 (43)	31·7 (32·7)

Datainspektionen (the computer inspection) have been compared with the total population in Sweden on the same occasion. The total population of Sweden is found in the *Register of the total population of Sweden* (*Register över Sveriges totala befolkning* = RTB) at the Swedish National Central Bureau of Statistics. In RTB, which is brought up to date every month, there is data on all registered people in Sweden and their national registration number. These national registration numbers have been obtained through the parish registers. By a comparison between the national registration numbers in our sample and the approximately 8 million in the RTB, we have found those probands who live in Sweden, and their addresses, civil status, previous domicile, national registration number of spouse, etc. Dead and emigrated probands cannot be found in this way. Regarding these 768 persons, we have had to go to the parish offices concerned. The majority of the people who have died were, at the time of their death, registered in Lundby. Concerning the 33 emigrants, we have obtained information from

TABLE 34.18

Point prevalence, 1 July 1957, of mental diseases

Age	Total population	Neuroses		Psychoses		Brain syndromes	
		N	Per cent	N	Percent	N	Percent
Men							
80+	47	3	6·4	—	—	10	21·3
70–9	70	1	1·4	—	—	—	—
60–9	99	3	3·0	2	2·0	—	—
50–9	201	1	0·5	3	1·5	1	0·5
40–9	193	2	1·0	3	1·6	2	1·0
30–9	170	—	—	—	—	1	0·6
20–9	170	4	2·4	2	1·2	1	0·6
10–19	216	5	2·3	—	—	1	0·5
0–9	169	1	0·6	—	—	—	—
Total	1335	20	1·5	10	0·7	16	1·2
Women							
80+	32	5	9·4	—	—	5	15·6
70–9	82	10	12·2	—	—	6	7·3
60–9	123	2	1·6	3	2·4	—	—
50–9	172	11	6·4	1	0·6	2	1·2
40–9	189	14	7·4	1	0·5	1	0·5
30–9	150	9	6·0	2	1·3	1	0·7
20–9	149	6	4·0	—	—	—	—
10–19	209	2	1·0	—	—	—	—
0–9	171	—	—	—	—	—	—
Total	1277	57	4·5	7	0·5	15	1·2

TABLE 34.19

Point prevalence, 1 July 1957, of psychopathy. Men and women

	Men					Women				
		Total number of psychopaths		Those with an absolutely positive diagnosis of psychopathy			Total number of psychopaths		Those with an absolutely positive diagnosis of psychopathy	
Age	Total population	N	Per cent	N	Per cent	Total population	N	Per cent	N	Per cent
80+	47	2	4·3	2	4·3	32	—	—	—	—
70–9	70	1	1·4	1	1·4	82	2	2·4	1	1·2
60–9	99	2	2·0	2	2·0	123	1	0·8	1	0·8
50–9	201	6	3·0	5	2·5	172	1	0·6	—	—
40–9	193	6	3·1	4	2·1	189	5	2·6	3	1·6
30–9	170	12	7·1	7	4·1	150	3	2·0	3	2·0
20–9	170	23	13·5	13	7·6	149	4	2·7	1	0·7
10–19	216	8	3·7	5	2·3	209	4	1·9	3	1·4
0–9	169	—	—	—	—	171	2	1·2	—	—
Total	1335	60	4·5	39	2·9	1277	22	1·7	12	0·9

TABLE 34.20

Point prevalence, 1 July 1957, of impairment

		Mild		Medium		Severe	
Age	Total population	N	Per cent	N	Per cent	N	Per cent
Men							
80+	47	1	2·1	2	4·3	7	14·5
70–9	70	—	—	3	4·3	1	1·4
60–9	99	—	—	2	2·0	3	3·0
50–9	201	—	—	1	0·5	5	2·5
40–9	193	2	1·0	1	0·5	4	2·1
30–9	170	1	0·6	—	—	—	—
20–9	170	4	2·4	1	0·6	2	1·2
10–19	216	4	1·9	2	0·9	—	—
0–9	169	1	0·6	—	—	—	—
Total	1335	13	1·0	12	0·9	22	1·6
Women							
80+	32	1	3·1	1	3·1	6	18·8
70–9	82	6	7·3	6	7·3	4	4·9
60–9	123	1	0·8	—	—	4	3·3
50–9	172	4	2·3	4	2·3	6	3·5
40–9	189	7	3·7	6	3·2	3	1·6
30–9	150	3	2·0	2	1·3	7	4·7
20–9	149	2	1·3	3	2·0	1	0·7
10–19	209	—	—	2	1·0	—	—
0–9	171	—	—	—	—	—	—
Total	1277	24	1·9	24	1·9	31	2·4

TABLE 34.21

Psychophysiological symptoms in Lundby 1 July 1947–1 July 1957

		Gastrointestinal				Endocrine			
		B†		C†		B		C	
Age	Total population	N	Per cent	N	Per cent	N	Per cent	N	Per cent
Men									
80+	47	2	4·3	—	—	—	—	—	—
70–9	70	7	10·0	2	2·9	—	—	—	—
60–9	99	12	12·1	1	1·0	1	1·0	—	—
50–9	201	32	15·9	3	1·5	—	—	—	—
40–9	193	33	17·1	6	3·1	—	—	1	0·5
30–9	170	32	18·8	5	2·9	1	0·6	—	—
20–9	170	16	9·4	3	1·8	—	—	—	—
10–19	216	9	4·2	5	2·3	—	—	—	—
0–9	169	1	0·6	4	2·4	—	—	—	—
Total	1335	144	10·8	29	2·2	2	0·1	1	0·0
Women									
80+	32	1	3·1	—	—	1	3·1	—	—
70–9	82	8	9·8	2	2·4	1	1·2	—	—
60–9	123	13	10·6	4	3·3	—	—	—	—
50–9	172	16	9·3	5	2·9	3	1·7	—	—
40–9	189	33	17·5	2	1·1	2	1·1	—	—
30–9	150	19	12·7	4	2·7	2	1·3	—	—
20–9	149	8	5·4	2	1·3	—	—	1	0·7
10–19	209	8	3·8	5	2·4	—	—	—	—
0–9	171	6	3·5	9	5·3	—	—	—	—
Total	1277	112	8·8	33	2·6	9	0·7	1	0·0

† The ABCD scale stands for a four-point rating expressing the evaluator's confidence that he is dealing with a psychiatric case (the D.C. Leighton Confidence Scale).

A = almost certainly psychiatric;
B = probably psychiatric;
C = possibly psychiatric—borderline;
D = no evidence of any symptoms of psychiatric significance.

TABLE 34.22

Point prevalence, 1 July 1957, of subjective complaints

Age	Total population	Restless N	Per cent	Optimistic N	Per cent	Tired N	Per cent	Nervous N	Per cent	Cry easy N	Per cent	Forgetful N	Per cent	Anxious N	Per cent	Vegetative sweating N	Per cent	Brooding N	Per cent	Do people treat you all right N	Per cent
Men																					
80+	47	—	—	—	—	7	14·9	2	4·3	—	—	9	19·1	1	2·1	—	—	1	2·1	1	2·1
70–9	70	1	1·4	3	4·3	9	12·9	1	1·4	3	4·3	12	17·1	2	2·9	—	—	1	1·4	1	1·4
60–9	99	1	1·0	2	2·0	9	9·1	11	11·1	4	4·0	5	5·1	6	6·1	5	5·1	3	3·0	1	1·0
50–9	201	7	3·5	4	2·0	10	5·0	28	13·9	3	1·5	3	1·5	20	10·0	29	14·4	9	4·5	5	2·5
40–9	193	4	2·1	2	1·0	7	3·6	15	7·8	5	2·6	1	0·5	14	7·3	16	8·3	5	2·6	4	2·1
30–9	170	3	1·8	2	1·2	4	2·4	17	10·0	1	0·6	—	—	7	4·1	22	12·9	2	1·2	1	0·6
20–9	170	11	6·5	1	0·6	3	1·8	22	12·9	3	1·8	2	1·2	6	3·5	18	10·6	5	2·9	2	1·2
10–19	216	10	4·6	—	—	1	0·5	15	6·9	—	—	—	—	3	1·4	9	4·2	—	—	—	—
0–9	169	3	1·8	—	—	—	—	8	4·7	—	—	—	—	3	1·8	1	0·6	—	—	—	—
Total	1335	40	3·0	14	1·0	50	3·7	119	8·9	19	1·4	32	2·4	62	4·6	100	7·5	26	1·9	15	1·1
Women																					
80+	32	—	—	1	3·1	8	25·0	4	12·5	1	3·1	6	18·8	2	6·3	—	—	—	—	—	—
70–9	82	2	2·4	4	4·9	23	28·0	21	25·6	11	13·4	6	7·3	14	17·1	7	8·5	6	7·3	—	—
60–9	123	3	2·4	4	3·3	25	20·3	33	26·8	20	16·3	7	5·7	38	30·9	21	17·1	8	6·5	2	1·6
50–9	172	9	5·2	3	1·7	18	10·5	48	27·9	22	12·8	2	1·2	38	22·1	28	16·3	8	4·7	7	4·1
40–9	189	6	3·2	3	1·6	29	15·3	59	31·2	39	20·6	5	2·6	47	24·9	47	24·9	22	11·6	3	1·6
30–9	150	11	7·3	—	—	13	8·7	48	32·0	17	11·3	1	0·7	31	20·7	43	28·7	17	11·3	7	4·7
20–9	149	8	5·4	—	—	8	5·4	25	16·8	15	10·1	1	0·7	18	12·1	22	14·8	6	4·0	1	0·7
10–19	209	7	3·3	—	—	3	1·4	19	9·1	9	4·3	—	—	6	2·9	11	5·3	3	1·4	1	0·5
0–9	171	—	—	4	2·3	—	—	—	—	10	5·8	—	—	—	—	2	1·2	5	2·9	—	—
Total	1277	46	3·6	19	1·5	127	9·9	257	20·1	144	11·3	28	2·2	194	15·2	181	14·2	75	5·9	21	1·6

TABLE 34.23

Forts. Point prevalence, 1 July 1957, of other traits

Age	Total population	Anxious N	Per cent	Tense N	Per cent	Tired N	Per cent	Lachrymose N	Per cent	Dysphoric N	Per cent	Semi-depressed N	Per cent
Men													
80+	47	1	2·1 (—)	1	2·1 (—)	16	34·0 (10)	4	8·5 (2)	—	—	1	2·1 (1)
70–9	70	3	4·3 (1)	3	4·3 (3)	15	21·4 (8)	11	15·7 (8)	—	—	3	4·3 (1)
60–9	99	—	—	11	11·1 (4)	14	14·1 (6)	10	10·1 (3)	2	2·0 (2)	1	1·0 (—)
50–9	201	12	6·0 (5)	29	14·4 (10)	19	9·5 (4)	10	5·0 (3)	7	3·5 (5)	13	6·5 (5)
40–9	193	10	5·2 (1)	29	15·0 (9)	4	2·1 (1)	3	1·6 (3)	12	6·2 (7)	9	4·5 (4)
30–9	170	8	4·7 (3)	18	10·6 (3)	1	0·6 (—)	3	1·8 (—)	7	4·1 (3)	4	2·4 (1)
20–9	170	10	5·9 (4)	15	8·8 (8)	5	2·9 (3)	4	2·3 (1)	6	3·5 (2)	7	4·1 (—)
10–19	216	3	1·4 (2)	2	0·9 (1)	2	0·9 (1)	—	—	4	1·9 (—)	1	0·5 (—)
0–9	169	—	—	—	—	—	—	—	—	—	—	—	—
Total	1335	47	3·5 (16)	108	8·1 (38)	76	5·7 (33)	45	3·4 (20)	38	2·8 (19)	39	2·9 (12)
Women													
80+	32	1	3·1 (1)	2	6·3 (—)	14	43·8 (9)	1	3·1 (1)	—	—	—	—
70–9	82	8	9·8 (2)	5	6·1 (1)	31	37·8 (17)	14	17·1 (6)	6	7·3 (3)	4	4·9 (2)
60–9	123	16	13·0 (5)	12	9·8 (2)	20	16·3 (11)	13	9·8 (7)	3	2·4 (—)	1	0·8 (1)
50–9	172	21	12·2 (7)	20	11·6 (10)	29	16·9 (17)	17	9·9 (11)	8	4·7 (3)	3	1·7 (1)
40–9	189	43	22·8 (20)	36	19·0 (16)	35	18·5 (13)	19	10·1 (8)	16	8·5 (7)	5	2·6 (2)
30–9	150	25	16·7 (13)	25	16·7 (11)	17	11·3 (6)	10	6·7 (4)	13	8·7 (7)	2	1·3 (1)
20–9	149	21	14·1 (14)	13	8·7 (3)	10	6·7 (3)	3	2·0 (1)	6	4·0 (4)	4	2·7 (2)
10–19	209	5	2·4 (3)	3	1·4 (2)	5	2·4 (2)	1	0·5 (1)	9	4·3 (5)	3	1·4 (—)
0–9	171	—	—	—	—	—	—	—	—	—	—	—	—
Total	1277	140	11·0 (65)	116	9·1 (45)	161	12·6 (78)	78	6·1 (39)	61	4·8 (29)	22	1·7 (9)

the parish offices and from relatives. Information concerning the probands who have died has been collected from the next of kin who have looked after the proband during his last living days, or from other people who knew him well, and from hospital case records, etc.

TABLE 34.24

Lundby study 1972

Population	Men	Women	Total
Alive (on cross-section date)	1425	1403	2828
Deceased (1947–72)	398	337	735
Total	1823	1740	3563

The personal examination of the proband has mostly been carried out in his home by one of the participating psychiatrists. This has partly consisted of an interview, and partly of an observation of the proband and of the environment.

The interview is focused on mental disorder. A part of the interview is a free conversation to make the interview as flexible as possible. The interviewer has been able to adjust in accordance with the situation, person, and other conditions.

In the field study, the investigator is given the task of, to the best of his ability, establishing if the proband has or has had any mental disorder. This is done through interviews and observations. The investigator must consequently adapt himself to each proband, and also to the various situations in which he will find himself. After that, the investigator is to complete a schedule prepared in advance, and make his own comments.

Between 98 and 99 per cent of those living have been interviewed.

When evaluating the third Lundby study we use both Hagnell's method from the 1957 study and other systems, e.g. I.C.D.

In addition we are using various single items that have a close connection with mental disorder such as: having been hospitalized because of mental disorder, consulting a doctor concerning mental disorder, reported sick according to the social insurance office, receiving sick compensation/sick pension for mental disorder, suicide, criminality according to the criminal register.

Psychosomatic diseases, personality deviations, and alcoholism are coded separately. Table 34.25 presents the point prevalence of alcoholism in the Lundby 1947 cohort on 1 July 1972 (Öjesjö and Hagnell 1980).

The Lundby study with its great amount of information now constitutes a 'psychiatric epidemiological laboratory'.

TABLE 34.25

Point prevalence of alcoholics in Lundby, 1 July 1972.
1947 cohort of men aged 25 +

Age 1972	N	Abus. N	Per cent	Addict. N	Per cent	Chron. N	Per cent	Alc. total N	Per cent
25–9	111	3	2·7	3	2·7	1	0·9	7	6·3
30–9	169	8	4·7	7	4·1	2	1·2	17	10·1
40–9	204	8	3·9	4	2·0	7	3·4	19	9·3
50–9	162	3	1·9	6	3·7	11	6·8	20	12·4
60–9	184	5	2·7	4	2·2	7	3·8	16	8·7
70+	122	6	4·9	4	3·3	2	1·6	12	9·8
Total	952	33	3·5	28	2·9	30	3·2	91	9·6

2. Non-representative populations
a. Normal birth cohort studies

35. Longitudinal study of the mental and social development of the child (Belgium)

E. ALFRED SAND

The Belgian project was begun in 1955 under the joint direction of Professor Marcel Graffar (Director of the Laboratory for Epidemiology and Social Medicine in the Faculty of Medicine at the Free University, Brussels) for the somatic and social aspects, and Professor E. Alfred Sand (Chairman of the School of Criminology of the Free University, Brussels) for the psychological and psychosocial aspects of child development. These persons are still in charge of the project.

The original objective was to follow from birth to adulthood, if possible, the growth and development of a sample of 'normal' children born in a suburb of Brussels. The aim was, and remains mainly, to establish longitudinal correlations between variables at

different levels of the child's life. Both sides of the research project have yielded numerous publications and reports.

The research was started with help from private funds. However, later the Ministry of Education of the Belgian Kingdom took over financial responsibility for the project. During its first stages the Rockefeller Foundation supported the project. Since January 1977 we have been living on a last-year subsidy which might enable the research team to analyse a certain amount of the rich harvest of longitudinal data available.

The index sample was recruited at birth through the registers of the local authority (commune) of Saint-Gilles, Brussels. The only bias at that time was related to the voluntary participation of the family. The original number of children was 265. The children were born between April 1955 and April 1958.

The drop-outs were more numerous in the first years of the study. The distribution by social class was, at the start, representative of that of the population of young families living in the commune of Saint-Gilles. Later on, the extreme social class groups I and V (social classification after Graffar, based on the American Warner Classification) left the study, and the actual distribution is a rather central one.

The sample was contacted through personal visits with the families, the objectives of the project being clearly explained. No information feedback, except for very casual information (height, weight, etc.) was supposed to be given to the families. In certain special circumstances the members of the team gave some information to the parents (e.g., a severe case of scoliosis not detected by the family physician). On the psychological side any sort of counselling was carefully avoided. As a 'reward' the children, from certain age levels, received a small amount of money (100 B. Fr., approximately $2 at that time). Photographs of the child were offered as well. The subject's anonymity was absolutely preserved.

The children of the cohort have been examined on somatic and psychological dimensions at the following age levels: 1, 3, 6, 9, 12, 18, and 24 months, then each year between ages 3 and 15, and again at 18 years. As foreseen, the number of subjects decreased with the progress of the research: at birth, 263; at 3 years, 179; at 6 years, 151; at 10 years, 135; at 18 years, 120. At each age, the mothers and/or the children were interviewed; psychological tests and projective techniques were used. Most of the subjects who were still participating in the project at the age level of three years remained very co-operative. The team intends to make it possible to follow

the subjects later on. For the time being, the 21-year-olds have been sent a questionnaire concerning their actual life circumstances and projects. The background information has been recorded extensively. A detailed list would be too long to be mentioned here. However, the complete data are on tape, including all data from birth to 18 years of age, and certain data from age level 21 years.

No doubt, the longitudinal approach is a particularly fruitful one, given that a certain number of conditions are fulfilled. It appears to us that it is useful to work on some clearly outlined hypotheses and that there may be a risk of collecting data of limited value if one does not define the objectives of the data collection.

In 1966 a book was issued (Sand 1966) which gives a summary of data relevant from birth to the age of six. For the time being, the psychological team is busy analysing data longitudinally from birth almost to adulthood. The objective of the present study is to determine whether some final variables (at ages 18–20) may be predicted from information collected earlier.

The variables collected during the whole life cycle of the children include:

(1) Social class (plus details about level of education, etc.);
(2) Family planning (wanted or unwanted child?);
(3) Breastfeeding; separations from family;
(4) Behaviour of the child: eating, sleeping, aggression, crying, affectionate behaviour, school success and adjustment to peers, autonomy;
(5) Data about the family: possible problems (divorce, separations, etc.);
(6) Attitudes and personality of the mother.

Plans are under way for the final analysis.

36. Longitudinal follow-up study of somatic, mental and social development in a sample of Prague children from birth to the age of twenty (Czechoslovakia)

M. PROKOPEC, M. HAVLÍNOVÁ, and M. NOVOTNÁ

The Czechoslovak research programme was launched by V. Kapalín and M. Prokopec in 1956. This programme was part of the standardized research project of the Centre Internationale de l'Enfance in Paris which, since 1949, had gradually been accepted in several European countries as well as in Africa and the United States. Some objectives and methods of this standardized project had to be modified because of different living conditions and specific problems characteristic of Czechoslovakia.

Since its very beginning, this research programme has become part of long-term governmental research in the field of school and adolescent hygiene. The team of investigators consists of a clinician, anthropologist, psychologist, statistician, social worker, and technical assistants. The team is concurrently led by Prof. F. Janda, M.D., Dr. Sc., Mrs Novotná, M.D., who is now responsible for programme organization and clinical studies, M. Prokopec, Dr.Sc., who is in charge of physical growth and development, and Dr M. Havlínová, who investigates the mental and personality development of the children under study.

Sample under study

The children involved in the study were selected at random from Žižkov, a district of Prague, which has about 100 000 inhabitants. Only children born on Wednesday were included in the group. A social worker visited the parents of these children, informed them of

the purpose of the study, and asked whether they would be prepared to call regularly at the health centre for children. The first visit took place one month after birth, then at the ages of 3, 6, and 12 months. After the first year of age the children and the parents were invited twice a year, i.e., exactly at each birthday and 6 months after that.

The examination of the child at the centre begins with a talk between the social worker and the mother, and then later with the child alone. Questions about the nutrition of the child, his behaviour in the family, and any changes since the last visit are discussed in detail. The intent is not to overlook any factor that might influence the development of the child. The information obtained is entered onto questionnaires especially designed according to the directives issued by the C.I.E. The child is examined by the psychologist who ascertains his mental and personality development; in early childhood motoric development is also observed. The pediatrician makes a detailed clinical examination concluded by taking anthropometrical measurements and photographs.

Children were recruited gradually until in the course of the first four years the number of children being studied reached 287. Table 36.1 presents the distribution of these children according to age, etc. The lack of bias of the method of selection is proven by the fact that the group consists of 50 per cent girls and 50 per cent boys although no attention was paid to the factor of sex. The composition of the sample corresponds well to the general structure of the population in Prague–Žižkov, including occupational representation both of the parents and later of the children. Topographically,

TABLE 36.1

Composition of the longitudinal group from Prague according to age groups in each year of the follow-up

Year of birth	1956	1957	1958	1959	1960	
Year of follow-up						
1956	0†	—	—	—	—	
1957	1	0†	—	—	—	
1958	2	1	0†	—	—	
1959	3	2	1	0†	—	
1960	4	3	2	1	0†	—group at full number
1961	5	4	3	2	1	N = 287 children
1962	6	5	4	3	2	
1963	7	6	5	4	3	
1964	8	7	6	5	4	
1965	9	8	7	6	5	
1966	10	9	8	7	6	
1967	11	10	9	8	7	
1968	12	11	10	9	8	
1969	13	12	11	10	9	
1970	14	13	12	11	10	
1971	15	14	13	12	11	
1972	16	15	14	13	12	
1973	17	16	15	14	13	
1974	18	17	16	15	14	
1975	19	18	17	16	15	
1976	20	19	18	17	16	
1977	—	20	19	18	17	—beginning of gradual
1978	—	—	20	19	18	decrease of the
1979	—	—	—	20	19	number, then decrease
1980	—	—	—	—	20	each year by about 1/5.

† 0 = birth.

the homes of the individual families are evenly distributed over the entire district.

The recruitment was practically 100 per cent successful. The first drop-outs occurred in the first year of life and were the most numerous. The second wave of an increased number of drop-outs occurred when the children went through the period of puberty. At present between 180 and 200 attend examinations regularly. All of them have passed the age of 16. The age levels under research in 1977 were 17, 18, 19, and 20. We are aware that among those children who have ceased to attend the examinations there are extreme cases from the socio-economic point of view which would deserve increased research attention.

Study objectives and methodological approach

Until recently our knowledge of the growth and development of children was based on cross-sectional investigations, in which each age group was represented by different children. It was expected that the means of height or other dimensions, such as IQ and DQ values in children of a certain age, will progress in a year to be the same as that of children one year older. Whereas cross-sectional research yields 'untrue' growth curves, the results of longitudinal studies are true growth curves of the individual children. When these true growth curves are complexly assessed, they demonstrate the variability of the course of growth, and the variability of the onset and termination of the acceleration of pubertal growth. It is possible to derive from these curves the so-called velocity curves constructed by means of yearly increases. These demonstrate the greatest and smallest velocity achieved in the course of adolescence and the age at which the individual nodal points occurred in the respective individual. A further specific contribution of the longitudinal studies which cross-sectional investigations cannot duplicate, is the determination of the variability of yearly increments in

the individual periods of age. The information thus obtained can be useful, for example, in decisions of future occupation. The future occupation of the child is often being decided at a time when his/her final bodily height, or other physical and possibly even psychological characteristics are not yet known. Yet these characteristics may be of decisive importance for the given occupation.

Without having individual curves from birth until termination of growth, we are unable to reliably predict growth values. Prognosis of individual growth is therefore a further contribution of longitudinal research for education, adult and industrial medicine, and for the classification of talented individuals in sports into the individual sports disciplines.

Our study was conceived on the assumption that the growth and development of children is primarily determined by congenital factors, with its realization depending upon the concrete living conditions of the child. Therefore, we had to include in the study the living conditions of the child and the family and all measurable somatic and psychological indicators of development.

In the conclusion to this paper we have applied several different methodological approaches and techniques in an attempt to assess individual factors (in their mutuality and unity) in the living conditions of the children. Until now we have not always been able to define them reliably. The mutual influence of external and internal factors, their temporal variability during different periods of age or development, and the changing reactivity of children does not allow us to include the individual factors separately.

Experience gained in the course of solving this task shows that we are in a position to select from the number of factors studied some dominating relations, although proof of the causality of these factors continues to remain problematic due to the variety of internal life phenomena in the course of the growth and development of children.

From the psychological aspect, the longitudinal study aims at ascertaining data from short- and long-term prediction of psychosomatic development, level of intelligence, behaviour and personality traits. All these predictions may be applied for the following purposes:

(1) To aid parents and educators in deriving the respective educational measures;
(2) To ensure normal physical and mental development and to decide the corresponding hygienic criteria;
(3) To aid parents and children themselves in making decisions on the vocation which would best suit their own interests and abilities.

It is not possible to consider one aspect only when testing the child (e.g., the hygiene aspect or the aspect of vocation), resulting from a single variable during one specific age. The position of the child in the population is best given by a long-term view by means of repeated examinations applying various methods.

From the point of view of the clinician, long-term study aims at systematic recording of the health status of each child during the entire period of growth, as completely as possible. Evaluation of the physical and health status of a child for whom we possess complete medical records since birth, bears far more weight than evaluation of a child after a single examination. At any deviation from norms or at the development of any kind of clinical syndrome, it is possible to examine former records for preclinical signs; these signs may have been within normal limits at that earlier time. This is why regular photographic documentation acquired at each visit of the child to the centre is of invaluable help.

An objective view back upon the social conditions of children in families records their gradual improvement until the time when the young couple set up a family. We can roughly evaluate the socio-economic conditions up to the age of 15 from information about the family and its environment; after the child reaches the age of 15 we may evaluate socio-economic status from the information of the subject himself. The betterment of the total living standard of the population in the past 20 years is reflected in the increased living standard in the families of the children studied. It is nevertheless not possible to uncritically compare the living conditions, family environment, and housing level making use of the categories formed (for example, by Prof. Graffar of Belgium for use by the C.I.E. teams). For our conditions it was necessary to establish our own criteria.

Research methods and techniques

A separate file is kept for each child and it contains all records and photographic documentation. In the anthropometric part of the study the following indices were ascertained at each visit: body height (until age of 18 months body length was measured in a lying posture), sitting height (the lying child was measured in length from the crown of the head to the buttocks, at bent lower extremities in the pelvis and in the knees at right angles), circumference of the head in front over the glabella and in the back over the greatest bulge of the back of the head, circumference of the arm in the centre between acromion and ollecranon point, maximal circumference of the calf, biopicondylar width of femur and humerus, maximal width of pelvis (bicristal), biacromial width, thickness of skin folds above biceps and triceps (in both cases in half the length of the arm, in the spot where circumference was measured), under the shoulder blade on the back (subscapular) and supra–cristal (suprailiacal), length of the head (glabella-opistocranion), width of head (maximal), circumference of neck, and abdominal circumference. Also, at each visit of the child (up to the age of 12) eruption of permanent dentition, and colour of the eyes and hair is ascertained; from the first month until the age of three years the Martin and Schultz scales are used for comparison of the colour of the eyes. The norms for the colour of the hair are according to Fischer and Saller. At each visit photographs, in standard posture according to Sheldon, are taken. An exact description of the dimensions is contained in the publication by Kapalín et al. (1969).

Clinical examinations, case histories of the health status and socio-economic living conditions of the children at home are also followed up twice a year, at each visit of the child. For the clinical examination a standard record is available in coded form taken over from the International Child Centre in Paris. Morbidity and case history data are recorded in descriptive form and transformed to numeric form so as to facilitate statistical processing. For the studies of the socio-economic conditions of the children, we used the modified method recommended by Grafar for all C.I.E. centres; this method has been adapted for our conditions and verified on a number of transversal as well as semi-longitudinal research.

Psychological examination of all children in the study was carried out at the ages of 6, 9, 12, 18, 24, and 30 months. Beginning with the age of 3 years the examination takes place within 14 days of the child's birthday. Mental development is studied according to the C.I.E. conception solely by means of standardized IQ tests. Changes of behaviour and development of the personality are studied by means of normal projective techniques and standardized personality tests, as well as by means of compiled scales of assessment, guided conversations, and questionnaires designed for long-term follow-up. Each individual examination is processed, recorded, and evaluated immediately after taking place.

Data analysis

The processing of the individual data takes place in several cycles:

(1) Transversal processing of data obtained by each method is usually carried out after each year of the study;

(2) Comparison of the results between the individual age groups of a certain complete period of development within each method (0–6 years, 7–15 years, 16–20 years) and also between different methods;

(3) Comparison of the results between selected age groups of different periods of age within each method;

(4) Comparison of results between selected indices obtained by different methods.

The values obtained by individual examination and its processing are either coded or are stored in absolute numbers on punchcards. The calculations are made on the Hewlett-Packard 2.116C computer according to programs we prepared. A report on results is submitted to the co-ordinator of governmental research. As a rule an extensive progress report is prepared each five-year period and this report is defended as a scientific paper. The team workers are currently publishing articles on specific questions. The results for the period from birth to six years have been published as a complex and the second part from six to 12 years is presently being prepared.

Some preliminary results

Some of the results published so far can be summarized as follows:

Growth in the individual age periods

Age 0 to 18 months. First the data collected in the course of research were processed cross-sectionally for each age group separately. The means and standard deviations were calculated. The physical development of each child was then evaluated in consideration of the whole group. In comparison with the published data of similar investigations of child groups in London, Paris, Zurich, and Dakar (Falkner 1958) the Prague children from 0 to 18 months ranged among the longest and heaviest, with especially large gains in the first year of life.

Age 0 to 36 months. The trend of the height and weight curves of children of the group under investigation was slightly above the curves of Prague children from the cross-sectional investigation reported by Šobová in 1959. A morphogram was constructed from the means and standard deviations of the studied indices in the individual age groups (the means were on the vertical in the centre of the morphogram); on the left of it the limits −1, −2, and −3 were marked and on the right of it the standard deviations +1, +2, and +3. The individual values of the children were plotted in the morphogram and connected into a curve. This characterized the deviation of the individual from the mean values in a clear form, so that by one look all the measured indices could be evaluated. If this curve is plotted on a transparency and gradually placed on the morphograms of the higher age groups, the curves plotted on the transparency and marked by age, indicate the change which the child underwent in the course of growth. Correlation tables were also constructed which indicate the weight for each centimeter of the child's height in all age groups, i.e. after three months until one year, and after each half of a year until the age of three.

Age 0 to 6 years. Further processing yielded the means and standard deviations from birth to six years. The mean curves demonstrated the change in growth velocity at different ages. The most rapid growth occurs from the first month until the end of the first year of life. The greatest change of rapid growth to slow growth was noted in the circumference of the arm, the abdominal circumference, circumference of the calf and the thorax, and in the width and length of the head. Much slower initial growth, earlier slow-down of growth rate, and gradual changes to even slower growth rates of the index after the first year of life were observed with the width of humerus and femur, as well as with the biacromial and bicristal width. With regard to the circumference of the head, a rapid initial growth and large increases with a long transition from rapid to slow growth, was observed. Development of height, height in sitting posture, length of trunk (occiput-coccyx) and weight were much slower.

The average girl reached half of her probable final height (present mean in adults) 81·3 cm., at 1·5 years, and the average boy reached 87·5 cm. at the age of two years. There are differences between the averages of boys and girls in all dimensions (those of the boys being higher) excepting the thickness of the skin folds and circumference of the calf, which are higher with girls after the second year of life. The trend of the curve of mean skin fold thicknesses is significantly uneven, the greatest mean is around the age of half a year, then it decreases and slowly rises again later. The coefficients of variation of the studied anthropometrical indices vary from 3·5 per cent for the dimensions of the head, to 50 per cent for the thickness of the skin folds. The height and weight norms of our group exceed the national anthropometric norm obtained in 1961; this is to be expected with city children who continue to have a higher mean height than children from the country.

The relative growth was evaluated by indices based on two dimensions. Some of these indices appeared to be suitable for estimation of the harmonic physical development, for the definition of pathological growth, and for studies of endocrinopathies. A change in the velocity of growth in the period from the age of one month until six years was ascertained between the growing width of humerus and femur, and biacromial and biiliocristal width.

The increases of the individual indices from one measurement to the other were calculated for each individual, and the means and standard deviations of these increases were calculated for the entire group. The shape of the curves of the mean increases from birth until the age of six years, resemble the letter L or the reversed letter J; the curves in the shape of L occur for abdominal circumference, arm, and width of head; those shaped like a reversed J are for the circumference of the calf and the thorax. The curve of the increase in the width of humerus and femur showed a similar trend. The curve of the increase of the biiliocristal width differs in shape from the biacromial curve.

The largest growth velocity from the age of one month until six years was ascertained for the abdominal circumference and the width of the head. These dimensions reach a quarter of the entire increase from the first month until the age of six already by the age of three months. Half of the total increase was reached at the lowest age, six months, for the circumference of the arm, and then between the sixth and ninth month for the width of the head and the circumference of the thorax, calf, and abdomen. The length of the head reaches half of the total increase between the tenth and eleventh months of life. The width of the humerus and femur, height in sitting posture, biacromial width, length of trunk and biiliocristal width each reach half of the total increase up to the age of six years, between the first and second year of life. After the second year of life, height and weight reach half of the total increase they will attain by six years. Girls reach the same sectors of total increase later than boys.

The growth of the Prague children from birth to the age of six years could be compared with the longitudinal groups studied in Paris and Zurich. It appeared that the Swiss children resemble the Prague children more than the children from Paris.

Age 0 to 18 years. In 1975 all the collected material was processed for the progress report. All active members of the group had already passed the age of 15, so that the school age was represented by final numbers. The numbers of the higher age groups were still incomplete. The results demonstrating the change in the individual dimensions and the physical structures of the body with age, their differences between both sexes, etc., were presented in tables and diagrams. For the majority of dimensions the means for the boys at

first exceed the means of the girls (neutral phase), then the girls temporarily exceed the mean values of the boys (steroid phase), whereupon the body growth of the girls slows down and ceases. In general, the boys, who grow for a longer time than the girls, reach higher mean values. Another growth programme was ascertained for the dimensions of the head (length, width, and circumference), and for the dimensions of robustness of the skeleton (biepicondylar width of femur and humerus) which, during all the time of growth, are higher in average for boys than for girls. This was also true in part for the abdominal circumference; the mean of girls between the age of 10 and 14 years does not exceed the mean of the boys, but rather fuses with it. Higher means for thickness of skin folds were found for the girls during the entire period of growth.

Stability of the somatic type

We tried to ascertain the earliest period in which one could reliably determine the physical type, which develops for the respective individual in adolescence. For this purpose we selected the photographs of 60 boys from the Prague group and determined physical types at the ages of 14 and 15 years, according to the method by Sheldon. We then attempted to retrospectively ascertain for each individual in the younger age groups, whether and when it is possible to determine this final type with certainty.

It appeared that this would be possible for purely ectomorphic and endomorphic types (only 11 cases) from the age of four years onwards. The determination was difficult with mesomorphic types, because it was not possible to distinguish them very well from the mixed types.

In the next phase we also attempted to estimate physical types by an objective method applying five indices: ponderal, cormic, sexual, width-height, and sum of skin folds. The physical type was determined by means of a five-digit formula at the ages of six and 14 years, and the results were mutually compared. In one third of the cases no change occurred in the somatotype from six to 14 years. A small change in direction towards endomorphy was ascertained in 7 per cent and a significant change in 22 per cent. A slight change towards ectomorphy from six to 14 years was ascertained in 17 of the children, and a significant change was found in 5 per cent of the cases. Changes in physical type from age six to 14 years in the direction to endomorphy were more frequent than changes towards ectomorphy. This study was undertaken jointly with J. Vácha.

Prediction of height

Using the data from our long-term group we verified jointly with Šrámková and Železný the method of height prediction suggested by Walker (1975) and Bayer and Bayley (1959). Using the Walker and Bayer and Bayley prediction equations we calculated the final height for each child, using the height at the age of 18 as the adult height for girls and at 19 years for boys. Whereas the means of the predicted height were rather close to reality, the results differed much for individuals. In 60 per cent of the cases, however, the predicted values did not differ from the real values by more than ±3 cm. Next, according to Walker's coefficients (Walker 1975), the constants for the Prague youths were computed in order to substitute them in the equations for prediction of the final height from measurements of height at younger age.

Mathematical expression of the growth curves

In co-operation with B. Meisnarová and J. Tošovský we applied simple mathematical functions for the expression of the relation between anthropometrical characteristics in the period of growth and the different types of curves, Gompert's curve, logistic and 'normal' curve according to Tošovský. These curves were applied to the individual physical dimensions in the course of ontogenesis. It appeared that the 'normal' curve presented the best agreement with the empirical values.

Analysis of the growth curves. The individual height curves were drawn into an orthogonal network of format A3 and smoothed out. From these straightened curves we subtracted the yearly increments, which we had used for the construction of the velocity curves, for the ages from one to 18 years. From these curves we deduced the peak of the highest growth velocity and its corresponding age; we also calculated the smallest yearly increment and the corresponding age, and some further characteristics of the individual velocity growth curve. The results coincided well with the data of the Swiss group of children from Zurich. All the anthropometrical data are punched on cards. When the members of the group attain a specific age, the statistical values of new tests are calculated. Further processing is planned for the time when all the members of the group will reach the age of 18 years.

The influence of socio-economic conditions upon growth values of children

We studied the values of growth age in relation to some socio-economic indices. We selected the following four factors as indicators: the level of education of the parents, their occupation, the mean monthly income per person, and the housing level. The sum of the partial factors determined for us the socio-economic situation of the family.

The results which we obtained were of statistical significance in respect to the socio-economic level and in some partial indices (occupation, education, and income). The differences in housing were insignificant. The analysis disclosed that in order to have an objective situation it is necessary to use the values of both parents' occupation and education.

The results of growth age of six-year-old children according to the number of children in the family, sequence of their birth, and income groups of the studied families. There were higher values of growth age for first-born and single children if they were classified in a higher category of income. This was true although their birth-weight, and for first-born, their length was lower. The differences were statistically significant.

The influence of care by the family and by social agencies upon the developmental level of pre-school children. Boys from kindergarten were slightly somatically retarded when compared to boys cared for by the family. Morbidity (infectious diseases and diseases of the upper respiratory pathways) was higher by almost 50 per cent in children from kindergarten. The other diseases occurred equally in both groups.

The dependence of the height of parents and their children at each age. The difference between the mean heights of children at each age level, classified in groups according to height categories of their parents were highly significant.

IQ in the same subjects at the ages of 3 to 11 years

The final purpose of the analysis of the trends of IQ development in children and adolescents is to make use of the specific contribution of the longitudinally obtained psychological data for the elaboration of prediction methods. Early prediction of the future mental development of the child and of his entire personality from preceding developmental indices may afford the selection of suitable hygienic measures against possible damage to the mental health of the child, and may affect the direction of the normal mental development of the child.

The basis for the analysis of the group trend of IQ development was established by using the results of the IQ examination (Terman–Merrill) over the course of eight years, at ages, 3, 5, 8, and 11 years. This is a continuation of the data from the early age period of 6, 9, 12, 18, and 24 months, measured by the Brunet–Lézin test. The IQ data also affords a prognosis for the period of adolescence, age 14, when IQ is measured by the WISC test. In order to make

this analysis on the basis of true longitudinal measurements, only those subjects were selected from the entire group for whom all measures from six months to 14 years were carried out and valid. The group selected consists of 70 children, 40 girls and 30 boys.

The entire IQ group trend rises from six months onwards, from a mean value of 106·00 to 113·10, until the age of five years. Thus the peak of the group trend is at the age of five. Other groups of children studied longitudinally with the same developmental test (in Zurich and Stockholm as well as in Brno, where they had a group of 500 children) report similar results. The scores of the Prague and Brno children are the highest of all.

The statistically significant decrease of the group trend starts between the fifth and eighth year. The IQ value decreases steeply (from 113·00 to 102·16) and the difference between the initial (at the age of five) and the subsequent (at the age of eight) value of the trend is significant ($p < 0.005$). The trend continues to decrease, although statistically insignificant, until the age of 11 when it reaches 99·21. When looking at the further developmental trend, after examining the groups at age 14 years, it is possible to estimate that the IQ remains more or less at about 100. The group trend from the age of 11 (99·21) rises at age 14 only insignificantly to 101·00.

The longitudinal method of follow-up affords unique possibilities of analysing individual developmental trends in the same subjects; accordingly, especially detailed curves of the individual IQ values were constructed. It was first ascertained that the individual trends are not stable; rather, they vary from age to age upwards and downwards even after the standard errors of measurement are deducted. Further analyses will be conducted to ascertain the correlates of the individual trends. In comparison with the group trend, several different courses of the individual trends of IQ development were ascertained.

We attempted to analyse the peak of the trend of IQ development of the entire longitudinal group at the age of five according to these social conditions: the number of children in the family, the sequence of birth of the studied child, the education of the father, the education of the mother, and the occupation of the mother.

According to the mentioned ascertainments the highest IQs at the age of five are in single children, in children first and third in the sequence of birth, children of fathers and mothers with university and grammar school education, children of mothers with a qualified occupation of all types in contrast to mothers in an unqualifed occupation or mothers in the household. The relation between the investigated social conditions and the IQ level of the children will be analysed further at the age of eight when it reaches a statistically significant difference ($p < 0.005$) from the IQ at age five.

For the time being we are only in a position to afford a quite hypothetical explanation for the rising group trend from birth until the age of five, as well as for the steep decrease at the age of eight and its relative stabilization around the mean of the population at the ages of 11 and 14. The explanations we tentatively propose are:

(1) It may be the consequence of outdated test standards, since all over the world the capability of small and pre-school children is being improved by more effective development of their mental capacity;

(2) It may be the consequence of better elaboration of the norms for children of school age in comparison with pre-school children;

(3) It may be the consequence of the composition of the longitudinally studied groups. In spite of their initially strictly random selection, the groups gradually changed according to parental interest in the health and development of the child. This circumstance may result from the fact that in pre-school children, the parents stimulate the child. Later, however, many of the parents seem to become satisfied when the mental development of the child is handed over to the care of the school. Thus a considerable

differentiation between the individual children takes place. This last hypothesis tends to also be supported by the fact that when the IQ value of the entire group decreases almost to the mean of the population, the individual differences simultaneously increase;

(4) It may be the consequence of the peculiarity of the longitudinal method which was still further exacerbated by our selection of 70 subjects. Studies of these subjects present a different perspective on the development of the child than does the data on age groups

measured in a single historic year (as in cross-sectional measurement). Since the norms of the intelligence tests are calculated on the basis of cross-sectional measurements, and in our study we calculated according to the IQ of longitudinally studied children, we are actually comparing values obtained by two different approaches. It is therefore necessary to be aware of this fact when analysing longitudinal data, until we find a more appropriate method of mathematical expression.

37. The development of children in a Swedish urban community: a prospective longitudinal study

GUNNAR KLACKENBERG

Introduction, design, and aims of the study

This study forms a link in an international project, co-ordinated by the Centre International de l'Enfance (C.I.E.) in Paris. Similar studies, listed in the order in which they started, have been in progress in London, Paris, Zurich, Stockholm, and Brussels. Developmental, behavioural, social, and somatic growth data are recorded for child samples at various stages on uniform lines and using the same methods. Continual, comparable data for the first years of life have also been obtained from children in two African centres (Kampala and Dakar).

An account of this internationally co-ordinated study, with regard to its aims, design, and methods, has been given in Vol. V of *Modern problems in pediatrics*, with Frank Falkner as co-ordinator and editor, and with contributions from team members in the different centres (Ferrel and Karlberg 1960).

The general aims of these studies have been formulated as follows:

Within each country:

(1) To chart the course of physical and psychological development of children, in terms of a number of important variables;

(2) To obtain reasonably comprehensive life histories, which will be applicable to a considerable variety of problems;

(3) To employ a sufficiently large sample to permit statistical analysis;

(4) To relate important features of development to other important variables, as, for example social background, size of family, parental methods, health, etc.;

(5) To study the interrelationship of one feature of development with another, as, for example of physique and health, behaviour problems and previous experience, intelligence and physical health, or of physique and behaviour.

Between countries:

(1) To determine to what exent the developmental process, and interrelationships between variables, show similar or different features in different countries;

(2) Where clear differences exist, to attempt to explore the possible reasons for them.

The aim of the Swedish investigation is to study children in a Swedish urban community in the Stockholm region according to the above-mentioned principles. Our primary objectives are:

The physical investigations should be so designed as to give a broader picture of the growth of normal children than is available at

present in Sweden. This can be achieved owing to the increased number of body measurements that are taken and to the longitudinal approach adopted for the evaluation for various age periods. Our purpose is to develop also a more detailed method of evaluating skeletal maturation from a smaller number of X-ray examinations than are made at present in Sweden.

The primary aim of the psychological investigations is the elucidation of those points which physicians, teachers, psychologists, parents, and other persons who have to deal with children every day are compelled to take into consideration. These are, for example, variations in sleep, sleep disorders and sleep requirements, time for cleanliness and toilet training, eating habits and eating problems, jealousy of siblings, different forms of fears, etc. Our knowledge is very limited with regard to the variations in children's behaviour, attitudes, and emotional reactions. Furthermore, in the psychological investigations we endeavour to get a picture of emotional and intellectual maturation and the development of the child's personality in his interaction with the other members of his family. In connection with this we are interested in studying the identification process and the child's adaptation to society and its value norms.

Through the composition of the sample the study gives a contribution to the discussions on the distribution of the intellectual, testable ability levels in different social groups. By testing children from infancy up through the years when the influence of the cultural environment probably becomes stronger, the investigation may furnish information regarding possible shifts in the level of ability. This study may also assist in elucidating whether it is possible to predict, at an early stage, a child's vulnerability and later adaptation.

The organization of the Swedish study

The Swedish study was initiated in 1954 by the late Professor Arvid Wallgren. His warm interest in both somatic and psychic development of children facilitated the gathering of a research team, composed of paediatricians, child-psychiatrists, psychologists, and nurses. In January 1955 a Clinic for the Study of Children's Development and Health was established at Karolinska Sjukhuset in the Children's Hospital. This clinic and the five original researchers are still working with the project. These are P. Karlberg, paediatrician, head of the team; G. Klackenberg, child psychiatrist; I. Klackenberg-Larsson, psychologist; H. Lichtenstein, paediatrician; I. Svennberg-Redegren, nurse. During delimited periods in past years various psychologists have been taking part in the study. Since 1963 I. Johannesson, psychologist and since 1965

I. Engström, paediatrician, have been committed to helping organize the future design of the study.

In planning, conferences and discussions the somatic and psychic sides are kept together, but due to economical reasons as of 1975, they have parted in searching for funds to work through the rich scientific material.

The index sample

The index sample is taken from the town of Solna in the inner suburban area of Stockholm. Recruitment started during 1955 with a pilot group comprised of 29 children. In these cases the first contact was made either antenatally or neonatally. The children were mainly recruited from the Obstetrical Department of Karolinska Sjukhuset. After December 1955 subjects were recruited exclusively from the Solna Antenatal Clinic. Every fourth expectant mother, according to her registration number, was asked whether she was willing to allow her prospective child to participate in the investigation. In a longitudinal study which, on account of repeated, time-consuming, and comprehensive investigations, may prove burdensome to the family, it is inevitable that already at the onset some of the randomly selected participants should withdraw. The number of these cases was small, however, amounting to only 3 per cent of all those who were invited to take part in the investigation. The time for sampling was finished in April 1958. Thus the children were born between April 1955 and March 1958.

Of the 198 mothers from the antenatal clinic who stated that they were willing to participate, 15 dropped out or were excluded (six abortions, four on account of the child's neonatal death, and five premature births with weight below 2000 g). The remaining 183 plus 29 from the pilot group composed the index sample of 212 children. Its representativeness was tested with respect to socio-economic grouping, mother's age, the percentage of children born out of wedlock, the time when the children were born in relation to the time when marriage was contracted, the children's successional number, the stated period of pregnancy in weeks, and the children's birthweight. In all those respects there was a good agreement between the index sample and comparable figures for Stockholm and Solna, the suburban town of Stockholm where Karolinska Sjukhuset is situated. We have considered it important to carry out these analyses since the more similarities that can be established, the stronger are the reasons to assume that the study will furnish data that have a wider application than merely to the group investigated. Hence where we have subsequently presented frequencies and tendencies we have done so with this degree of confidence that can be based on the above-mentioned considerations and with the working hypothesis that the sample represents not only itself but also a greater area, a Swedish city community.

Losses

Up to and including 3 years of age, 3 children had dropped out = 1·4 per cent.
Up to and including 8 years of age 12 children had dropped out = 5·6 per cent.
Up to and including 13 years of age 24 children had dropped out = 11·3 per cent.
Up to and including 18 years of age 37 children had dropped out = 17·5 per cent.

In consideration of the sampling method and the longitudinal nature of the study the losses are small. The drop-outs have affected all social groups. They have not resulted in any statistically significant changes in the social composition. In general the interest shown by the families must be mentioned as satisfactory. It has been possible for the Clinic to keep in touch also with representatives of more extreme social, economic, and psychological conditions, for whom participation might have been expected to be a burden. Thus the drop-out rate for the original 23 children born out of wedlock

was proportionally the same as for the sample as a whole. The educational level of the group of mothers who have ceased to take part in the study corresponds very closely to that which is representative of the original sample. However, the losses do not only depend on removals to remote areas in Sweden or abroad, but also on lack of interest or other reasons. Four cases have died. One was given up owing to synostosis cranii with serious mental retardation.

Each case repesents not only an economic but also an emotional investment and each loss has implied a scientific weakening of the sample.

Contact of sample

No governmental approval was needed for starting the study. Permission was given by the authorities of the antenatal clinic in Solna. As mentioned before, every fourth expectant mother was questioned about co-operating. Then she was personally contacted by the psychologist in the mother's home one to two months before the estimated time for delivery in order to establish contact and introduce the study. The purpose was described in plain words as a contribution to the widening of our knowledge about the development of children through following each child and his family through the years. The long-term aspect was put into focus. A short interview was taken concerning the mother's attitude towards the delivery, her former experiences of children, and what sex she wished. Since the children were recruited irrespective of their order of sequence the sample represents a mixture of primiparae and multiparae. In a Lying-In interview the psychologist then continued the contact, and at the maternity hospital the paediatrician commenced his field work.

During these first contacts it was clearly stated to the parents that the growth study centre was not a substitute for the well baby clinic. It was recommended to the mothers that they visit the well baby clinic, as was the case with other children in town, to get advice about child care. Those who were in need of medical consultation were encouraged to visit their family doctor or an out-patient department.

The only material rewards given to the participants were payment of travel expenses and a print of one of the photographs taken at each visit. In later school years the children received 10 Swedish crowns as encouragement. When they had started working, lost earnings were compensated.

Ethical considerations

The subjects' anonymity was guaranteed. Each research record was given a registration number; the number code with names and addresses was kept in a locked cupboard. Our data register is subject to special strong regulations prohibiting misuse. The team members do not divulge any information to institutions, authorities, or colleagues without explicit permission from the parents and the child.

Background information

Every year from one to 18, a comprehensive social interview was arranged covering parent's civil status, number and order of siblings and other members of family, parent's occupation, educational level, sources of revenue, and dwelling conditions (type, space, access to modern conveniences). For some of these important variables (housing, income, education, and profession) a 5-point scale was used. By adding the figures of these different variables for each family, one obtains the total figure indicating the socio-economic level of the family. As the range in each variable is from 1 to 5 the variability of the total score is from 4 to 20. In this way we obtained a measure of the socio-economic standard according to the Graffar system, applicable to international comparison.

Further information was obtained on the family history including hereditary diseases, the mother's antenatal and obstetric history, the course of labour and delivery, the child's condition immediately after delivery and during the subsequent time in the maternity hospital.

During the consecutive yearly interviews, information was gathered about major changes in the health and social conditions of the parents and in the family composition. Social deviances, divorces, abuse of alcohol, and criminality are noted if they are mentioned in the interview. We have not yet applied for permission from the social authorities to get access to registers.

Assessment of the cohort

After the maternity hospital period the children were examined at the clinic at the following ages: 1 month (4 weeks), 3 months (13 weeks), 6 months (26 weeks), 9 months (39 weeks), 12 months, 18 months, 24 months, and thereafter once a year up to 18 years of age. At each visit both somatic and psychological investigations and observations were made. The physical examination comprised a general appraisal of health since the last visit and the present condition of health status, body measurements for 16 different parts of the body area, estimation of skeletal development, and photographs in different positions (with exceptions for ages 14 and 15).

The extent and contents of psychic information has changed at different years, but always it comprised a structured interview (or in school years a structured questionnaire), various ability or personality tests and ratings of personality traits. Up to three years of age these interviews took place with the mother only, but when the child was four years old the father as well was interviewed (at home). Both parents filled in an attitude scale (abridged Schaefer–Bell). They were even asked about their attitudes to their own upbringing. The fathers were again interviewed when the children were 12 to 13 years old, but it was rather difficult for fathers to find time; therefore the interviews are incomplete. From 15 years of age, the youths themselves gave information.

Each of the three interview forms (four at 4 to 5 years, two at later years) concerning the child's behaviour in general and in special circumstances (e.g. separations, accidents) contains 80 items. The alternative answers are rarely confined to the categories 'yes' or 'no'. Usually the mother being interviewed was offered a range of alternative answers enabling her to make graded or qualified statements concerning the child's symptoms together with their frequency and duration. The basic information of interviews and questionnaires—a minimum of data-gathering—has step-by-step been agreed upon at the regularly arranged C.I.E. conferences. At some ages the Swedish team has added special interviews for parents or children, for example, about punishment, sexual education, sleep patterns, and sleep disturbances. During puberty ages and up to 18 a comprehensive interview was taken with the youngsters concerning their habits in using alcohol, tobacco and narcotics, and their experiences of sexual relations. A summary of ability and personality test methods, which have been applied at various ages, is available from the author.

The co-operation of the subjects has shown some variations through the years. The most difficult ages to keep the children and mothers motivated to continue in the study were during puberty. In all about 4600 investigations have been achieved and about 280 have been missed. This amounts to 6 per cent of the 4600 possible planned opportunities in remaining cases. The yearly missed investigations ranged from 1·4 per cent at 3 years of age to 10·9 per cent at 15 years.

Status of the data

The collected information has been transferred to computer cards and then to magnetic computer tape. Since the investigation has been in progress for several years various types of computers have been used. The consequences of this have been a successive transfer

of data as better machines have been available. Data from the investigations accomplished last year are not yet fully on tape, as well as some of the personality test data from earlier years, but up to age 16 the tape recorded information has been used in programs treating the material. A few items of the psychic data have not been suitable to code without special adaptation, and thus must be taken directly from written forms in working through the special topic.

Analysis and reports

A list of publications emanating from the longitudinal study group in Stockholm is available from the author. At present it compromises 50 items, including three doctor's theses in different disciplines (child psychiatry, psychology, and paediatrics) and five papers by psychologists for gaining higher degrees. In the list are also to be found comprehensive essays on longitudinal mental development, measured by ability tests on disciplinary methods through the years, and upon somatic growth and maturity.

Special problems encountered

If a longitudinal follow-up is to be a practical proposition it must take into account the visiting frequency for which parents and children can be motivated. Another limitation is imposed by financial considerations. A project which sets out tracing individual development from birth to adulthood is bound to be expensive and the scientific return must be reasonable in proportion to the financial outlay. From the very beginning it was intended that the first financial aid from C.I.E. should be taken over by national research funds. Through the years it has been so. During several years the Swedish Medical Research Council and the Bank of Sweden Tercentenary Fund have granted means towards the study along with various generous private foundations and the Child Welfare Committee in Stockholm. Periodically, however, we have been faced with financial difficulties. The feeling of insecurity about funding for the next year has many times affected future planning in a disturbing way. It is pleasant to be able to state now, when the collection of data has been finished, that the staff has maintained its calm and stayed with the study in spite of uncertain circumstances. The staff has invested a great deal of emotional capital in the study, helping over troublesome passages.

By the age of eighteen, 96 children together with their families or the children themselves moved from their original homes in Solna. Mostly they still live in Stockholm or in the suburban areas. Some families have by and by come to live outside Stockholm and its suburbs. In spite of distance difficulties we have found it important to follow these subjects.

The five people on the staff who began the study 23 years ago are still working on it. During the past years some additional persons, mainly psychologists, have made valuable contributions. The stability of the composition of the staff has given a favourable consistency for all contacts.

Through organizing data-collection from the very beginning in coded forms, punch cards, and tape records (Karlberg), the study has been preserved from burdening data problems with difficulties of accessing data for analysis. The co-operation with the local university organ in the Karolinska Institute which administered our varying funds has been frictionless.

Advantages of the psychological project

The main purpose has been the longitudinal aspects. However, through good sampling and the continuation of contact with families of different social origins, we have been able to get many additional cross-sectional pictures of behaviour distribution. When we have compared those pictures with the results from some big cross-sectional studies in our country regarding special developmental and behavioural traits we have found good agreement. It has strengthened us in our opinion that even cross-sectionally obtained results from a small, well-documented, longitudinal sample, treated with care, might have a wider application than merely to the group investigated. At least, it will be valid until the loss of cases reaches considerable dimensions and distorts the composition of the original sample.

The most essential aim of the study is the longitudinal follow-up, with its possiblilities for referring early signals in behaviour to later traits. The working through of this aim is still partial but is in full progress. Several interesting findings have emerged:

(1) Single emotional symptoms in pre-school ages often seem to be of episodic occurrence;

(2) An accumulation of deviation in the individual child at age four implies a high risk of having correspondingly high symptom load of the tested variables in later years;

(3) The symptom load in groups of children at ages four and eight, whose mothers had had regular employment when the children were small (1–3 years old), proved to be as great as in children whose mothers never had had gainful employment at that time;

(4) Developmental tests for infants have little long-term predictive value for normal children, but predictability increases with age;

(5) Differences in mean quotients between infants from lower and higher social groups shift over to significant differences in the opposite direction when they grow older in favour of the higher social group. When the children in the higher social group begin to be more developed this is first noticed in the language quotients and is linked with mother's higher educational level;

(6) Speech-retarded 3-year-old children (in the so-called normal sample) should be regarded as children at risk, because these children compared at ages 3, 8, 14, and 17 with other children were still definitely inferior in ability tests. The highly significant differences in IQ means between groups were practically unchanged when the children had started school.

The evaluations of the persistence of various variables (e.g. sensitivity and fears, temper, aggressiveness, sleep disturbances, school achievements, and so on) are now carried on parallel to data of parental personality traits, parental methods, and social conditions. With this part-project we hope to be able to elucidate the relationship between parent's and children's personalities.

When the time is ripe we want to widen the horizon by exploring the relations to the contemporary registered data on somatic development. One of the aims of the international co-operation, according to the general considerations at the beginning of our work, was a determination of the extent to which the developmental processes and interrelationships between variables show similar or different features in different countries, and an exploration of the possible reasons for any differences. Some interesting collaborative evaluations have been done concerning the development of the capacities for feeding, walking, bladder control, and tested intellectual ability. In spite of a common base line for data-gathering there are obvious difficulties in doing comparative studies on psychic and functional domains. They are complicated and time consuming and are in need of wholehearted and devoted contributions. The English team has led this part of the study. Much more data are resting in our data banks awaiting initiative.

Conferences

Conferences have been held alternatively every second or third year under the sponsorship of the Children's International Centre in Paris. At these recurrent conferences representatives of other types of longitudinal studies both in Europe and abroad have participated.

Administrative considerations

The group unit of researchers of the Clinic for the Study of Children's Development and Health is responsible for the project. The permission to utilize data must be given by this study group. The responsibility for raising money from funds is the duty of the same group. The payments of salaries, taken from the obtained fund-means, are managed by the financial department of the Karolinska Institute. There are no long-term guarantees of funding. We have the use of several rooms at the paediatric clinic at Karolinska Sjukhuset.

Impact of project

One of the main practical fields for the application of growth diagrams is in prophylactic and diagnostic work with children. For several years the Swedish medical authorities have accepted data from the longitudinal study for use at child care centres and at children's hospitals, including both the diagrams from the somatic part of the study with weight-, length-, and head-circumference data, and milestone data from the psychic development during pre-school years. They are put in as delimited fields on the corresponding time-axis with borderlines at ±1 standard deviation. Thus the doctor can follow the deviations in individual cases during growth and react early enough in suspicious risk cases.

b. Specialized cohort studies
i. Twin cohorts

38. The Finnish twin registry: a preliminary report

JAAKKO KAPRIO, MARKKU KOSKENVUO, SEPPO SARNA, and ILARI RANTASALO

Introduction

The Finnish Twin Registry was established in 1974 to conduct epidemiological studies of chronic diseases. In the first phase, all living adult twin pairs of the same sex have been gathered. For the determination of zygosity, and collection of base-line data on various environmental factors, a questionnaire study was carried out in 1975. Twin zygosity has been determined to a high degree of accuracy by a combination of deterministic and stochastic methods. Longitudinal studies, which have been started, form the main part of the research programme of the Finnish Twin Registry.

Twin studies offer a simple and powerful instrument for studying the role and interactions of genetic and environmental factors in human disease. In a WHO report (Report of WHO meeting of investigators 1966), investigators recommended the twin method for use in epidemiological studies. These twin studies are based on large twin registries made possible by recent developments of statistical and data-processing facilities together with the existence of a nation-wide personal identification system. Sufficiently reliable, efficient, and generally applicable methods enable the results of epidemiological studies to be internationally comparable.

An International Symposium (Cederlöf 1971) reviewed the principles of the twin method in the research of chronic diseases. After a meeting of twin investigators in Miami in 1973, it was decided to establish a Finnish Twin Registry. The Finnish Twin Registry has been in operation since 1974 at the Department of Public Health Science, University of Helsinki. In the first phase of the formation of the Registry, a cohort of all adult twin pairs of Finnish citizenship was formed.

The main emphasis of the Finnish Twin Registry will be on longitudinal follow-up studies on chronic diseases. A particular feature of twin studies is the need for accurate determination of zygosity. For this purpose and to provide base-line data, a questionnaire study has been carried out.

In this paper the formation of the Registry, the questionnaire study, the determination of zygosity, and planned follow-up studies will be described.

Formation of the registry

A file of all Finnish adult like-sexed twin-pairs born before 1958 was created for those cases in which both members of the twin pair were alive in 1967. This twin population was picked from the computer files of the central population register, which includes all Finnish citizens, both those living abroad and those dependent on institutional care. No variable indicating twinship was available, so the twin candidates (i.e., persons who satisfy the selection criteria) were picked when two or more persons satisfied the following criteria:

(1) Same sex;
(2) Same date of birth;
(3) Same commune of birth;
(4) Same surname at birth.

A number of pseudotwin (not biological twin) pairs were included by these criteria. These 7388 singletons serve as controls in some of the studies. A basic file of 34 730 twins was formed. A detailed description of the compilation procedures is given by Sarna et al. (1976). The size of the basic file corresponds to an a priori estimate of the numbers of same-sexed adult twins using natality, mortality, migration, and twinning rate data.

The basic file contained information on various socio-demographic variables. Current address data were also available and were used in the mailing procedures of the questionnaire study. Information on the parents of the subjects is limited to knowledge in some cases of the date of birth of parents. This information was used to determine whether some unclear cases of twin candidate pairs were actually twins.

Questionnaire study

A questionnaire study has been carried out for two main reasons. Firstly a questionnaire method of determining zygosity was applied and verified as described in the next section. Secondly base-line data on many variables relating to medical, sociological, economic, and psychological factors were obtained. The questionnaire used was based on that designed for epidemiological twin studies at the International Meeting of Twin Investigators (1973). The question-naire was sent to all twins with adequate address data. Four mailing rounds were carried out, with answers from each mailing identified to be able to assess the effect of the date of response. In an accompanying explanatory letter the broad aim of the questionnaire was explained to be an investigation on health, and the importance of answering promptly and accurately was explained. No direct feedback information was promised, and no honorarium was used. No mass media contact was considered necessary, as in Finland it is well known that the response rate would be high. A total of 97 questions on the following main topics were included:

(1) Twinship and zygosity;
(2) History of angina pectoris according to Rose (1962), and modified by Reunanen, Aromaa, and Pyörälä (unpublished);
(3) History of illnesses diagnosed by a physician;
(4) Coronary heart disease history of relatives;
(5) Smoking history, modified version of the Swedish Twin Registry questionnaire (Cederlöf 1966);
(6) History of alcohol use (Myrhed 1974);
(7) Drug usage history;
(8) Physical activity history;
(9) Education and employment history;
(10) Three series of psychological questions:
    Nervosity scale
    Abbreviated Eysenck personality inventory;
    Bortner scale.

Basic characteristics of these variables, and the questionnaire have been documented (Kaprio et al. 1978a, b, 1979; Koskenvuo et al. 1979). Responses from both members of 12 074 pairs, and from one member of 2419 pairs have been received. This corresponds to a response rate of 89 per cent of twins who have received the questionnaire, and a rate of approximately 83 per cent of all twins in the Registry. Respondents who live abroad (mainly in Sweden) comprise 3·1 per cent of the sample.

Determination of zygosity

Zygosity diagnosis in large-scale epidemiological twin studies cannot, for practical reasons, be done by blood marker tests, which are considered the most accurate method of zygosity determination. For this purpose questionnaire methods offer an alternative that previous studies have shown to be reliable and sufficiently accurate (Cederlöf et al. 1961; Nichols and Bilbro 1966).

In the Finnish Twin Registry, the questionnaire method has been further developed. Deterministic and stochastic methods have been applied both to twin pairs where both members have replied, and to twin pairs in which only one member has replied.

A deterministic decision tree was constructed for classifying twin pairs on the basis of the responses of both co-twins to questions on confusion and similarity in childhood (Sarna 1977). The decision tree contains two levels of certainty of diagnosis, which provides two different groupings of the twins for use in different studies. The use of the stricter criteria leaves a larger group of twins unclassified by zygosity, and may include a bias relating to the selection of the twins. The less strict criteria might misclassify a slightly larger number of twins, but will include more cases in the studies. When using the less certain level, the deterministic decision tree classified 92·7 per cent of the twins. A sample of 156 twin pairs randomly chosen from those twins living in and around Helsinki was taken for the verification of the zygosity determination procedures by blood marker tests. Eleven blood markers were determined for all pairs and the blood marker results were compared with the questionnaire classification. The probability of misclassification of a blood marker concordant pair was 0·0169 (Sarna 1977). The blood marker system tests were in 100 per cent agreement with the classification results for the samples tested by the decision tree.

The classification of twin pairs unclassified by the decision tree was done by multivariate methods. The decision tree classified all cases correctly, but left unclassified 7·3 per cent of cases. The classification by multiple discriminant analysis and multiple logistic analysis showed that 75 per cent of these cases were classified correctly (Sarna 1977). Thus subsequent multivariate analysis improved the classification of the decision tree. The additional cases classified decrease the proportion of unclassified cases, still maintaining a very low probability of misclassification. A total of 98·2 per cent of respondent twin pairs could be classified with almost 100 per cent accuracy by a combination of the two methods of analysis.

In the Finnish Twin Registry there are a certain number of twin pairs of whom only one member has replied. The zygosity of these twin pairs cannot be verified using blood marker tests. For the purposes of the twin registry, the assignment of zygosity in these cases is considered necessary. This has been done by modification of the decision tree and by multivariate methods (Kaprio et al. 1977).

Studies of the Finnish twin registry

The broad aim of studies performed involving the material of the Registry is to elucidate the role environmental factors play in the manifestation of diseases. The four main sources of information to be used are the questionnaire data, additional questionnaire studies, data from other registries, and the results of clinical examinations of twins.

The questionnaire data has now been collected and is under analysis. Further questionnaire studies will be carried out:

(a) To measure longitudinal changes in various variables;
(b) To study in detail various subsamples. These could then be followed by clinical studies.

In addition to further questionnaires, follow-up studies based on cross-linking of data from other registries will be carried out. This is feasible in Finland because every Finnish citizen has a unique personal identification number. At the same time, safeguards for protecting the information from misuse have been taken. All the registries with medical information are official and permission to use them must be obtained. Follow-up studies based on the following sources are possible:

(1) *Death certificates*. Source and responsible unit: The Central Statistical Office. Permission to use the data has been obtained and death certificates up to 1977 collected. Non-natural causes are also recorded. A separate suicide register does not exist.
(2) *Hospital records*. Source and responsible unit: The National Board of Health. Contents: All persons who have died in or left a general, mental, or tuberculosis hospital. Permission to use these records has been obtained.
(3) *Data of the Finnish Cancer Registry*. Analysis of cancer incidence data for 1967–74 indicated risk of cancer in co-twins of affected probands is increased only for basal cell carcinoma.

(4) *Registries of the Social Insurance Institution*. These include information on persons receiving fully reimbursable drugs or on disability pensions for various chronic, including mental, illnesses.

All the above registries are computerized and the information is on magnetic tape files.

As the basic file of the Finnish Twin Registry has only recently been compiled, longitudinal studies are only now commencing.

Data-processing procedures

The register is computerized and the data is on magnetic tapes. A special program package has been created for the formation of the registry, control of the mailing procedures, statistical analyses of paired data, and for the cross-linking of data from follow-up studies.

Comments

The Finnish Twin Registry is administered by the Department of Public Health Science, University of Helsinki, which bears responsibility for the project and the public use of the findings. A committee of senior research workers gives consultant advice on research activities. Post-graduate work is carried out as part of the research project.

The importance of using unselected populations in epidemiological and twin studies is well recognized (e.g. see Report of WHO meeting of investigators 1966). The use of only like-sexed twins has been chosen because of the general purpose of the Registry, that of study of chronic disease. A bias of the population under study is the condition that both members of a twin pair had to be alive in 1967. By studying twins who have died between 1967 and 1976, the effect of this bias can be estimated to some degree. In future prospective studies, this effect will be less meaningful as the mortality of younger age groups, where broken twin pairs are rarer, grows.

Approximately one-third of the twins in the Registry are monozygotic, as classified by the methods of zygosity determination. This corresponds to *a priori* estimates (Koskenvuo et al. 1976) by Weinberg's rule.

The methods used in zygosity diagnosis are applicable in other national studies.

The Finnish Twin Registry is able to participate in research on chronic diseases, including mental health problems. The use of internationally comparable methods and the unnecessary duplication of efforts is considered important.

Acknowledgement

This study has been supported by a grant from the Council for Tobacco Research, USA, Inc.

39. The Danish twin register

MOGENS HAUGE

Introduction

During the last decades research in medical genetics has, to an increasing extent, turned its interest from the very rare, fully hereditary abnormalities to the more common diseases and disorders which constitute a significant burden to society as well as to individuals and families. The number of these disorders is high in most developed societies and it seems difficult to control them. Thus public health authorities must devote more and more time and resouces to the elucidation of their causes and possible preventive measures, rather than just to a reduction of their symptoms and sequelae.

Although the control and prevention of the rare, hereditary disorders are, of course, extremely important, especially to the patients and their families, the results are not likely to influence the morbidity or mortality figures for the total population to any conspicuous extent. Medical geneticists are now becoming aware of the value of epidemiological and long-term studies, especially in disorders with a particular genetic background which have a prolonged period of manifestation. These studies help to elucidate the relative weight of genetic aetiological factors, and to detect environmental influences which bring the specific genetic predisposition to the surface, i.e. make the disorder observable, or, on the other hand, prevent the predisposition from becoming manifest. These types of research have their special methods, many of which have only recently been developed, especially as far as the analytical procedures are concerned. However, as early as the beginning of the 1950s Professor Tage Kemp, head of one of the very first institutes of medical genetics in the world (at the University of Copenhagen), realized that the potential value of long-term studies of twin pairs, a special subsection of the population, had never been fully appreciated. With substantial support from the National Institutes of Health, the Danish Twin Register was established in the Medical Genetics Institute by two of Kemp's staff members: Dr B. Harvald, M.D., and the author of the present report, who for the last ten years has been the Director of the Register now situated in the University Institute of Clinical Genetics in Odense. Since the 1920s studies of twins had been quite popular in human and medical genetic research, but mainly as collections of case reports; with few exceptions their possible contributions to epidemiological research had never been realized. Later on, twin registries analogous to the Danish were established, first of all in the other Scandinavian countries.

The twin study method

It is a characteristic and basic principle of the Danish Twin Register—in contrast to previous twin studies, at least of diseases—that investigations start from the total population of twins, who are followed as cohorts right from birth and through their whole life. In this way the well-known, but usually unavoidable biases of previous studies of diseases of twin patients selected from hospital files and similar sources, are largely prevented. Many methodological analyses have demonstrated the influences of these biases on the conclusions of such studies; furthermore, most previous investigations have been cross-sectional which, in cases of diseases with a long period of manifestation, adds to the problems of the general validity of the conclusions. It is also sometimes forgotten that exclusion of twin pairs in which one or both partners have died tends to make the sample more healthy than the average.

When twin populations are sampled and followed, it is possible to collect epidemiological data concerning more common diseases, their distribution, incidence and prevalence, and their relation to sex, place of birth, place of living, occupation, etc.; such a method also permits more refined analyses of associations between an abnormality or disorder and a specific environmental factor, e.g. by penetrating studies of genetically identical pairs (monozygotic) carrying the same predisposition, in which only one has been exposed to the specific factor. By application of recently developed statistical methods the classical comparisons between the two types of twins (monozygotic (MZ) with complete identity of their genetic set-up, and dizygotic (DZ) with no more genes in common than ordinary sib pairs), provide estimates of the extent to which the variation in a given population with respect to a certain trait is gene dependent. The careful scrutiny and comparison of the life history of MZ twins will, hopefully, give some leads to environmental

influences which caused one of the two copies of the same genotype to develop a trait at a later date than did his co-twin, to a milder degree, or perhaps not at all. This may provide information about interactions between special genotypes and special environmental agencies and assist in finding high risk groups which should be informed about possible preventive measures.

The Danish twin register

The Twin Register serves as a unit, providing material and special methodological assistance to research workers who conduct projects which may find significant extensions by these special types of analyses.

The practicability in Denmark of long-term studies of a total population group is determined by a number of very essential, technical facilities available. All births, marriages, and burials have been registered for centuries; total population censuses have been performed at regular intervals; death certificates have since about 1920 nearly always been filled in by doctors; medical care including hospital services, special examinations, also on an out-patient basis, are free or nearly free; the distance to the nearest doctor or hospital is short; the standard of the medical services is fairly uniform, and only a few private clinics exist. Furthermore, all information from the above-mentioned sources is filed, and medical records may be perused and information from general practitioners and practising specialists obtained without limitations when needed for medical research purposes. A number of special nation-wide registers exist: for example, a National Population Register dating back more than 50 years permits one to trace and follow any person irrespective of how often he moves and, to be informed about the date and place of death, which makes it possible to get a copy of the complete death certificate. Individuals known to be mentally retarded or who have at any time been admitted to a psychiatric ward have been centrally registered for the last 30 to 40 years or more, and similar regional registers of admissions to somatic wards are now being established. All law offenders may be found in a Central Police Register which dates back to the turn of the century. Various checks give reason to believe that all the registers and files mentioned are very complete, but no detailed studies of this aspect have so far been made to permit numerical estimates. Finally, it should be mentioned that the population is ethnically very homogenous; the socio-economic conditions have generally been quite good, at least for the last 50 to 60 years, and the understanding and co-operation of the population is very good.

The Register contains data on all twin births which have taken place in Denmark since 1870; it is still under construction, more pairs are being traced, and new decades will be added when funds permit an extension. Right now, the Register is very close to having data on the total population of twins born up to and including 1930 in its files. The Danish population from which the Register draws its information included about 1·8 million inhabitants in 1870 and 3·5 million in 1930. The annual number of twin births has been rather constant over this period, amounting to 900 to 1000 pairs per year.

The basic data has been obtained from the birth registries kept loyally by the parishes; these have been searched for all twin births. For the period 1870 through 1910, like-sexed as well as unlike-sexed pairs were recorded and included in the sample. It was decided to start registration in 1870 in order to obtain a sample of individuals who, at the time of registration, would have passed the major part of the risk period for a high number of disorders. It is then intended to follow all the individuals recorded from birth until the time of registration or to their death without paying any attention to the presence or absence of diseases or to their zygosity. Various checks support the view that the registration of twin pairs may be considered virtually complete.

Procedure for the follow-up

The first step in the follow-up of the twins has been to make use of the register of deaths in the parishes. This provides the date of death of all those who died in the parish where they were born. The next step is to ask the National Population Registers to provide any information they may have or have had about the twins or their close relatives. Since 1924, when these registers were established by law, it has been compulsory to report any change of address to the municipality. This implies that any person whose place of living in 1924 or later is known may at any moment be traced through these registers. Before 1924, many towns and cities had annual censuses in addition to the nation-wide censuses carried through every five years. The reports of these detailed population surveys are still available and have been important sources of information. The same applies to the archives of the local probate courts where names and addresses of relatives of deceased persons may be found, provided the day and place of death are known. Through these channels more than 90 per cent of the twins have been traced so far.

A questionnaire is sent to the twins as soon as they have been traced. If they are not alive at the time of registration an attempt is made to locate their closest relatives who then receive the questionnaire. The intent is to obtain the medical history by asking the informants to list all stays in hospitals and to indicate the presence or absence of symptoms of a number of specified diseases mentioned in the questionnaire. In the case of twins belonging to like-sexed pairs, specific questions are included about the degree of similarity between the partners which would permit an evaluation of the zygosity diagnosis as described below.

It was soon found to be impossible to get reliable information about medical events, including the cause of death, and especially about the zygosity diagnosis in twins dying at an early age. As like-sexed pairs of unknown zygosity are useless in most studies, it was decided at an early stage to stop the collection of information about a pair as soon as it was found that one partner had died before attaining the age of six years. Thus in principle the working material comprises all twin pairs born in Denmark between the years 1870 and 1930 in which neither partner is known to have died prior to the day on which he or she attained the age of six years.

To ensure the most economic use of the funds it was decided that after 1911 only like-sexed pairs would be considered, since pairs with partners of different sex are of lower value in the majority of studies.

Zygosity diagnosis

The size of the material and the fact that one or both twins had in many cases died prior to the time of registration, called for methods of zygosity diagnosis other than the most reliable which are based on the extensive use of blood and serum group determinations. All questionnaires sent to like-sexed twins or their relatives contained questions about the degree of similarity between the partners, and about the difficulties, if any, experienced by parents, friends, and other acquaintances in distinguishing between the two partners; on the basis of the answers given, all pairs were classified as probably monozygotic (MZ), probably dizygotic (DZ), or of doubtful zygosity or unclassifiable (UZ).

The class of *MZ pairs* includes all those pairs in which the partners were described as strikingly similar in appearance, i.e. more similar than ordinary sibs, and to such an extent that even people who knew the twins well found it difficult to distinguish one from the other.

The class of *DZ pairs* comprises such pairs where the partners were stated to present no striking similarity and where identity difficulties had never appeared.

Unclassifiable pairs constitutes the remaining part of the like-sexed pairs. This group includes all pairs where no reliable information was available or where the informants disagreed about the similarity. Pairs in which the partners themselves claimed to be strikingly similar in appearance although they had never been mixed up, would be placed in this class. The same applied to pairs denying any striking similarity but where it was stated that the partners had now and then been mistaken for one another. About 5 per cent of the same-sexed pairs are found in this class.

This method of classification has been used in all cases, but when more intensive studies are carried through the practice is to include serological examinations in all like-sexed pairs with both partners being alive. The serological approach has a very high degree of reliability which may be expressed numerically. In principle, any difference between two partners with regard to any well-defined serological character is taken as a proof of dizygosity. With the systems employed now it is calculated that about 99 per cent of all DZ twin pairs may be expected to show some serological difference proving their dizygosity. Thus, the class of serologically discordant pairs will include DZ twins only. The remaining like-sexed pairs with complete blood group concordance will comprise all MZ pairs plus an extremely small proportion of DZ pairs. In a given series, the actual number of DZ pairs in the group of serologically concordant pairs may be estimated, and the conclusions of the study may be considered in the light of this specified error of classification.

The validity of zygosity classification based on answers to the questionnaires has been evaluated by a comparison with the results of later blood group determinations in 383 like-sexed pairs selected for more detailed medical examinations, which in some cases was intended to comprise MZ pairs only. The results of this comparison were as follows:

(1) Pairs initially classified as MZ: 193 out of 196 pairs in this class were subsequently found to be serologically concordant. Two of the remaining three pairs were brought up apart, which may have limited the value of their answers to the question about experiences of identity difficulties. The results give good reasons to believe that pairs in this class have an MZ probability exceeding 95 per cent.

(2) Pairs initially classified as DZ: 172 out of 175 pairs in this class presented some blood group discordance proving their dizygosity. The remaining three pairs showing complete concordance with respect to the systems studied may or may not be DZ. This number of serologically concordant pairs in the DZ class is in agreement with the expected number according to the calculations mentioned above. Thus, the DZ probability of pairs placed in this class also seems to exceed 95 per cent.

(3) Unclassifiable pairs: The answers from 18 pairs contained some internal inconsistencies which made them unclassifiable:

(a) The partners from seven pairs, all showing some blood group discordance, gave conflicting answers concerning their similarity;

(b) Five pairs described themselves as strikingly similar in appearance, but they had on the other hand never experienced being mistaken for one another. Three of these five pairs were serologically discordant;

(c) Six pairs stated that people who knew them had now and then found it difficult to distinguish between them in spite of the fact that they considered themselves clearly different in appearance; five of these pairs showed some blood group discordance.

The total results of this analysis indicate that the general reliability of the classification method used here is high, with a frequency of misclassifications which is probably below 5 per cent. The group of unclassifiable pairs constitutes a problem, but the size of this group will be reduced in most intensive studies where an interview with the informants will provide more details regarding the similarity of the partners, thus permitting valid classification in an additional number of cases.

Current state of the study

Tables 39.1 and 39.2 give the details concerning the working material as it stands in March 1980. It must be mentioned that the 1911–20, and especially the 1921–30 groups, have been added rather recently and have not yet been thoroughly searched. In these tables the pairs born in the period 1870–80 have been discarded because they are not being followed any longer, for obvious reasons; the losses have been quite pronounced in this decade. Separate analyses have shown, as expected, that female/female pairs are more difficult to trace than male/male pairs. It may be noted that the proportion of pairs not yet traced has been below 10 per cent since 1895, and only about 5 per cent in 1910. The proportion of unlike-sexed pairs born in the period under study was about 36 per cent at birth and about 38 per cent in the working material. The difference between these two figures is probably fully explained by the higher infant mortality in twins belonging to like-sexed pairs.

TABLE 39.1

Survey of the Danish Twin Register (March 1980). Like-sexed twin pairs

| Years of birth | Total no. born | Traced | | Untraced |
		Survived age 6	Broken or lost before age 6	
1881–90	5660†	1082	3822	756
1891–1900	6145†	1427	4169	549
1901–10	6737	2051	4283	403
1911–20	7056	2754	4055	247
1921–30	6653†	2580	3262	811

† Estimated values (not given in the official statistics).
All figures refer to pairs.

TABLE 39.2

Survey of the Danish Twin Register (March 1980). Unlike-sexed twin pairs

| Years of birth | Total no. born | Traced | | Untraced |
		Survived age 6	Broken or lost before age 6	
1881–90	3354†	629	2223	502
1891–1900	3446†	784	2146	516
1901–10	3779	1135	2212	432

† Estimated values.
All figures refer to pairs.

The sample is followed up at intervals through new questionnaires sent to the twins who are still alive. Once a year copies of death certificates of all those who have died in the preceding year are received from the Central Register of Deaths, irrespective of whether the pair has already been traced or not.

The most conspicuous difference between the group of traced pairs and the small group of pairs still untraced is likely to be that the latter includes a higher number of pairs which moved from their place of birth at an early age. Areas with a relatively low rate of emigration would, therefore, be expected to show a higher proportion of retrieved pairs. This view is supported by the finding that among pairs born in Copenhagen in the years 1896–1910 only 3 per

cent of male/male pairs and 5 per cent of female/female pairs have so far remained untraced, compared with 7 and 9 per cent respectively, for the remaining part of the country. There seems to be no reason to expect an undue proportion of a specific zygosity type or with a specific disease among those pairs who moved from their place of birth at the decision of their parents. Twins moving at a later age would be expected to leave some family member behind which in most cases will lead to the ultimate tracing of the pair.

It seems justified to conclude that it is possible to obtain a representative twin sample by basing the selection of index cases on the material found in the Danish Twin Register, and once found it is no problem to follow the twins continuously. Regional or national files of individuals with specific disorders and abnormalities may be matched with the Twin Register, and thus a fully unbiased twin sample is obtained which may be kept under continuous surveillance for any length of time. The study of disorders for which no central registers exist have to be based on the material ascertained primarily through questionnaires. This implies that those who refuse co-operation will be omitted from this type of material; they constitute, however, less than 2 per cent of the total material, and may be searched for in the central files of hospital admissions, from death certificates, etc., and from information obtained from their doctors.

Some of the main results of the research based on the Twin Register have been surveyed earlier (Hauge *et al*. 1968). All previous publications including material from the Register may be found in the list of references.

Advantages of longitudinal studies

A few examples illustrating the special advantages of longitudinal studies in twin populations will be given in the following. The research devoted primarily to an evaluation of the relative importance of genetic factors in the development of a given trait will at the same time provide answers to many other important questions. Thus, studied 122 like-sexed female pairs in Holm *et al*. (1980) which at least one twin presented cancer of the breast, and in which the partners without cancer had been followed for at least ten more years. Holm demonstrated, first of all, a limited significance of specific genetic factors in this common type of cancer. Thus, the question which is often raised by a healthy MZ partner of a twin who has recently contracted cancer of the breast is whether this implies that she too will develop a malignant tumor. This may be answered with reasonable confidence: her risk of developing breast cancer is about five times that of the general population whereas her risk of cancer at other sites seems to be the same as it is for anyone else in the general population. Furthermore, long-term follow-up of the pairs permits an evaluation of the possible importance of exogenous factors which have often been supposed to influence the risk of developing cancer of the breast. The detailed examinations of 45 MZ breast cancer pairs showed that neither marital status nor number of deliveries and age at the first delivery was significantly associated with the appearance of the cancer; these results would have been difficult to obtain in other types of material because it is only here that the patients and their controls have been completely matched not only for sex, age, place of birth, etc., but also for the total genetic equipment (as they are MZ pairs). This is a unique situation in medical research. Similarly, in diabetes, fully matched controls (i.e. non-diabetic MZ twin partners of female diabetics), followed for many years after the appearance of diabetes in the first partner, have shown no differences with respect to number of pregnancies. This reduces the weight of the assumption that pregnancies *per se* increase the risk of developing diabetes. On the other hand, in MZ pairs known to have the genetic liability to develop diabetes, the heavier partner seems to be likely to manifest the symptoms first (Raebild 1967).

In a study over a period of twenty years of the influence of tobacco consumption on health, MZ twin partners with different smoking habits have shown that, given the same genotype, the partner who smokes more develops respiratory, cardiovascular, and gastroduodenal (ulcer) symptoms earlier and more often than the partner who smokes less (Hauge *et al.* 1970).

In the present Register, the classical type of twin study aiming primarily at an estimate of the relative contribution of genetic components to the variation within a population with respect to a given disease, has quite often shown this contribution to be smaller than postulated previously in studies based on samples with an overrepresentation of severe and concordant cases. When the investigations start from the total population of twins, as is the case in the Twin Register, one gets a more representative sample and a better impression of the situation generally prevailing (Fischer *et al.* 1969; Fischer 1971, 1973; Gotlieb Jensen 1972).

Turning to the psychological and psychiatric disorders, the same pattern has also been observed. Twins followed through the major part of their lives show less concordance with respect to law offences than previously postulated (Christiansen 1968). The special registration systems found in Denmark make possible a rather complete ascertainment of law offenders, and the total twin population may be taken into a study of this type. No previous investigation has been based on an unselected sample representative of the general population. The size of the material and the prolonged observation will permit detailed analyses of possible associations with social class, upbringing, occupation, etc.

The studies of some of the major psychoses, schizophrenia, and manic-depressive disorders, as well as other types of depressions have among other things provided information on the range of symptoms manifested by persons carrying the same 'sensitive' genetic predisposition and on the extent to which external factors determine age of onset, course, severity, response to treatment, etc. (Fischer *et al.* 1969; Fischer 1971, 1973; Bertelsen *et al.* 1977; and Shapiro 1970).

It has been observed repeatedly that twins are more prepared to co-operate in research and to continue to do so. Thus, the opportunity exists to get highly valuable knowledge from a rather unique group of individuals, i.e. the still healthy partners of MZ twins affected by a given disorder. By continuous observation and examination, new information may gradually be revealed about early signs and symptoms of the disorder, and about minor indications of the responsible, underlying but invisible, 'sensitive' gene-constitution, known to be there as inferred from the affected twin partner. This may be of essential value in the early detection and prevention of important, common health problems and maladjustments.

The value of longitudinal twin studies based on twin populations in epidemiology has only recently been appreciated. Beyond doubt more will be learned in this way about the significance of genetic equipment in response to the increasing amount and number of environmental influences which may affect the health of the individual and the population. This new knowledge may thus permit preventive measures to be directed towards the most sensitive groups. This tool should, therefore, be taken into consideration in the general efforts to improve the health of human populations.

40. Psychomotor and cognitive development of twins from birth to six years (Belgium)

WILLIAM DE COSTER, ANDRÉ VANDIERENDONCK, MIEKE DE ZUTTER, MICHEL THIERY, and ROBERT DEROM

Introduction

Twin studies have often been considered as an important means to settle the nature–nurture controversy. All differences between the members of monozygotic (MZ) twin pairs are due to environmental influences, whereas the differences between the members of dizygotic (DZ) twin pairs can be attributed to heredity as well. The ratio of the intrapair variances of MZ and DZ twins yields a simple and straightforward index of the relative importance of genetic factors (h^2). However, there are several objections against such a measure (e.g. Bodmer and Cavalli-Sforza 1970; Ginsburg and Koslowski 1976). In the first place, the measure is based on the assumption that a test score is the algebraic sum of a hereditary and an environmental score (test score = heredity + environment). An alternative model includes a component score expressing the interaction of heredity and environment (test score = heredity + environment + interaction). The rationale behind this interaction component is the idea that certain genotypes are more suited to some kinds of environments than to others. However, if the latter model is correct, by necessity the idea of measuring the relative importance of heredity leads to oversimplification.

A second, and more serious problem with h^2 is the generalizability problem. As far as the twin situation is concerned, it must be remarked (see Bodmer and Cavalli-Sforza 1970):

(a) That the amount of environmental intrapair variability in twins is only part of the total amount of variability possible;

(b) That the amount of hereditary intra-pair variability in DZ twins is only part of the amount of hereditary variability between people.

Moreover, the twin situation is not comparable to any other situation in several important respects:

(a) Physical identity or resemblance might be a cue for parents to induce psychological identity;
(b) In the first years of life, parental care must be divided among the twin partners;
(c) From the beginning on, both members of the pair are frequently together, to such an extent that parental intervention is less often called for.

All these factors—and possibly many more—are specific to the twin situation and might confuse the issue.

These considerations, namely the impracticability of solving the nature–nurture issue on the basis of twin studies and the possibility of equalizing effects in the twin situation itself, lay at the basis of the presently reported studies of twin development.

The main purposes of this research project were:

(a) To investigate the impact of some important covariates of twin characteristics, such as birth weight, gestational length, socio-economic class, educational care, and parity;
(b) To get more insight into the specific dynamics of the twin situation;

(c) To replicate the findings of other investigators, so as to find some order in the rather contradictory evidence and to see whether the findings from other studies can be extrapolated to the local situation (province of Flanders, more specially district of Ghent).

To realize these purposes the longitudinal approach seemed appropriate for the following reasons:

(a) The number of new-born twins is rather small, so that it is advantageous to follow a relatively small sample over a certain period of time;

(b) To obtain the exact zygosity of the twin set, it is necessary that this diagnosis be made at the time of birth, i.e., on the basis of placental morphology, blood typing, etc.; therefore collaboration with a hospital is essential, a fact which inevitably will restrict the sample size;

(c) Spreading the study over several years, the sample may be enlarged so as to reach more reliable conclusions;

(d) Follow-up research is a very suitable method to depict the course of psychological development, although other approaches are equally effective.

Nevertheless, the method has some drawbacks which should be mentioned:

(a) Successive administrations of the same test, which is sometimes inevitable, leads to retest effect. Even when test–retest reliability is high, such effects do occur.

(b) Drop-out is inevitable, and it is often not possible to test whether this drop-out is selective or not.

(c) Administration of a test on repeated occasions is often done by different examiners, and because developmental tests tend to be susceptible to experimenter effects (see Chapter 13, this volume), the validity of the results is often degraded. Of course, similar effects may be obtained in transversal studies, but a careful planning in such studies permits a separation of experimenter and age effects. This is not possible in longitudinal studies because the assessment of the test at a certain age level must be done by an experimenter who is available at that time.

Method

Subjects

Subjects were twins born at the Department of Obstetrics, University Hospital, Ghent, Belgium. Only twins living in the district of Ghent were included in the sample. The sampling covered several years, so that by now 36 MZ and 43 DZ pairs have already been observed at the age of 6 months, and 13 MZ and 20 DZ pairs have been observed at the age of 5 years. A control group of singletons born at the same hospital was matched with the first born twin partner for age, sex, socio-economic class, and parity. There are currently no data available on the representativeness of these samples.

A second sample of twins was drawn from the first year of elementary schools (age about 6 years) in the city of Ghent. Eighty-seven twin children were attending these schools. A control group of 87 singletons was randomly selected from the same schools.

Procedure

Zygosity was diagnosed on the basis of foetal blood examination and analysis of the placenta and membranes. In cases of doubt, supplementary analyses were carried out, such as zymograms of the placenta.

The children of the first sample were observed in their home environments at the ages of 6 months, 2, and 4 years. In addition, the twins were also observed at the ages of 1, 3, and 5 years. A slightly modified version of the Bühler–Hetzer Entwicklungstest (BH) was administered. This test yields a general development quotient (DQ), and scores on six subscales measuring sensory and motor capacities, social adjustment, learning, manipulatory skills, and intelligence. By summation of all item scores of items which involve the use of language by the child, a language score was obtained. From the age of three on, information was also gathered from the nursery school staff. From the age of four on, the Leiter International Performance Scale (LIPS), an IQ test, was also administered. Socio-economic class was measured in three levels, based on a classification of parental occupations. Educational care was measured also in three levels on the basis of a questionnaire administered to the parents of the twins.

The twins and singletons of the second sample were administered the Nijmeegse Schoolbekwaamheidstest (NST—Mönks et al. 1969), a school readiness test, and a Dutch adaptation of the Primary Mental Abilities (PMA—Knops 1967). These tests were administered at school.

Results

Developmental and intelligence quotients

In contradistinction with evidence reported by Zazzo (1960) and Koch (1966) on the average, singletons did not differ from twins. Moreover, no differences between the first- and second-born twin partners reached significance.

In general there were no significant differences between MZ and DZ pairs, although some exceptions have been noticed at the ages of 3 and 4 years (De Coster et al. 1977). These data suggest that although there are certain systematic differences between MZ and DZ pairs, in general they are small. However, when DZ pairs of same (DZ=) and DZ pairs of different sex (DZ ≠) are compared to MZ twins, there is a clear tendency for differences to increase with age. The picture presented by these data is, however, not very clear. Nevertheless, DZ= pairs tend to perform better than MZ and DZ≠ twins, and the difference between MZ and DZ≠ twins seems to be rather small and unsystematic. These findings are not entirely consonant with the evidence presented by Zazzo (1960) and Koch (1966).

There appears to be a strong tendency for twins from higher socio-economic classes and from a more stimulating environment (high educational care) to show higher developmental and intelligence quotients, and higher language scores (see Table 40.1). The effects of parity are, on the contrary, rather unsystematic, whereas gestational length and birth weight have a deleterious effect on development in the first two years of life; from the age of two on, no significant differences attributable to these factors appear (Table 40.2).

Intrapair differences in developmental and intelligence quotients

MZ pairs tend to show smaller intrapair variance than DZ= pairs, which in turn show less intrapair variance than DZ ≠ pairs. The differences between these three groups tend to increase with age. The effects are observed in IQ scores as well as in DQ scores and language scores (Table 40.3). These findings are consonant with those of other investigators (Koch 1966; Vandenberg 1968; Zazzo 1960).

Socio-economic class, educational care, and parity were not found to affect intrapair variance of twins, in either of the dependent variables studied. This finding is at variance with evidence reported by other investigators.

Scores on NST and PMA

Comparison of twins and singletons of the second sample on NST

TABLE 40.1

Mean DQ, IQ, and language scores of twin pairs as a function of socio-economic class and educational care

	Socio-economic class				Educational care			
Age	I	II	III	F[b]	I	II	III	F[b]
DQ								
0;6 (2,76)[a]		103·6[c]	99·2	0·32 ns	94·6	92·7	114·0	3·50*
1;0 (2,66)		104·0[c]	109·5	1·75 ns	105·9	101·8	114·8	7·78*
2;0 (2,48)	93·5	97·3	102·8	3·94*	80·9	96·3	103·9	34·38*
3;0 (2,43)	97·4	101·1	107·2	4·00*	89·1	97·1	110·3	24·78*
4;0 (2,38)	101·5	100·6	112·4	9·47*	96·2	99·2	111·7	16·99*
5;0 (2,30)	103·4	96·7	109·1	11·76*	96·7	102·5	104·6	3·37*
IQ								
4;0 (2,38)	94·7	95·1	109·9	7·39*	87·2	93·7	108·4	12·45*
5;0 (2,30)	94·7	94·9	111·9	10·26*	88·8	97·2	105·6	5·35*
Language								
2;0 (2,48)	0·6	1·0	1·2	5·40*	0·4	0·7	1·3	19·80*
3;0 (2,43)	2·6	3·2	3·8	6·59*	1·8	2·9	3·9	23·69*
4;0 (2,38)	4·4	4·6	5·9	9·55*	3·9	4·6	5·6	9·06*
5;0 (2,30)	6·5	6·7	7·4	6·24*	6·5	6·4	7·2	7·41*

[a] The numbers in parentheses indicate the degrees of freedom of the corresponding F-value.
[b] ns stands for 'non-significant at the 5 per cent level'; an asterisk indicates significance at least at the 5 per cent level.
[c] For these data degrees of freedom for the F-test are (1,77) at 0;6 and (1,67) at 1;0.

TABLE 40.2

Mean DQ and IQ of twin pairs as a function of gestational length and birth weight

	Gestational length[a]				Birth weight[a]			
Ages	I	II	III	F[c]	I	II	III	F[c]
DQ								
0;6 (2,76)[b]	88·6	106·9	112·6	4·05*	82·9	108·6	110·4	5·81*
1;0 (2,66)	102·6	107·4	112·3	3·74*	99·7	106·7	113·6	9·14*
2;0 (2,48)	100·5	94·8	95·3	1·39 ns	96·6	100·4	93·9	1·88 ns
3;0 (2,43)	102·2	101·4	99·6	0·30 ns	97·5	102·2	103·5	1·79 ns
4;0 (2,38)	107·9	102·7	101·0	2·64 ns	98·9	106·3	104·9	3·04 ns
5;0 (2,30)	99·7	105·5	102·4	2·04 ns	99·6	105·9	101·0	2·65 ns
IQ								
4;0 (2,38)	103·7	93·9	98·9	2·18 ns	92·6	100·8	100·4	1·73 ns
5;0 (2,30)	99·0	98·8	100·6	0·04 ns	91·7	105·1	99·9	4·15*

[a] Gestational length is measured in three levels: I: < 259 days; II: pair 259 to 266 days; III: > 266 days.
[b] The numbers in parentheses indicate the degrees of freedom of the corresponding F-value.
[c] ns stands for 'non-significant at the 5 per cent level'; an asterisk indicates significance at at least the 5 per cent level.

TABLE 40.3

Mean intrapair differences in DQ, IQ, and language scores of MZ, DZ =, and DZ ≠ twins

	DQ				Language			
Age	MZ	DZ=	DZ≠	F[b]	MZ	DZ=	DZ≠	F
0;6 (2,76)[a]	4·8	10·0	8·4	3·21*				
1;0 (2,66)	10·1	11·5	9·5	0·16 ns				
2;0 (2,48)	4·6	4·0	6·2	2·32 ns	0·1	0·3	0·2	3·02 ns
3;0 (2,43)	6·5	8·7	13·9	8·22*	1·6	0·5	1·2	2·04 ns
4;0 (2,38)	4·2	4·2	8·1	7·67*	0·8	0·4	1·2	7·20*
5;0 (2,30)	4·3	3·8	7·4	3·56*	0·5	0·4	1·1	6·33*
IQ								
4;0 (2,38)	15·5	8·8	12·7	1·76 ns				
5;0 (2,30)	12·5	8·5	18·0	3·62*				

[a] The numbers in parentheses indicate the degrees of freedom of the corresponding F-term.
[b] ns stands for 'non-significant at the 5 per cent level'; an asterisk indicates significance at at least the 5 per cent level.

scores reveals a general difference in favour of the singletons. With the exception of two subtests (concepts of size, quantity and proportions, and critical perception) the differences on the subtests did not reach the conventional level of significance of 5 per cent. Scores on the PMA differed only on the verbal factor, again in favour of the singletons (Table 40.4).

In general intrapair differences of the 40 twin pairs in the sample (16 MZ, 13 DZ=, and 11 DZ≠) did not vary over the three twin categories. Only one significant difference was observed (on a motor subtest of the NST), and this might as well have occurred by chance (1 observation out of 15). Intrapair differences showed up for the total score of the NST, and the verbal factor of the PMA (Table 40.4).

TABLE 40.4

Mean scores and intrapair differences on NST and PMA of the children in the second sample (6 years of age)

	Mean scores[a]			Mean intrapair differences[b]			
Tests[d]	Singletons	Twins	F[c]	MZ	DZ=	DZ≠	F[c]
NST 1	104·7	103·5	1·27 ns	1·3	0·9	1·8	1·10 ns
NST 2	100·9	99·9	0·52 ns	1·6	1·1	1·9	1·03 ns
NST 3	101·7	98·3	6·63*	1·3	0·9	1·9	2·49 ns
NST 4	106·1	104·5	1·34 ns	1·3	2·2	2·3	1·53 ns
NST 5	104·1	100·0	13·54*	1·7	1·6	1·9	0·15 ns
NST 6	102·5	101·7	0·45 ns	1·7	1·6	1·8	0·02 ns
NST 7	102·6	101·6	0·72 ns	2·4	2·8	3·2	0·33 ns
NST 8	99·7	97·8	1·37 ns	1·5	1·1	2·0	1·92 ns
NST 9	103·1	101·3	1·50 ns	1·3	2·1	2·0	1·70 ns
NST 10	98·4	98·4	0·00 ns	1·1	1·3	1·6	0·41 ns
NST total	102·2	98·2	6·17*	5·4	6·8	12·6	3·33*
PMA V	104·5	100·6	4·24*	2·4	2·7	6·1	7·68*
PMA P	112·7	109·1	2·12 ns	3·9	4·7	5·3	0·34 ns
PMA Q	114·0	112·9	0·09 ns	2·3	3·3	5·0	3·06 ns
PMA S	92·1	88·1	1·94 ns	3·4	3·0	5·1	1·77 ns

[a] Degrees of freedom for the F-term in this analysis are (1,172).
[b] Degrees of freedom for the F-term in this analysis are (2,37).
[c] ns stands for 'not significant at the 5 per cent level'; an asterisk indicates significance at at least the 5 per cent level.
[d] Scores are given for the 10 subtests of the NST, the total NST score, the PMA factors: V (verbal), P (perceptual), Q (quantitative), and S (space).

Discussion

In general, our results are in agreement with those of other investigators. However, some exceptions should be mentioned:

(a) In our study, performance level of MZ and DZ≠ pairs is lower than that of DZ= pairs, whereas Zazzo (1960) found that DZ≠ pairs perform better than MZ pairs, but less well than DZ= pairs. Koch (1966), on the contrary, found no differences between DZ= and DZ≠, but both groups performed at a higher level than MZ pairs.

(b) Although socio-economic class and educational care were found to correlate with DQ and IQ, they did not affect the intrapair variance of the several twin types. In the literature, generally, such differentiating effects are reported.

(c) No significant differences whatsoever, were found between the first- and second-born twin partners, whereas Zazzo (1960) reported such differences.

(d) Comparison of a random sample of singletons with twins leads to the traditionally reported difference between both groups. However, when the singletons are matched with the first-born twin partner for age, sex, and parity, this difference does not obtain.

Our sample is small, but it proved large enough to detect some major inter-group differences. However, such a sample leads to *non-significant* differences between groups *whenever the observed differences are rather small*, relative to the error variance. As Zazzo (1960) worked with larger samples, it is not surprising that he found significant differences between first- and second-born twin partners. It is clear that such differences exist, but they are surely small. Besides, as was pointed out in an earlier research report:

A tentative explanation of this divergence may be that very few of the twins sampled had suffered from birth complications. Moreover, if as a rule the first-born twin is more endangered by mechanical stress during labor and delivery, it is less affected by biochemical noxae, mainly hypoxia. [De Coster *et al.* 1977]

The sample size argument seems also to be valid in the interpretation of the effects of socio-economic class and educational care. Moreover, there are several differences between the studies in this respect, such as:

(a) Method of sampling;
(b) Operational definition of socio-economic class;
(c) Measurement of educational care;
(d) Time of research, and concomitant modification of the common educational style of the parents, etc.

Concerning the differences in the general level of performance of the different twin types, it should be remarked that the differences between our findings and those of Zazzo and Koch, might well be due to random fluctuations in the samples. Although it might be tempting to exaggerate this discrepancy, in our opinion, the general picture is the same, but because of the smallness of the differences relative to the sample size the picture is not always that clear; it is manifest that this remark does not only concern the present study.

Discussing the agreements and disagreements between our data and those of other investigators does not release us from the duty to interpret the data. This interpretation concentrates on two points:

(a) The influence of perinatal factors;
(b) The influence of the specific twin situation.

It is generally known and accepted that gestational length and birth weight are important factors in physical and psychological development. As twins have on the average a shorter period of gestation than singletons, it may be expected that they show the same symptoms as prematurely born singletons, i.e., a slightly lower level of performance on developmental and intelligence scales.

Analogously a lowered birth weight may have consequences for psychological development.

On the basis of this reasoning it is expected that the DQ of twins is slightly lower than that of singletons (born on term). This is exactly what has predominantly been reported by investigators. Moreover, gestational length and birth weight should differentiate further within the twin group, such that the shorter the period of gestation or the smaller the birth weight, the lower the DQ. Furthermore, it might be expected that within certain limits, the influence of these perinatal factors is only temporary and may be compensated for by optimal biological functioning in a normal environment. Hence, with growing age, the effects of gestational length and birth weight should disappear, and this is exactly what appears to happen in our sample of twins.

This rather simple hypothesis can account for a large part of the data. Nevertheless, it does not apply to differences observed between MZ, DZ=, and DZ≠ twins. In our opinion, however, the typical twin situation is an important determinant of parental behaviour. Often, due to the circumstances, twin partners are thrown on each other's society so that they are less frequently confronted with adult models of behaviour and especially of adult language. Thus, it may be expected, if this analysis of the twin situation is right, that systematic differences in language development appear, such as the following:

(a) Singletons have on the average a higher language score than twins (confirmed only in the second sample, at the age of six with a more reliable test);
(b) The language score of MZ twins is on the average lower than that of DZ twins (confirmed only at the level of three years).

Furthermore, extending the reasoning, as adult models of language are assumed to be generally more favourable in higher socio-economic classes, it is expected that there is a positive relationship between socio-economic class and language performance (confirmed). Analogously, higher types of educational care involve more frequent intervention of adult verbal models, so that the same pattern of results is expected (confirmed).

If it is assumed that the presence of adult models of language is a principal factor, it is evident that the model may be assumed to be equally effective for both twin partners; consequently, language modelling is not a difference-provoking factor and it is manifest that—if it is a principal variable—the intrapair variance of all twins should remain rather small, at least in language scores (confirmed).

The argument developed so far for the case of language performance may be extended to performance in general. As a consequence, the same pattern of results is expected for DQ and IQ. This interpretation is, at least in part, in agreement with the data. However, a difficulty should be mentioned. The fact that the DQ and the language score show the same pattern of results cannot imply with any degree of confidence that these results extend beyond the language items of the BH scale. With a conventional test, it would be relatively easy to analyse the relationship between the scale and its language items, but because of a rather clumsy technique of associating to each item a certain value in 'days', such an analysis is difficult to perform and almost impossible to interpret.

The data of our second sample suggests that the effect of the twin situation is to a high degree restricted to verbal intelligence: on the PMA only the verbal factor discriminated between twins and singletons, and one of the NST subtests may be suspected of high verbal loadings. On the other hand, the intrapair differences in this sample seem to be somewhat larger, although on the whole still small.

In summary, there appears to be evidence in favour of the hypothesis that a smaller frequency of encounters with adult language models is responsible for the divergent development of several types of twins and singletons as far as verbal performance is concerned. It is not yet clear whether this hypothesis may be extended to other types of adult modelling as well. As far as the IQ scores on the LIPS suggest this extension seems to be called for, especially as this test is generally described as a culture-free test.

However, the hypothesis is not completely confirmed by the present data, namely, the ordering of MZ, DZ≠, and DZ performances is not as predicted. But this does not imply that the hypothesis is completely incorrect. For one thing, the trend of MZ twins scoring less on the average than DZ twins is present, but contrary to prediction, DZ≠ twins tend to score less than DZ=. This might be due to the presence of certain situational factors which are not yet studied. Therefore, future studies of twin development, if they are deemed necessary, should start with a thorough analysis of the social situation, and the specific parental behaviour and attitudes. From that moment on, twin studies become more relevant for educational sciences and social welfare (advice to parents concerning educational interventions, attitudes, behaviour, etc.).

In this context some remarks on the desirability of twin studies are in order. Twin studies are rather expensive, due to the relative rareness of twins and the absolute necessity to invoke the co-operation of medical workers to arrive at a reliable diagnosis of zygosity. Furthermore, in studies of twin development one is often urged to use the follow-up method, which, on account of certain drawbacks, is apt to lead to doubtful interpretations, at least for part of the data. A third point concerns the existence of a specific twin situation: if such a situation exists, it implies that findings from twin studies cannot be extrapolated to singletons.

To sum up, anyone who wishes to study twins should know that such research is especially fitted to the nature–nurture issue. However, if psychology intends to solve this problem, it should try to do so by proving or disproving the inheritance of very specific miniature abilities or skills. The larger the units studied, the more complex the structure of inherited and acquired components becomes, and the less probable it is to find an acceptable answer to the problem.

Acknowledgements

The authors are indebted to all persons who have collaborated in this research project, which was sponsored by the *Fonds voor Collectief Fundamenteel Onderzoek*. The authors wish to thank especially M. C. Dutoit, J. Lerou, K. Verheyden, and T. Monsecour for their invaluable cooperation. The project was executed in collaboration with the department of Obstetrics and Paediatrics. Their co-operation is kindly acknowledged. André Vandierendonck was responsible for the statistical treatment of the data.

ii. Adoptee cohort

41. The Danish adoption register

BJØRN JACOBSEN and FINI SCHULSINGER

The idea of using adoptees and their families is not a new one. For practical purposes this method has been the only one where it was possible to obtain samples of sufficient size, the number of monozygotic twins reared apart being too small. Roe (1945) made a study on children of alcoholic parentage raised in foster homes, and Heston (1966) and Heston and Dunney in a now classic study (1968) examined genetic factors in schizophrenia and the effect of being brought up in a foster home versus in an institution. Hitherto, the method had mostly been used in retrospective studies but potentially the design could also be used for longitudinal studies and follow-up studies. This is one aspect of Heston's and Dunney's study (1968) and of the study by Eldred et al. (1976). Bohman's (1973) big study of adopted children and their families by using 10-year-old probands has created a cohort he is using for follow-up studies.

The method could be described as quasi-experimental using 'nature's own design' which can be varied in different ways as shown so elegantly by Rosenthal (1974a). The renewed interest in the use of adopted populations was due to Kety (1959) who pointed out the potential value of using adoptees and their families for research into the factors causing schizophrenia.

In 1963 the major adoption studies carried out at the Psykologisk Institut, Kommunehospitalet, Copenhagen were initiated by Seymour S. Kety, H. Wender, and David Rosenthal in collaboration with Fini Schulsinger. Denmark was chosen because of its relatively stable, homogeneous population with a low emigration rate. Thanks to different public registers (Adoption Register of the Department of Justice, Folkeregistret, the Central Register of Psychiatric Admissions at the Institute of Psychiatric Demography at the state hospital, Risskov; Professor Erik Strömgren and Dr Annalise Dupont from the Institute of Psychiatric Demography, the Psychiatric Hospital near Århus, are gratefully acknowledged for their kind co-operation. Without the extensive service of this institute it would not have been possible to carry out the adoption studies described later in this article. It was possible to trace all adoptions during a selected period and to find adoptees' relatives through the Folkeregister. Through the Institute of Psychiatric Demography at the state hospital, Risskov, (Dupont et al. 1974) it was possible to check all psychiatric admissions of the adoptees and their relatives.

Originally, a pool of nearly 5500 adoptees from adoptions which had taken place in the city and county of Copenhagen from 1924 through 1947 were selected. There were three reasons for limiting the sample to this period:

(1) The Folkeregister began in 1924 and it would be much more time-consuming to trace all relatives (biological parents, siblings, half-siblings, adoptive parents, and -siblings) without it.

(2) 1947 was chosen because we wanted the adoptees to have lived for so long that most of them would have traversed at least part of the calculated risk years for the outbreak of schizophrenia because the first study concerned schizophrenia.

(3) Finally, the number of adoptions in Denmark began to show a sharp decrease after the Second World War.

Later, the pool was extended to cover all Denmark from 1924 through 1947. This pool consists of approximately 14 500 adoptees; it is planned to extend some studies to cover all these adoptees and in other studies the whole pool has already been used.

Because of the lack of adequate standard background information for the adoptees a special sample (the K-Sample) has also been selected. It consists of approximately 5500 non-adopted children and their families from the greater Copenhagen area who have been matched pairwise with the Copenhagen adoptees. They have been selected to match the adopted Copenhagen pool. So far this sample, however, has been used very little.

Before describing some of the more important results of the studies finished so far it is necessary to take a look at the methodological problems involved, since the design has disadvantages as well as advantages.

Methodological disadvantages

It is now well known that adoptees and their families represent a screened group. Adoptive parents are in general older, often rather much so, than the biological parents and the average age for parents in the population at large. When they get their often only adopted child it may be after many years of frustration and because of their own inability to get children. The screening procedures that precede adoption are in themselves somewhat unpleasant and might influence the attitude of the adoptive parents to their future child in a negative way. It wouldn't be surprising then if many people after going through screening procedures and waiting in vain for a biological child might have too high expectations about getting an adoptive child. When problems then set in after the child has arrived they may overreact because of their disappointment. How this has affected studies using adoptees is difficult to evaluate but it is counteracted by the use of adopted control groups.

People with obvious health problems, known mental illness and/or mental deficiency, and criminal records for the last five years, above a certain age and single, would in general not be accepted as adoptive parents by the Danish authorities. Also children with a known genetic load of mental illness and/or deficiency, with chronic physical injuries, etc. would often be screened out of the pool offered for adoption. Instead they might be brought up in children's homes or only offered for adoption with a warning to the adoptive parents about the risks involved. Mednick and Hutchings (1977) have discussed these problems of labelling (see also Bohman 1973). It is difficult to say how much possible knowledge about behaviour disorders in the biological parents influences the attitude of the adoptive parents. If a child had developed clear-cut signs of retardation and of mental illness he would generally not be offered to prospective parents. However, neither the adoptive index nor control probands selected for our studies had parents whose mental illness had started before the adoption procedure had taken place.

People who gave away children for adoption obviously did not represent a cross-section of the population. The mothers were often young, younger than mothers in general, the fathers perhaps more antisocial in their behaviour. Both mothers and fathers showed more criminality than the population in general. Most of the biological parents were so young that they had lived for too short a time for an effective screen for mental illness. This fact in various ways might work in the opposite direction of the screening procedure for adoptive parents mentioned above.

Hutchings and Mednick (1974) state that the adoption agencies (Mothers' Aid) seemed to follow a procedure which resulted in a correlation between social class in the biological and adoptive fathers. They may have matched for more general characteristics such as educational background, intelligence, and to a certain degree appearance (no children with brown eyes and black hair to fair-haired and blue-eyed people). We have earlier (Schulsinger and Jacobsen 1975) questioned the use of the biological father's social class in this way because of his peripheral role in the adoption situation. Bohman (1973) in his study of 10–11-year-old adoptive children and their families found it very difficult to get exact information about psychopathology, drinking, and criminality in the biological fathers in his material. His study, however, was not aimed specifically at uncovering genetic influences.

In genetic studies the use of adoptees and their families, such as has been done in the Family Study (Kety et al. 1968, 1975), presents some problems because the largest group of persons examined are half-sibs. Besides not being first-degree relatives they also carry a genetic load from a person (mother or father) not examined by us. In the co-parent study by Rosenthal (1974b) assortative mating occurred very often. We don't know if that has been the case in other studies but some comfort may be had from the fact that the paternal and maternal half-sibs in the Family Study didn't differ with respect to schizophrenic disorders.

The way that adoptees and their families have been used in research until now may also have other weaknesses. The studies have all been retrospective; this may mean that it is impossible to trace some factors contributing to schizophrenia or other behavioural disorders. We don't think that information on 'skewed' messages and 'double binds' can be dug up in such a retrospective investigation.

Many other poorly defined variables might influence people in choosing children for adoption. It is known for instance that girls are preferred to boys, being considered easier to bring up. A certain connection might also exist between some forms of psychopathology especially in the adoptive mother and the appeal that some prospective adoptive children with perhaps striking features might have to her.

Methodological advantages and experimental designs

As already mentioned the advantages of using adoptive samples can be summarized as follows: the researcher works with 'nature's own setting' in a quasi-experimental design. Laboratory conditions such as used by geneticists when studying behavioural disorders in animals are, of course, not possible to establish where a human being is the focus of our study.

Depending on the material used and the aims of the investigation, it is possible to devise follow-up studies or longitudinal studies. Bohman's (1973) population could easily be, and has been, used in this way; the differences he has found might be much clearer and easier to interpret with repeated follow-up studies and increasing age of his probands. Using a longitudinal design provides a greater possibility of uncovering environmental factors of importance, and thereby increases the possibility of some kind of primary prevention.

Rosenthal (1974a) has described some experimental designs using adoptees and their families. Some of these designs have already been used by this Institute. At this point we can indicate some of the advantages which are offered by these methods. The researcher can be kept blind with respect to the status of his subjects, and thus selective bias is avoided. Under ideal but hardly practical circumstances the experimenter could even be blind as regards the aim of the investigation. Furthermore, with these designs it is possible to treat heredity and environment as relatively independent variables.

The designs can be varied in a number of ways. One way is to begin with the adoptees as probands and make their families the focus of study (see Table 41.1). This method has been employed by Kety et al. in the Family Study (1968, 1975). The preliminary results of this study will be described below. With this design we can test the hypothesis that if schizophrenia is heritable, then schizophrenic spectrum disorders should cluster among the biological relatives of the index cases. Conversely, if schizophrenia develops

TABLE 41.1

Adoptees' families design (after Rosenthal et al. 1974)

Probands (Adoptees)	Relatives	
	Biological	Adoptive
Schizophrenic		
Control (Non-schizophrenic)		

because of environmental factors, we would expect that the adoptive parents of the index cases would have schizophrenic spectrum disorders in greater numbers than the adoptive parents of the controls.

The design can be altered so that the focus becomes the adoptees themselves. This design is referred to as the Adoptees' Study (see Table 41.2). If we find that a significantly higher number of the index cases (i.e. adoptees with a schizophrenic biological parent) than of the controls (i.e. adoptees who do *not* have a schizophrenic biological parent) are given a diagnosis within the schizophrenic spectrum, this would support a theory of the heritability of schizophrenia. This design has been used in a study of adopted-away offspring of schizophrenics (Rosenthal *et al.* 1974).

TABLE 41.2

Adoptees' study design (after Rosenthal et al. 1974)

	Biological parents	
	Schizophrenic	Non-schizophrenic
Adoptees	1	1'
	2	2'
	3	3'
	4	4'
	.	.
	.	.
	.	.
	.	.
	n	n'

The cross-fostering design has been used in some studies by the Psykologisk Institut (Wender *et al.* 1974; Hutchings and Mednick 1974; Rosenthal *et al.* 1975; Eldred *et al.* 1976). This design is depicted in Table 41.3. Here the two opposing hypotheses are tested at the same time. If it is desired to test the two variables independently other designs will have to be used (see Tables 41.4 and 41.5).

Goodwin *et al.* (1974b) has used the so-called half-sib method (see Table 41.6), in a study of men with alcohol problems. The method is less precise than those mentioned above, with greater environmental variance and a genetic factor which is not so well defined. For longitudinal purposes, however, the method may prove useful.

TABLE 41.3

Cross-fostering design (after Rosenthal et al. 1974)

Parents	
Biological	Adoptive
Schizophrenic	Schizophrenic
Non-schizophrenic	Non-schizophrenic

TABLE 41.4

Design to test the 'pure' environmentalist hypothesis (after Rosenthal et al. 1974)

	Biological Parents Non-schizophrenic	
	Rearing parents	
	Schizophrenic	Non-schizophrenic
Adoptees	1	1'
	2	2'
	3	3'
	4	4'
	.	.
	.	.
	.	.
	.	.
	n	n'

TABLE 41.5

Design to test the effects of a hypothesized environmental variable coacting with the genetic variable (after Rosenthal et al. 1974)

	Biological parents Schizophrenic	
	Rearing parents	
	Schizophrenic	Non-schizophrenic
Adoptees	1	1'
	2	2'
	3	3'
	4	4'
	.	.
	.	.
	.	.
	n	n'

TABLE 41.6

Biological parents alcoholic

Rearing parents

Biological parents alcoholic	Adoptive parents
1	1'
2	2'
3	3'
4	4'
.	.
.	.
.	.
.	.
n	n'

A short review of some of the more important results from studies published to date using the adoptive material

In a study by Rosenthal *et al.* (1974) concerning the adopted-away offspring of schizophrenics, the adoptees themselves were the focus of the study. Index cases were selected from the pool who had a parent with known schizophrenia, borderline schizophrenia, or, in some cases, with manic-depressive psychosis. Controls were adoptees whose biological parents at that time had no known record of mental illness. The two samples were matched with respect to demographic variables. The index and control probands had a very thorough and careful examination which included psychological and psychophysiological testing, and an intensive and extensive psychiatric interview. The diagnostic evaluation was then done by several independent raters. Throughout, examiners and diagnostic raters were kept blind as to the subject's status as an index or control case. This blindness has also been maintained in the other studies using the adoptive material. The data which have been analysed so far indicate that heredity plays a significant role in the transmission of schizophrenic spectrum disorders. It was also found that 17·8 per cent of the controls received a diagnosis within the schizophrenic spectrum. Hanne Schulsinger (1976) discussed this problem thoroughly. It may be that when examining a population so intensively as has been done in these studies, many more people with schizophrenic spectrum disorders will be found than has been the case in previous, more extensive population examinations. The findings may also reflect the fact that a sample consisting of adoptees and their families has a greater amount of psychopathology than the population at large. In all the studies reviewed here, not only has schizophrenia occurred more often than expected, but also, non-schizophrenic behavioural disorders, as can be seen for example in the controls of the Family Study (Kety *et al.* 1968, 1975).

The cross-fostering design has been used in two studies (Wender *et al.* 1974; Rosenthal *et al.* 1975) where the same pool of adoptees and their parents was the basis of the study. In both cases adopted-away offspring of normal biological parents who were reared by schizophrenic adoptive parents were compared with a group of adopted-away offspring of normal biological parents reared by normal adoptive parents, and adopted-away offspring of schizophrenic biological parents reared by normal adoptive parents. The study by Wender *et al.* (1974) found a greater prevalence of psychopathology among the adopted-away offspring of schizophrenics, while no such increase was seen among the cross-fostered group. The tentative conclusion was that genetic factors play a role in the aetiology of the schizophrenias while familial psychopathology (as measured by psychiatric diagnosis of the parents) does not. In the other study by Rosenthal *et al.* (1975) the parent–child relationship was examined using the same method. The quality of relationship between the child and his adoptive parents was assessed in four groups of subjects:

(1) A group consisting of index adoptees with a biological parent who was schizophrenic or had a manic-depressive disorder;
(2) A group of controls who were similarly adopted but whose biological parents had no known psychiatric illness;
(3) The cross-fostered subjects who had a biological parent with schizophrenic or manic-depressive disorder but were adopted by persons who didn't have such disorders;
(4) Non-adoptees who had a schizophrenic or manic-depressive parent and were reared in the parental home at least during the first 15 years of life (see Table 41.7).

The degree of illness in the child was correlated with the quality of the parent–child relationship. It was found that the quality of rearing and hereditary input both affected the development of psychopathological disorder, but the amount of variance explained by rearing was low.

In the study by Eldred *et al.* (1976) many of the same subjects were again used as index and control groups. In addition, the cross-fostering group was included. Again these subjects were people with an adoptive parent who was schizophrenic or manic-

TABLE 41.7

Type of rearing

Genetic background	Unspecified adoptive	Non-schizophrenic adoptive	Schizophrenic and manic-depressive biological
Schizophrenic and manic-depressive	Index adoptees (Group 1)	Cross foster (Group 3)	Non-adoptees (Group 4)
Non-schizophrenic	Control adoptees (Group 2)		

depressive while the biological parents had no history of psychosis. The aim of this study was to clarify some aspects of adoption to see if some of the common assumptions about what to do or not to do in the adoption procedure could be confirmed. The findings in some cases were somewhat surprising. It has in general been said that agency adoptions are preferred to independent adoptions; but with respect to psychopathology and parent–subject relationships of the adoptees, no such difference was found. It is also said that the child should be placed early in life. However, age and separation from the biological mother, age of placement, number of homes prior to placement, and time in institutions prior to placement were not related to the variables of psychopathology and parent–subject relationship of the adoptees. Nor was the age at which the subject learned about the adoption related to the outcome measures of adoptee psychopathology and the parent–child relationship. There seemed, however, to have been a correlation between having learned early about the status as an adoptive child and having a positive relation to the parents. The assumption that the child should be told about the adoption by his adoptive parents seems to be confirmed by the study, but it didn't seem to be true that learning about being an adopted child is nearly always problematic. The adoptees in general had not much interest in their biological parents nor were they concerned about the possibility of hereditary predispositions.

In a study by Rosenthal (1974b) the co-parents of the index cases in the above-mentioned study were used as probands. The idea behind this study was to see if assortative mating took place at an appreciable rate and if the genetic input from co-parents (including diagnoses in the 'soft end' of the schizophrenic spectrum such as schizoid and inadequate personality) might increase the percentage of spectrum diagnoses in the adopted-away offspring. In this study a very high percentage of psychopathology was found among the co-parents, and the percentage of schizophrenic spectrum disorder was also very high. Among the fathers many sociopathic personalities were found. In the cases where one parent had a diagnosis of chronic schizophrenia the genetic input from the co-parents with diagnoses including the whole schizophrenia spectrum increased the percentage of spectrum diagnosis in the adopted-away offspring to approximately 50 per cent. Because of the rather small number of families in this study the results should perhaps be viewed with some caution, but there seems to be some genetic evidence for the existence of a schizophrenic spectrum.

The family study

Kety and his co-workers have done two studies (1968, 1975) using the adoptees' families design. A total of 33 persons from the adoption pool with different types of schizophrenia were selected as index cases. Thirty-four subjects with no psychiatric record but otherwise similar to the index cases with respect to demographic variables and age at adoption, were selected pairwise as controls.

All siblings, half-siblings, foster siblings, and biological and adoptive parents were traced whenever possible. In the first study only information from institutional records were used, but later a full psychiatric interview was obtained for about 90 per cent of the available subjects. In both studies the persons with schizophrenic spectrum disorders clustered significantly among the biological relatives of the index cases. The interview study showed many more individuals with psychopathology than did the study based simply on hospital record material. In some respects the environment didn't seem to be of great importance. As has been mentioned earlier the paternal half-siblings who didn't even share the intrauterine environment with the schizophrenic index cases turned out to have just as high a prevalence of schizophrenic spectrum disorders as the maternal half-siblings. There were no significant differences in psychopathology among the two groups of adoptive parents. With regard to psychopathology diagnoses outside the schizophrenia spectrum, it was found that these were distributed evenly among the four groups of relatives. The prevalence of affective disorder was lower in the index biological relatives than in the control biological relatives. No significant difference in prevalence between index and control relatives was found for the other diagnostic categories.

In a study based on the same group of interviews, Rimmer et al. (1979) have studied the personal and social characteristics differentiating between adoptive relatives of schizophrenics and non-schizophrenics. The results of this study are only preliminary. It was found that of the 467 variables from the interview form, only a few were seen to differentiate between the groups. On the basis of chance alone, 46 variables would be expected to differentiate the groups, given the number of variables and the level of significance employed; not even this many were found to be significant differentiators. The variables thus selected did not appear to conform to any consistent or apparent theoretical hypothesis or point of view; i.e., no single variable was selected for mothers, fathers, parents, or siblings. There may be many explanations for these findings. One may be that there is no basis for the many theories concerning the characteristics of persons who have reared a schizophrenic. Another and perhaps a more reasonable explanation is that the rearing and parental variables involved in schizophrenia may be unique to each case and too complex for the evaluation instrument used in this study, i.e., a retrospective interview.

Another study, by Kinney and Jacobsen (1978), uses the Family Study interview design and investigates environmental factors in schizophrenia. This study was based upon Mednick and Schulsinger's idea that the study of differences within samples of persons at high risk for schizophrenia is more likely to yield relevant results than studies of the differences between schizophrenic samples and matched samples at low risk for schizophrenia. The schizophrenic index probands were divided into two groups, those with a high genetic risk for schizophrenia (i.e. the schizophrenic proband had a biological parent, sibling, or half-sibling who was schizophrenic) and those with a low genetic risk for schizophrenia (i.e. with no relative identified as schizophrenic). The data seem to indicate that among those individuals with a low genetic risk for schizophrenia there were more with postnatal brain damage than in the group with a high genetic risk for schizophrenia. Differences were statistically significant for those who were born during the May–December period. Earlier studies (for example, Dalén 1975), which had found an excess of schizophrenics born in the first three months of the year, seem to be confirmed by this study. Among the 34 schizophrenic 'index probands' there is a significant association between season of birth (January–April) and low genetic or postnatal risk (brain injury). This was not true for the schizophrenics at high risk. The seasonal birth distribution of the biological relatives of the 'low risk' probands did not show such a pattern.

The proportion of 'index cases' at high genetic risk for schizophrenia or postnatal brain damage who were also born from January to April is relatively low, as compared with all non-schizophrenics. Compared with their non-schizophrenic biological relatives the difference reaches statistical significance.

Studies about non-schizophrenic disorders

Psychopathy

We will now shift the focus to studies concerning behavioural disorders other than schizophrenia but which still use the same adoption material from the Copenhagen area. Schulsinger (1974) has carried out an epidemiological study of psychopathy using essentially the same method as Kety et al. (1968). Schulsinger established an operational, reliable definition of psychopathy before selecting his cases. After that it was possible to find 57 psychopathic probands from the 507 adoptees with a known mental disorder. A control was selected pairwise for every index proband using the same criteria as in the Family Study. Then all case record material of the biological and adoptive relatives was examined and diagnoses were given blindly. An excess of psychopathic spectrum disorders was found among the biological relatives, while there was no difference between the percentage of spectrum disorders in the remaining three groups—the biological control group, and the index and control adoptive groups. When only psychopathy was considered, the same overrepresentation was found among the biological relatives of the index probands. This overrepresentation was most marked in the biological fathers, and the whole study showed a tendency for the psychopathic spectrum disorders and core psychopathy in particular to appear more frequently among the male than among the female relatives. Sex differences were, however, not so consistent and marked when examining the sibling and half-sibling subgroups. From these findings it could be concluded that genetic factors seem to play an important role in the aetiology of psychopathy. Schulsinger also tried to examine environmental factors such as deprivation during early infancy as expressed in length of institutionalization in early childhood. In order to test this factor it had to be assumed that psychopathic spectrum disorders would be less frequent among biological relatives of index probands who were transferred late to their adoptive homes than among those transferred at an early age. There were no statistically significant differences in the frequency of psychopathic spectrum disorders among the biological family members of these two subgroups. Another possible aetiological factor in psychopathy is brain damage. As the case material didn't permit an evaluation of this factor Schulsinger had to be content with examining the cases for pregnancy and birth complications, which could be done by using midwife reports. The analyses from these midwife reports gave no support for a hypothesis that brain damage from birth complications plays any role in the aetiology of psychopathy in this sample.

Alcohol

Goodwin and co-workers have done some studies on alcohol problems using a modified version of the adoptee study. In the first study (1974a) the sample consisted of an index group of probands with biological parents who had been hospitalized primarily for alcoholism. Only male probands were selected because men are known to be at higher risk for alcoholism than are women. In selecting the controls the above criteria were again applied with one exception: none of the controls had a biological parent with a hospital record indicating alcoholism or alcohol abuse. Two control groups were established, one where none had a biological parent with a record of psychiatric hospitalization, and a second control group where a biological parent had at one time been hospitalized for a psychiatric condition other than alcoholism. Schizophrenics, however, were also excluded. After the interviews had been carried out, an analysis of the data revealed no significant differences between the two control groups and they were combined into a total control group. Index probands were four times more likely to develop alcoholism than their controls. The total psychopathology rate exclusive of alcoholism was almost identical in both groups. The two groups, however, differed significantly with respect to psychiatric treatment and hospitalization. The index probands had five times the rate of psychiatric hospitalization compared to the controls. When comparing the probands and the controls on a list of drinking problems it was found that on nearly all items the index probands had more problems, and on five items the results were statistically significant (hallucinations, loss of control, morning drinking, treatment for drinking, and ever alcoholic). The two groups of adoptive parents were very similar. The probands' parents tended to have more depression than the parents of the controls, but the differences were not significant. Altogether, the study seems to lend some support to the theory that genetic factors have an aetiological role in alcoholism, at least among men.

In a later study by Goodwin *et al.* (1977) of alcoholism and depression in the adopted daughters of alcoholics, 65 women from the adoption pool with a parent who had been hospitalized for alcoholism, were compared with 65 women whose biological parents had no record of psychiatric hospitalization. Otherwise the procedure was the same as used in the study above. The results showed that daughters of alcoholics didn't differ from daughters of non-alcoholics with regard to problem drinking, depression, or other psychiatric disorders. Alcohol problems were rare in both groups with one exception: 22 per cent of probands had experienced alcoholic black-outs, usually severe, and sometimes frequent. Only here was there a hint that daughters of alcoholics differed (but not significantly) from daughters of presumed non-alcoholics with regard to alcohol problems (black-outs).

In a third study (Goodwin *et al.* 1974b), drinking problems in adopted and non-adopted sons of alcoholics were compared. Twenty adopted sons of alcoholics were found who had brothers who had been raised by their alcoholic parent (the half-sib method). Some of these were full sibs. To avoid bias, interviews were also conducted with 50 non-adopted control subjects, so that the interviewer wouldn't know whether he was interviewing index subjects or controls. It was found that both groups who had alcoholic parents had high rates of alcoholism, 25 and 17 per cent in the adopted and non-adopted sons respectively. But the difference was not statistically significant. There was a comparable frequency of alcohol problems in the two groups, but the non-adopted sons were older and belonged to a lower socio-economic class. The length of exposure to the alcoholic parent was not associated with the development of alcoholism, but the severity of the parent's alcoholism was positively related to alcoholism in the offspring. The results suggested that environmental factors (in the form of paternal alcoholism) contributed little to the development of alcoholism in sons of severe alcoholics in this sample.

Criminality

The last study to be described using the adoptive sample is by Hutchings and Mednick (1974). They have made an epidemiologi-

cal study of registered criminality in the biological and adoptive fathers of 1145 males drawn from the original pool of adoptees. A control group of 1145 male non-adoptees were selected from old census lists. Denmark has a central police register that makes it easy to find people with criminal records (Rigsregistraturen). It was found that the 1145 adoptees showed markedly more registered criminality than their non-adopted controls or a comparable part of the general population. A significant correlation was found between criminality in the biological fathers and the adoptees; this was also the case with the adoptive fathers. It was also found that the index biological fathers were worse criminals than those fathers of the controls who had criminal records. Mental illness among the adoptees was considerably greater than in the controls. Among the adoptive parents there were no differences in the psychiatric histories of the index and control groups. Psychiatric illness in the biological parents just reached statistical difference, with the biological parents of the index probands being more often registered for admissions to psychiatric hospitals. It was also found in a selected pool of 92 index cases and 93 controls, that the midwife reports didn't differ with respect to the course of pregnancy or delivery nor to the nature or extent of the ensuing complications. In a cross-foster analysis 52 adoptees who were born to biological fathers not known to the police but with criminal adoptive fathers were compared with another group of 219 adoptees with criminal biological fathers adopted by fathers who were not known to the police. This analysis, though not statistically significant, shows that the hereditary effect might be more important than the environmental effect with respect to predicting criminality in the adoptees. In the discussion of the results Hutchings and Mednick warn that it may not be possible to draw conclusions from this investigation that will generalize to other national situations. They emphasize that the amount of environmental variability in a stable homogeneous country such as Denmark would tend to unmask genetic factors more than in most other countries and not show the influence of environmental factors to the same degree as in other populations.

Conclusion

We have described the Danish adoption sample and a number of methods for its use. By this we hope to have proved that adopted populations are suitable for studies of behavioural disorders when the aim is to disentangle genetic and environmental factors. The use of adopted populations is a method well suited for studies with longitudinal aspects, i.e. prospective ones. Our own population of adopted persons (approximately 14 500) is so old that prospective studies can only be realized to a relatively small extent.

The ideal way to exploit adopted populations when regarding adoption as nature's own experiment would be to make a prospective study of such populations with maximum knowledge about both biological and adoptive parents. Bohman (1973) comes near to this ideal, but working in Sweden he has had less ideal conditions than we in Denmark when examining variables on the biological side.

iii. First-cousin study

42. Mental disorders in children of first-cousin marriages in Iceland: a preliminary report

TÓMAS HELGASON and HÓLMFRÍDUR MAGNÚSDÓTTIR

Introduction

The Genetic Committee of the University of Iceland initiated this study of the children of first-cousin marriages in Iceland in collaboration with the Department of Psychiatry and the Blood Bank in Reykjavík. The purpose of the study is to investigate various genetic markers among these families as well as their fertility, morbidity, and mortality for comparison with that of the general population. The collection of data and some preliminary results regarding psychiatric disorders will be described here.

Shields and Slater (1956), Nixon and Slater (1957), and Ödegaard and Herlofsen (1955) have studied psychiatric patients who were born to cousins and compared them with control groups of patients. The data from England showed that schizophrenia was more frequent in the groups which were selected because the patients were children of cousins than in the control group of patients. In the Norwegian study affective syndromes were more predominant among the patients whose parents were first-cousins. The present study differs from those mentioned by including *all* first-cousin marriages and their children in a certain population.

Subjects and method

Our sample is comprised of all first-cousin marriages in Iceland from 1917 to 1964 and their children. The children were retrieved from the birth register by computer linkage with the marriage records. The material includes two sets of data:

(1) Linkages between the first-cousin marriage families and a file of all known psychiatric cases;
(2) A more intensive clinical and biochemical study of 109 families, selected on the basis of their living in Reykjavík and vicinity and being most recently married.

From these families approximately 500 individuals have been studied clinically. A comprehensive medical and psychiatric anamnesis has been obtained, partly by personal examinations and partly from information from key members of the families. Information has also been collected from hospitals and general practitioners. Members of the families, age 14 years or more, have responded to the Cornell Medical Health Index Questionnaire. For those who were dead before 31 December 1975, information has been obtained about the date and cause of death. Blood samples from the majority of those still living have been studied biochemically with regard to various genetic markers. In order to increase the number of individuals for the biochemical study, 36 additional families have been studied carefully. The spouses in these families are closely related, although not first-cousins.

All the relevant data have been punched on cards. The intensive clinical study has been supervised by Hólmfrídur Magnúsdóttir. Tómas Helgason has organized the more extensive study. The preliminary results of the study by Helgason are presented here; these results need considerable further analysis and interpretation.

There are 378 first-cousin marriages registered in Iceland during this period of 48 years. The rate of consanguinity has decreased with the increase of the population and with improved means of transportation within the country. Table 42.1 shows consanguinity of spouses for five-year periods during 1941–60. The decreasing number of first-cousin marriages can also be seen from Table 42.2. Table 42.2 shows the number of families without children as well as the total number of children born to the first cousins.

During the 24-year period 1917–40, there were 256 first-cousin marriages compared with only 122 first-cousin marriages in the following 24-year period (1941–64). In the earlier period the couples had 860 children (3.3 children per couple) while 16 per cent of the couples had no children. In the latter 24 years there were 335 children (2.7 children per couple) whereas 18 per cent were childless.

TABLE 42.1

Consanguinity per 100 marriages, 1941–60

	1941–5	1946–50	1951–5	1956–60
First cousins	0·8	0·5	0·3	0·3

TABLE 42.2

Number of first-cousin marriages, their children, and families without children, 1917–64

Period	No. of years	No. of first-cousin marriages	Families without children	Total no. of children
1917–25	9	127	21	454
1926–40	15	129	19	406
1941–64	24	122	22	335
Total	48	378	62	1195

Results

The first-cousin families have been linked to the psychiatric registry in order to get a comparison of the psychiatric morbidity in these families and the general population. Out of the total of 378 first-cousin marriages studied, 316 had a total of 1195 children, with an average of 3·8 children per fertile marriage.

Table 42.3 shows the distribution of psychiatric diagnoses among these parents and their children. Of these parents, 15·6 per cent were found in the psychiatric register; there were more women than men. Of the children, 10·5 per cent were found in the register; these were almost evenly divided between male and female. There seems to be an excessive number of children with organic mental disorder and mental deficiency when compared to our study of 535 families of the normal population of parents born from 1918 to 1924. In that study only 2 children with mental deficiency were found in the registry. It is known that the registry is still incomplete with regard to mental retardation, but there is no reason to expect that this affects these studies in any selective way. The morbidity among the children is not directly comparable between these two studies since a considerable number of the children of the first-cousin marriages have reached a higher age than the children of the general population sample.

TABLE 42.3

Psychiatric diagnosis of parents and children in first-cousin families

Diagnosis	Parents		Children	
	M	F	M	F
Psychoses	8	20	13	15
Organic mental disorder	11	9	3	5
Neuroses	18	40	28	45
Alcoholism	10	2	10	2
Mental deficiency	—	—	6	3
Total	47	71	60	70

In Table 42.4 a comparison is made between expectancy of psychoses in the first-cousin families to that of married persons born 1918–24. As can be seen from Table 42.4, the expectancy of the first-cousin couples is similar to that found among married persons born 1918–24. These rates are slightly higher than those found for the population born 1895–7 (Helgason 1964). The higher rates reported here may partly be explained by the increasing tendency to diagnose minor depressive illness as endogenous depression. However, these would affect the children of the first cousins to the same extent. Other methodological problems may be involved, and the data will be further examined.

TABLE 42.4

Expectancy (per cent) of psychoses in first-cousin families and among married persons in the general population born 1918–24

	M	F
First cousins, married	2·6	6·1
Children of first cousins	6·4	7·5
Married persons born 1918–24	4·0	6·1

Table 42.5 shows the linking of the psychiatric diagnoses of husband and wife in the first-cousin marriages. The tendency seen in the earlier study (1964) for both partners in the marriage to have a psychiatric diagnosis, is not as marked among the first cousins in the present study.

Table 42.6 shows the number of children in the first-cousin marriage families according to the parent's mental health and the proportion of children with psychiatric diagnoses. This is fairly similar to what we found among the children of married parents in general born 1918–24 (see Table 42.7). For technical computer reasons we did not trace more than approximately two-thirds of the children in this latter series. Therefore the fertility in the two series

cannot be compared from these tables. The rates in Tables 42.6 and 42.7 are not age-corrected. Therefore, it is premature to draw any conclusions from them. They are only used here for preliminary comparison, until data from a matched control group are available. In the near future we hope to be able to present the results of the analysis using a control group in which the marriages are matched by year of marriage and age of partners at that time.

TABLE 42.5

Linkage of spouses' psychiatric diagnoses in first-cousin marriages

Male	Female					
	Psychoses	Organic mental disorder	Neuroses	Alcoholism	No diagnosis	Total
Psychoses	1	2	1	1	3	8
Organic mental disorder	—	1	1	—	9	11
Neuroses	—	1	1	1	15	18
Alcoholism	1	—	3	—	6	10
No diagnosis	18	5	34	—	274	331
Total	20	9	40	2	307	378

TABLE 42.6

Total number of children and children with diagnoses in first-cousin families where neither parent, either, or both have psychiatric diagnoses

Parents diagnosis	Families with children	Number of children		Children with diagnoses	
		Total	Average per family	N	Per cent
Both without diagnosis	232	904	3·9	91	10·1
Mother with diagnosis	51	171	3·4	27	15·8
Father with diagnosis	25	96	3·8	8	8·3
Both with diagnosis	8	24	3·0	4	16·7
Total	316	1195	3·8	130	10·9

TABLE 42.7

Total number of children and children with diagnoses in families where neither parent, either, or both have diagnoses (parents born 1918–24)

Parents diagnosis	Families with children	Number of children		Children with diagnosis	
		Total	Average per family	N	Per cent
Both without diagnosis	214	429	2·0	32	7·5
Mother with diagnosis	78	158	2·0	23	14·6
Father with diagnosis	63	127	2·0	20	15·7
Both with diagnosis	30	56	1·9	11	19·6
Total	385	770	2·0	86	11·2

iv. Birth difficulty, neonatal brain damage

43. Neurological syndromes, disturbances of speech and language and/or perception at five years of age in a neonatal high risk group (Finland)

MÄRTA DONNER, ANNELI YLINEN, and KATARINA MICHELSSON

This is a prospective study which started at the Institute of Midwifery, Helsinki, Finland, in 1970–1. The aim is to elucidate the prognosis of the children belonging to a high risk group in the neonatal period, especially with regard to the occurrence of slight neurological syndromes—and to test certain screening procedures used to identify these syndromes at the age of five years.

The sample

The criteria for including the child in the high risk group were the following:

(1) Diabetes of the mother;
(2) A birth weight of 2000 g or less;
(3) Apgar points 6 or less at 5 min after delivery or later;
(4) Hyperbilirubinaemia with two or more values higher than those allowed before exchange transfusion is made;
(5) Hypoglycaemia with two or more values of the same level or below the level used as criterion for neonatal hypoglycaemia considering weight and age;
(6) Neurological symptoms in the neonatal period;
(7) Respiratory difficulties necessitating assisted respiration;
(8) Other serious diseases of the newborn such as sepsis.

If we were to start the project anew we would also include 'small for date' children. The children we studied were born in the years 1971 to 1974. Mostly they come from the city of Helsinki and its neighbouring communities. Data about the mother's age, parity, social and marital status, health and illness during pregnancy, treatment given, and working load were collected as well as data about the delivery and the state of the new-born child. The number of children belonging to these groups was about 5 per cent of the 5500 to 6000 children born each year at the Institute.

The method

The children are followed up at the child welfare clinics as usual in this country. They are not called risk children; rather, the mother and the health nurse are informed that the children had some difficulties as new-borns. Special forms are sent to the child welfare clinics to be filled in when the children are 6 months, 1, 1½, 2, and 4 years of age. In these forms the normal motor and speech development is described. If the child fails to keep up to the level described the nurse is instructed to contact the neuropaediatricians taking part in the study. This plan has not been completed in a satisfactory way because of too much work in the child welfare centres. However, those children who have been reported were examined and appropriate measures were taken.

The examination of the five-year-old children

In 1974 and 1975 this examination was planned by a team consisting of neuropaediatricians, paediatricians, a speech therapist, and a psychologist. The screening test decided upon consisted of the following items:

(1) A neurodevelopmental test described by Bax and Whitmore (1973) including tests of gross and fine motor function, co-ordination and balance, upper-motor neuron function, sight and strabismus, speech and language, perception and imitation of gestures, concentration and behaviour;
(2) Tests of speech and language development which examine motor function, articulation, and concentration, using the Illinois Test of Psycholinguistic Abilities (ITPA), especially the auditive and language items (Kirk *et al.* 1968);
(3) Psychological tests using Frostig tests (1963) and ITPA items;
(4) The filling in of a questionnaire by the parents with the help of a nurse (the questionnaire has been compiled with the aid of CIBA Foundation and has been translated into Finnish and Swedish by our team). This concerns the profession of the parents, housing, stability of the environment and family, mental and physical illness in the family, the development and illnesses of the child, daily care of the child, and hereditary disorders;
(5) Audiometry.

In 1975, between 100 and 300 normal children in Helsinki not belonging to the risk group were tested using the neurodevelopmental test and the tests of speech and language. The other tests had earlier been standardized for Finnish children. In 1976, 220 children born in 1971 and belonging to the high-risk group underwent the above-mentioned screening procedure. The children born in the first six months of 1971 were examined during March and April 1976, and the other children during October and November 1976. Each child participated in two sessions lasting two hours each time. About 80 per cent of the primary group participated in the examination. The examination of the children born during the first part of the year 1972 was made between February and April 1977.

In each case the results of the tests are discussed afterwards by the team; the information and advice that should be given to the parents is discussed, and also, possible additional examinations that should be made and possible treatment or training that should be given are evaluated. Information is given to the parents in the form of a meeting with lectures and discussions, as well as personally by one of the doctors of the team.

Since 1975 there have been negotiations with the authorities of the city of Helsinki concerning the possibility of starting a special preschool class for 8–12 children from the risk group who would benefit from a special programme. In the autumn of 1976 this class began. The personnel consists of a special preschool teacher and her assistants, a speech therapist, a consulting physiotherapist, a psychologist, a paediatrician, and ADB-therapist. A training programme developed as part of the ITPA-test series is also used.

Results

The results of the work done so far have not yet been published. They are being prepared for data processing. It is planned to continue with this programme until all the risk children born between 1971 and 1974 are tested at the age of five years. If possible a follow-up examination will be made when the children are eight years old. However, future work depends on possibilities of financing the project. Until now, the project has been made possible by the generosity of the Association of the Insurance Companies of Finland and the Gyllenberg Foundation.

We hope that if this relatively short screening procedure to identify children with neurological, speech, and/or perceptional difficulties at the age of five could be standardized it could be used for risk groups. Children needing special education could be given this as early as at the preschool age (children start school in Finland at age seven), and parents and teachers could be informed of the difficulties of the child. In this way neurotic reactions due to school failure could be largely prevented.

In the future we hope that the screening procedure would especially be used routinely for children treated in neonatal intensive care units, so that those planning this treatment could be given feedback about its results.

44. Screening and evaluation of the high-risk pregnancy and labour as related to the perinatal mortality and morbidity of the infant (Czechoslovakia)

Z. ŠTEMBERA, J. ZEZULÁKOVÁ, J. DITTRICHOVÁ, and J. TOMANOVÁ

Background

This work began in 1968 at the Research Institute for the Care of Mother and Child, Prague-Podolí, Czechoslovakia. At present it continues as a part of a long-term state project entitled *Care for the health of the new generation*. The aims of the work are to identify the most important causes (risk factors) leading not only to perinatal mortality, but especially to perinatal morbidity, and to work out, on the basis of quantification of these risk factors, a simple screening that would make possible:

(a) A selection of women with high risk pregnancies for intensive prenatal and intranatal care in specialized institutions;
(b) A selection of high risk new-borns for a further specialized psychoneurological follow-up and for early specialized rehabilitation;
(c) A selection of the neurological symptom manifestations that very early and most frequently signal a neurological deviation.

In 1968 a retrospective analysis of perinatally dying foetuses and new-borns with lowered Apgar scores was performed in cases delivered in the Institute in the years 1966 and 1967 (326 cases). The aim of this study was a preliminary selection of the most important risk factors.

In 1969 a test prospective study was performed with all pregnant women who delivered that year in the Institute (total number 1099). The infants were followed up to the age of 18 months. The aims were:

(a) To work out criteria for the selection of high risk pregnancies for the study;
(b) To try the most suitable forms of data recording;
(c) To work out and test the optimal methodological procedures (obstetric, paediatric, neurological, psychological, and sociological);
(d) To develop the optimal system of mutual co-operation among the quoted experts;
(e) To choose a suitable program for processing the obtained data.

The proper prospective study was started in 1970. In the course of the years 1970 through 1972, 1103 women with high risk pregnancies and 150 control cases were selected according to desig-nated criteria. These women were selected out of 3613 deliveries during these years. The first preliminary evaluation was performed in 1975 according to the clinical condition (paediatric and psychoneurological) of the infants at the age of 18 months. The second evaluation, according to the clinical condition of the children at three years of age, was performed in 1977. The workers responsible were as follows: Štembera, for the obstetric part; Zezuláková, for the paediatric and neurological parts; Dittrichová, for the psychological part; and Tomanová, for the sociological part.

The project

In addition to perinatal mortality, perinatal morbidity has recently become a criterion of the quality of care of the population. Retrospective studies which have shown that damaged infants originate more frequently from high risk pregnancies and deliveries than healthy ones, are being replaced by prospective studies. The prospective method is more exacting; it records dynamics of development, shows that perinatal complications adversely influence development (particularly in the neuropsychic component), and enables an early therapeutic intervention.

The prospective method in the long-term follow-up studies has been utilized for years in our Institute when solving problems of the development of infants. A causal correlation between different pathological conditions of the mother in the course of pregnancy and labour and the foetal condition has been shown in an obstetric–paediatric study by Horský and Znamenáček (1956). A group of low-birth-weight infants was followed up to the age of three years, and their somatic and psychic condition evaluated by Stanincová and Dittrichová (1964). A group of infants of diabetic mothers was followed up to the age of three years. A model of development of infants with good or bad prognosis was established on the basis of a correlation of the infant's neuropsychic condition with risk factors complicating foetal development (Zezuláková 1974).

All these experiences were of great value to us when planning and starting our prospective longitudinal project.

Method of processing

It was necessary to arrange a set of information concerning the pertinent population that would bring about new knowledge of the correlation between perinatal factors and long-term development. Analyses were done to assess the weight of individual risk factors or of groups of risk factors, and to lay the foundations for identification and quantification of these factors. The subject of our present study is a scanning of the dependence between cause and result, i.e., between the complex of risk factors and long-term prognosis. For this decision-making, the method of sequential multilinear discriminant function, developed at UTIA-CSAV in Prague, is used.

The weight of individual neurological phenomena or of groups of phenomena to be used in designing the neurological screening, was determined by the method of informational measure of dependence, worked out at the computer centre UHKT in Prague.

Selection of subjects

Out of the total number of 3613 deliveries from the years 1970 to 1972, 1013 high risk pregnancies were included in the experimental group. There were also 150 control cases. In our Institute there is a cumulation of pathologic pregnancies. Consequently this group cannot be considered a representative sample of the population. In addition, our material was characterized by the fact that only 5 per cent of the infants exhibited signs of a deteriorated postnatal adaptation without having risk factors in the personal history of the mother, in the course of pregnancy, or during labour. The control group consisted of new-borns without any risk. Every week the first two new-borns of this type were included.

In all cases the following procedures were carried out: gathering of a detailed personal history; observation during the course of the whole pregnancy and labour; neonatal and neurological examination during the first seven days of life; further neurological examinations at 3, 8, 18, and 36 months of life; psychological examinations at 12 and 36 months of life; and an ongoing evaluation of the social situation of the family. All infants with congenital malformations were excluded from the experimental group.

Obstetric examination

Method. Prenatal care for all pregnant women under study was ensured at the Institute in a special out-patient clinic. The average number of examinations was 10 for the control group and 15 to 20 for the women with high risk pregnancy. Frequently, women with high risk pregnancies required hospitalization for several weeks or even months. All deliveries were accomplished in the Institute. The registered risk factors, whose importance for our population has been assessed in the preliminary work, can be divided into three groups:

1. Personal history:
   (a) General: age; height; pre-pregnant weight.
   (b) Previous illnesses: diabetes mellitus (duration, therapy); hypertensive disease; cardiopathies; diseases of the urinary tract; endocrinopathies; sterility.
   (c) Previous pregnancies: deliveries (number, time elapsed to present pregnancy); spontaneous abortions (number, time elapsed to present pregnancy); legal abortions (number, time elapsed to present pregnancy); perinatal mortality (number, kind); perinatal morbidity (number, kind).
2. Present pregnancy:
   Length of pregnancy;
   Weight gain;
   Blood pressure (in relation to the length of gestation);
   Proteinuria;
   Oedema;
   Rh isoimmunization;
   EPH gestosis (kind, duration, length of therapy);

Diabetes mellitus only in pregnancy (duration, therapy);
Bleeding in the first, second, and third trimester;
Imminent premature labour (time, kind of therapy);
Placenta praevia;
Premature separation of the placenta;
Smoking (how long during pregnancy, how much);
Multiple pregnancy.
3. Delivery:
   Duration:—first stage in hours
             —second stage in minutes;
   Amniotic fluid: stained
             —how long
             —time from escape to delivery;
   Change of foetal heart rate:
             —absolute value (tachycardia, bradycardia);
             —duration of the change
             —first or second stage of labour.
Foetal malposition;
Umbilical cord complications;
Intrapartal fever;
Operative delivery: forceps (high, midforceps, low):
   Caesarean section (elective, during labour);
   breech extraction (complete, incomplete).

Results. The most important risk factors were identified (anamnestic, during pregnancy and labour). Their preliminary quantification was carried out in relation both to perinatal mortality and to serious perinatal morbidity. It has been shown that the majority of the risk factors contribute different weights for perinatal mortality and morbidity. Risk factors leading to the onset of acute foetal hypoxia predispose to perinatal mortality, whenever risk factors leading to chronic foetal distress represent a greater risk for the onset of perinatal morbidity.

The practical utilization of these risk signs was tested through screening of the most serious cases of risk pregnancies, with the aim of early transfer of these women to specialized clinics and institutions for risk pregnancies (Štembera *et al.* 1975). There is no doubt that the absolute values of this scoring system are valid and applicable only for the population from which they were gained. The absolute and relative weight of individual risk factors depends on a series of other influences, e.g. extent and quality of prenatal, natal, and neonatal care, health condition, and consciousness of the population, etc. Nevertheless we feel that the principles we used in this scoring system have a broader validity, and that after modification corresponding to the local conditions the system could be used in any population.

Paediatric examination

Method. In our Institute the new-born is examined immediately after delivery by a paediatrician–neonatologist. A paeditrician–neonatologist is present in the obstetric theatre during deliveries on a 24-hour schedule. Each case selected for the long-term follow-up was examined daily by an obstetrician and a paediatrician. From the point of view of the condition of the new-born immediately after delivery, and in the course of the first week of life, all the cases were selected in whom some of the following paediatric criteria were found:

(a) Small-for-dates newborn;
(b) Excessive birth weight (more than 4000 g);
(c) Apgar score in 1 minute less than 8 points,
              in 5 minutes less than 9 points,
              in 10 minutes less than 10 points;
(d) Duration for longer than one hour of any pathological clinical signs, including respiratory and circulatory deviations, motor manifestations, changes of tone and basic reflexes of the newborn;
(e) Respiratory distress syndrome;

(f) Peripheral trauma;
(g) Infection of the neonate;
(h) Icterus;
(i) Other complications.

All the new-borns were observed daily by a paediatrician in the usual way in departments for new-borns or in intensive care units. During all further observations (at 3, 6, 18, and 36 months of life) the somatic condition and basic anthropometric data were evaluated, and any illnesses, hospitalizations, or injuries occurring since the last examination were registered.

Before being discharged from the Institute, the mothers whose infants were included in the follow-up were informed of the reason for regular observation of their infants. A worker was put in charge of organizing the examinations and corresponding with the mothers. In spite of the fact that a large number of the infants lived outside of Prague the number of infants in individual age groups who were not followed up varied between 3 and 12 per cent. It was possible to obtain information about these infants from their local health care institutions. When an infant was discovered to have some deviation he/she was immediately given therapy (rehabilitation and movement stimulation) or was transferred, according to the kind of deviation, to a special institution. Due to these reasons approximately one-quarter of the infants visited our out-patient clinic more frequently than scheduled. Local infant clinics were informed of the results of our examinations. When requested, transportation costs for infants and their parents living outside of Prague were covered by the health centre.

Results. The reliability of prognosis for the infant increases if the paediatric criteria of the new-born are supplemented by the obstetric risk factor occurring in maternal personal history, during pregnancy, and in the course of labour. This complex represents the personal history of the new-born. The paediatric criteria of the new-born were analysed in a way similar to the pregnancy factors.

The results have shown that Apgar scores evaluated one minute after delivery were of no prognostic significance. Only lowered values found five and ten minutes after delivery combined with persistence of pathological signs for a time longer than three days had a significant effect on the prognosis. The time factor was of decisive importance for assessment of weight. The longer the clinical signs persisted after delivery, the greater was the probability of permanent consequences. Serious complications in the neonatal period such as RDS, sepsis, meningoencephalitis, etc., influenced development very adversely. Transient retardation of psychomotor development (during the ages of 3 to 18 months) was found to be related to such factors as dysplasia of hip joints, intercurrent illnesses, etc.

Neurological examination

Our aim was to draw up an examination code covering the developmental and the neuropathological component. We chose tests which we considered to be essential for evaluating infants from high-risk pregnancies. Our examination code is comparatively short, but its purpose is to detect the neurological development of individual infants. When studying high-risk infants we want to detect in a relatively short time only the essential deviant features by a qualitively and quantitatively standardized simple method, to enable the results to be processed by computers. In principle we have used our own neonatal and infant examination technique, which was verified by years of experience. We have chosen tests by which the infant's development and any pathological signs in the neonatal period and subsequent trimesters can be assessed. In further follow-ups we have tried not to omit a single test from the series; for later phases of development we were naturally obliged to add a number of tests.

Method. During the examination we try to proceed as naturally and gently as possible, so as not to affect the child's behavioural state. We are interested in:

1. The child's condition and appearance;
2. Position of head, trunk, and limbs;
3. Motility: spontaneous, passive, and provoked.

We begin with observation, which is followed by palpation, auscultation, and percussion. Lastly we test exteroceptive reflexes by tactile stimulation.

We examine the infant in the following sequence:

   I. First in the position in which the mother places the infant on the examining table, i.e. on his back;
  II. Traction response: we next take the infant by the hands and slowly raise him to a sitting position. When the trunk is at an angle of about 60 degrees to the table, we record the position of the head and trunk and of the upper and lower limbs. In the full sitting position we also test a number of reflexes;
 III. Prone position: to turn the child on to his abdomen we use the neck-righting reflex on the trunk and the rolling reflex. We again examine appearance, posture, and passive and provoked motility;
  IV. Suspension: we lift the infant from position III above the level of the table into horizontal suspension. We examine a number of postural reflexes (e.g. Landau's reflex, the rolling reflex in suspension, lateral suspension, and others). We next examine the infant in vertical suspension and then try to swing him, etc.;
   V. In the vertical position we examine the positive supporting reflex, the walking reflex, spontaneous standing, walking etc.;
  VI. At the end we test some irritating and upsetting reflexes (e.g. the Moro's reflex).

Spontaneous motility, tremor, hyperkinesia, and opisthotonus are evaluated and registered only at the end of the examination, when we are better able to assess them.

Our examination technique is thus standardized. Its standardization is not rigid, but can be partly varied according to circumstance. In principle, it corresponds to the requirements of Prechtl's school. We standardize the external environment, the infant's state, and the intensity of stimuli and responses. We also standardize the sequence of the examination, not only as regards the examination positions and their sequence, but also the initial positions of the individual body segments, i.e. of the trunk and limbs, and the sequence of reflexes and other phenomena in the various positions. (A detailed description of this technique can be obtained from the authors.)

Results. Some of the partial results from the neurological examinations performed by the above-mentioned method are here presented. On the basis of an analysis of the neurological data, we determined in every infant its neurological condition for each examination period. We then divided the infants into groups as follows:

Those with normal neurological conditions;

Retarded infants (psychomotorically retarded without neurological deviations). Those infants who were behind by more than six months were considered as retarded;

Those with neurological deviations (primarily changes of tone, asymetric findings, sporadic pathological reflexes). At three years of age we annexed to this group infants with clinical signs of minimal brain dysfunction;

Those with expressive neurological findings. In the new-born period this group was characterized by expressive derangements of tone connected with a serious general condition, such as seizures, etc. In the course of further examinations this group consisted of those infants with signs suggesting the syndrome of cerebral palsy or some other morphologic lesion of the CNS.

TABLE 44.1

Neurological examination findings of children of high-risk pregnancies and control group

| Evaluation | Children of high-risk pregnancies | | | | | | | | | | Control group | |
| | 1 week | | 3 months | | 8 months | | 18 months | | 36 months | | 36 months | |
	No.	Per cent	No.	Per cent	No.	Per cent	No.	Per cent	No.	Per cent	No.	Per cent
Normal	532	59·5	398	42·1	446	46·5	491	53·3	757	78·3	138	93·9
Developmental retardation	—	—	250	26·5	390	40·7	382	41·5	142	14·6	7	4·7
Neurological deviations	340	38·1	279	29·6	107	11·2	33	3·6	34	3·5	1	0·7
MBD	—	—	—	—	—	—	—	—	23	2·5	1	0·7
Cerebral palsy	21	2·4	12	1·2	15	1·6	15	1·6	11	1·1	—	—
+	—	—	6	0·6	—	—	—	—	—	—	—	—
Total	893	100	945	100	958	100	921	100	967	100	147	100

Table 44.1 shows a relatively small percentage of infants with an expressive neurological finding. With increasing age the percentage of infants in whom neurological deviations were found tended to decrease (that is, children tended to 'grow out' of their neurological symptoms).

The development of these infants was no doubt slowed, but in the majority of cases the development of some of the forms of cerebral palsy did not take place. The percentage of developmentally retarded infants increased up to the age of 18 months, whereas the percentage of normal findings at the same age did not differ substantially from the neonatal period. At three years of age 78 per cent of the infants were healthy, and in 23 per cent of the cases there was a pathological neurological finding.

In comparison with the situation at age 18 months, the percentage of infants with neurological deviations at three years of age practically did not change. The group of infants with minimal brain dysfunction was composed partly of infants in whom neurological deviations were found; however, also included were those who exhibited a normal neurological finding up to the age of 18 months, or who were only retarded. A difference in the percentage of normal and retarded infants can be seen when compared with the control group at three years of age. Particularly striking is the difference in the percentage of occurrence of neurological deviations. In the control group five times fewer infants were afflicted. In addition, there was no serious neurological damage in the control group. The premature infants, small-for-dates, and infants of diabetic mothers—infants with a serious pregnancy risk—constituted nearly half of the group.

In Table 44.2 one can see the absolute and percentage occurrence of infants with neurological deviations, minimal brain damage, and expressive neurological findings at three years of age. In addition, all other categories of risk infants are included. It can be seen that, from the prognostic point of view, those infants who are both small-for-dates and premature (SFD+P) represent the most serious group; 33 per cent of them exhibited a pathological neurological finding. The infants of mothers treated for diabetes mellitus by insulin (IDM) or by diet (DDM) did not differ substantially in the occurrence of deviations. In the IDM group, which is prognostically more serious, there is one infant with a serious neurological deviation. In our series there was only a small number of premature infants of diabetic mother (IDM+P)—14 cases. In two of these, minimal brain damage (MBD) was diagnosed. When compared with other groups, the infants of mothers suffering from diabetes had a substantially greater developmental tendency towards MBD manifestations.

Dynamics of the development of individual infants in the course of 36 months were analysed in some groups with serious pregnancy risk. According to the results they were directed into the appropriate diagnostic group in each age group. Figures 44.1 and 44.2

TABLE 44.2

Neurological examination at three years of age

| | | Neurological deviations | | MBD | | Cerebral palsy | |
	No.	No.	Per cent	No.	Per cent	No.	Per cent
P	128	5	3·9	4	3·1	4	3·1
SFD	91	3	3·3	1	1·1	2	2·2
P + SFD	15	5	33·3	—	—	—	—
IDM	74	3	4·1	4	5·4	1	1·3
DDM	98	4	4·1	5	5·1	—	—
IDM + P	14	—	—	2	14·3	1	7·14
OR	547	14	2·6	7	1·2	3	0·5
Total	967	34	3·5	23	2·5	11	1·1

P   = Low-birth-weight infants.
SFD = Small-for-date infants.
IDM = Infants of insulin dependent diabetic mother.
DDM = Infants of gestational diabetic mother.
OR   = Other infants 'at risk'.
MBD = Minimal brain dysfunction.

show the shifts of individual infants from one diagnostic group to another over the course of development. Models of the development of premature and small-for-dates infants having normal neurological findings in the neonatal period are demonstrated as examples. In both instances only half of the infants at the age of three months remained in the normal diagnostic group. The others shifted among the retarded infants or to the group of infants with neurological deviations. At the age of eight months a normal neurological finding prevailed among the small-for-dates infants; in the prematures, on the other hand, retardation was prevalent. At 18 months retardation was found in 47·5 per cent of the prematures,

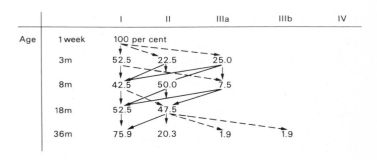

FIG. 44.1. Shifts of low-birth-weight infants having normal neurological findings in the neonatal period from one diagnostic group to another over the course of development.

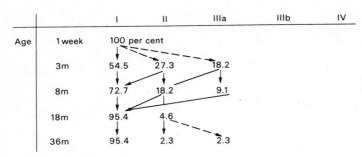

FIG. 44.2. Shifts of small-for-date infants having normal neurological findings in the neonatal period from one diagnostic group to another over the course of development.

but only in 4·6 per cent of small-for-dates infants. At three years of age the percentage of normal cases among small-for-dates was the same as at 18 months. In half of the retarded cases, neurological deviation developed. In prematures at three years of age there was a striking increase of infants with normal neurological findings and a decrease of cases with retardation. The figure also shows the prognostic value of neurological examinations after delivery for the given groups: if the neonatal neurological finding is normal, then small-for-dates infants have, under the precondition of good care, a 95 per cent chance that development at three years of age will be normal. The neurologically normal premature newborn has, under the same precondition, a 75 per cent chance. If neurological deviations occur in the neonatal period, the risk groups can be analysed by the same procedure, as demonstrated in Figs. 44.3 and 44.4. The infants were grouped as follows: I—normal; II—developmental retardation; IIIa—neurological deviations; IIIb—minimal cerebral dysfunction; IV—cerebral palsy (see figures).

Later in our research we tried to determine the neurological signs from our series of tests that would detect neurological deviations as early as possible and in the majority of afflicted cases, so that we

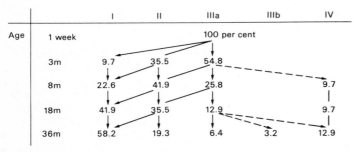

FIG. 44.3. Shifts of low-birth-weight infants showing neurological deviations in the neonatal period from one diagnostic group to another over the course of development.

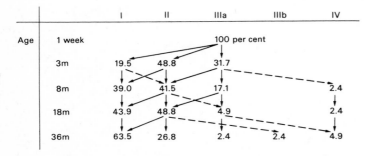

FIG. 44.4. Shifts of small-for-date infants showing neurological deviations in the neonatal period from one diagnostic group to another over the course of development.

might develop a screening test. We aimed at decreasing the number of examinations to a minimum while maintaining their diagnostic value. Up to now we have only analysed the data on the first supine position. The results show that the diagnostic importance of this group decreased with increasing age. Certain phenomena have been found in all age groups, although not always in the same place of sequence; i.e., the phenomena have a different validity at different ages of the infant. However, with continued analysis of other data we expect to be able to choose the appropriate examinations to compose a shorter, yet diagnostically valuable, procedure.

The above-mentioned results are not final by far. They suggest the trend of further detailed analyses and show a possibility for the solution of the daily problems which a paediatric neurologist meets.

Psychological examination

Method. The infants were examined at the ages of one and three years. In the first year the Gesell test was used; at three years of age we availed ourselves of the Terman–Merill test. The Terman–Merill test was extended by evaluation of fine motor co-ordination (building a tower of cubes, copying of further images, drawing a line). We further devised rating scales for evaluation of the infant's activity during the examination, and for concentration problems. We feel that this amplification is important for detection of soft deviations in the development of the central nervous system (MBD).

Results

A. *Control infants:*

The quoted parameters—IQ, number of points attained in the tests of fine motor co-ordination, place in the scale of activity, and concentration—were first evaluated in the group of control infants.

It was found that the IQ test we use overestimated the three-year-old infants: the average IQ score was 120·0 with a significant deviation of ± 12·62. An IQ score under 100 was considered to be below average and was found in 12·5 per cent of the infants; with the exception of one case the IQ in these infants averaged between 91 and 100. An IQ score of 140 or higher was attained by 11·0 per cent of the infants.

In the tests of fine motor co-ordination the infants were able to obtain a maximum of 14 points. On the average the control infants obtained 9·5 ± 2·95. Five to three points were considered to be a less than average result, two and less points a serious deviation. From the control group 16·8 per cent of the infants were found to be under the average; a serious deviation was discovered in 3·3 per cent of them.

The evaluation of motility of the infant was aimed at selection of infants with hyperactivity, considered to be one of the symptoms of MBD. According to our evaluation hyperactive infants were those who were restless, unable to sit in the course of the examination, and who got up and ran away from the examination table. The mothers of these infants also complained of their restlessness. In the control group 9·3 per cent of the infants were of this kind.

A striking inability of the infant to focus attention is also considered as one of the signs of MBD; in the control group this was found in a considerably high percentage—16·2 per cent. These results show that in a three-year-old infant it is not possible to accurately infer minimal brain damage from only one sign, such as poor motor co-ordination, hyperactivity, or inability to concentrate.

B. *Infants with risk factors:*

At present, IQ, fine motor co-operation, activity, and concentration problems are being evaluated in infants with different pregnancy and perinatal risk factors. The preliminary results show that some groups of infants with risk factors differ significantly at the age of three years from control infants. For example, a group of 31 infants who experienced respiratory distress in the early neonatal period differed significantly, from control infants, at the age of three years in IQ and fine motor co-ordination ($p < 0.01$). Further analyses are being performed and are not yet finished. It appears that it is very important to evaluate pregnancy and perinatal risk factors along with social factors, because they can make themselves felt either independently or dependently to biological factors in the psychical development of the infant.

Socio-economic examination

Complex care for mother and child requires, both in clinical–preventive and in research fields, a knowledge of the family environment in which the child develops. Family environment is an important factor in an analysis of causes producing a risk pregnancy. The significance of an inquiry into the social and economic conditions of high risk pregnancy infants consists of:

(a) The need to characterize the infants and families from the social aspect;
(b) The possibility of discovering factors specific to a given population which might play a role in the development of certain conditions.

It is not easy to investigate the social environment as we do not yet possess any uniform criteria for its evaluation. Socio-economic influences, however, frequently share in perinatal mortality and morbidity as well as in the occurrence of premature deliveries. Because of this we have investigated socio-economic factors of infants delivered from high risk pregnancies. This allows us to verify the effect of social, economic, and family factors upon the onset, and course of high-risk pregnancy as well as upon the development of the delivered child. The aim is to evaluate the effect of these factors on the development of the infant, and to separate these effects from those of the biological factors.

Method. Our questionnaire enquired about basic socio-economic characteristics, i.e. age of parents, education, occupational status and income of the infant's parents, data on family structure, number of brothers and sisters, living conditions, and health situation of the family. We also recorded information about the course of the mother's pregnancy, her mental and physical working stress, quality of the work place and its distance from home, and possible stress situations during pregnancy. The above data were obtained directly from the mother in the maternity hospital by means of an interview conducted by one worker (the same interviewer for all cases). Further enquiries were conducted when the child was 18 months and three years old. At six years of age a final evaluation took place. The purpose of the interviews was to determine changes in basic socio-economic data, such as in the family structure, birth of more infants, changes in the family life style, changes in education, in profession and income of parents, resumed employment of the mother after delivery, changes in living conditions, in the type of care for the infant, and in the family environment of the infants. Repeated examinations made it possible to get in touch with the mother quite closely and to obtain reliable data.

Characteristics of the group. At the moment of delivery of the infant there was a nearly equal representation of 'complete' families (parents and children)—46 per cent, and of 'enlarged' families (parents, children, and additional relatives)—45 per cent. Six per cent of the families were 'incomplete' (one parent absent). In 68 per cent of the cases the studied child was the first one in the family; 30 per cent of the infants already had one or more siblings.

In 44 per cent of the cases the mother had 'lower' primary school or handicraft education; 54 per cent of the mothers had attended high school and/or university. Due to socio-economic factors, an adverse influence during pregnancy was found in 56 per cent of the mothers. Eight per cent of the mothers were occupied in the household during pregnancy. Most of the infants (86 per cent) lived in good family conditions; however, 11 per cent of the infants were endangered in their milieu by such factors as incomplete families, bad care, or insufficient hygienic conditions.

Basic factors selected for assessment and evaluation. These were: structure of the family, number of children in the family, education and profession of both parents, living conditions, type of care for the child (e.g. mother, grandmother, nursery), evaluation of the family environment, presence of an adverse influence during pregnancy. The following situations were considered adverse: shift working hours, long working time with a midday break, journey to work by some means of transportation if one way lasted longer than 45 minutes, a high risk working environment, physical or mental strain imposed by employment, stress situations during pregnancy.

Results. The preliminary results show that the degree of maternal education correlates with the neurological situation of the infant at 18 months of life. In the group with normal neurological findings, 28 per cent of the mothers had a lower level of education. In the group with some neurological deviation 47 per cent of the mothers had a lower level of education. A further factor found to influence the development of the infant is the family environment. For infants living in a non-harmonic family environment the neurological condition at 18 months of life was normal in 5 per cent of the cases and pathological in 11 per cent. In order to reduce the complexity of the analysis of individual social and economic factors within the context of the many medical and psychological data we were analysing, we instead evaluated by means of a cumulation of three negative social signs (lower educational status of the mother, adverse influences during pregnancy, adverse environment for the infant) against three positive social signs (higher educational status of the mother, no adverse influence during pregnancy, a good environment for the infant). The two resulting groups exhibited differences in many other factors as well: anamnestic (obesity), during pregnancy (severe gestosis), obstetrical (hypoxia during labour), in the course of long-term development (severe psychic retardation at the age of 12 months). These differences were always in favour of the group with positive social signs.

The preliminary results from the data gathered at 18 months and three years of life afford us a deeper knowledge of the relationship of the socio-economic environment to high risk pregnancy and high risk infancy.

Employment of the obtained preliminary results in clinical practice

I. The most consequential of the risk factors identified in pregnant women were used for a screening of women with a high risk pregnancy in the prenatal clinic, so that they might be transferred to selected institutes for special care. With the aim of a practical nation-wide application of this specialized care, the following measures were performed:

1. A 'passport for pregnant women' was designed with a list of the most serious risk factors, so that screening could be performed uniformly in the whole country. This new type of passport was introduced in Czechoslovakia by the Ministry of Health in 1973.
2. The leading doctors responsible for the realization of this screening were informed of the main principles and the mode of execution in postgraduate courses organized by the Institute for postgraduate teaching.

II. A neurological procedure for examination of high-risk new-borns was worked out. It is now being introduced in special clinics where these infants are cared for.

III. The most serious groups of high-risk new-borns can be identified, and their psychomotoric development examined as needed in the first three years of life.

45. Effects of labour induction with prostaglandin $F_2\alpha$ on the psychomotor development of the child in the first 30 months: a follow-up study of risk cases (Belgium)

WILLIAM DE COSTER, ANITA GOETHALS, ANDRÉ VANDIERENDONCK, MICHEL THIERY, and ROBERT DEROM

Introduction

An aetiological relationship between intrauterine oxygen deprivation and irreversible damage to the foetal CNS is commonly postulated (Hellman and Pritchard 1971). A variety of specific obstetric factors have been proven to be hazardous or are at least suspected in this respect (Thiery 1969).

This longitudinal study was planned within the framework of a systematic investigation of potentially hypoxygenic factors.

The follow-up was devised to determine whether any deleterious effect of labour induction, using prostaglandin $F_2\alpha$ (PG), on the neurological state of the neonate and the psychomotor evolution of the child could be demonstrated.

It was decided to plan a follow-up study because of:

(a) The possibility that certain effects appear early in life but disappear after some time;

(b) The possibility that certain effects emerge only at a later stage;

(c) The expensiveness of and the deontological problems associated with a large sample of children born under these circumstances.

Subjects and methods

Our subjects comprised 80 mature (gestational age 38–42 weeks) children born to clinically normal women between March, 1972, and March, 1973, at the Department of Obstetrics of the University of Ghent. The parents of all children lived within a 10-km radius of this city. The children were assigned at random to an index and a control group. The 40 index group children were born from women in whom labour had been induced by low amniotomy and intravenous infusion of prostaglandin (PG)$F_2\alpha$. The mothers of the 40 control children had gone into labour spontaneously. The design was a $2\times2\times2$ factorial, with the factors: birth circumstances (index vs. control group); parity (first-born or not); and sex (boy or girl) as independent variables. There were 36 children from nulliparous and 44 children from parous women. Fifty-four of the children were boys and 26 were girls.

On day 4 or 5, all of the children were subjected to a neurological examination according to Prechtl and Beintema (1964). At the ages of 3 and 6 months, the Bayley Developmental Test (Bayley 1969a, b), consisting of a mental and a motor scale, was applied. At 30 months of age, both groups were tested with the Stutsman Intelligence Test for Preschool Children (Smulders 1963). The raw scores of the Bayley scales and the raw and language scores of the Stutsman test were analysed in a three-way analysis of variance design (Winer 1962). The sample was personally contacted, first in the hospital (day 4 or 5 after birth), and at 3, 6, and 30 months in the home environment. This contact was made by a social worker.

Results

On day 4 or 5 all children were found to be *neurologically* normal.

From the data concerning the psychomotor evolution (Tables 45.1 and 45.2) the following conclusions can be drawn:

At 3 months of age there were no significant differences between the two groups;

At the age of 6 months, we found a significant effect only for parity; children of nulliparae scored significantly better on the mental scale than children from parous women ($p < 0.05$);

At 30 months, compared to the controls, the PG-group scored significantly better on the intelligence test ($p < 0.05$), and children born from nulliparae obtained higher intelligence scores than children from parous women ($p < 0.01$). With respect to language development too, the index group scored higher than the control group ($p < 0.001$). Furthermore, the girls obtained higher scores than the boys ($p < 0.001$) and children of nulliparae were advanced in language development at 30 months compared with children of parous women ($p < 0.01$). Index children tended to originate from higher socio-economic classes than the controls. However, this difference was not statistically significant, neither on the Kolmogorov–Smirnov Two-sample test (cf. Siegel 1956) nor on a χ^2-test. It is evident from this analysis, that socio-economic class is not responsible for the difference between the index and control groups. Nevertheless, socio-economic class cannot be ruled out as a possible factor, because it could have worked in addition to other causal factors.

Discussion

The general conclusion from this investigation appears to be that elective induction of labour at term with intravenous $PGF_2\alpha$ has no untoward effect on the psychomotor development of the baby and toddler up to the age of 30 months. An interpretational difficulty arises, however, at the age of 30 months. PG children appear to perform better than control children. Certainly, this should not be interpreted as a demonstration of the utility of labour induction with PG. In our opinion, it is more probable that this statistical difference is rather accidental. For one thing, although the examiner was blind with respect to the condition the children he was testing belonged to, the mothers were not. As the mother was present when the child was tested, it is almost inevitable that the examiner would receive cues relevant to the difference between index and control groups. Furthermore, there was a small but not significant tendency for PG children to originate from higher socio-economic classes than control children. These factors together, perhaps in addition to other factors, might well be responsible for a statistically significant difference in favour of the PG children.

Another interesting finding concerns the difference between children of nulliparae and children of parous women. As similar

TABLE 45.1

Cell means of the raw mental and motor scores at 3 and 6 months, and of the raw intelligence and language scores at 30 months

Age (months)	Score	PG-children				Control children			
		Male		Female		Male		Female	
		NP	P	NP	P	NP	P	NP	P
3	mental	39·58	34·81	34·83	35·50	37·90	36·87	38·12	39·83
3	motor	16·33	15·69	15·00	16·00	16·10	15·12	16·12	16·67
6	mental	73·67	68·69	74·17	67·17	74·40	71·56	72·12	72·33
6	motor	26·67	25·19	25·83	25·00	27·00	24·87	25·87	26·83
30	raw score	29·42	26·37	37·33	29·33	28·00	19·87	31·37	18·33
30	language score	18·33	13·12	22·17	21·17	11·40	4·62	20·62	12·50
	N	12	16	6	6	10	16	8	6

NP = nulliparae; P = parous.

TABLE 45.2

Cell means of the raw mental and motor scores at 3 and 6 months, and of the raw intelligence and language scores at 30 months. Statistical significance indicated

Variable	3 months mental	3 months motor	6 months mental	6 months motor	30 months raw scores	30 months language scores
PG-children	36·18	15·76	70·93	25·67	30·61 ⎱ *	18·70 ⎱ ***
Controls	38·18	16·00	72·60	26·14	24·39 ⎰	12·29 ⎰
Male	37·29	15·81	72·08	25·93	25·92	11·87 ⎱ ***
Female	37·07	15·95	71·45	25·88	29·09	19·12 ⎰
Nulliparae	37·61	15·89	73·59 ⎱ *	26·34	31·53 ⎱ **	18·12 ⎱ **
Parous	36·75	15·87	69·94 ⎰	25·47	23·48 ⎰	12·85 ⎰

* = significant $p < 0.05$; ** = $p < 0.01$; *** = $p < 0.001$. Effects not indicated by an asterisk are not statistically significant at the 0·05 level.

findings have been reported in other studies (e.g. De Coster *et al.* 1977) it is clear that this finding is not accidental. There are at least two sources of variability which might be responsible for this difference:

    (a) Nulliparous women have often more time available for, and are often more concerned with the physical and mental welfare of their children than parous women;

    (b) Children from parous women are often in the company of other children, who supply entertainment but not necessarily education.

Considering these factors, the interpretation might be stated in terms of modelling behaviour, as follows: children from nulliparous women are very often confronted with good adult models whereas children of parous women have less experience with such good adult models, but more with models which are in some respects less stimulating. This interpretation is a special case of a general hypothesis of the effects of modelling which has also been applied to the twin situation (see chapter 40, this volume). Thus far this hypothesis opens up some promising lines of investigation. However, further research will be necessary to determine its value.

Acknowledgements

This research was supported by grants from the United Cerebral Palsy Research and Educational Foundation, New York (No. R-192-68 C), the Fonds voor Geneeskundig Wetenschappelijk Onderzoek, and the Fonds voor Fundamenteel Collectief Onderzoek (Belgium). The PGF$_2\alpha$ was kindly supplied by J.-M. Decoster, M.D., Medical Director, Upjohn-Belgium. This research report is a more elaborated version of an earlier report (De Coster *et al.* 1976).

v. Follow up studies of deviant groups
a. Epidemiological studies

46. A study of incidence of mental disorder in Iceland

LARUS HELGASON

Introduction

This chapter is a short review of a study of all 2388 first admission psychiatric patients in Iceland for the years 1966 and 1967 (Helgason 1977). The description of the patients in this study covers general demographic data and some possible precipitating factors with special emphasis on the difference between those who were admitted to mental hospitals and those who were not. The study also includes a 6 to 7 year follow-up and evaluation of outcome, with a special emphasis on the relationship between mental illness and changes in socio-economic status. Hospital admissions, some demographic factors registered from 1956 on, and changes in estimated income from 1962 on, were used to observe possible changes before and after seeking psychiatric services.

Iceland and its medical system

Iceland lies close to the Arctic Circle. The country is rather mountainous and the total area of 103 000 km² includes about 20 000 km² of land covered by vegetation and 11 800 km² of land covered by glaciers. The mean temperature in January is only −0·4°C but in July 11·2°C.

Since 1937 Iceland has had a comprehensive system of statutory national insurance basically similar to that in other Nordic countries. Medical care by general practitioners is almost free. The National Insurance System covers three-fourths of the cost for care by specialists to out-patients; it also covers half to full cost of medicine, and pays for hospitalization and treatment in hospitals.

Since 1960 there has been no waiting list for out-patient treatment, but a severe shortage of beds makes it impossible to accurately assess the actual need for hospitalization. The ratio of psychiatrists to the population is about 1:20 000, with a ratio of 1·4 psychiatric beds to 1000 inhabitants. The policy of the hospitals has been to discharge the patients as quickly as possible and then continue treatment in out-patient clinics. The number of admissions has increased steadily during the survey period.

More than half of the population of Iceland lives in the capital, Reykjavík, and the adjoining towns. At the time of the survey employment and income were stable, and other social circumstances were favourable.

Method

The investigation is based on first-ever arrival at all psychiatric services in Iceland between 1 January 1966 and 31 December 1967. All the services were located in Reykjavík. The available services during the survey were as follows:

Two mental hospitals, one with an out-patient psychiatric clinic;
Two out-patient clinics for alcoholics;
Psychiatric services at an old people's home in Reykjavík;
Psychiatrists in private practice;
Psychiatric consultations in general hospitals in Reykjavík and vicinity;
A child guidance clinic.

We examined a psychiatric case register of all patients admitted to mental hospitals, those treated in out-patient clinics, and also many treated by psychiatrists in private practice. Further information came from perusal of files of every psychiatric service in Iceland. Inclusion of all patients not in the register and exclusion of those with recorded evidence of previous use of psychiatric services was thus made possible. The National Insurance System (compulsory for every citizen) and the National Register gave further data on different demographic factors. Information was also gathered by perusal of files of practically all hospitals and disablement insurance documents from 1 January 1956 to 31 December 1973. The project could not have been completed without the full co-operation of all psychiatrists and other physicians working in the country.

The patients were divided into three groups.

Patient group A: Those admitted to a mental hospital the same calendar year they first consulted a psychiatrist. About 85 per cent of the patients in this group were admitted within 4 weeks of arrival at the psychiatric services.

Patient group B: Those admitted to a mental hospital after the first calendar year of consulting a psychiatric service until 31 December 1973.

Patient group C: Those never admitted to mental hospitals during the survey period.

The division of admitted patients is meant to give information about those admitted more or less directly to mental hospitals as compared to those who were planned to be treated as out-patients but were admitted to hospitals later. About 40 per cent of the patients were self-referred.

Results

Only a brief summary of the results will be presented here. Of the 2388 patients studied 1957 obtained treatment outside of mental hospitals only; of these, 1587 patients were treated by psychiatrists in private practice. There were 1009 men (42·3 per cent), and 1379 women (57·7 per cent). The incidence rate for all ages for males was 506 per 100 000 per year and for females 707 per 100 000 per year; the total incidence rate was 607 per 100 000 per year.

Age

Table 46.1 shows the incidence of mental disorder as a function of age where age is defined as age at first arrival for psychiatric services.

Patient Group A. In this group there were 253 patients, 114 males and 139 females. The admission rate for males age 15 and over was

TABLE 46.1

Incidence per 100 000 per year, by age, sex, and patient groups†

Age	Group A	Group B	Group C	Total
Males				
–14	0 (0)	4 (3)	168 (116)	172 (119)
15–44	87 (71)	70 (57)	523 (427)	680 (555)
45–64	102 (34)	60 (20)	536 (179)	697 (233)
65–	59 (9)	39 (6)	566 (87)	668 (102)
Females				
–14	2 (1)	3 (2)	122 (80)	127 (83)
15–44	88 (69)	86 (67)	923 (720)	1097 (856)
45–64	138 (46)	54 (18)	591 (196)	783 (260)
65–	126 (23)	28 (5)	836 (152)	990 (180)

† Number of patients in brackets.
M: $X^2 = 32·29$; d.f. = 6; $p < 0·001$.
F: $X^2 = 37·92$; d.f. = 6; $p < 0·001$.

88 per 100 000 per year and for females 106 per 100 000 per year. The difference was not significant. Attention should be drawn to the fact that the admission rate for patients in group A did not mean the total first admission to hospital rate, as patients treated by psychiatrists outside hospitals before the study period were not included. The highest incidence for both sexes occurred at the ages of 45–64. The incidence at the ages of 15–44, however, was practically the same for both sexes.

Patient Group B. In this group there were 178 patients, 86 males and 92 females. During the 6 to 7 year follow-up the late admission rate for males age 15 and over was 64 per 100 000 per year and for females 70 per 100 000 per year. The highest incidence for both sexes occurred in the age range 15–44.

Patient Group C. In this group there were 1957 patients, 809 males and 1148 females. The rate for not-admitted males age 15 and over was 532 per 100 000 per year and for females 825 per 100 000 per year. The highest incidence for males occurred at age 65 and over but for females in the age range 15–44.

A higher percentage of the males in the cohort were hospitalized (19·8 per cent) than females (16·9 per cent) during the study. This could partly be explained by the fact that there were fewer males than females in the cohort and that there may have been a selection bias for more 'severe' cases among the males. The fact remains, however, that the actual number of hospitalizations was higher for females than for males.

Residence

Table 46.2 shows the incidence of mental disorder as a function of residence where residence in the present study was defined as

Urban	population of 10 000 and over;
Semi-urban	population of 1000–9999
Rural	population up to 999.

Even though the crude incidence of patients was three times higher for males in urban than in rural areas and 2·3 times higher for females, the percentage from either sex of those not admitted from these residences was nearly equal.

Figure 46.1 shows the higher number of patients under the age of 10 and over the age of 70 from urban areas. This is explained by the fact that all psychiatric services were located in the urban area. It can be seen that easier access to psychiatric services especially affects patients in those age groups.

Social class

Compared to many other countries status differences in Iceland are

TABLE 46.2

Crude incidence per 100 000 per year, by residence, sex, and patient groups†

Residence	Group A	Group B	Group C	Total
Males				
Urban	75 (76)	65 (66)	589 (604)	738 (746)
Semi-urban	52 (23)	18 (8)	216 (95)	286 (126)
Rural	27 (15)	21 (12)	198 (110)	246 (137)
Females				
Urban	83 (87)	64 (67)	812 (849)	959 (1003)
Semi-urban	68 (29)	35 (15)	300 (129)	403 (173)
Rural	47 (23)	21 (10)	350 (170)	418 (203)

† Number of patients in brackets.
M: X^2 value not significant.
F: $X^2 = 13·72$; d.f. = 4; $p < 0·01$.

minimal. Two main forms of scoring were used in the study. One of them was based on the occupational groups defined by the Statistical Bureau of Iceland and the other on the method devised by Helgason (1964).

Occupation was defined as the patient's main occupation in 1967. It was often not clear which one, if either, of the married couple was ill or whether the parents or the child were in most need of treatment. The anxiety or depression of the wife could be related to her husband's alcoholism, or a child could be disturbed because of difficulties between the parents. I therefore assumed it relevant to include married females and children with the husband's and the father's occupations. Table 46.3 shows ten major groups of the Icelandic occupational classification (The Statistical Bureau of Iceland). The highest crude incidence of mental disorders was found among service workers (maids, cleaners, and the lowest level of office workers). The main problems in this group were alcoholism and neuroses. The lowest incidence was found among agricultural workers. Most of these were farmers who owned their farms and had a relatively good income.

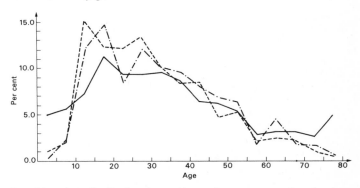

FIG. 46.1. Age distribution, by residence, in percentage; (——) urban; (----) semi-urban; (-·-·-) rural.

Marital status

Table 46.4 shows the incidence of mental disorder as a function of marital status where marital status in this study means the status of patients as listed in The General Population Register (Statistical Bureau of Iceland). The crude incidence rate for single and married males was fairly equal, but the rate for married females was somewhat higher than for single females.

Patient group A. The crude incidence rate for single males was nearly twice as high as for married males, but the rates for single and married females were nearly the same. The crude incidence for previously married patients was approximately twice as high as for single patients.

TABLE 46.3

Comparison between the economically active population, 1967, and the cohort, by occupation and patient groups, in percentage, and by crude incidence per 100 000 per year

	Population	Cohort	Group A	Group B	Group C	Crude incidence
Government and municipal employees, bankers, and social unions	15·9	15·7	11·9	17·4	16·0	1286
Agricultural workers	8·5	4·4	5·5	2·3	4·5	682
Fishermen and fish processing workers	12·2	11·6	17·0	10·7	10·0	1234
Manufacturers	12·7	8·2	6·3	5·6	8·7	843
Construction workers	9·5	10·8	12·7	11·2	10·5	1471
Sales workers	9·5	11·6	9·9	8·4	12·2	1591
Workers in transport/communication	6·5	7·3	5·5	9·6	7·4	1467
Service workers	4·8	6·5	4·7	7·3	6·7	1786
Disability pension and no income	17·2	20·9	24·5	25·8	19·9	1579
Workers not classified and workers at NATO air-base	3·2	3·0	2·0	1·7	3·2	1226
Total = 100 per cent	183 322	2388	253	178	1957	1303

TABLE 46.4

Crude incidence per 100 000 per year, by marital status, sex, and patient groups, age 15 and over†

Marital status	Group A	Group B	Group C	Total
Males				
Single	107 (54)	63 (32)	440 (223)	610 (309)
Married	62 (46)	62 (46)	535 (398)	658 (490)
Previously married	213 (14)	76 (5)	1097 (72)	1387 (91)
Females				
Single	97 (40)	58 (24)	727 (300)	882 (364)
Married	95 (71)	76 (57)	816 (609)	988 (737)
Previously married	183 (27)	61 (9)	1078 (159)	1322 (195)

† Number of patients in brackets.
M: $X^2 = 13·97$; d.f. = 4; $p < 0·01$.
F: X^2 value not significant.

Patient group B. The crude incidence rate for late admission was practically the same for single, married, and previously married males and females.

Patient group C. For both males and females crude incidence rates increased from single to married to previously married patients. The crude rates were practically the same for previously married patients of both sexes. The rates for those seeking psychiatric services were higher for both single and married males and females aged 30–44 than for those aged 15–29. The rates for previously married males and females aged 15–29 were more than twice as high as for those aged 30–44.

The incidence rate for previously married people from semi-urban and rural areas was much lower than the rate from urban areas. This may reflect the insufficiency of psychiatric services for semi-urban and rural areas, but it could also be a reflection of the greater acceptance and better health of the old persons in these areas.

Diagnosis

Diagnostic classifications were made according to the International Classification of Diseases, 8th revision, World Health Organization. Persons with epilepsy or mental retardation were only included when there was also a clear psychiatric diagnosis. Psychiatric services in Iceland do not primarily treat these patients as they are cared for by other resources. Patients in Iceland do not generally go to psychiatrists for psychophysiologic disorders only; thus, for those with an accompanying psychiatric syndrome, the diagnoses were made according to that syndrome.

The illnesses were divided into the following diagnostic groups:

(a) Senility, arteriosclerosis, and other organic diseases: 290, 292, 293, 294, 309 (WHO diagnostic classification numbers).
(b) Schizophrenia: 295.
(c) Affective psychoses: 296.
(d) Other and unspecified psychoses and paranoid states: 297, 298, 299.
(e) Neuroses, transient situational disturbances, behaviour disorders of childhood: 300, 307, 308.
(f) Personality disorders, sexual deviation: 301, 302.
(g) Alcoholic psychosis, alcoholism, and drug dependence: 291, 303, 304.
(h) Special symptoms not elsewhere classified (and unclassified symptoms): 306.

One of the questions posed was: What differences were there in psychiatric diagnosis between admitted and not admitted patients in the study?

Patient group A. In this group, 63 per cent of the males were alcoholics and 11 per cent were schizophrenic. About 43 per cent of the females were patients with affective psychoses, 16 per cent with alcoholism, and 15 per cent with schizophrenia.

Patient group B. About 49 per cent of the males were alcoholics, 15 per cent were males with affective psychoses, and 14 per cent with schizophrenia. About 30 per cent of the females had affective psychoses, 24 per cent neuroses, and about 19 per cent schizophrenia.

Patient group C. About 54 per cent of the males had neuroses, and 16 per cent were alcoholic patients. About 66 per cent of the females had neuroses, and 13 per cent affective psychoses.

An analysis of diagnosis according to residence provides the following data. The incidence rate per 100 000 per year for all ages is 34 for schizophrenic patients from urban areas, 13 from semi-urban areas, and 26 from rural areas. For patients with alcoholism the rates were, respectively, 116, 48, and 19; for patients with neuroses 434, 177, and 186; and for patients with affective psychoses 106, 56, and 55; and for patients with personality disorders 43, 12, and 12.

An analysis of diagnosis according to marital status (Table 46.5) showed that the crude incidence of organic mental disorders was nearly seven times higher for previously married than for married patients. Comparison by marital status for both sexes showed that the crude incidence rates for schizophrenia were similar for single as compared to married and previously married patients, the rate for single patients being somewhat higher. The crude incidence rate

TABLE 46.5

Crude incidence per 100 000 per year, by marital status, sex, and diagnosis, age 15 and over†

Diagnosis	Males				Females			
	Single	Married	Prev. marr.	Total	Single	Married	Prev. marr.	Total
Organic mental disorders	43 (22)	52 (39)	350 (23)	64 (84)	87 (36)	36 (27)	251 (37)	77 (100)
Schizophrenia	67 (34)	19 (14)	30 (2)	38 (50)	68 (28)	27 (20)	34 (5)	41 (53)
Affective psychoses	28 (14)	79 (59)	137 (9)	62 (82)	121 (50)	188 (140)	332 (49)	183 (239)
Other and unspecified psychoses	14 (7)	15 (11)	0 (0)	14 (18)	24 (10)	29 (22)	41 (6)	29 (38)
Neuroses	263 (133)	279 (208)	366 (24)	277 (365)	489 (202)	611 (456)	502 (74)	560 (732)
Personality disorders	49 (25)	20 (15)	30 (2)	32 (42)	51 (21)	44 (33)	34 (5)	45 (59)
Alcoholism	139 (70)	183 (136)	472 (31)	180 (237)	22 (9)	44 (33)	115 (17)	45 (59)
Special and unclassified symptoms	8 (4)	11 (8)	0 (0)	9 (12)	19 (8)	8 (6)	14 (2)	12 (16)
Total	610 (309)	658 (490)	1387 (91)	676 (890)	882 (364)	988 (737)	1322 (195)	992 (1296)

† Number of patients in brackets.

for affective psychoses was over four times as high for single females as for single males, and three times as high for married females as for married males. The crude incidence for neuroses was nearly equal for single and married males but higher for married than for single females. The distribution of patients with alcoholism shows the highest crude incidence for both sexes in the previously married group. The crude incidence was higher, however, for married patients of both sexes than for single patients. (Note that when reading Table 46.5, crude incidence does not correspond to the totals in each row. This is explained by the fact that each marital status in the cohort is compared to the same marital status in the population, but the crude incidence for the totals were compared to the respective sex in the population. Summary of each marital status should therefore show three times higher incidence than the total. For example, there were in Iceland 50 648 single males, 74 456 married males, and 6563 previously married males, or a total of 131 665 males age 15 and over for the years 1966 and 1967. Of the 50 schizophrenic males in the cohort 34 were single males; 34 divided by 50 648 gives 67 per 100 000 per year. The same calculation was made for married (14 divided by 6563) and previously married males, etc.)

Length of treatment

The length of treatment outside mental hospitals is expressed in 'treatment months' meaning each month in which there were one or more consultations. Treatment inside mental hospitals is expressed as duration of stay in calendar months.

Patient group A. Patients in this group had an average of 6·6 'treatment months' and an average of 4·4 calendar months inside hospitals. About 11 per cent of the males and 20 per cent of the females in this group became more or less chronic out-patients, and about 15 per cent of the males and 23 per cent of the females became more or less chronic in-patients. In 1973, 34 per cent were still receiving treatment.

Patient group B. On the average, patients in group B used 10·4 'treatment months' and 4·1 calendar months. About 22 per cent of the males and 35 per cent of the females in this group became chronic out-patients and 21 per cent of the males and 35 per cent of the females became more or less chronic in-patients. In 1973 44 per cent still were receiving treatment.

Patient group C. On the average the patients in this group used 5·9 'treatment months', and about 7 per cent were still receiving treatment in 1973.

Mortality

The mortality risk of the cohort was about 1½ to 2 times that of the general population. Table 46.6 shows the distribution of some

TABLE 46.4

Causes of death in the cohort compared with the population, 1966–73

Cause (disease classification numbers)	Cohort 1966–73	General population 1966–73	Cohort/ population
Heart disease (391, 392, 393–8, 402, 404, 410–4, 420–9)	47	3414	1·38
Neoplasms (140–209)	33	2311	1·43
Cerebrovascular disease (430–8)	63	1504	4·19
Arteriosclerosis (440)	19	194	9·79
Accidents (E800–949, E970–89)	6	935	0·64
Suicide (E950–9)	25	186	13·44
Other	30	2952	1·02
Total	223	11 496	1·94

causes of death in the cohort and in the general population during the years 1966–73; also shown are figures of the percentages of the population, for each cause of death, which are accounted for by patients in the cohort. Five of the nine most common causes listed in the Public Health Statistics of Iceland are given. The greatest number of patients from the cohort died of cerebrovascular diseases. Patients in the cohort accounted for 9·79 per cent of the deaths from arteriosclerosis in the general population, 4·19 per cent of the deaths from cerebrovascular diseases, 0·64 per cent of the deaths from accidents, 13·44 per cent of the deaths from suicide, and a total of 1·94 per cent of all deaths in the population. Of special interest is the low percentage in the cohort of deaths from accidents; three of these patients had organic mental disorders. Registration of the cause of death was according to the death certificates (The Statistical Bureau of Iceland). The standard mortality ratio of the cohort is shown in Fig. 46.2.

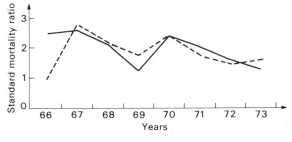

FIG. 46.2. Standard mortality ratio of the cohort 1966–73; (——) male; (----) female.

Outcome

The measurement of outcome was affected by the fact that each patient was not personally interviewed at the end of the follow-up period. Information was gained for each patient, however, and the measurement of outcome defined as much as possible in terms of objective rather than subjective factors. A rating scale was used for the three categories of function: working status, treatment, and mental status. The outcome was assessed for each of the years 1962, 1967, 1970, and 1973. 'Relatively good outcome' is defined as follows: the patient was working regularly or full time, was in out-patient treatment less than 2 months or had no treatment, and had mild mental symptoms or no complaint ('normal'). In 1973 a relatively good outcome was assessed for 31·6 per cent of the patients in group A, 28 per cent of those in group B, and 76·7 per cent in group C. The outcome was relatively good for 28·3 per cent of the patients with schizophrenia, 4·8 per cent of those with alcoholism, 46·8 per cent of those with affective psychoses, and 84·1 per cent of those with neuroses.

The Department of Internal Revenue publishes yearly a list of actual income tax for each economically active person. From this list it was possible to estimate gross income taking into account allowed deductions for self, spouse, and children, and also taking into account variations in the tax scale for each year. Income is also calculated annually by the Statistical Bureau of Iceland for each of 30 distinct occupational groups. We thus classified each patient according to his main occupation in each of the years 1962, 1967, 1970, and 1972. The information was collected both for economically active patients 16 years and over at arrival, and for the husbands of the married women in the cohort for the same years. The income was then grouped into a less than mean income group, a mean income group, and a more than mean income group. The mean income group is defined as those whose income is within the range of the mean ±25 per cent for each occupational group, or those whose income level was earned by 65–75 per cent of the population working in each occupational group. Since the patients were older in 1972 than in 1962, an increase in income was expected. It was therefore not possible to conclude whether the increase found in the study was due to increasing age or improved health; however, a comparison between the patient groups showed that the increase was higher for patients in group C than in groups A and B. The results also showed that persons with less than the mean income tended to seek more psychiatric services than did those who earned more.

Related studies

Incidence rates

One of the main characteristics of the study of first-ever psychiatric patients was the relatively high number of patients treated only on an out-patient basis, 80·2 per cent of the males and 83·1 per cent of the females. Very few studies have comparable results.

Hagnell (1966a, b) found, over a period of 10 years in the Swedish county of Lundby (population 2297) that the incidence rate for males of all ages was 434 per 100 000 per year and for females 707 per 100 000 per year; as compared to our study this is a slightly lower rate for males but an equal rate for females. In Hagnell's study about 68 per cent of the males were treated on an out-patient basis and 70 per cent of the females. Hollingshead and Redlich (1958) found the incidence in New Haven over a 6-month period to be 104, or approximately 208 per 100 000 per year. Adelstein et al. (1968) studied adult patients (age 15 and over) in Salford, England (population 150 000) who consulted any form of psychiatric service during the period 1959–63. The incidence they found for males was 296 per 100 000 per year and for females 360 per 100 000 per year, with a total incidence of 330 per 100 000 per year. Using the same definition of incidence as did Adelstein et al. (age 15 and over) the incidence rate for males would be 683 per 100 000 per year and for females 1001 per 100 000 per year, or a total incidence rate of 842 per 100 000 per year.

T. Helgason (1964) studied all 5395 Icelanders born in Iceland during the years 1895–7 and still alive in Iceland in 1910. He calculated the expectancy of mental disorders in Iceland up to the average age of 61 years. He also published a preliminary report (T. Helgason, 1973) on the follow-up of the cohort to the average age of 75 years. A comparison of expectancy found in his study with the expectancy found in the present study of first incidence psychiatric patients made it possible to estimate the difference between those seeking psychiatric services and those expected to be mentally ill according to various demographic and diagnostic categories. We can therefore give answers to some of the basic questions which are ideal both for epidemiological studies and for elaboration of programming the mental health services. What is the unduplicated count of patients arriving at psychiatric services in a whole country over a two-year period? Where do people initially contact the services? How ill were these patients? What are the results of treatment in a 6–7 year follow-up? What is the relationship between data on the mentally ill seen in psychiatric services and mental illness in the general population?

Age

Assuming that there have been no major changes in the expectancy of mental disorders and assuming that patients in the present study would be included in T. Helgason's categories, a comparison of the expectancies shows that about 25–30 per cent of the total expected mentally ill patients seek psychiatric services before the age of 63, with about 10 per cent doing so between the ages of 63 and 75. The psychiatric services in Iceland were more often used by those acquiring mental disorder at a younger age.

Tomasson (1938) studied all new patients applying for psychiatric services in Iceland during the years 1928–36. A comparison with the present study shows that there has been an increase in the number of patients aged 15–19, with a decrease in the age group 20–59. It is possible that patients now seek psychiatric services at an earlier stage of their symptoms than before.

Social class

T. Helgason (1964) grouped his probands into three large categories. I used the same categories to make a comparison possible (doubtful cases were discussed with Helgason). A comparison of the expectancy found in his study with the incidence found in the present study points to the fact that patients with mental disorders from social class 2 did seek psychiatric services in higher numbers than did those from the other two classes. The highest number of schizophrenic patients were in social class 3 but the greatest number of neuroses was from social class 2.

Marital status

Adelstein et al. (1968) found the incidence to be higher for single than for married patients. Hagnell (1966a, b) found, however, no apparent difference in incidence between married and unmarried men but a higher incidence for married as compared to unmarried women. These results were more in accordance with the results found in the present study. Essen-Möller et al. (1956) also found a slight predominance of mental disorders among married women. T. Helgason (1964) grouped marital status into single patients and ever-married patients. An analysis of his results shows that single females with mental illness seek more psychiatric services than do single males.

A comparison between T. Helgason's (1964) study and the present study shows that relatively fewer single schizophrenic males and females in Iceland seek psychiatric services than do married or previously married patients. The single may cope better with their symptoms than do the married. It is also possible that more of the schizophrenic people got married, and at a younger age, during the present study than during the period of T. Helgason's (1964) study.

Diagnosis

A comparison of results from this study and T. Helgason's 1964 study indicates that in Iceland 62·3 per cent of males and 52·9 per cent of females with schizophrenia seek psychiatric services.

As some new cases of affective psychoses were found in T. Helgason's (1973) follow-up (age up to 75), the expectancy rate expressed in Table 46.7 is a minimal figure. The results suggest, however, that females with affective psychoses sought more help from psychiatric services than did males. The high percentage of female alcoholics is partly explained by an increase in the use of alcohol by females, but it also reflects the possibility that female alcoholics seek psychiatric services more than male alcoholics.

Tomasson (1938) calculated the incidence of new patients during the years 1928–36. He found the incidence rate at age 15–70 to be 848 per 100 000 per year. The incidence for the same age period in the present study was 833 per 100 000 per year. Even though Tomasson included mental retardation and epilepsy in his study as well as some neurological cases, the results show that there was no significant change in the incidence of mental patients from the period 1928–36 to the period 1966–7. The so-called increase in number of patients and increased need of psychiatric treatment in Iceland is therefore probably caused by longer duration of treat-

ment, patients seeking help earlier, and more consultations being given than before.

It is impossible to give a clear answer to the question: How ill were those who did not use psychiatric services? A comparison with T. Helgason's (1964) study, however, shows that only half of the expected rate of psychotic patients in Iceland actually use psychiatric services. Many of those who did not probably had a substantially disabling health condition and should have been easily identified by general practitioners. Some of them are probably treated by the general practitioners, but it is also likely that some clearly psychotic patients were able to live and work in the community without the aid of either doctors or drugs.

TABLE 46.7

Comparison of expectancy rates (per cent) with Helgason's 1964 study

	Expectancy					
	Present study		Helgason's study		Present study	
					Helgason's study	× 100
Diagnosis	M	F	M	F	M	F
Schizophrenia	0·43	0·54	0·69	1·02	62·3	52·9
Affective psychoses	1·20	3·17	2·18	3·23	55·0	98·1
Neuroses	3·92	6·90	9·50	18·04	41·3	38·2
Personality disorders	0·34	0·48	2·35	2·36	14·5	20·3
Alcoholism	2·20	0·59	8·63	0·84	25·5	70·2

47. The three-county schizophrenia study: a study of the prevalence and incidence of schizophrenia and an assessment of its clinical and social outcome in the Republic of Ireland

AILEEN O'HARE and DERMOT WALSH

Introduction and historical background

For some time it has been known that statistics for hospitalized psychiatric illness in the Republic of Ireland have shown prevalence rates and admission rates that are amongst the highest in the world, particularly for schizophrenia (Walsh 1968). This observation has posed the question whether these hospital figures reflect a truly raised incidence of psychiatric illness, including schizophrenia, in Ireland, or whether they merely indicate that most if not all psychiatric illness in Ireland is hospital-treated by community psychiatric services. By the early 1960s the hospitalized prevalence for psychiatric illness in Ireland was 0·7 per cent and almost half that prevalence was due to schizophrenia. First admission rates for schizophrenia were approximately three times those of England and Wales and it was calculated that four out of every one hundred people in the Republic of Ireland could be expected to be admitted to a psychiatric hospital at least once with a diagnosis of schizophrenia before age 55 (Walsh and Walsh 1970).

The undoubtedly raised hospital prevalence of schizophrenia together with clinical impressions suggest that the outcome of schizophrenia in Ireland may be less favourable than in other Western countries. In the light of these considerations the Mental Health Section of the Medico-Social Research Board has implemented a number of research projects specifically designed to

examine these two questions (Medico-Social Research Board, Annual Reports 1970–6).

Associated projects

Since 1971 the Mental Health Section of the Medico-Social Research Board has been responsible for the National Psychiatric In-patient Reporting System. This is a record-linked system to which all psychiatric hospitals and units in Ireland report all admissions, discharges, and deaths. The system began with a census of all patients in psychiatric hospitals and units on 31 March 1971 and has been monitoring patient movement activities since then. It is partly on the basis of data returned by this system that the figures of high hospital prevalence and incidence emerged (O'Hare and Walsh 1975, 1977).

The first step towards looking at the 'real' incidence and prevalence of psychiatric illness in Ireland was the 'Three-County Psychiatric Case Register Project' which commenced in 1973. For this project three of Ireland's twenty-six counties were selected as location for the relevant research. These counties were selected because of geographical, demographic, and social considerations. One of them, in the east of the country, is relatively prosperous, has a high proportion of urban dwellers, little out-migration, and favourable economic circumstances. The second county selected is in the west of the country and has generally unfavourable socio-demographic conditions. Thus there is high out-migration, high unemployment, a low proportion of urban dwellers, and a high proportion of elderly and single people. The third county chosen was intermediate in these characteristics between the western and eastern counties.

A psychiatric case register was established in each of these three counties whose combined population of 150 000 is 5 per cent of the entire country. The psychiatric case register gathers information by trained interviewers on all patients entering psychiatric care of any form, whether out-patient, day care, or in-patient care, who reside in these three counties. In addition, data on patients ordinarily resident in these counties receiving private care are also being returned to the registers. These registers have been ongoing since 31 March 1973, when they began with a census of all patients in care and the results of that census are currently being analysed. Diagnoses on all patients coming to case register notification are supplied by the service psychiatrist in the area in accordance with the International Classification of Diseases. The psychiatrists have all undergone video-tape training in symptom rating and I.C.D. diagnosis kindly provided by the Institute of Psychiatry, University of London, (Drs J. Copeland and M. Kelleher).

The three county case registers will, it is hoped, answer some questions concerning whether 'first' admissions returned to the National Psychiatric In-patient System are really 'first' in fact, or whether some different interpretation, other than that directed, of 'first' admissions is being used. Furthermore the standardization of diagnosis by the methods already outlined will go far to answering the question whether any characteristic Irish fashion in diagnosis may be responsible for the 'high' rate of schizophrenia. In this context however the U.S./U.K. diagnostic team visited Ireland during the 1960s showing video-tape tapes to Irish psychiatrists and the findings indicated that Irish psychiatrists' diagnostic behaviour is very similar to that of United Kingdom psychiatrists (Copeland *et al*. 1971).

The St. Loman's Psychiatric Case Register is another psychiatric case register, established and operated for the Eastern Health Board by Dr Dermot Walsh, covering a mainly urban population of approximately 150 000 in west city and county Dublin. The St. Loman's Case Register has been operating in this service area for 5 years now. The combined Three-County and St. Loman's register population of 300 000 comprises 10 per cent of the Irish population (Butler and Walsh 1976).

Because schizophrenia as a condition in terms of prognosis often has an unfavourable outcome, because it constitutes over half the resident psychiatric population of the Republic of Ireland, and because the possibility exists that its social and clinical outcome in Ireland may be less favourable than in other Western countries, it was decided to supplement the Three-County Case Register Study with the Three-County 'Schizophrenia' Study.

The three-county schizophrenia study

Objectives

The objectives of this study are to investigate whether the incidence and prevalence of schizophrenia in representative Irish communities is any greater than appears to be the case in other comparable countries. It is a further objective of the study to test the hypothesis that the prognosis of individuals suffering from schizophrenia is less favourable in this country, in social and clinical terms, than is the case in other Western countries.

Location of project

The project will be located in the three Irish counties already

described and in the St. Loman's Psychiatric Case Register area. It thus provides a study population of approximately 300 000 persons with, assuming a minimum expectancy of schizophrenia of 0·1 per 1000 of population, an annual incidence of at least 30 recent onset first contact cases of schizophrenia.

Practical application of proposed research

It is envisaged that the proposed research will, according to its findings, indicate where service deficits exist in relation to the needs of schizophrenic patients and will indicate what medical and social measures, administratively and organizationally, are needed to improve the prognosis of schizophrenic individuals. It will also indicate which environmental–social factors are particularly associated with favourable or unfavourable outcome.

Methodology

This study consists of two phases. The first of these has been going on since April 1974 and will conclude on 31 March 1978. The methodology of this study is that all individuals within the combined Three-County and St. Loman's areas, given a hospital diagnosis of schizophrenia and in care on the census day which began the study, are subjected to a standardized interview, the Present State Examination, by a psychiatrist trained at the Institute of Psychiatry, London. The completed medical schedules relating to the Present State Examination are then forwarded to Professor J. Wing, Institute of Psychiatry, London, for processing and analysis. This instrument employed by the appropriately trained field research psychiatrist ensures that all individuals in care at one point in time (the census day) and formally diagnosed as schizophrenic by service personnel, are being examined by an objective interviewing technique, thus standardizing diagnoses. In addition, within the three counties, sample areas are being examined by means of the key informant method, to identify cases of schizophrenia either existing at the beginning of the study or occurring during its course and not presenting to the specialist psychiatric teams, so that as complete as possible a prevalence and incidence study of the condition can be undertaken. Following census day all new cases diagnosed as schizophrenia coming to the psychiatric service and those notified by key informants arising in the community but not coming to the psychiatric services, are examined by the research psychiatrist using the same instruments and schedules, i.e. the P.S.E. and supporting techniques.

In addition to the P.S.E. and the other medical content of the psychiatric examination, a sociologically based examination of schizophrenic patients identified in the study, their next-in-age siblings, and a matched control taken from the electoral register, is being carried out. The instruments being used were partly developed by ourselves, and they concern early life experience, recent role performance, and major life events within the year preceding contact with the psychiatric services.

From the combined Three-County and St. Loman's Register areas a cohort of first-contact schizophrenic patients has been assembled which, it is hoped, will be followed up at two-year and five-year intervals. Clinical and social outcome will be assessed by means of schedules which we ourselves are adapting to the Irish scene, though largely based on the K.A.S. and S.I.A.M.

The second phase of this Three-County Schizophrenia Study is simply an adaptation of the present study to utilization of the methodology being developed by the World Health Organization in its projected project entitled *Determinants of outcome of severe mental disorders*. This project has developed from the International Pilot Study of Schizophrenia and is an extension of that project to constitute a more rigorous epidemiological approach to the incidence of schizophrenia in the various participating field research centres. In addition to the core study concerned with incidence, the project will embody a number of substudies concerned with various subjects believed to be relevant to the outcome of schizophrenic illness. Among these is one known as the *Disability study*. It is projected that the Irish Three-County Schizophrenia Study in its second phase, as well as following the methodology of the core WHO study, will also carry out the Disability substudy.

For the purpose of collaboration with the WHO project as a satellite participant, Dr Walsh attended a recent meeting in Geneva of collaborating investigators for the WHO project. It is hoped to recruit a field research psychiatrist for this project very shortly and although the field work may not begin until July/August 1978,

training in the use of the ninth edition of the PSE and the Disability instrument will begin towards the end of 1977.

Estimated cohort size

It is anticipated that each year the combined Three-County and St. Loman's case registers should encounter between 30 and 40 new schizophrenics. As it is envisaged that the project will run for three years, there should be a final cohort of between 90 and 120 schizophrenic patients.

b. Patient studies

48. A 10-year prospective follow-up study of 2268 cases at the child guidance clinics in Stockholm, Sweden

HANS CURMAN and INGVAR NYLANDER

Introduction

The Child Guidance Clinics (CGC) in Stockholm came into being in 1933 as a result of the efforts of the Child Welfare Committee at that time. From its humble beginnings with 3 employees, the CGC has grown to its present position with 300 persons employed at about 20 clinics spread throughout the Stockholm County area. Child psychiatrists, psychologists, welfare officers, and special teachers collaborate in attempting to solve familial problems. The CGC thus functions as a child psychiatric counselling organization for out-patients with additional decentralized and sectorized facilities designed to facilitate local contacts between the family, the school, the social care authorities, and the other child welfare authorities who are empowered to act within their geographically defined regions. The CGC also possesses facilities for treatment on a semi-out-patient basis (therapeutic play schools, therapeutic schools, etc.). At the present time, about 10 000 families are in contact with the CGC annually.

When the investigation started in 1953, the CGC consisted of four counselling offices manned by about 40 employees. A statistics sheet was drawn up which, together with a manual containing instructions for its use, served as the basis for the investigation. Information was collected pertaining to family and social circumstances, school situations, investigations completed earlier and currently, symptomatology, diagnostic data, and therapeutic measures. Each single registration on the sheet was checked carefully by one and the same experienced psychologist.

The follow-up study described here is the result of a 10-year follow-up observation period of the patients who were discharged from the CGC during the years 1953–5.

A future publication is planned which will deal with a further 10-year follow-up period in a similar manner. With regard to this planned report and in view of the fact that the age distribution of the patients covers patients who had not yet reached adulthood by the end of the first 10-year period, it has been necessary to wait until the full 20-year observation period reached completion before subjecting the data to detailed analysis. The questions to be dealt with in the light of the information available to us today are:

1. What will happen to our patients in the coming years? How many of them will be in need of continued psychiatric care after having been discharged from the CGC? How many will require supportive measures from the community? How

many will, in time, be in contact with alcohol polyclinics and law enforcement authorities?
2. Is it possible to predict, on the basis of the investigation technique and the working methods that are used daily in child psychiatric care and from the information given by these procedures, which of our patients are likely to be in need of medical or social care facilities?

Subjects

The material studied covered 2364 patients aged up to 20 years, of whom 2268 could be followed up. In the vast majority of cases, contact with the CGC had been intiated by the families themselves.

Characteristics of the sample

With respect to social class levels, the clientele conformed to the average population of Stockholm according to the official population statistics valid for the years in quesiton. In 77 per cent of the cases, the child was living at home with both mother and father; in 20 per cent of the cases, the child lived at home with only the mother. The number of boys who applied to the CGC for care was very much greater than the number of girls. This was particularly noticeable during the school years. Above school age, however, the numbers were more or less the same for both boys and girls.

Symptoms

For the most part, the symptoms that had prompted the contact between patient and CGC were of a 'child neurotic' nature: anxiety, lack of contact, habitual manipulations (thumb-sucking, nail-biting, etc.), obstinacy, negativism, hyperactivity, tics, insomnia, and so forth. Symptoms of asocial behaviour were less common, as were symptoms of grave psychopathological conditions.

The pattern of symptoms shown by the boys differed from that shown by the girls in that the boys reacted more frequently with hyperactivity, disturbing behaviour at school, truancy, pilfering, etc., while the girls were predominant with respect to symptoms of depression, insomnia, anorexia, and anxiety. The data showed that the boys reacted to a very large extent with symptoms that were liable to affect their environment in a disturbing manner, particularly at school, whereas the girls reacted with symptoms that were more inclined to cause suffering to themselves rather than to their environment. Very probably, it is just this tendency on the part of the boys to behave in a manner that disturbs the environment that explains the prevalence of boys among the child psychiatric clientele. Furthermore, this particular reaction pattern is quite common even in boys generally in a normal school environment, at least in what is known as a 'Western-type' culture. This implies that our sample does not necessarily include a group of especially disturbed or deviant boys.

In fact, only a very few of the cases were noted as being psychotic, or having primary personality disturbances or being otherwise severely handicapped. In this respect it should be observed that diagnoses of these categories among the CGC patients are inclined to be somewhat less specific since considerable caution was exercised before definitely tagging a patient with such a grave diagnosis.

In summarizing, it can be stated that, on the basis of the case histories and the test results, the patient sample does not *a priori* appear to be particularly heavily burdened. During the course of the observation period, certain patients handled by the social assistance medical officer and the CGC children's homes were often found to be socially deteriorated but these individuals were not included in the patient sample covered by the study.

Procedure

In order to answer the first of our questions: 'What will happen to our patients in the coming years?', we kept track of each of the patients for 10 years after they had been discharged and written off from the registers in which they had been entered. The relatively few drop-outs have been accounted for. The number of deaths occurring during the follow-up period was no higher than the figures for the normal population in relation to the age and sex distributions.

A study has been made of the entries for each patient in one or more of the following registers:

(1) The Social Welfare Register (criminal offences);
(2) The Temperance Board Register;
(3) The National Swedish Board of Excise Register;
(4) The Register of Criminal Offences;
(5) The Register of the Recruitment and Replacement Office of the Swedish Armed Forces;
(6) The Mental Register (registers for adult and child psychiatric patients, both open and closed care).

Information from the registers

Entries were found in the Temperance Board Register for 13 per cent of the boys and 2·1 per cent of the girls. The risk for boys younger than 10 years was relatively small but was 20 per cent for 10-year-olds and older boys. For 45 per cent of the subjects, registration referred to only an occasional charge of drunkenness, while for 31 per cent there were 2 or 3 entries, for 21 per cent there were 4 to 6 entries, and for 4 per cent there were more than 10 entries. A calculated cumulative percentage reached 13 per cent by the end of the 10-year observation period after discharge from the CGC.

The entries in the Social Welfare Register referred to 33·8 per cent of the boys and 17·7 per cent of the girls, the boys being registered chiefly because of criminal offences, the girls for other reasons, usually a need of supportive measures. Criminality among the boys reached approximately 30 per cent in the 11·6- to 15·5-year age group, and was about 10 per cent for the lowest age group. The cumulative percentage for the boys was found to be 21 per cent at the end of the 10-year period. The measures taken by the Child Welfare Committee as a result of criminal offences are reported separately. For 20 per cent of the boys, these measures were confined to investigations only.

In the case of those who reached legal age during the observation

period, the Register of Criminal Offences contains entries for 13·2 per cent of the boys and 1·5 per cent the girls. The boys were mostly charged with illegal possession, i.e. theft. In the age group 6·6 to 11·5 years, registrations amounted to 10·1 per cent, followed by 21·4 per cent for the 11·6- to 15·5-year age group, and 21·1 per cent for the oldest group. Even among the boys who were no more than 10 years old at the time they were discharged, the frequency for those who were registered later corresponded to peak percentages. The cumulative frequency for boys (calculated from the total sample for the sake of comparison) rises steadily by 1 to 2 per cent per annum to reach 11·9 per cent after the conclusion of the 10-year observation period. Total registrations for criminality among the boys showed a frequency of 25 per cent with a maximum of about 36 per cent for the 11·6- to 15·5-year age group.

The Register of the Recruitment and Replacement Office of the Swedish Armed Forces showed that 1003 boys out of the total of 1477 had been inducted into the armed forces. Of the remainder, 13 per cent were freed from military service on the grounds of mental disability and 3 per cent on the grounds of physical disability.

Applications for mental care had been received from 32 per cent of the total number discharged; the figure was the same for both boys and girls. However, the frequency descended from the lowest age group to the highest in the case of the boys, whereas for the girls, this curve was reversed. With respect to hospitalization, the situation was the same for both boys and girls. Generally speaking, the boys had applied for child psychiatric care and the girls for adult psychiatric care, while a few required both types of facility. Approximately half the number of boys as well as girls applied for aid during the first two years following their discharge from the CGC. The pattern of diagnoses is more or less the same for both sexes. The most common diagnoses were *behavioural disorders, environmental reactions* (16 per cent boys and approximately 15 per cent girls). These are followed by *neuroses* (10 and 12 per cent respectively), *defective intelligence* (approximately 4 and 5 per cent respectively), and *sociopathy* (approximately 4 and 2 per cent respectively). A diagnosis of *psychosis* was arrived at for approximately 1 per cent of the boys and 2 per cent of the girls. In total this applied to 30 cases, 15 boys and 15 girls, who were given this diagnosis either during the time they were registered with the CGC or during the subsequent observation period.

The follow-up study thus showed that, altogether, more than half the number of boys and more than one-third the number of girls had applied for mental aid (at child or adult clinics as out-patients or in-patients) during the 10-year observation period, or had been registered in one or more of the various 'asocial' registers (the Social Welfare Register, the Temperance Register, the Customs and Excise Register, or the Register of Criminal Offences). As each individual patient has so far only been followed up for 10 years after his discharge from the CGC, and the cumulative frequencies for registrations show a steady upward trend, it is feasible to assume that these figures will continue to increase, especially as children who were at pre-school age during the observation period have not yet reached adulthood. The 20-year follow-up study that has been planned appears to be particularly important in that it may shed some light on certain disorders and background factors occurring during the pre-school years which may contribute some information of prognostic value relating to the methods that were used.

For various reasons, it has not been considered possible in this connection to arrive at any assessment of the results of the therapeutic measures employed in dealing with the families during the years 1953–5. Obviously, a choice has been made in selecting which children and families are to receive special attention in the form of more intensive psychotherapeutic aid. Furthermore, to assess the treatment results at this late stage would involve a completely different and extremely time-consuming methodology requiring personal interviews, assessment scales, and so forth.

Therefore, we do not know how many families would have suffered even greater worries and problems if they had not been the recipients of our efforts. However, the fact that a family whose contact with a clinic is experienced as positive, will contact that clinic again (or will approach an adult psychiatric clinic at a later date) when they are in need of help for some reason or other, can hardly be regarded as a poor result.

The preceding text shows clearly that there are very marked sex-linked differences in the material, apparent right from the start. Boys applied to the CGC at an earlier stage and with greater frequency than girls, and generally showed a different picture of symptoms.

Even more specific differences appeared during the 10-year follow-up period.

Information from the 10-year follow-up study

While the boys were totally predominant with regard to entries in the 'asocial' registers, the girls predominated on a steadily increasing scale with respect to applications for psychiatric care. Although the percentages for both sexes in the Mental Register were about the same, the figure for the boys was highest in the lowest age groups (implying registration under child psychiatry); the girls showed the opposite trend with a successively rising curve (implying dominance under adult psychiatry). No clear-cut reasons can be given for this sex-linked difference.

The differences in male and female reaction patterns as demonstrated above can nevertheless be assumed to play an important role. It has already been mentioned that the reactions shown by boys as early as in the pre-school years are more likely to affect the environment than the reactions shown by girls of the same age, the consequence being that a larger number of families apply for child psychiatric care for boys than for girls. This tendency culminates during the school years. Children who start school with mental handicaps and behavioural disorders run a considerable risk of being victimized by the alienation mechanisms at work in schools, despite continuous efforts to reform thinking among the pupils and to help the victim. The efforts made by the CGC through the introduction of the therapeutic play schools and therapeutic schools, and other forms of co-operation with the normal schools, can consequently be regarded as necessary but inadequate attempts to counteract this development.

A few of the patients who were discharged from the CGC during 1953–5 had been given diagnoses of child psychoses in connection with the primary examination of the child. The symptoms included withdrawal, lack of contact, delayed speech development, stereotypy, etc. Without exception, these cases had required long periods of institutionalization during the observation period. A few patients who had been suffering from uncharacteristic nervous symptoms at the time they applied for help from the CGC had been diagnosed during the subsequent observation period as suffering from schizophrenia or manic-depressive psychosis. In none of these cases did the picture of psychosis emerge before puberty. The patients who were diagnosed as neurotic at the time of their examination at the CGC were found to have good prospects insofar as they were not overrepresented in any of the registers in question, and as only a few of them turned up again under the diagnosis of neurosis in the adult psychiatric register.

In order to throw light onto the second of the questions posed earlier: 'Whether it is possible to predict, on the basis of the sum of the information obtained from child psychiatric sources and from the investigation techniques used, which of the patients are likely to be in need of psychiatric and social care facilities. . .', a study has been made of the relationships existing between data obtained from the initial examinations at the CGC during the years 1953–5 and the notations entered in the various official registers during the subsequent 10-year follow-up observation period.

Even here, circumstances relating to boys differed from those applying to girls. Thus, the frequency of boys living with only the marternal parent, and therefore not having a father or a permanent father substitute, was greater (on a highly significant level) among both those who had applied for psychiatric care and those who had been entered in one of the 'asocial' registers, than among those who were not noted in any of the registers. The boys who were to be found in the 'asocial' registers during the observation period came more frequently from lower class homes than non-registered boys. Furthermore, a greater number of them were 'illegitimate', had grown up in homes where the father or the mother was an addict, had more often responded with symptoms such as pilfering, lack of concentration, disruptive behaviour at school, etc. All these circumstances are well known from earlier investigations.

As only a very few of the girls in the study had been registered in one or other of the 'asocial' registers, a comparison could only be made between those who were not registered at all and those who had applied for psychiatric care during the observation period. The comparison showed that data deriving from the initial examinations were of the same magnitude for both groups. Strangely enough, among those children who later required mental care or who were registered in the 'asocial' registers, in comparison to the children who were not registered at all during the observation period, there was no evidence that a greater number of children came from homes with 'mentally sick' or 'neurotically insufficient' parents, or from homes where the parents' marriage was 'disharmonious'.

It can be said that, in the case of the boys, certain recorded background factors of a sociological and psychological nature, in combination with a special reaction pattern, give some indication of a risk of asocial development; however, these factors are not necessarily indicative of a risk of future psychiatric complications. In the case of the girls, the factors recorded did not provide any information of this nature which would lead to predictions of future development.

The differences in reaction patterns between boys and girls established in this report might indicate that the reactions displayed by the girls in the face of environmental stress factors follow a pattern which outwardly appears to be less emphatic than the symptoms displayed by the boys but which, with increasing age, leads to a progressively greater need of psychiatric care.

When it comes to predicting future psychiatric complications for the boys and girls in the present material, the background factors and their statistical treatment have not provided any leads. It is possible that a more detailed study employing a technique that is more sensitively attuned to registering disorders and complications, not only for the individual but also for family relationships, might be able to supply improved prognostic information.

One of the essential results of the present study shows quite clearly that the CGC clientele contains a large number of children who will be needing help and support from the community for a very long time ahead. The applies to the boys who act out their reactions and who will later become progressively involved in more and more serious conflicts with the norms of society, acquiring an ever-increasing burden of charges and registrations for alcoholism and criminal offences, and also to the children and young people who will later become increasingly handicapped because of mental troubles and psychiatric illness. There is no doubt that the investment of resources in prophylactic measures in the fields covered by both these categories is a matter of highest priority, with respect to both the humanitarian and the economic aspects involved.

In conclusion, we wish to point out that the 10-year follow-up study outlined above was published in full (Curman and Nylander 1976). A 20-year follow-up study of the same clientele has also been published (Nylander 1979).

49. A study of psychological symptoms and primary care (United Kingdom)

JACK INGHAM, PATRICK MILLER, and JOE KIFF

Introduction

The project has its roots in the coming together of two major lines of interest in the senior investigator's earlier work. These were

(1) The genesis of psychological illness from a much earlier stage than that at which it is generally encountered in hospitals or clinics;
(2) The selection of patients along various referral routes into different branches of the National Health Services, including the psychiatric services.

There was already much circumstantial evidence that the destination and labelling of patients (for example their declaration and acceptance as psychiatric patients by clinicians) was as much determined by non-illness factors as by the manifestations of the illnesses themselves (Robinson 1963; Wood and Elwood 1966; Robinson and Wood 1968; Ingham *et al.* 1972). The development of an illness from its earliest beginnings through various stages until the patient becomes a clinically declared psychiatric case, involves a continuous process of interaction between two causal networks, one of them directly influencing the genesis of symptoms, the other determining selection into various parts of the Health and Social Services.

Procedure

We decided to enter this complex system at the point of self-referral to primary care, looking first for factors other than illness that influence people in deciding whether or not to consult their general practitioners. Psychological complaints were obviously of special interest, but the investigations were not restricted to psychological illness. It was necessary first to measure symptom severity in the population of non-consulters to determine how many people experience symptoms as severely as those who consult their doctors (Ingham and Miller 1976). The second objective was to look for non-illness factors associated with the occurrence of symptoms themselves (Miller and Ingham 1976); for example, pilot studies have indicated an association between the occurrence of stressful life events and psychological symptoms such as anxiety and depression, and it has been necessary to confirm these findings in a larger sample.

Following the pilot studies a survey was started in a new town health centre providing the only general practitioner services in one clearly defined district, having a population of approximately 10 000. A sample of about 1100 patients, who attended the health centre with new episodes of illness from March 1976 to March 1977, is being compared with the same number of non-attenders selected at random from the list of patients registered. Data collection for this phase of the operation is almost complete, and we are now proceeding to the second phase which is a one-year follow-up (Interview II) on a subsample of about 800 people. This aims to predict, on the basis of the results of Interview I:

(1) Further self-referrals;
(2) The genesis of psychological symptoms in people who were previously well;

(3) The maintenance or remission of psychological symptoms in those who were previously ill.

These three aims overlap to some extent in their requirements, and in all of them we shall be trying to make the best predictions possible using information already collected during the first interview. We are confident that we have reliable and generally satisfactory methods of assessing some relatively stable characteristics which can be related both to future attendances at the health centre and also to onsets and/or remissions of symptoms. The predictive variables include:

(a) Self-disclosure, i.e. the extent to which the subject is willing to talk about his problems to other people;
(b) Availability of social support;
(c) Life stress;
(d) Denial of, or sensitization to psychological stress.

Characteristics (a) and (b) have been assessed by questionnaires in Interview I and there is no problem in using the data in a straightforward predictive study. Characteristics (c) and (d) are more complicated. A life event interview adapted from the techniques of Brown *et al.* (1973) has enabled us to discriminate people who have suffered one or more threatening life events during the three months prior to Interview I. This is a variable that is likely to change, however, and it could not be used as a predictor on events during the subsequent year without re-interviews to find out whether the stresses involved have been resolved or not, or whether any new stresses have appeared. We propose to adopt a more economic procedure, namely to examine all the life events interviews carefully, and to decide on the basis of evidence available which subjects are most likely to have suffered continued stress during the following year. We will identify these as subjects who suffer from either (1) chronic long-term difficulties; or (2) events likely to lead to long-term difficulties; or (3) events likely to lead to further threatening events. We shall re-interview a small subsample to validate a predictive assessment.

With regard to characteristic (d), a sensitizer–denier division has been described by other workers, including Caplan (1974), Goldstein (cited in Averil 1973), and Fenz (1975), and has been claimed to affect the outcome of some traumas, such as major surgery. Sensitizers are people who 'focus attention on threatening events, search for cues regarding potential harm, and emphasize the affective quality of experience'. Deniers are people who avoid thinking about seriously threatening events and/or suppress their anxiety about them. We propose to define as a denier a person who has experienced apparently threatening life events (at least one in the previous three months) and who yet denies the presence of anxiety or depression.

It is convenient to consider the three aims of the follow-up study separately.

A prospective study of self-referral

When the results of the 1976–7 survey have been analysed we expect to have clear correlational evidence of a number of individual characteristics associated with the act of deciding to consult the general practitioner. As with all correlational enquiries, however, association does not necessarily imply causation, and we shall be seeking confirmation from the predictive study. The dependent variable will be the number of episodes of contact with a general practitioner during the follow-up period.

The natural history of psychological illness with particular reference to its genesis

One of the advantages of studying patients when they are seeking primary care is that illnesses can be observed much sooner than is possible in hospitals or specialist clinics. The difficulty lies in recognizing and diagnosing the illness at this stage when the symptoms and signs may be minimal and may overlap with those of other illnesses or with normal psychophysiological reactions. It is not, of course, suggested that all those seeking primary care come into the 'early illness' category. Some are relatively advanced and clearly recognizable, but the early cases are of special interest and are rarely to be found elsewhere.

The fundamental difficulty with most prospective community studies is that huge samples are required to produce enough cases of any one disorder within a reasonable period of time. Two ways of overcoming this are to select illnesses with high incidence and to pick out groups of high-risk individuals. We are therefore concentrating the enquiry on psychoneurotic and psychosomatic disorders, rather than psychoses which are relatively infrequent. We are mainly concerned with the problem of selecting high-risk groups in order to be able to study small samples more intensively over a long period.

The *theory* we base this section of our study on involves the following factors:

(a) *Individual differences*. Neurosis is a process rather than a constant that differentiates one individual from another throughout life, but there are long-term or even lifelong interindividual differences in susceptibility. We have included one questionnaire amongst our predictor variables (E.P.I.) that has been claimed as a provisional index of susceptibility; self-disclosure and denial of distress may also be relevant.

(b) *Life stress*. Noxious stimuli and stressing situations are a natural and inevitable part of living, and do not in themselves lead to pathological changes, though they do lead to some degree of distress. Under some circumstances (varying with the susceptibility of the individual) and under continuing stress, the individual may undergo a qualitative change and become 'ill'. Leaving aside the question of whether the change involved is illness in any of the senses in which that term is used in the context of physical disease, its essential nature is a breakdown of existing relationships between the individual and his environment, chiefly his social environment (personal illness; see Foulds 1976). This means that the modes of adjustment and coping that had previously served to keep him functioning within the behavioural boundaries set by the relationships he has held in the social system of which he forms a part, no longer work. He either succumbs and virtually ceases to function, or extraordinary changes (e.g. symptoms, abnormal illness behaviour, etc.) take place that keep him functioning to some degree.

There is great difficulty in differentiating clearly between 'normal' distress and the distress of 'personal illness'. Many would argue that there is no qualitative difference and that it is only a matter of degree. Nevertheless, the acutely neurotic individual himself experiences his condition as qualitatively different from his normal state, and from the outsider's point of view, there are, for example, patients whose anxiety levels are quite incommensurate with their known sources of stress, even after exhaustive investigation. This is not to say, however, that all patients coming to the doctor with severe anxiety are suffering from pathological anxiety states.

(c) *External support*. Vulnerability to stress (i.e. susceptibility to neurotic illness under stress) is also modified by circumstances outside the individual. Support from other people protects against personal illness, even when the stress is severe. There is a conceptual difficulty here in deciding whether to think of such support as actually reducing the stress, or as helping the stressed person to cope with higher levels of stress.

Objectives. The importance of understanding the transition between normal distress and personal illness cannot be overestimated. Our ultimate objective is to define this transition, to understand the circumstances in which it occurs, and to describe how it occurs. If this could be achieved it would have profound implications for a theory of psychogenesis, and also for the handling of psychological distress and illness, particularly at the level of primary care. Our immediate objective is to devise a method of selecting from a given population a sample of people who are not ill at the initial interviewing but with a high risk of developing a personal illness during a subsequent period (one year is a convenient interval).

Methods. The assessments of predictive variables have already been described. The dependent variable presents a problem. Ideally it should be an established validated criterion of personal illness. This is not possible within the limitations of the proposed study. There are, however, a number of indices that are available to us related to the ideal criterion in the sense that individuals suffering an onset of a personal illness would be likely to show increased values. These indices will be reassessed at Interview II. It would also be possible to use existing health centre records for evidence of psychological disturbance. Although such records could hardly be accepted as a criterion of personal illness, a sample selected from them would certainly be expected to show a prevalence higher than chance.

The dependent variables to be assessed one year after the initial interview are:

(a) Increase in psychological symptom severity since initial interview as measured by the symptom scales used in Interview I;
(b) Increase in score on Foulds's scale since initial interview (available for a subsample).

Both (a) and (b) are assessed by established validated procedures. We also propose to explore the use of:

(c) Recall of increased psychological symptom severity during the intervening year, elicited by a questionnaire already used in Interview I;
(d) Records of diagnosed psychological illness and/or prescriptions of psychotropic drugs recorded in the case notes.

None of these is an entirely satisfactory method of diagnosing personal illness, but nevertheless reasonably accurate predictions of them or a suitably weighted combination of them would represent substantial progress towards developing a screening procedure. This could then be used to select a sample small enough for detailed longitudinal study in the future, yet likely to produce a sufficient number of personal illness onsets.

The maintenance of psychological symptoms

The same sort of analysis can be made using subjects who had high scores on symptoms/personal illness indices at the initial interview. Here the prediction would be of persistence or further increase of symptoms rather than onset, but the design is the same and the same predictor variables will be used.

50. Prognostic factors in socio-psychiatric rehabilitation (Switzerland)

L. CIOMPI, J. P. DAUWALDER, AND C. AGUÉ

Introduction

Until recently large populations of chronic and deteriorated patients were the logical outcome of the custodial form of care for mental illness born simultaneously with the Industrial Society during the nineteenth century. Isolated most of their lives from the reality of the outside world, these patients could hardly be expected to adjust to it in the unlikely situation of a discharge from their institution. These problems having been forseen in some few exceptional circumstances, work and social interactions in the hospital were used more or less intuitively as a form of social therapy. However, it is only during the last 20 years that psychopharmacological advances and the concomitant changes in social attitudes toward mental illness allowed some newly developed theoretical frameworks to be put into practice. Thus, to provide essential psychiatric services to such a varied population, the need for specific rehabilitation units were deemed necessary in most of the industrialized countries, set within a clearly defined sector of inhabitants of a given area. These goals having been reached in most of the canton of Vaud, the need for systematic research into the most decisive factors, psychiatric or otherwise, upon which any rehabilitation efforts depend, were the basic reasons for the creation of a Socio-psychiatric Research Unit at the University Clinic of Cery. The project to be described hereunder, is the first undertaking of such a group.

Overall data on the project

The project is financed by the Swiss National Fund for Scientific Research for a period of three years, which began in 1975. The project is to be carried out within the newly created Socio-Psychiatric Research Unit at the University Psychiatric Clinic of Cery.

The rationale behind this research group was the unavoidable need to improve everyday clinical practice through scientifically sound principles. The first step in this direction was to create circumstances in which:

(a) Clinical routine could be controlled by standardized methods;

(b) Some of the putative variables which influence any rehabilitation procedure either positively or negatively, could be controlled;

(c) The patients' input for rehabilitation measures could be selectively studied in order to maximize its chances of success.

This research group is run basically by two psychiatrists, Prof. L. Ciompi and Dr C. Agué, one psychologist, Mr J. P. Dauwalder, and a secretary. Other members include part-time psychology students who investigate partial questions and perform *ad hoc* tasks according to some of the specific needs arising from various aspects of the project.

Socio-psychiatric framework in which the project is set

The Lausanne rehabilitation services are included within the overall psychiatric organization of the central sector of the canton of Vaud. These have a centralized medico-psychiatric supervision under Prof. Ciompi since 1974, both at the Psychiatric Clinic itself and at several half-way institutions supported by the Society for Mental Hygiene of the canton of Vaud, and in close collaboration with the Out-patient Services (Policlinic) and the Invalidity Insurance Regional Office.

Basically, the structure of the rehabilitation services are as follows:

Within the hospital:
A rehabilitation unit, functioning also as a night hospital according to needs (24 places);
A day hospital unit (24 places);
A preparatory work shop (6 places), used mainly for assessment purposes.

Outside the hospital:
A centre for professional rehabilitation, providing both readaptation and supervised work shops (approximately 60 places). They include mechanical, assembly, bakery, and clerical sections;
Two supervised hostels (26 places);
Two supervised flats (8 places).

The catchment area includes the town of Lausanne and areas in its vicinity. The total population is about 280 000.

General structure of the project

The project followed the chronological steps below:

(1) *A preparatory phase* in which:
(a) Various methodological approaches existing in the field were reviewed, discussed, and worked through (Agué *et al.* 1977a, b, c);
(b) The basic aspects of the project were specified and its goals defined functionally;
(c) Various methods of assessment were studied and compared (i.e., for psychopathological status, for subjective ratings) and a final choice decided upon;
(d) When needed (i.e., working/social behaviour assessment) special instruments were constructed, the reliability and validity of which was studied in various *ad hoc* pilot studies.

This phase was completed during the year 1975.

(2) An *experimental phase* consisting of:

(a) A *transversal study*, in which a selective long-term population of chronic in-patients was assessed upon various general and specific parameters of social, work, and psychological performance, in view of their likelihood of eventual future rehabilitation (Ciompi *et al.* 1977).

(b) A *longitudinal study*, throughout one year, of all patients attending the rehabilitation services with a similar methodology and with the specific goal of identifying putative prognosis variables, especially with reference to their social and working levels of performance. The basal assessment was carried out during 1976 and final data should be available during 1977;

(c) *Pilot studies* concerned with the comparative efficiency of rehabilitation procedures within the various agencies available. They are intended as short term. Protocols for such studies are still in the working-through phase and it is still unclear if they will fit within the original deadlines of the general project.

General design

The variables used in this study are divided into six headings: general, socio-professional, premorbid handicaps, primary handicaps, secondary handicaps, and overall assessments. These variables have been described elsewhere (Ciompi *et al.* 1977). (Forms presenting an outline of the assessment procedure, the questionnaires that were developed for this project in their original French version, and the code for the assessment of the results of the rehabilitation procedures are available from the authors.)

Treatment of data. All data is collected in individual files containing all the corresponding variables. These are coded and put either on punched cards and/or magnetic tape memory. In this way, any desired transformations of data and/or *ad hoc* analyses are made possible and any data retrievable throughout the course of the project. Computer facilities both at the University of Lausanne Computer Centre (Miss E. Brooke) and at the Clinic of Cery are to be used.

State of the project—1978

1. *Transversal study*
The following is a summary of results. For further elaboration see Ciompi *et al.* (1978a, b).

(a) *General data.* Of the 340 places available within the Lausanne Psychiatric Services, 110 were filled by persons whose basic duration of stay was more than one year. Of these, only 40 patients (40 per cent) were also of less than 60 years of age and had an IQ over 75. This number represents about 0·66 per cent of the total population within the central sector of the canton of Vaud. There were 21 males and 19 females. The average age was 40 and the main diagnoses were: schizophrenia (21), psychopathic/neurotic states (12), and epilepsy and manic-depressive psychosis (7). The duration of hospitalization ranged from 1 to 30 years with an average of 8·5 years, nearly half of these ranging between 1 and 5 years. Within the hospital, 63 per cent lived in open wards and 70 per cent worked for more than 25 hours per week in the various hospital departments. Of these patients, 65 per cent had been away from normal social life for more than five years; 32 per cent were found to have no contact whatever with the outside world in the form of visits and/or correspondence, during the month prior to the investigation.

(b) *Assessment.* Taking into account intelligence, school attendance, and professional education, the following assessment of *pre-morbid handicaps* was made: low (32 per cent), relatively low (20 per cent), relatively high (13 per cent), and high (5 per cent). Regarding *primary handicaps* (psychopathology), only 40 per cent had a clearly defined psychopathological status, but frequently occurring symptoms were: affective flattening (23), verbal restriction (14), suspicion (12), loss of confidence (14), feelings of inadequacy (11). Systematized delusions occurred in only 5 cases. About 47 per cent of the population was judged as having moderate to severe *secondary handicaps* (institutionalism), as judged by their overall satisfaction in the hospital, plans for their future and wish for discharge.

(c) *Correlations.* Although no significant correlations were found between the overall assessment of handicaps, various significant correlations between single variables permitted a hierarchy of factors of prognostic importance, i.e., type of occupation in the hospital, contacts with the outside world, duration of hospitalization and of social isolation.

(d) *Rehabilitation potential.* This was judged to be moderately good in 22 per cent, and moderately poor in 37 per cent of the cases.

(e) *Conclusions.* Despite its relatively small sample, this study has confirmed the importance of specific social factors appearing to perpetuate a long-term hospital admission. These social factors seem to influence hospitalization length to a greater extent than factors reflecting psychopathological status and/or socio-professional experience. In this sense, the lack of contact with the outside world, the duration of stay and of social isolation constitute first-order factors of a syndrome of 'institutionalism' evident in such a population. Such persons seem unlikely to benefit from standard measures of rehabilitation, especially in view of such a long period of social isolation. However, the relatively small number of long-term chronic patients in relation to the global population of the catchment area appears to confirm the overall efficacy of prompt measures of treatment and discharge.

2. *Longitudinal study*
The first assessments of a population of 80 patients attending the various Rehabilitation Services of the canton of Vaud on the target day (4 January 1977) have already been made, coded, and put into memory. The remainder will be performed 12 months later. Although as compared to the transversal study some variables have been modified or altogether eliminated, the basic structure presented remains unaltered. Furthermore, special parameters such as social and work behaviour, for use in psychodynamic evaluations, have been purposely developed for this study. The overall assessment of rehabilitation prognosis is to be compared and correlated with the corresponding level reached by the subject on the second evaluation, both on the habitat and work continuum. Some methodological problems have not yet been satisfactorily resolved, such as the overall assessment of psychopathological status. Basically, the study will explore the influence of the social variables found in the long-term chronic population upon patients submitted to standard rehabilitation procedures for at least one year. It is hoped that such results may allow the identification of a hierarchy of prognostic variables to be used in the clarification and selection of rehabilitation techniques appropriate for the subject at the earliest clinical moment possible.

51. Follow-up studies of patients admitted to the state mental hospital in Iceland

JÓN G. STEFÁNSSON

Introduction

The State Mental Hospital in Iceland, Kleppsspítalinn, was opened in 1907. It was the only psychiatric hospital in Iceland until 1956 when the city of Reykjavík opened a small psychiatric unit which in 1968 became a part of the City Hospital. In 1951 Kleppsspítalinn had a bed capacity of 240 for acute and chronic patients, but now it only has 235 beds. Of these beds 125 are occupied by chronically ill long-term patients, 40 beds are for patients whose main problem is alcohol or drug abuse, and 70 beds are for short-term patients. Since 1968 the city of Reykjavík has had 121 psychiatric beds available, 31 for the more acutely ill, 30 for rehabilitation, and 60 for chronic care. In addition, there are now 10 psychiatric beds available in the town of Akureyri in the northern part of the country. Changes in the number of first admissions and length of stay at Kleppsspítalinn during the 20-year period 1951–70 have been described by Thorsteinsson (1974). He found the number of first admissions to have increased greatly and the average duration of hospitalization to have decreased considerably during this period.

A retrospective follow-up study of patients admitted for the first time to Kleppsspítalinn in the years 1953 to 1957 was done from 1966 to 1968 (Stefánsson and Helgason 1969).

Method

Patients admitted for the first time to Kleppsspítalinn between 1953 and 1957 were identified in the hospital files, their hospital records were reviewed, and record review forms were filled out. This was done by a psychiatrist in training supervised by a senior psychiatrist. A senior psychiatric nurse made a visit to the patients' homes to gather information about the patients from the patients themselves, and their relatives, friends, or neighbours. The nurse's written report about the home visits, as well as hospital charts, were then used by the psychiatrists to make the follow-up assessments.

Outome was assessed in terms of the following:

(1) A broad psychiatric assessment: a global assessment by the investigator of the patient's mental health on follow-up;
(2) Information on culturally appropriate self-support: living on one's own income or contributing to the family's productivity at the time of follow-up;
(3) Functional state during the follow-up period: the social and work performance during the follow-up period as compared to the culturally expected norm.

Results

In the years 1953 to 1957 there were 281 first admissions to the Kleppsspítalinn, but in 1957 the general population of Iceland was 166 831. The majority of these admissions (166) were men admitted because of alcoholism. Ten years after admission 18 patients had never been discharged, 14 with the diagnosis of schizophrenia and 4 with the diagnosis of manic-depressive psychosis. Seventy-one of the patients were dead on follow-up and 34 patients had disappeared without being known to be dead. These patients were included in the study and their functional state from first admission until time of death or disappearance as well as mental state and self-support prior to that time were assessed.

The hospital diagnosis by age and sex is shown in Table 51.1. Marital status of the patients on admission and the change in their marital status during the follow-up period as it relates to self-support on follow-up is shown in Tables 51.2 and 51.3. It appears that being married or becoming married, legally or by common law, is associated with being self-supporting. Those who are divorced or separated on admission also appeared more likely to be self-supporting on follow-up.

Occupation and zone of residence on admission as it relates to outcome in terms of culturally appropriate self-support is seen in Tables 51.4 and 51.5. Patients living rurally and those who have no occupation, an unknown, or 'other' occupation, appear from these tables to do rather worse than others. The duration of illness was estimated from the data available in the hospital chart when pos-

TABLE 51.1

First admissions to Kleppsspítalinn 1953–7—ten-year outcome survey. Diagnosis by age and sex

Diagnosis	0–19 years		20–39 years		40–59 years		60–		Total		Total
	M	F	M	F	M	F	M	F	M	F	
Toxicomania	3	0	104	7	57	6	6	0	170	13	183
Schizophrenia	1	2	20	8	7	4	2	4	30	18	48
Psychosis manic-depressiva	2	4	4	9	7	19	6	6	19	38	57
Psychosis psychogenica	0	0	1	7	5	7	0	1	6	15	21
Other	10	0	20	9	11	11	5	6	46	26	72
Total	16	6	149	40	87	47	19	17	271	110	381

TABLE 51.2

First admissions to Kleppsspítalinn 1953–7—ten-year outcome survey. Marital status on admission by outcome in terms of culturally appropriate self-support

Marital status on admission	Not self-supporting	Partially self-supporting	Self-supporting	Not assessible	Total
Single	75	32	87	4	198
Legal marriage	24	15	48	3	90
Common-law marriage	3	2	1	2	8
Divorce or separation	18	13	31	2	64
Widowed	11	2	5	2	20
Unknown	1	0	0	0	1
Total	132	64	172	13	381

TABLE 51.3

First admissions to Kleppsspítalinn 1953–7—ten-year outcome survey. Change in marital status during follow-up by outcome in terms of culturally appropriate self-support

Change in marital status during follow-up	Not self-supporting	Partially self-supporting	Self-supporting	Not assessible	Total
No change	115	53	114	10	292
Legal marriage	2	2	27	0	31
Common-law marriage	2	1	15	0	18
Divorce or separation	12	6	16	2	36
Widowed	0	2	0	0	2
Unknown	1	0	0	1	2
Total	132	64	172	13	381

sible, and its relationship to broad psychiatric assessment and self-support on follow-up is seen in Tables 51.6 and 51.7. Although diagnosis is not considered in these tables it should be noted that most of the patients with the diagnosis of toxicomania had a long duration of illness prior to admission. From these tables it appears that patients with duration of illness less than 6 months and particularly less than 4 weeks prior to admission, do better both regarding mental state and in terms of self-support on follow-up.

TABLE 51.4

First admissions to Kleppsspítalinn 1953–7—ten-year outcome survey. Occupation on admission by outcome in terms of culturally appropriate self-support

Occupation on admission	Not self-supporting	Partially self-supporting	Self-supporting	Not assessible	Total
Professional, technical, and related workers	10	3	10	0	23
Managerial, administrative, clerical, and sales workers	10	7	22	0	39
Farmers and farm labourers	14	6	12	0	32
Fishermen and workers in sea transport	11	13	34	4	62
Craftsmen, production process workers, and labourers	42	23	69	5	139
Service workers and chauffeurs	24	7	24	3	58
Others, unknown, and unoccupied	21	5	1	1	28
Total	132	64	172	13	381

TABLE 51.5

First admissions to Kleppsspítalinn 1953–7—ten-year outcome survey. Zone of residence on admission by outcome in terms of culturally appropriate self-support

Zone of residence on admission	Not self-supporting	Partially self-supporting	Self-supporting	Not assessible	Total
Capital city	78	49	114	11	252
Other towns	32	9	42	2	85
Rural	21	5	16	0	42
No stable residence	1	0	0	0	1
Unknown	0	1	0	0	1
Total	132	64	172	13	381

TABLE 51.6

First admissions to Kleppsspítalinn 1953–7—ten-year outcome survey. Duration of illness prior to first admission by broad psychiatric assessment on follow-up

Duration of illness prior to admission	Psychosis	Borderline psychosis	Neuroses or personality disorders	No abnormality	Not assessible	Total
0–14 days	3	1	9	9	1	23
2–4 weeks	3	2	3	12	1	21
1–6 months	6	7	8	6	0	27
6–12 months	8	1	3	4	1	17
12–24 months	8	5	11	5	2	31
2–6 years	11	5	25	4	4	49
6+ years	18	6	63	6	4	97
Not assessible	15	7	83	9	2	116
Total	72	34	205	55	15	381

TABLE 51.7

First admissions to Kleppsspítalinn 1953–7—ten-year outcome survey. Duration of illness prior to first admission and outcome in terms of culturally appropriate self-support

Duration of illness prior to admission	Not self-supporting	Partially self-supporting	Self-supporting	Not assessible	Total
0–14 days	3	4	15	1	23
2–4 weeks	3	5	13	0	21
1–6 months	9	5	13	0	27
6–12 months	7	1	8	1	17
12–24 months	10	7	12	2	31
2–6 years	20	7	18	4	49
6+ years	31	14	48	4	97
Not assessible	49	21	45	1	116
Total	132	64	172	13	381

When the diagnostic groups are examined as in Tables 51.8, 51.9, and 51.10, it can be seen that 72 of the patients (19 per cent) are considered to be psychotic on follow-up. The majority of these (42) are persons diagnosed as schizophrenic, that is, 87 per cent of those receiving this diagnosis. In spite of this, 13 of the schizophrenic patients are self-supporting and 4 are partially self-supporting, so that 36 per cent of patients diagnosed as schizophrenic are completely or partially self-supporting on follow-up. Four schizophrenic patients were not known to have ever been disabled during the follow-up period. The prognosis is better in manic-depressive psychosis and in psychogenic psychosis than in schizophrenia, both in terms of mental state and in terms of self-support on follow-up.

Discussion

These results are in agreement with other research results which show that besides diagnosis other variables are also important in predicting outcome (Astrup and Noreik 1966; Strauss and Carpenter 1974). Married patients have been found to be more likely than single patients to be employed following hospitalization (Markowe *et al*. 1955). Previous social relationships and the duration of symptomatology have been found to help predict outcome (Kringlen 1970; Noreik 1970; Strauss and Carpenter 1974a, b). Variables such as these that are not included in diagnostic criteria and help predict outcome have been suggested by some investigators to represent important processes in psychopathology that transcend the usual diagnostic categories (Zigler and Phillips 1962).

The following variables are particularly likely to be predictive of outcome for patients with functional mental disorder:

1. Diagnosis (Astrup and Noreik 1966);
2. Type of symptoms (Albee 1951; Astrup and Noreik 1966; Strauss and Carpenter 1972);

3. Disruptiveness of symptoms (Brown *et al*. 1966; Freeman and Simmons 1963);
4. Previous duration of disorder (Strauss and Carpenter 1974a, b);
5. Patterns of personal relationships (Phillips 1953);
6. Employment function (Monck 1963; Brown *et al*. 1966);
7. Family living situation including roles, family structure, and relationships (Brown *et al*. 1962; Freeman and Simmons 1963);
8. Social class (Myers and Bean 1968);
9. Precipitating events (Brown and Birley 1968);
10. Family history of cetain types of psychiatric disorder (Vaillant 1964; McCabe *et al*. 1972);
11. Treatment received (May 1968).

Present studies

At the present time two follow-up studies are in progress. One is a retrospective follow-up study of patients whose first psychiatric hospitalization was to Kleppsspítalinn in 1965 or 1966. The method used is the same as in the study described above. Its primary aim is a comparison between the 1953–7 and 1965–6 groups of patients (Thorsteinsson 1974).

The second is a prospective follow-up study where the variables mentioned above are considered as likely to be predictive of the outcome for patients with functional mental disorders. This study uses as a model a study in progress since 1973 at the Department of Psychiatry, University of Rochester, New York with Professor John S. Strauss, M.D. as the principal investigator.

The patients included in the second study are those admitted to Kleppsspítalinn who consent to participate in the study and who fulfil the following criteria:

TABLE 51.8

First admissions to Kleppsspítalinn 1953–7—ten-year outcome survey. Diagnosis on admission by broad psychiatric assessment on follow-up

Diagnosis	Psychosis	Borderline psychosis	Neurosis or personality disorders	No abnormality	Not assessible	Total
Toxicomania	5	5	149	18	6	183
Schizophrenia	42	5	1	0	0	48
Psychosis manic-depressiva	10	14	8	22	3	57
Psychosis psychogenica	1	6	5	8	1	21
Other	14	4	42	7	5	72
Total	72	34	205	55	15	381

TABLE 51.9

First admissions to Kleppsspítalinn 1953–7—ten-year outcome survey. Diagnosis on admission by functional state during the follow-up period

Diagnosis	Continuously disabled	Periodically disabled	Never disabled	Not assessible	Total
Toxicomania	27	131	18	7	183
Schizophrenia	32	12	4	0	48
Psychosis manic-depressiva	17	27	10	3	57
Psychosis psychogenica	4	9	8	0	21
Other	29	21	19	3	72
Total	109	200	59	13	381

TABLE 51.10

First admissions to Kleppsspítalinn 1953–7—ten-year outcome survey. Diagnosis on admission by outcome in terms of culturally appropriate self-support

Diagnosis	Not self-supporting	Partially self-supporting	Self-supporting	Not assessible	Total
Toxicomania	48	34	95	6	183
Schizophrenia	31	4	13	0	48
Psychosis manic-depressiva	19	15	21	2	57
Psychosis psychogenica	5	2	14	0	21
Other	29	9	29	5	72
Total	132	64	172	13	381

1. Have their residence in Iceland;
2. Have never been admitted to a psychiatric hospital before;
3. Are 15 to 54 years of age;
4. Have a functional mental disorder as the main reason for hospitalization.

Patients admitted because of organic disease or alcohol or drug abuse will not be included in the study. The decision about who will be included will be made after considering the information available during the first days of hospitalization.

For the initial evaluation three interviews will be used which were developed as part of the data collection techniques for the International Pilot Study of Schizophrenia sponsored by the World Health Organization. These instruments evaluate a wide range of psychiatric symptoms, history, and demographic variables and have demonstrated reliability (World Health Organization 1973). These interviews include:

(1) The Psychiatric Assessment Interview (PAI)—a standardized interview for evaluating psychiatric symptoms and signs. This schedule was derived from the eighth edition of the Present State Examination (PSE) (WHO 1973) and is used with the same instructions and rating system. PAI data are readily converted to the PSE format (Carpenter *et al.* 1976);
(2) The Standard Psychiatric History—an interview for obtaining psychiatric and medical history;
(3) The Social Data Interview—an interview for obtaining information on patients' social, educational, and occupational background and performance.

To obtain data on possible precipitating events, the Life Event Scale (Holmes and Rahe 1967) will be administered. This scale includes a list of events that have been judged to be upsetting by many groups and which records the number of these events that have occurred at different time spans prior to the patient's admission to the hospital. For an evaluation of the patient's functioning intelligence, selected subtests of the WAIS will be given.

The patient and each member of his family will be asked to engage in a procedure designed to give information about relationships in the family. This procedure, the Inventory of Family Feelings (Lowman 1975), is a self-report measure of the quality and intensity of emotional involvement between family members. A family member will be asked to complete the following forms:

1. Social Effect of Behaviour Scale II—a description of the degree to which the family perceives the patient's symptoms interfering with family functioning (adapted from Freeman and Simmons 1963).

2. Katz Adjustment Scales R1 and R2—ratings by a family member regarding symptoms and functional levels of the patient for comparison with the data collected from patient interviews (Katz 1968).
3. Family Expectancy Scale (adapted from Katz Adjustment Scale R3)—a scale to determine the family's anticipation of the patient's functioning over the follow-up period.

After reviewing these data and the patient's hospital record the following scales will be completed by the investigators:

1. Menninger Health–Sickness Rating Scale (Luborsky 1962)—a unidimensional measure of degree of psychopathology in terms of overall psychological disorganization;
2. Phillips Scale of Premorbid Social Adjustment (Phillips 1953)—a measure of premorbid social functioning that has demonstrated ability to predict outcome.
3. Prognostic Scale (Strauss and Carpenter 1974a, b)—including items such as previous level of work function, duration of symptoms, and social class.
4. Social Effects of Behaviour Scale I (adapted from Freeman and Simmons 1963)—a scale to evaluate the disruptive influence which patients' symptoms appear to have on their families;
5. Diagnostic Assessment—a standardized diagnostic form adapted from the International Pilot Study of Schizophrenia;
6. Level of Function Scale (Strauss and Carpenter 1972)—a scale that rates patients' levels of functioning in several areas including social function, occupation, symptoms, and need for hospitalization.

The follow-up evaluation will be done two years after first admission and will include:

1. The Psychiatric Assessment Interview;
2. Follow-up Psychiatric History and Social Data Interview.

The patient's relatives will be asked to complete:

1. The Social Effect of Behaviour Scale II;
2. The Katz Adjustment Scales.

The patient and his family will be asked to complete the Inventory of Family Feelings.

A team consisting of a psychiatrist, two psychologists, and two social workers has been trained to use and administer the instruments. A pilot study of 20 subjects has been completed. The initial evaluation period is planned to last for two years during which about 220 patients are expected to meet the study criteria.

The number of drop-outs (e.g. non-co-operation, death) is expected to be 20 per cent.

52. Studies in functional psychoses (Switzerland)

J. ANGST and CHR. SCHARFETTER

The study of functional psychoses (Schizophrenia and the affective psychoses) is centred on the question of their homogeneity or heterogeneity. It deals with the following main fields:

(1) Psychopathology and the problems of psychiatric assessment and documentation;
(2) Hereditary studies of index case families;
(3) Studies of index case personality and first degree relatives (and spouses) by application of personality inventory tests;
(4) Studies of the course of the psychoses.

Index cases are in-patients of the Psychiatric University Hospital Zurich with the ICD-Diagnoses 295 and 296, including first admissions as well as readmissions. Sampling from the daily admissions is taken at random by a special key. Between 1971 and 1976, 273 index cases were studied.

Psychopathology

The psychopathology of the index cases is studied in an extensive clinical interview according to the present state examination (PSE) scale by J. K. Wing *et al.* (1974); it is documented by three means:

(1) WHO's psychiatric assessment schedule (after the 8th revision of the PSE);
(2) In-patient multidimensional psychiatric rating scale (by Lorr and Klett 1966);
(3) AMP-System (Scharfetter 1972).

This permits comparative studies of the different rating scales. By factor analytic studies one can find the dimensions which are common to all these rating scales. Discriminant analysis should demonstrate how far it is possible to separate the traditional diagnostic subgroups (hebephrenia, catatonia, etc.) in each rating scale. In case of good congruence in clinical subgrouping and the results of discriminant analysis, the possibility of quantification of the clinical criteria for separation of diagnostic subgroups is supported. In addition, new subgroups may be found by the application of taxometric procedures (cluster analysis, factor analysis of the Q-type) to the syndrome patterns of the rating scales. In this section of the study we deal with the problem of diagnostic assessment without previous mental history.

Hereditary studies

Sources of information for the hereditary studies are the index cases, personal interviews (in the clinic or by house visits) of first degree relatives, registrar's offices, and the files or case reports of the hospitals in those regions from where the index cases originate or where their families live. In this way we hope to gain as much information as possible about characteristic personality features and, possibly, about secondary cases in the families. The diagnoses of the secondary cases with hospital records, which constitute the majority, are evaluated blindly, i.e. by an expert not knowing the diagnosis of the index case.

We cannot expect that the re-evaluation of morbidity risk figures will bring results differing grossly from the figures known at present. Also we cannot hope that such traditional hereditary familial research will answer the question of the genesis or even the mode of inheritance of the psychoses. But the material studied most thoroughly in a population of high stability and in a region with relatively uniform psychiatric education (Bleulerian school), should make it possible to study other related areas, such as: the problem of genetic homo- or heterogeneity of the psychoses, their subtypes in respect to psychopathology, age of the onset, course, and personality characteristics.

Personalities of the index cases and the relatives

As the traditional diagnosis of personalities and personality disorders is questionable, we have conducted a diagnostic assessment of the personalities by application of two personality inventory tests: the MPI (Maudsley Personality Inventory, Eysenck 1970), and the FPI (Freiburger Persönlichkeitsinventar). These have been administered to the index case and to all first degree relatives (and spouses). The index case is asked to fill out the inventory after remission of the present psychotic episode. This is expected to permit the study of two problems:

(1) Correlation of personality and psychosis, subgroups of psychopathology, age of onset, sex, dependence on precipitating factors (a method based on an inventory in which we used Brown's investigations as a pattern);
(2) Correlation of the personalities of the index cases and the relatives with relation to the question of family similarities of personalities.

Furthermore we try to get an estimation of the premorbid personalities of the index cases, judged by an adjective check list (developed by von Zerssen 1973; von Zerssen *et al.* 1969, 1970) which the relatives of the index cases are asked to fill out. The results can be compared with the conventional personality classification.

Course of the disease

Special sheets provide documentation of every single episode (duration, age of onset, interval, degree of remission, psychopathology, precipitating factors, and some social psychiatric data) and of the hospitalization data. Thus we can study, among other problems in the course of the illness, stability or change of psychopathology with increasing age of the patient, number of psychotic episodes, duration of the interval, and hospitalizations. After an interval of 5 to 10 years, catamnestic re-evaluation of the outcome is in order (prospective longitudinal method).

Current status of the project

Data collection was finished in the summer of 1976. At present the data evaluation is still in process. The first results of the analyses were prepared for publication in 1977. A diagnostic comparison has been published between the Zurich clinical diagnosis and a computerized (CATEGO, see Wing *et al.* 1974) diagnosis (Scharfetter *et al.* 1976), based on PSE and SCL (Syndrome Check List, Wing).

53. The course of monopolar depression and bipolar manic-depressive psychoses and schizoaffective psychoses (Switzerland)

J. ANGST, R. FREY, W. FELDER, and B. LOHMEYER

Introduction

Our interest in longitudinal studies of endogenous psychoses is based on the tradition of our hospital, mainly on the studies of Eugen and Manfred Bleuler in schizophrenia. Follow-up studies have been shown to be extremely fruitful for the evaluation of the efficacy of treatment, for testing the influence of independent variables that could modify the course, and for testing the hypothesis of prognostic indicators. Finally, studies on the course of the illness are of great theoretical interest in respect to the formation of a model of the disorder. Despite the many studies in this field, we are still suffering from a great lack of knowledge as to the spontaneous course of endogenous psychoses. The lack is mainly due to the fact that it is impossible to study untreated natural courses and that many investigators were less interested in quantative variables than in the quality of the course and were more interested in the outcome than in the careful study of each episode.

Our own interest was originally strongly connected with the introduction of new psychotropic drugs in the 1950s and our follow-up of the patients after cessation of treatment. Previously neglected in favour of schizophrenia, the interest in affective disorders has been strongly stimulated by the progress of psychopharmacology.

The present investigation on the course of affective and schizoaffective disorders is based on a monograph (Angst 1966) entitled *The etiology and nosology of endogenous depressive psychoses. A genetic, sociological, and clinical study*. It was partly translated into English in 1973. The patients were studied by the author between 1959 and 1963 and since then followed up personally or by the co-authors until 1975. The co-authors are Dr R. Frey (monopolar depression and bipolar manic-depressive psychoses), Dr W. Felder, and Dr B. Lohmeyer (schizoaffective disorders). The aim of the study is to develop a model on the course of affective psychoses and to re-examine the original genetic findings that lead to the conclusion that manic-depressive psychoses have to be split into monopolar (unipolar) depression and bipolar manic-depressive psychoses, a hypothesis that was later confirmed independently by Carlo Perris in Sweden. The study deals also with the question of whether schizoaffective psychoses should also be divided into monopolar and bipolar subgroups.

Subjects

The index sample of patients consists of all hospital admissions to the Psychiatric University Clinic, Burghölzli, in Zurich during the years 1959–63. All patients with a diagnosis of ICD 296 and ICD 295·7 were selected for the study. First and readmissions were included. The cohort is representative only of a hospitalized sample of patients with affective or schizoaffective illness. It is not representative of milder cases that are treated as out-patients or of untreated disorders. The sample was originally examined between 1959 and 1963 during the subjects' stay in the hospital. Since then, the subjects were followed up at least every fifth year by Angst by telephone calls with the patient and the nearest relatives, as well as by letters to the doctors who were in charge of the patient. A further investigation was carried out by Frey and Felder in 1975. At each follow-up a standardized set of questions was asked about the necessity of treatment, capacity of work, and about any manifestation of new secondary cases in the families. The patients were not informed of the aim of the study. It was explained to them that we were interested only in their further mental and physical condition.

In all cases we obtained personal information from the patients or from a close relative, and in all cases we obtained the results of the treatment by the doctors. We had no difficulties in collecting records about hospitalizations and treatments in other institutions. For about 50 per cent of the patients we collected records from other hospitals, for another 50 per cent information was obtained from close relatives, and in one-third of cases from the family doctors.

The information was kept secret, especially during data processing, and every patient was given a code number.

Beginning with birth registers, we collected background information about first degree relatives (parents, siblings, children) of the index cases. The register is complete. The information includes only age, social deviance, mental illness, and type of treatment. In all cases we collected medical records if the secondary cases had been treated in any institutions.

During the follow-up study we had very few drop-outs (less than 2 per cent) due to the fact that we followed only Swiss patients. We had to exclude foreign labourers because it was impossible to follow them in a reliable way.

Assessment of the cohort

The first assessment, based on personal examinations of the patients, took place between 1959 and 1963. There was a second assessment in 1965, a third in 1970, and a fourth in 1975. The latter were only done by telephone calls listing treatments during the follow-up period with names of doctors, drug treatment, and so on. Patients who were known to be less co-operative were first informed by a letter that they would get a telephone call. The telephone interview of the patients and the close relatives was conducted in the following way:

(a) General information was provided to the patient or the relatives regarding the aim of the interview;
(b) Facts about the patient's previous history were repeated to show the patient that his history is known, and to begin a discussion about the follow-up;
(c) An unstructured interview was conducted with the patient with regard to obtaining follow-up history;
(d) Specific questions were asked to complete the history.

The doctors who were in charge of the patients received a letter with 11 questions about follow-up history and treatment. All information was recorded on data sheets for punching. The patients and their relatives were usually highly delighted to receive a telephone call asking them about their well-being. They were extremely co-operative. Until 1975 we only had one drop-out in 238 cases.

Data analysis and preliminary results

All information was first punched and then organized on a magnetic tape for data analysis. The data analysis has almost been completed and several publications are in print (see Angst 1978, 1980; Angst and Frey 1978). The preliminary results are based on the following samples:

Bipolar affective illness	(ICD 296·1, 296·3)	$N=\ 95$
Monopolar affective illness	(ICD 296·2, 296·0)	$N=161$
Schizoaffective psychoses	(ICD 295·7)	$N=150$

Some of the results deal with the following areas:

(1) Comparison of early and late onset cases of depression (before 40 and later);
(2) The change of diagnosis from monopolar and unipolar depression to bipolar affective psychoses or schizoaffective psychoses;
(3) The change of diagnosis from bipolar to schizoaffective psychoses;
(4) The heterogeneity of bipolar psychoses from a clinical point of view;
(5) An analysis of differences between bipolar males and females in respect of frequency of syndromes;
(6) The development of a mathematical model based on a multiple regression analysis and on path analysis to describe the course and the influence of intervening variables.

The model should provide a base to test the efficacy of long term treatments like lithium (Angst and Weis 1967).

Methodological problems, special problems encountered

A follow-up investigation is a lifelong task for a group of

investigators who frequently show a shorter half-life than the sample to be studied. In a follow-up study like ours of more than 10 years the staff undergoes changes. Only one investigator (Angst) was permanently involved in the project. The others, even the administrative staff, changed. During the last three years there was a permanent secretary and during one year there were two doctors who collected data in a full-time position. For such longitudinal studies it is of paramount importance that the project is not funded by short-term grants. In our case funding was provided by the University of Zurich, who sponsors the research department. Follow-up studies of endogenous psychosis and genetic studies in this field can be carried out for as long as possible.

In our case, where we already knew the patients personally and where they were used to getting telephone calls or letters from time to time to ask them about their mental condition, we got the impression that we collected most of the necessary information in a reliable way. That was confirmed by written reports from the doctors, by records of other hospitals, and by the information from close relatives. Of course we may have lost information on milder manifestations of the illness, but this is a basic difficulty in all prospective studies. If we would attempt to exclude this error, we would be forced to examine the patients personally at intervals of one month over the course of ten to twenty years. Of course this task is impractical.

Another methodological difficulty lies in the definition of a pathological affective episode, i.e., when does it start and when does it end. In particular, the end of the episode is very frequently altered by an intervening drug treatment and consequently becomes extremely difficult to define. Therefore, our analysis is mainly based on the onset of an episode.

Another source of error is that we did not examine the patients personally. We think that one should not overestimate the additional information that can be gained in this way. The cross-sectional impression of a patient's condition is not representative of a longitudinal course and a present state can be strongly misleading. We think it is very important to collect information from close relatives and family doctors, rather than just from patients alone. In this way we frequently collected more information about the patient and his family than he knew about personally. The interview of a patient is mainly valid for a judgement of the present state.

Some special problems arise with the statistical analysis of the material. It is absolutely necessary to organize the data on a magnetic tape and to use multivariate statistical procedures. Some time is also spent on the analysis of distribution of data (they are frequently logarithmically distributed). Multiple regression analysis and path analysis have been shown to be the most useful models.

Future plans

The study will be ongoing for the next ten years and will continue to be supported by the University of Zurich. The sample of schizoaffective psychosis is still increasing because we are going through all the records of schizophrenia index cases that were admitted between 1959 and 1963.

We are attempting to study all of our sample patients until their deaths and to collect complete lifelong histories of their illnesses. Thus, we should be able to know more about the definitive course of these disorders, the efficacy of long-term prophylactic treatment, and outcome including suicide rates. We especially hope to know more about the heterogeneity of affective disorders from the perspective of genetic information as external criteria for classification.

54. Growing up as a mentally subnormal young person: a follow-up study (United Kingdom)

STEPHEN A. RICHARDSON

Introduction

The primary purpose of the study is to describe the life courses from age 10 to 22 of a total population of young people living in a city in Great Britain who were administratively defined as mentally subnormal during childhood. There is a remarkable dearth of knowledge about young people who are mentally subnormal during the transition from childhood to adulthood. Yet there are a number of critical issues related to mental subnormality dealing with social policy, the planning and evaluation of services, and the lives of young people who are mentally subnormal and their families, which cannot be properly examined without a longitudinal study.

A unique opportunity was available for the pursuit of the present research in the form of a well defined community population of young adults with the whole range of subtypes of mental subnormality who were identified and studied when they were eight to ten years of age (Birch et al. 1970). Various psychometric, neurological, reading, and psychiatric measures were obtained through individual examinations. In addition, a detailed home interview to obtain information on the social environment of each child, his health, education, and social history was carried out when the child was ten to twelve years of age. Because of the unusual stability of

the community where the studies were undertaken, over 80 per cent of this now-adult population still live in the community. The existing research records on the total population of the five-year cohort make it possible to study all who were classified as mentally subnormal in childhood and also to carefully select an appropriate sample for comparison who were not classified as mentally subnormal. Further, because group intelligence tests were given to all children in the community at age 7 and 9, the borderline subnormal children who remained in regular classes can also be identified. Given the scope of the present research, the selection of the aspects of the young person's life history which are most salient for research was guided by knowledge that already existed, and by specific questions and issues which arose from research and social policy. The following section deals with the specific research issues and questions.

Research issues

Young people who cease to be officially considered as mentally subnormal after leaving school

Many children who are administratively classified as mentally subnormal when they are at school do not continue to be officially considered as mentally subnormal after they leave school. Gruenberg (1964) has pointed out that in a number of epidemiological studies, the prevalence of mental subnormality after the age of 14 is only half as high as at the age of 14. These findings pose critical questions for understanding the nature of mental subnormality and for decision-making in public policy. Gruenberg suggests for example,

. . . For this drop in prevalence to occur, a large group of people regarded as retarded at fourteen must improve in their functioning to the point where people no longer regard them as retarded and also must succeed in escaping their history of earlier unsatisfactory performance (p. 274).
. . . Either these individuals are continuing to be extremely handicapped in later life and are unknown because the services they need are unavailable to them (in which case society is failing to do its duty toward them and ought to learn how to find and help them) or they have stopped being retarded in any real sense at all and do not need any special protection, help or services, in which case one had better change one's concept of what 'real' retardation 'really' is (p. 274).

The phenomenon 'cries out for investigation' (p. 274). The present study will provide the answers to this issue. Children who attend the special schools for the educable and trainable mentally subnormal generally end their schooling at age 16. Following up these young people to the age of 22 provides a six-year period to study those who, after school, do not continue in any services for the mentally subnormal and thus would no longer be administratively defined as such. Inevitably some young people continue to receive special services for the mentally handicapped and the study provides an opportunity to compare these young people with those not receiving special provision. By comparing the life histories from 16 to 22 years of age of all these young adults with comparisons of the same sex, age, social class, and area of residence in the community, we shall determine to what extent and how the lives of these two sets of young people are similar or different in their vocational careers, spare time interests and activities, social relationships, and their subjective evaluations of their lives and themselves.

Mental subnormality and stigma

The responses of people to those who are mentally handicapped may be influenced by the stereotypes and general values associated with mental subnormality. Goffman (1963) characterizes stigma in the following ways:

While the stranger is present before us, evidence can arise of his possessing an attribute that makes him different from others in the category of persons available for him to be (pp. 2–3).
. . . an individual who might have been received easily in ordinary social intercourse possesses a trait that can obtrude itself upon attention and turn those of us whom he meets away from him, breaking the claim that his other attributes have on us (p. 5).
We tend to impute a wide range of imperfections on the basis of the original one (p. 5).

These characteristics also have consequences for the person who is handicapped. For the person who is stigmatized, Goffman suggests he

. . . tends to hold the same beliefs about identity that we do (p. 7).
. . . he may perceive . . that whatever others profess, they do not really 'accept' him and are not ready to make contact with him on 'equal grounds'.

In a study of adults who had been in a residential institution and who were then released and living in the communty, Edgerton (1967) was so impressed by the problems of stigma for the adults in his study that the concept is included in the title of his book, *The cloak of competence. Stigma in the lives of the mentally retarded.* He found that those he studied went to great lengths to conceal the fact that they had been institutionalized and thus labelled as mentally retarded by society. They also desperately tried to conceal their various forms of incompetence so as not to appear different from others. In this study we wish to determine for a total population of

young adults with various subtypes of mental subnormality whether the concerns associated with stigma that Edgerton reports for his very special group, are also expressed in the community under study and, if so, how frequently and with what intensity.

The study of stigma will be restricted to the phenomenological view of the young adults and their parents. We wish to find out the extent and type of prejudice that young people at different ages and levels of functioning have experienced and remember. Have the mentally subnormal been bullied, teased, made fun of, exploited, or ostracized by peers in their neighbourhood? What difficulties have parents experienced with their own families, friends, and with adult neighbours with regard to their child? How do children feel about attending special schools for the retarded? Do young adults who were in special schools feel they have been discriminated against when trying to find jobs? For those who have been or are employed, what problems have been encountered? In seeking recreational facilities after leaving school, are there organizations and clubs that young people feel are congenial and meet their needs, and others from which they have withdrawn, having felt unwanted or rebuffed?

What new perspectives can be gained from the experiences of young people who are mentally subnormal and their parents?

(a) *Assessment of services.* The Warnock Committee (1978) of enquiry into special education has the following terms of reference: 'To review educational provision in England, Scotland, and Wales for children and young people handicapped by disabilities of body or mind, taking account of the medical aspects of their needs, together with arrangements to prepare them for entry into employment; to consider the most effective use of resources for these purposes; and to make recommendations'. The present study provides a comprehensive view of these issues from the viewpoint of the consumers—those who are mentally subnormal and their parents. In the United States, the President's Panel on Mental Retardation (1962) emphasized the need for a 'continuum of care' in developing a comprehensive programme for the retarded (p. 73). The continuum needs to be considered not only with reference to differing stages of individual development, but also to the relationships among services at any particular stage of development. Assessment of services both during the school years and afterwards has been largely fragmentary based on the view and experience of professionals in the field of mental retardation. The assessments have been of particular services and the unit of study is generally the institution or organization and how it provides the service. Relatively little attention has been paid to the consumer's viewpoint and experiences and how the various forms of services effect a young person as he or she progresses from childhood to adulthood. Investigation of the consumer's viewpoint provides a method of directly studying how effectively a continuum of care is being provided and the interrelationships among various services. An important element in consumer research is to determine whether there are unmet as well as met needs and whether there may be alternative forms of service consumers would prefer to those now given. By obtaining both a factual account of services received by young adults with various subtypes of mental subnormality and their parents, and their assessment of these services, we can gain a fresh perspective and new knowledge on the issue of continuity of care and forms of services which are satisfactory and unsatisfactory to consumers.

(b) *Learning from the experiences of parents in bringing up mentally subnormal children.* For most minority groups the experience of coping with their problems and disadvantages can be shared within and between families and passed on from one generation to the next. In this way a body of knowledge develops in the minority group which cumulates and can assimilate ingenious social inventions discovered by members of the group. Parents of children who are mentally subnormal are a minority group which does not have this advantage. They are generally unprepared for their role of rearing intellectually impaired children and have limited sources to turn to for help in socializing their child. A heavy emphasis in the literature on mental subnormality is on the tragedy and problems associated with having, caring for, and rearing a child who is mentally subnormal. There is the widespread assumption that the experience of having a mentally subnormal child is negative and punitive. In our interviews with parents who have raised mentally impaired children we obtain their views and determine whether there are also positive and rewarding experiences associated with being the parent of a handicapped child. A purpose of this study is to draw on and cumulate the knowledge parents have gained in rearing and socializing their mentally subnormal children. This should be of great value in the future to parents of intellectually impaired children.

(c) *Encouraging young people who are mentally subnormal to speak for themselves*. It has not been customary to let people who are mentally subnormal speak for themselves about their experiences or to obtain from them an evaluation of their experiences. Spokesmen for the mentally subnormal have generally been professionals in the mental retardation services and sometimes parents of mentally handicapped people. Yet, we know from our experience and the reports of other investigations (Edgerton 1967) that for all but the most profoundly retarded, it is possible with time, patience, and skill to obtain an account of their lives in considerable detail. The form of interview we have developed for use with the young adults who were classified as mentally subnormal as children provides unique points of view which will contribute to almost all the stated purposes of the research. Moreover, our early experience suggests that additional interviewing of carefully selected young adults can form the basis for biographies which will have great value in their own right. They will provide hitherto unknown insights and understanding into the day-to-day lives of people from whom we have much to learn.

The identification of variables which may predict the level of adult functioning for children who are mentally subnormal

'What will my child be like when he is grown up?' is a question of profound concern to all parents of children who are mentally subnormal. At a more general level the same question is equally important to those responsible for the planning and operation of services for the mentally subnormal. In very broad terms some prediction can often be made for the profoundly retarded, especially when there are associated severe functional handicaps. But for most children with mild and moderate degrees of mental subnormality as measured by intelligence tests very little is known about what factors provide indicators for prediction. It is known that IQ, which was a measure developed and intended for the prediction of school performance only, is not necessarily a reliable predictor of future adult functioning (Cobb 1966).

From the earlier study made of mentally subnormal children in the community, it is clear that any prognosis must take into account biological and social experiential factors and the ways in which these biosocial factors interact. There are no longitudinal studies of a total population of mentally subnormal children spanning the first 22 years of life, so the present research is largely exploratory. Using children who were relatively homogeneous in their level of functioning at age eight to ten, the association between various social and biological experiential histories and variation in adult level of functioning in the society is being examined to attempt to identify what factors influence development after the age of eight to ten.

School and post-school careers of young people who are borderline mentally subnormal

The recent concern over the possible effects of labelling a child as mentally subnormal has primarily focused on the stigmatizing aspects (e.g. Mercer 1970). Evidence supporting the deleterious consequences has been derived from studies of children with IQs in the borderline and mild mental subnormality range who were placed in special classes. There has not been sufficient recognition that this evidence is one-sided and has not taken into account children of comparable IQ who are not labelled and remain in regular classes. These children have been largely ignored in research. It is true that they avoid the stigma attached to being labelled as mentally subnormal. They are, however, deprived of the protection, special care, and concessions given to those in special education. Some educators believe that the borderline children in regular schools may experience severe difficulties in achieving any form of legitimate status or success at school and that their poor work performance is often interpreted as the result of inattention, laziness, or poor study habits. They can easily become the scapegoats of teachers and peers and develop resentment against authority figures. They may also seek to achieve some status among peers through delinquent and deviant behaviour.

No follow-up studies have been done of a defined population of borderline subnormal children in regular schools. One purpose of the present research is to compare the post-school careers and the quality of life of this group with young people who had the same IQ levels at school but who were administratively defined as mentally subnormal and placed in special schools. In addition, the special school group is also being compared with peers of comparable age, sex, and social class in regular schools who were not subnormal. These comparisons will be of value for considering the consequences of labelling children as mentally subnormal. They will also provide evidence to determine how justified is the concern of educators that the borderline children experience severe difficulties in their post-school careers.

Methods

Selection of subjects

The methods used in determining which children are administratively defined as mentally subnormal differ from one community to another. It is thus critical to appreciate the selection procedure used in the community in order to understand and interpret the results of the study.

All children in the community were group tested at the ages of 7, 9, and 11, and those whose IQ was below 75 were referred for individual psychometric evaluation by a psychologist. The child could subsequently remain in a regular school or could be recommended for special educational placement after his case had been fully reviewed by the Director of Education. Parents had the right of appeal against the recommendation.

The kind of placement of the mentally subnormal children provided, then, an administrative assessment of subtypes of mental subnormality. The forms of placement were:

1. School for educable children;
2. School for trainable children;
3. Child not able to benefit from school placement and living at home under parental care;
4. Child in care in a residential institution.

After the initial placement by authorities changes were made in light of experience with the placement. Some children were transferred back to regular schools if this appeared to be in their best interests.

We are fortunate in the proposed study in having, in addition to a very careful administrative selective procedure, an independent evaluation by our research team in 1962 of the total population of children administratively defined as mentally subnormal born in the years 1952–4. The independent research team who examined these children was made up of psychologists, paediatricians, neurologists, and psychiatrists. The psychological, neurological, and psychiatric assessment of each child provides the basis for subdividing the total population of mentally subnormal children into clinical subtypes at the age of 8–10. In every case, the research team judged the children to be in need of special placement for mentally subnormal children.

Definition and size of the study population

The study population was selected from all persons who were born in the years 1951 through 1955 and who were residents of the community in 1962. The oldest study subjects were 22 years of age in 1973. From this total population, the following subsets of subjects were selected:

1. Children administratively classified as mentally subnormal by the education and health authorities and placed in special educational placement or residential care at any time during the school years (5–16 years of age). There follow estimates of the numbers of children in different forms of care who meet the study definitions for inclusion:

At school for educable children	201
At school for trainable children	20
Not at school—cared for at home	6
In residential care	31
	258

To increase the number of more severely subnormal young people, the study has included those born in 1950 who were in all forms of special placement except the school for educable mentally subnormal children. This provided 12 additional cases of more severe subnormality.

2. Borderline subnormal children, defined for the purpose of this study as:

(a) those born in 1951 through 1955;
(b) who remained in regular classes throughout their schooling;
(c) at both 7 and 9 years of age scored below 80 on the group intelligence test given all children at these ages.

It is estimated that there are 61 young people who fulfil these criteria.

3. For each child administratively defined as mentally subnormal and born in 1951–5, a comparison child was selected from a 20 per cent random sample of all children who were in regular schools, had IQs of over 75, and were at no time administratively defined as mentally subnormal. This 20 per cent random sample was selected in 1964. From the 20 per cent random sample which contains approximately 2500 cases, for each mentally subnormal child, a comparison was selected using two steps:

(a) All children from the 20 per cent sample were selected who have the same age, sex, social class, and same geographic area of family residence as the mentally subnormal child, and
(b) of the children who meet these matching requirements, one is randomly selected.

The total number of mentally subnormal, borderline, and comparison children is approximately 589 cases.

Data collection methods

The information being used in the present study consists of new information being collected through interviewing and observation, and data that has already been collected for research and administrative purposes.

Interviews. The primary method used in obtaining the life histories from 10–22 years of age is interviewing. One interview is conducted with the young adults and the other with their parents or guardians. In most cases, the parent interview is with the mother, and at times, also the father. The main outline of the young adult's life history is obtained from both the parent and young adult. This provides for cross-checking of the information between the two interviews. The overlap is also necessary because the most severely subnormal young adults are limited in their ability to give information. The remainder of the two interviews focuses on data each informant is better or uniquely qualified to give. For example, the parents are asked about their experiences in rearing their child, the forms of help they sought and found, the kinds of help received from various community services, and their evaluation of these experiences. The young adult, if he has been employed, can best provide information about his jobs, his experiences at work, and his evaluation of these experiences.

The young adults in the study span almost the entire range of intelligence from severely subnormal to some very high IQs among the comparison population. As a result, they have followed widely varied life courses both during and after school age. They may have been in regular schools, special schools for the mentally subnormal, the deaf, or other forms of handicap, or in residential or home care for the most severely subnormal. After leaving school, the young people follow life courses which may include further education or training, jobs, unemployment, living at home with little possibility of getting any job, being a full or part-time housewife, attending a day care centre, or being in a residential institution. In the development of standardized interviews , it was necessary to cover any one or any combination of these various contingencies over time. Exploratory and pretest phases of interviewing provided the knowledge necessary for contstructing the two standardized interviews.

An important concern was to develop interviews in which the informants are not asked inappropriate questions which may cause embarrassment or which may hurt the informant. To prevent this from happening, a summary overview of the life history is obtained early in the interview. Then, depending on the particular life course the young person has taken, appropriate sections of the standardized interview are selected and used. The basic methods and principles used in the exploratory interviewing and in the development of the standardized interviews are described fully in the book *Interviewing: its forms and functions* (Richardson *et al.* 1965).

Observation. After each interview, the interviewer completes a schedule of observations. The major purpose is to record anything about the appearance, movement, dress, hygiene, speech, vision, hearing, language use, and behaviour of the informant that is sufficiently atypical to attract unusual attention and possibly influence other behaviour in a negative way toward the informant, e.g., obesity, adventitious or uncontrolled movements (e.g. athetosis or ataxia), drooling, physical stigmata associated with some cases of mental subnormality (e.g. facial characteristics common in Down's Syndrome, microcephalia).

Research design and conceptualization

The research purposes provided the major guides for selecting what information should be obtained in the life histories of the study population. The unique opportunity provided by the population available for study provides an exciting research opportunity but also one fraught with hazard. The study requires steering a careful course between the Scylla of trying to obtain excessive information at the cost of losing the co-operation of informants, overburdening interviewers, and amassing a body of data that will not be fully analysed, and the Charybdis of being so limited and specific in research design that the research opportunity is inadequately exploited. To find and hold a middle course has been and continues to be a central concern of the study. The study has been discussed with numerous scientific colleagues and with a wide range of professional personnel who have had long experience providing help and services for young people who are mentally subnormal and for their families.

Dependent and independent variables

The primary purpose of the research is to describe the life courses of young adults in the transition from childhood to adulthood and to begin to fill a serious gap in knowledge. We may consider these the dependent variables. But in order to gain some understanding and insights into these lives, it is also essential to consider some of the factors which at different ages influence their life courses. These may be considered as independent variables. The distinction between dependent and independent variables provides a helpful guide in ordering classes of data that are being used in the study. It must be recognized, however, that dependent variables when considered longitudinally and ecologically at a later point in time may become independent variables; e.g., placement of a child in a residential institution at the time of placement may be considered a dependent variable, but the experience of several years of life in an institution may, at a later point, be considered as an independent variable. Some of the variables then which will be placed as independent or dependent in the following sections may shift between these categories depending on the particular question being asked.

Dependent variables

In Western industrial societies there are general customs and practices, norms, and values which enable one to define in general terms the behaviours expected during childhood and young adulthood. To organize the array of behaviours over time we have used the three general concepts used by Homans (1950, 1961) of activities, interactions, and sentiments.

Activities

1. *Educational and vocational activities.* There is a general expectation in the community being studied that for five days a week children aged 5–16 will be engaged in educational activities. Beyond the age of compulsory education it is expected that people will engage in a vocational activity, or continue for some time in further education or training in preparation for an adult vocational role. Included in vocation is the role of housewife which may or may not include bearing and rearing children. For those who cannot meet these expectations certain special educational, day and residential care facilities are provided.

2. *Leisure time activities.* During waking hours, in time not used for educational or vocational activities, there is a wide variety of activities which are customary and acceptable within the society. These include pursuit of personal and social interests, hobbies, and sports. These may be solitary or shared and take place outside or inside an organizational or institutional context. There will also be some activities which are sanctioned either formally or informally by the society as a whole or within particular subcultures.

Interactions. It is generally expected that children and young adults will be involved in a variety of interpersonal relationships and will develop friendships and affectional ties with others. The particular interactions stem in part from the activities outlined above.

Sentiments. Sentiments expressed include personal reaction to judgements toward, and evaluation of activities and interactions, self-evaluation, fulfilled and unfulfilled goals and aspirations. In general, in obtaining the life histories, a distinction will be maintained between obtaining an account of activities and interactions (evidence) and the personal evaluation or subjective reaction to the particular happening (inference and subjective reaction). A specific example of sentiments is the parent's and young adult's evaluation of the various kinds of help and service they have received from educational, vocational, and health authorities.

Independent variables

The administrative designation of a child as mentally subnormal is made because the authorities believe the child is different in some respects from those not so defined. The belief of difference deals with kinds of educational needs and possible special needs after school age. It also implies a different life course from other children. The presence or absence of mental subnormality as defined in this study is a major independent variable.

Within the broad definition of mental subnormality there are various ways in which the total population so defined may be subdivided. These may be socially, clinically, or genetically determined. These subtypes are used in part because assignment to a subtype is expected to be related to different kinds of life histories for each subtype. The subtypes that are being used are:

1. Forms of placement during school years. These may be attending a regular school, a school for educable or trainable children, being judged unable to benefit from education and being cared for at the child's home, or placement in some residential institution for care. To view placement as an independent variable for considering outcomes at post school ages it will be necessary to consider the various combinations of placement between age five and sixteen that each child experiences during this time period.
2. The provision of services because of mental subnormality, after school-leaving age and up to the age of 22 (e.g. placement in a day centre, living at home with outside assistance in meeting the special needs of the young adult, placement in a residential institution for the retarded). Again, such services may, over time, be continuous or intermittent, and may change with time. Patterns of service over time will be considered. These subgroups may be compared internally with those who are mentally subnormal and receive no services after school and the subgroups from the comparison population based on matched pairs.
3. Clinical subtypes of mental subnormality based on the detailed examination made when the 1952–4 population of mentally subnormal children was examined at age 8–10.
4. A particular subtype of mental subnormality about which there is no longitudinal information for a defined population is Down's Syndrome. There should be about 15 cases.

So far we have considered different classifications of mental subnormality. The following independent variables deal with experiences which may influence the life histories and which may not be related to mental subnormality.

Health history. Attention is being confined to accidents and illnesses that required hospitalization, chronic illnesses, seizures and whether or not they were controlled with medication, physical, motor, and sensory handicaps, and psychiatric disturbance. In addition to the health of the study subjects another variable is the presence of health problems in other members of the primary family which have interfered with the care and rearing of the child. These include chronic illness, handicaps, alcoholism, behaviour disturbance, and death. Defining health problems broadly they also include severe dislocations and social pathology in the primary family of orientation.

Stigma. Recurrent reports of experiencing teasing, bullying, being made fun of, being taken advantage of, together with the young adult's interpretation of these events as being related to his mental subnormality, will be used to infer stigma. Avoidance or negative behaviour towards others who were defined as mentally subnormal and attempts on the part of the young adult to conceal the fact of his mentally handicapped classification or forms of incompetence will also be considered as evidence of stigma. Because of the importance given to stigma in the lives of the mentally subnormal we want to examine it both as an outcome and as a dependent variable influencing later activities, interactions, and sentiments.

The sex of the study subjects, their social class, and area of residence will often be used as control variables. Their use as controls is based on their being considered as independent variables. For certain questions, these variables will be used then as independent variables. For example, will those young adults who were in the school for educable children have vocational careers which differ by social class background when IQ, psychiatric disturbance, and neurological damages are held constant?

Data analysis

No amount of sophistication or effort in data analysis can turn poor data into sound results. Because of this belief we have given primary attention thus far to the organization and conduct of data collection. Because of the intimate interplay between data collection and analysis it has been essential to think through the analytic steps and begin developing methods for coding and organizing the data for computer storage and retrieval and for the analytic procedures required by the various research purposes.

The coding and digestion of the parent and young adult interviews entails a variety of procedures. A considerable number of questions are formulated so that the coding of the data can be worked out in advance of seeing the response. Precoding of questions has been done whenever possible using the general principles that have been well worked out in survey, behavioural science, and epidemiological research. Some questions call for descriptions which cannot be meaningfully precoded. Only after a number of interviews have been completed will it be possible to do a content analysis of responses and begin developing a set of categories. These initial categories will reflect the most usual responses and continued analysis of the remaining contents is necessary to develop additional categories.

The observational schedules are largely precoded. A detailed code book with instructions is being prepared and pretested and the interviewers will be taught coding procedures. The coding experience sensitizes the interviewer to the need for obtaining complete and unambiguous data. Interviewers will code responses to questions requiring special local knowledge. The reliability of the coding will be determined and, where unsatisfactory, the reasons will be explored. Samples of all coded interviews will be checked for accuracy. Additional personnel will be trained especially for coding.

All the quantified data from the coded interviews and the observational schedules will be placed on tape or disc so that it can be used for computer analysis. The chapter 'Reaction to Mental Subnormality' by S. A. Richardson in the book, *The mentally retarded and society* (1975), deals with some of the conceptual issues related to the analysis of data in the present study and also gives some of the insights and impressions derived from experience with the study.

Progress to date

The study has been planned, organized, and directed at The Albert Einstein College of Medicine, Bronx, New York, USA by Stephen A. Richardson, Ph.D., Professor in the Departments of Paediatrics and Community Health. In the United Kingdom, Mrs Janice McLaren, Research Fellow, is responsible for the supervision of data gathering and coding when Dr Richardson is in the United States. Valuable administrative and scientific support and consultation for the study has come from Professor Raymond Illsley and the staff of his Institute of Medical Sociology, Medical Research Council, Professors Herbert Birch, Michael Rutter, and Jack Tizard. Financial support for the study has come from the Foundation for Child Development, New York; The Grant Foundation, New York; The National Institutes of Child Health, Washington, D.C.; The Social Science Research Council, London; and the Easter Seal Research Foundation, Chicago.

Feasibility and pretest studies began in 1971 and the formal study began late in 1972. Data gathering was completed in 1979. The coding of the data is proceeding and initial analyses have been carried out (Richardson 1978, in press; Richardson *et al.* in press a, b). Any correspondence related to this study should be addressed to: Stephen A. Richardson, Ph.D., Professor of Paediatrics and Community Health, Albert Einstein College of Medicine, 1300 Morris Park Ave. Bronx, New York, 10461.

55. Longitudinal studies of autistic children (United Kingdom)

MICHAEL RUTTER

Introduction

There has been a long-standing interest in infantile autism at the Maudsley Hospital. The first studies were carried out by James Anthony and Kenneth Cameron in the 1950s and for the last 15 years there has been a programme of research directed by Michael Rutter. The programme has involved a variety of research strategies summarized in Rutter (1974, 1979b). However, this chapter will concentrate exclusively on the three main studies which have utilized a longitudinal design.

The first project involved a follow-up into adolescence and adult life of the psychotic children originally studied by Anthony and Cameron (together with a matched control group). Attention was paid to behavioural characteristics (Rutter and Lockyer 1967; Rutter *et al.* 1967) and psychological features (Lockyer and Rutter 1969, 1970) as well as to neurological aspects. The same group was reassessed six years later when most were young adults (Rutter 1970a); a third follow-up is currently being planned now that all the group are in their 20s and 30s.

The second project provided a systematic appraisal of the relative value of different educational approaches. Three units with contrasting philosophies and policies were studied in detail and the autistic children's progress in each unit was followed over a 4-year period (Bartak and Rutter 1971, 1973, 1975; Rutter and Bartak 1973).

The third project also focused on the benefits of therapeutic intervention. A home-based approach to treatment, which utilized behavioural techniques in a developmental context, was compared in terms of both short-term and long-term effects with two control groups treated along more conventional lines (Howlin *et al.* 1973a; Hemsley *et al.* 1978; Rutter *et al.* 1977).

Naturalistic follow-up

When the first follow-up study was planned (in the early 1960s) there was uncertainty over the validity of the concept of the syndrome of infantile autism. The investigation was planned by the author, together with Linda Lockyer, to examine this issue by making a systematic comparison between autistic children and children with other non-autistic psychiatric disorders attending the same psychiatric hospital. The study was supported by a grant from the Medical Research Council. The main points of the follow-up into adolescence and early adult life were:

(a) To determine whether the diagnostic differentiation was of any value for long-term prognosis (the approach first followed by Kraepelin in his studies of schizophrenia and manic-depressive psychosis);
(b) To describe the 'natural history' of the development of autistic children;
(c) To find out whether the changes over time in symptomatology and pattern of handicap threw any light on the nature of the autistic syndrome.

Sampling

For this purpose it was necessary to have as well diagnosed a group of children with infantile autism (or infantile psychosis) as possible. Cases were chosen on the basis of first attendance during the years 1950–8 and having received an unequivocal diagnosis of child psychosis, infantile autism, schizophrenic syndrome of childood (a term used for infantile psychosis at the time of the study), or any synonym of these, which had been agreed by all Maudsley Hospital consultant psychiatrists who had seen the child. Sixty-four such cases were found. In all the onset was before $5\frac{1}{2}$ years and in all but 5 the onset was before 30 months.

The choice of comparison group was crucial. First, it had to include children with a psychiatric condition (as the differentiation to be tested was that between autism and other psychiatric disorders). Second, both the cases and controls should come from the same hospital (to diminish referral biases) and both groups should have been assessed through the same standard procedures (so that the base-line data were comparable). The Maudsley Hospital Children's Department patient population met both these criteria. Third, the groups had to be closely matched for age, sex, and IQ—features known to be associated with differences in symptomatology (see Rutter *et al.* 1970b). This was essential in order to be sure that any differences found were specific to autism and not merely an artefact of age, sex or IQ associations. Accordingly, controls were chosen on an individually matched basis. For each autistic child the next child–patient meeting the criteria was taken (i.e. of the same sex, attending the clinic within the same year, within 12 months of age); in the event 14 controls had to be chosen in which the age difference was 13–24 months, and within 10 points of IQ.

Base-line assessments

The case records of both cases and controls were gone through systematically according to a standard schedule which listed a comprehensive set of defined symptoms and behaviour, psychological test findings, developmental data, neurological examinations, and medical investigations.

In addition, each case record was searched for any information which might be of value in tracing. This included the names and addresses of all agencies involved at any time, of all hospitals contacted, of the family doctor and all relatives noted in the case file. Any possible leads (such as the fact that a relative was a doctor thus enabling tracing through the medical register) were recorded. Previous studies (see Robins 1966; Douglas *et al.* 1968b) had shown the value of having as many sources for tracing as possible and certainly we found that this paid off richly when it came to the detective work of locating cases and controls as long as 5 to 15 years after their hospital referral.

Tracing and contact. A wide range of sources was used to trace the children in both groups. This involved a high degree of persistence over a period of nearly two years but finally all psychotic children were located and personally examined. No detailed information was available for one control child who had emigrated to Australia and one control child had died. Otherwise all controls (i.e. 97 per cent of the initial group) were seen and tested.

Follow-up assessment

The children in both groups were individually seen at follow-up in 1963/64 and were given neurological, psychiatric, and psychological examinations. The mean age of autistic children at follow-up was 15 years 7 months, the mean duration of follow-up being 9 years 8 months. The mean age of controls was 16 years 5 months with a mean follow-up of 10 years 3 months. Each child was given a standardized neurological and psychiatric examination and was observed in an unstructured situation with other people. A detailed account of the child's past and present behavioural state (together with an account of illnesses at treatment, health of the rest of the family, etc.) was obtained from a parent or a parent surrogate. A specified list of behaviours was covered, each being rated on a 5-point scale. The individual psychological examination included the WISC or WAIS, Peabody Picture Vocabulary Test, Schonell Graded Word Reading Test, and the Vineland Social Maturity Scale. Where appropriate, a report of the child's behaviour and attainments was obtained from the school or training centre attended by the child.

Later follow-up. The autistic children were studied again in 1970 by means of a postal questionnaire to parents and reports from hospitals and clinics. At that time the age range extended from 15 to 29 years with a mean of 21 years 8 months. Information was obtained on 63 (98 per cent) of the 64 children. The control group was not reassessed in this second follow-up.

Findings

The results showed a host of differences between the autistic children and their controls, amply demonstrating the validity of the diagnostic differentiation. The follow-up also showed that about a quarter of autistic children developed epileptic fits during adolescence (Rutter *et al.* 1967; Rutter 1970a). This was important because in most cases there had been no suggestion of an organic component up to that time. The strong implication was that the autistic syndrome had arisen as a result of organic brain dysfunction.

Previously, most clinicians had considered that the IQ scores of autistic children had little meaning and that the poor cognitive performance shown by many merely reflected social withdrawal or lack of motivation. The longitudinal data clearly demonstrated that this view was mistaken. Three findings were crucial:

(1) Even when the children were greatly impaired in their social involvement and awareness there was little change in IQ level;
(2) The IQ score showed much the same association with later educational attainment as that found in other children;
(3) Not only did the mentally retarded autistic children have a worse social and academic outcome than autistic children of normal non-verbal intelligence, but also their incidence of epilepsy was seven times as high (see Rutter 1978b; Bartak and Rutter 1976).

Only three measures obtained in early childhood were significantly related to social outcome in adolescence and adult life. These were: the initial IQ, the degree of language impairment, and the total symptom score (reflecting general severity of disorder). However, apart from language, no single symptom predicted outcome and, in particular, social abnormalities did not. The findings strongly suggested the importance of a basic cognitive deficit in the development of autistic children—and possibly also in the genesis of the autistic syndrome itself. All the findings have since been replicated in other prospective or follow-up studies (see Lotter 1978). Longitudinal data were crucial in producing a shift of view about the nature of autism.

The only treatment measure related to outcome was the children's experience of schooling. It was necessary to test this effect through a prospective study in which there was direct assessment of the educational process. That constituted the second longitudinal project (see below).

Status of data

As noted above, a further follow-up of the same group of autistic children is now being planned. All the initial and follow-up interview and psychological test protocols have been retained and are available for further analysis. The data remain in raw form and are not on punchcards or tape.

Three units study

In order to study the effects of education, Lawrence Bartak and the author selected three well established units which took sizeable groups of autistic children and which differed markedly in both theoretical orientation and therapeutic practice (Bartak and Rutter 1971, 1973, 1975; Rutter and Bartak 1973). One unit (A) was primarily a psychotherapeutic unit with little emphasis on teaching; the second (B) provided a permissive classroom environment in which regressive techniques and an emphasis on relationships were combined with special educational methods; and the third (C) provided a structured and organized setting with a focus on the teaching of specific skills. The study was funded through grants from the Department of Education and Science and the Calouste Gulbenkian Foundation.

Sample

Children were selected for inclusion in the study if they had a disorder beginning before the age of 30 months in which all three autistic features (a profound and general failure to develop interpersonal relationships, delayed and deviant language development, ritualistic or compulsive phenomenon) were present (see Rutter 1971b, 1978b). There were 50 children in the sample: 8 at unit A, 18 at unit B, and 24 at unit C, with an average age of 7–9 years (varying slightly according to unit). The children were roughly comparable across the three units but there were some differences at the extremes of the ranges of age and IQ which needed to be taken into account in assessing the progress of the children.

Assessment of units and children

The units were assessed through questioning of staff and by detailed time-and-event-sampled direct observations in the classroom and elsewhere. Staff-child interaction was systematically measured in terms of type of interaction (acts of instruction, acts of approval, etc.), affective style, and contingencies in relation to various kinds of child behaviour. Interrater reliability was tested and shown to be high for all observational measures.

All children were assessed on measures of intelligence, language, social behaviour, and educational attainment. Intelligence was assessed on the Merrill–Palmer and Wechsler scales; language on the English Picture Vocabulary Test and through audio—tape-recorded speech in a standardized free play situation; social

behaviour through time-sampled observations in the classroom and in a play situation, ratings of behaviour during testing, and parental interview; educational attainment on the Neale Analysis of Reading Ability and the Staffordshire Arithmetic Test.

Measurements were taken at the start of the study in 1967, at a first follow-up in 1969, and finally at a second follow-up in 1970–1, some $3\frac{1}{2}$ to 4 years after the initial baseline assessment.

Findings

The direct observation measures showed that the three units not only differed in theoretical orientation, but also they differed significantly in the amount and in the character of staff interactions with the children. These differences seemed to have implications for the children's progress in that the children at unit C fared best in terms of scholastic attainment, co-operative behaviour in a free-play situation, and on-task activity in the classroom. It was concluded that large amounts of specific teaching in a well-controlled classroom are likely to bring the greatest educational benefits.

However, the results also showed large individual differences between autistic children in the progress made. A longitudinal design was essential to take account of these initial differences in assessing school progress. As in the first study, the autistic children of low IQ did least well, and the special educational treatment made no significant difference to the IQ level. A further finding with implications for both research and practice was that changes in one situation tended not to generalize to others. This observation influenced the design of the third longitudinal study (see below).

Status of project. The data are stored on punchcards and the subjects could be identified for a further follow-up. However, no further contact is planned at the moment.

Home-based treatment project

The third study was a $6\frac{1}{2}$-year project initiated in 1970 by the author, William Yule, Michael Berger, and Lionel Hersov on a grant from the Department of Health and Social Security. Rosemary Hemsley and Patricia Howlin were the chief investigators and Daphne Holbrook and Fraida Sussenwein served as consultant social workers.

The treatment programme to be evaluated consisted of treatment *at home* with parents acting as the principal therapists. A wide range of behavioural techniques formed the main basis of treatment but these were applied in an individually tailored fashion relevant to each child's developmental level and home situation, and the techniques were combined with counselling to help with family problems and practical help with housing, holidays, and the like when this was needed (see Howlin et al. 1973a; Hemsley et al. 1978; Rutter et al. 1977).

Sampling

Previous studies had all shown that severely retarded autistic children had a fairly uniformly poor prognosis. It seemed desirable, therefore, to exclude very low IQ children in order to reduce individual differences and hence to highlight possible treatment effects. The experimental group, therefore, consisted of 16 boys, aged 3 to 11 years, without overt neurological or sensory impairments, with a non-verbal IQ of 60 or above, who lived within a 60-mile radius of London.

Two different control groups were used. First, there was a *short term* group consisting of autistic children group-matched with the cases for age, language level, and IQ. These children were receiving no consistent form of treatment. Changes in the children and *in their parents* were compared with changes in the experimental group children and parents over a 6-month period. This comparison provided a test of whether the treatment could lead to systematic short-term changes in the way the parents dealt with their children and in the behaviour of the children themselves.

However, autism is a chronic condition and in order to make policy decisions about the value of different therapeutic approaches, it was essential to have a much longer follow-up. We considered it unethical to withhold treatment from a control group for a period of longer than 6 months, so the first group could not be used for this purpose. We had hoped to compare the home-based treatment programme with another and different form of treatment. However, in spite of very active searching, we could not locate a sufficient sized group treated in a markedly different way. As a result, we had to modify our plans somewhat. For the *long-term* control group we used autistic children seen as out-patients at the Maudsley Hospital but not included in the experimental programme because they lived too far away. They had received similar advice but had been seen only sporadically.

The timing of the decision to use this group meant that it was not possible to study the children prospectively in the same way as the cases. Most of the controls had first attended some years ago (which incidently created the problem of a longer follow-up period for controls than for cases—necessitating statistical manipulation of the data to take account of the difference). However, because the controls had attended the same clinics, they had been similarly assessed, thus providing adequate data for matching. Cases and controls were closely matched on a child basis according to their age, non-verbal IQ, and language level at the time of first attendance.

Assessments

Systematic assessments were made prior to starting treatment, after 6 months of treatment, and then again after 18 months. The children's language was assessed in terms of a standardized analysis of audio-tape recordings (Cantwell *et al.* 1977), parental interview, and the Reynell Developmental Language Scales (at follow-up only). The children's behaviour was evaluated on the basis of systematic time-sampled observations in the home and parental interview data. In addition, all children had cognitive testing using the Merrill–Palmer or Wechsler scales.

Parental behaviour and parent–child interaction assessments included a standardized audio-tape analysis of maternal communication (Howlin *et al.* 1973b), other interview measures, and a specially devised measure of parental coping skills (at follow-up only). No cases or controls were lost from the study. One child in the experimental group moved abroad but a special visit was made to complete the follow-up measures.

Findings

The results showed that the treatment programme was effective both in causing parents to modify their interaction with their autistic children and in reducing the children's level of behavioural disturbance. Treatment was also associated with a significant short-term improvement in the autistic children's communication. However, the long-term follow-up was crucial in demonstrating that the final language gains associated with treatment were much less marked. This was not due to any later regression but rather reflected the immense individual variation in extent of cognitive and linguistic handicaps. Within the IQ range of 60 and above, IQ did not predict outcome but the initial language level did. These findings, with their important theoretical and practical implications, could only have emerged with a longitudinal design.

Status of project. The study came to an end in 1977. However, all the data are available (mostly on punchcards), the subjects are identifiable for research purposes, and a further follow-up is planned.

Conclusions

Any assessment of the public impact of these studies is complicated by the fact that they constituted part of a more extensive research programme and by the fact that there were comparable investigations of autistic children from other centres in this country and elsewhere. It has been important that the findings from all over the world have generally been closely similar, providing powerful evidence of their validity. (Of course there are also some vital differences which still require investigation).

No one investigation does (or indeed should) in itself lead to a change of theoretical concept or practical policy. On the other hand, the various longitudinal studies of autistic children have played a crucial role in the change of view of autism from a motivational disorder (as once thought) to an organically determined condition in which a serious cognitive deficit is basic (as now thought). The three units study was influential as part of the move to an increased emphasis on a structured educational approach for autistic children; and the home-based project led to the Maudsley Hospital establishing the treatment as part of the generally available services for autistic children.

56. Psychiatric sequelae and cognitive recovery after severe head injury in childhood (United Kingdom)

OLIVER CHADWICK, GILLIAN BROWN, DAVID SHAFFER, and MICHAEL RUTTER

Introduction

Approximately a quarter of all people who receive hospital treatment for head injury in England and Wales are school-age children (Field 1976). These injuries may be classed as accidental, and amongst children who are admitted to hospital for an accident of any sort, 'intracranial injury' is the most common diagnostic category (Department of Health and Social Security 1977). The number of children receiving hospital treatment for head injury has shown a steady annual increase since the 1950s (Craft *et al.* 1972). However, there has been little change over the years in the total number of patients staying in hospital for longer than a day (Field 1976). Thus the additional numbers of children who receive hospital treatment for head injury each year are likely to have suffered relatively minor injuries. Of those children who have had severe head injuries, the increased availability and sophistication of treatment methods have probably resulted in a decrease in the number of deaths due to head injury (Field 1976), and, at the same time, an increase in the number of disabled survivors (Jennett 1975).

Alongside the material improvements in treatment facilities, there has been a recognition of the importance of the social and psychological problems which follow head injury in both children and adults. This recognition has been reflected in the choice of measures which have been used to assess outcome. Whilst the high prevalence of 'mental symptoms' and behaviour problems has been acknowledged for many years, it is only recently that attempts have been made to study these systematically in relation to other sorts of problems which may arise. Thus, Bond (1975) found that for adults the most important component of handicap is to be found in the patient's psychological and social adjustment. Problems in these areas of functioning were more prevalent and more likely to be a cause of difficulty in posttraumatic adjustment than sensory or motor defects.

The importance of psychological and social difficulties in children with brain injury has been indicated in a number of studies. High rates of psychiatric disorder and low levels of scholastic attainment have been shown in children with a variety of types of damage to the brain or epilepsy (Rutter et al. 1970a), and for children who have sustained a localized head injury (Shaffer et al. 1975). These high rates of disturbance and low levels of attainment do not appear to be a consequence of the physical handicaps which may result from brain injury (Seidel et al. 1975). Rather, it seems likely that brain injury itself has the effect of making the child more vulnerable to psychiatric disturbance and educational failure (Rutter 1977b).

A prospective longitudinal approach

The majority of studies of psychological disorders in children who have suffered brain injury have been retrospective in design. Although such studies have been useful in showing associations between injury and impairment, there are several ways in which a prospective longitudinal design provides a much more powerful framework for the investigation of these relationships.

In studies of human brain injury, any attempt to assess the cognitive and behavioural difficulties which may have been present prior to injury will almost inevitably be retrospective. However, by employing a prospective design in which cases are assessed shortly after head injury occurs, it is possible to reduce the unreliability of such retrospective assessments. The investigation of the effects of childhood head injury is particularly well-suited to prospective study because it is possible to specify precisely when injury occurred. In contrast to many other causes of childhood brain injury, such as infection or progressive disease, there is seldom any appreciable delay between the occurrence and diagnosis of head injury. As a result, the assessment of the child's condition prior to injury can be carried out relatively soon after injury and before the child has shown any substantial degree of recovery. This minimizes the likelihood that the assessment of pre-injury behaviour will be influenced by knowledge of outcome.

Similar considerations apply to the measurement of the severity of injury. With retrospective studies, there may be inaccuracies or omissions in the recording of information about the injury simply because such data were not a primary focus of concern at the time. The accuracy, validity and completeness of such data can be greatly improved by the use of a prospective design in which standard methods of assessment are applied to all cases at the time of injury.

Whilst the primary strength of a prospective strategy lies in its potential for improving the quality and validity of the measures used, the advantage of a longitudinal method of study lies in the scope it provides for examining changes in outcome over time. With childhood head injury, a research design of this kind allows a number of issues to be considered which cannot be approached satisfactorily by cross-sectional studies. By carrying out assessments at successive intervals after injury, the speed and extent of recovery can be examined and their relationship to the severity of injury can be expressed in the form of recovery curves. In addition, the causal pathways between injury and later impairment can be examined in detail to identify the role of possible intervening factors. This is especially important in considering educational and psychiatric outcome where changes in the child's environment after injury may be expected to play an important mediating role. For example, physical handicap or problems in school performance or adjustment may arise as a result of head injury. This may lead to the child being placed in a special school. The change in school (or uncertainty about whether such a change should be made) may itself contribute independently to any subsequent adjustment or educational problems. Alternatively, changes in the child's behaviour after injury may lead to disagreement between the parents about appropriate forms of supervision. If discord is severe, the child's behaviour problems may be exacerbated. In both cases, a longitudinal design provides a powerful basis for *causal* inference by allowing the possibility of establishing the temporal sequence of such events.

There have been relatively few studies which have used a prospective longitudinal design to study head injuries in children. Black et al. (1969, 1971) reported that psychological disturbance developed afresh in approximately a fifth of their consecutive series of childhood head injuries. The prevalence of different behavioural and emotional problems after injury appeared to show separate patterns of development and recovery over time, but generally returned to their estimated pre-injury levels within three years after injury. Intellectual level showed a small but gradual improvement over the five years of follow-up. Unfortunately, in the absence of a control group, it is unclear to what extent this improvement reflects the effects of practice on the tests rather than recovery from brain injury.

Klonoff and his colleagues (Klonoff and Paris 1974; Klonoff et al. 1977) reported a five year longitudinal study of 231 children admitted to hospital following a head injury. Each was matched for age and sex with a child referred by a paediatrician. Gradual improvement on a large battery of cognitive tests was observed over the course of the five year follow-up period. However, there was a progressive loss of cases during the course of the study such that by the end of the follow-up less than half of the original sample remained, and it is not clear how far the progressive drop in sample size contributed to the decreasing likelihood of observing statistically significant differences between groups at successive assessments. Behavioural sequelae usually took the form of 'personality changes', headaches, fatigue, learning difficulties, poor concentration and irritability. They showed a marked tendency to subside during the first two years after injury.

The present study

The primary purpose of the present study was to examine the course of psychological recovery following head injury in school age children and also to determine the nature of any resulting cognitive or behavioural impairment. Three groups were collected for study, each consisting of children aged between 5 and 14 at the time of injury.

Severe head injury group

In order to examine the course of recovery, it was essential to study head injuries of sufficient severity such that most children would show at least some initial impairment. To meet this requirement, a sample of children who had sustained a head injury resulting in a **post-traumatic amnesia (PTA)** of at least a week was collected. Preliminary piloting showed that most children with a head injury of this severity are admitted to a Regional Neurosurgical Unit. Six of these Units serving the southeast of England were used as a basic sampling frame. Cases were identified by weekly telephone (or personal) contact with the ward staff and administrative offices of each unit to monitor suitable cases which had been admitted during the previous seven days. The aims, scope and inclusion criteria had previously been explained to the relevant staff so that they could serve as screening agents. Methods of case identification differed from hospital to hospital so that the most systematic and reliable method of case identification could be utilized. Usually the ward admissions book proved to be the most satisfactory source of information. Where possible the same member of staff was contacted each week. Where information from the hospital staff left doubt about the suitability of inclusion, supplementary information was obtained from the child's parents or any other appropriate source.

Control group

In seeking to identify the contribution of *brain* injury to psychological outcome, a control group was needed for several reasons. Firstly, it is clear from previous studies that children who sustain head injuries are not a random sample of the population. Such injuries occur more commonly in boys (e.g., Rowbotham *et al.* 1954; Partington 1960) and the injured are more likely to come from socially and economically disadvantaged families (Backett and Johnston 1959; Klonoff 1971). It was therefore important to control for these background risk factors. Secondly, it was also necessary to control for the non-neurological consequences of head injury which may influence the child's later behaviour and adjustment. Amongst these are the child's experience of hospitalization, separation from his parents, absence from school and the residual physical handicaps resulting from injury. Thirdly, because outcome was to be assessed by repeated administration of the same tests, it was essential to examine a comparison group in an identical way in order to differentiate practice effects on the tests from improvements due to recovery from brain injury. Also, since a variety of unstandardized tests were included in the assessment battery, data were needed from a comparison group matched on those background factors, such as age, sex and social class, which were likely to affect test performance.

For these reasons, a control group was included consisting of children receiving hospital treatment for orthopaedic injuries which did not involve damage to the head or central nervous system. Each was individually matched with a child from the severe head injury sample for age (divided into two year age blocks), sex, and occupation of the main family breadwinner (classified according to three categories: non-manual, skilled manual, and semi- or unskilled manual). Difficulties in obtaining suitable matches from children who had received in-patient hospital treatment necessitated the inclusion of five with orthopaedic injuries who had received out-patient treatment only. The controls were obtained from five local hospitals serving southeast London.

Mild head injury group

A sample of children who had sustained mild head injuries was also collected in an attempt to determine the threshold level of severity above which psychological deficits might be expected. This consisted of children who had received hospital treatment after head injury giving rise to a PTA of at least an hour but less than a week. Resources did not permit the collection of a matched control group for this sample.

Only a minority of children with head injuries of this severity are admitted to Regional Neurosurgical Units. As a result, cases in this group were collected primarily from the five local hospitals from which the controls were collected. A quarter of the mild head injury group, however, were cases from Neurosurgical Units, who were initially thought to have suffered severe injuries, but who were reclassified as mild on the basis of more detailed information.

Assessment of severity of head injury

If a head injury is severe enough, one of the immediate consequences of trauma is a disturbance of consciousness. The degree of disturbance may vary from deep unresponsive coma to a slight reduction in alertness. Even when the patient has emerged from coma to the extent of being responsive and speaking, there usually remains a period during which recent events are not remembered reliably. This period of post-traumatic amnesia (PTA) usually lasts considerably longer than the duration of coma. Jennett *et al.* (1977) found that 91 per cent of patients with a coma duration of at least 6 hours have a PTA of more than seven days.

Posttraumatic amnesia was preferred as a measure of severity in the present study because it allowed rough quantification along a single continuum of both severe and mild head injuries. The measure has also been shown to be a reasonably good predictor of long-term mental and physical recovery (Russell and Smith 1961; Russell 1971; Jennett 1976). The degree and extent of amnesia improves during the course of recovery, and it is common to measure the duration of PTA up to the point at which memory for ongoing events of daily life becomes continuous (e.g., Brooks 1976). In the present study, rough estimates of PTA were obtained for screening purposes from the hospital staff who initially identified the cases. The measures used in classifying the severity of the injury were the estimates of PTA obtained at interview with the child's parents.

The distribution of cases according to their severity is shown in Table 56.1 alongside Jennett's (1976) classification of severities. The labels used in the present study are generally less grave than those of Jennett because PTA ratings were obtained from the child's parents who were probably in a better position than the hospital staff to recognize persisting subtle defects in ongoing memory.

TABLE 56.1

Distribution of cases according to severity

Jennett (1976)		Present study	
PTA.	Label	*N*	
<5 min	Very mild		
<1 h	Mild		
1–24 h	Moderate	19	} Mild
1–7 days	Severe	10	
>7 days	Very severe	23	} Severe
>4 weeks	Extremely severe	8†	

† Included if testable within 3 months of injury.

The choice of control group

In seeking to identify the contribution of *brain* injury to psychological outcome after head injury, it is necessary to control for two types of factors which may contribute to outcome. Firstly, there are *predisposing* factors which may put the child at risk for accident or injury. For example, Backett and Johnston (1959) found that children involved in pedestrian road traffic accidents are more likely than matched uninjured controls to come from families living in overcrowded homes where protected play facilities are limited or absent, and maternal supervision and care is restricted because of pregnancy, work, or ill health. Secondly, there are *consequences* of the accident, not specific to brain injury, which may affect later behaviour and adjustment. Amongst these are the experience of separation from the family and absence from school, and the residual physical incapacities resulting from injury.

In order to control for the effect of these factors, it was considered essential to study a group of children who had been involved in accidents requiring hospital treatment, but amongst whom there was no evidence of damage to the central nervous system. Ideally, it would have been desirable to control for the circumstances of accident also, since it may be anticipated that the circumstances giving rise to the accident will be related to background social and psychological characteristics of the child. The severe head injuries were individually matched with controls for age, sex, and parental occupation, but resources did not permit the inclusion of this additional control variable. The control group was assessed on the same measures and at the same time intervals since accident as the severe head injuries in order to control for the effects of readministration of the measure as well as developmental changes in the child.

Contact with the sample

After being informed of a patient suitable for inclusion in the study, contact was made with the child's parents as soon as survival seemed certain. When it was possible to see the parents on the hospital ward, an introduction was effected through a member of the nursing staff. Otherwise a letter was sent to the parents of the child outlining the purpose of the study, and where the family lived locally permission was sought for one member of the research team to visit their home and explain what would be involved. With children living outside London, this explanation was given in the letter of introduction and the parents were asked to indicate on a prepaid reply postcard whether the appointment suggested was convenient. Parents of all three groups were told that we were interested in how quickly children recovered from different kinds of accidents and whether they have any problems afterwards. It was also mentioned that we were particularly interested in how children react to hospitals, and how families are affected by the problems that accidents create. Parents of the (orthopaedic) control group were also told that one of our aims was to study children who had had head injuries, and for this purpose we were interested in studying a comparison group of children whose injuries did not involve the head.

It was made clear to parents that the research workers were not in a position to offer advice or treatment themselves. Where significant problems were encountered, and the parents expressed a wish for some form of action to be taken, the matter was referred to the child's hospital consultant—or, after discussion with the hospital, to the child's general practitioner, school, local authority social service department, or other appropriate body. At later follow-ups the parents were asked how satisfied they were with any practical help which had been offered. Where problems remained or new difficulties had developed, the appropriate authority or agency was contacted again. All parents were given the telephone number of the office from which the research was being co-ordinated, so that if problems developed between follow-up assessments, advice could be sought about whom to approach for help.

Outcome measures

Timing

Initial assessments were carried out as soon as the child's clinical condition had improved sufficiently to allow psychological testing. In cases of very severe head injury, the parental interview took place after survival had been assured, rather than before recovery had progressed to this stage, in order to avoid a lengthy delay in the collection of information concerning the child's pretraumatic state. The mean duration of time between injury and initial psychological assessment was approximately 36 days for the severe head injuries and 18 days for the controls and mild head injuries. Further assessments were carried out at 4 months, 1 year, and 2–3 years after injury.

Nature

Information from the parents. The parental interview was adapted from that described by Rutter and Graham (1968) and included sections designed to identify psychiatric disturbance in the child, disturbance in either parent, and the quality of family relationships. Detailed enquiries were made about the type of treatment intervention received, the parents' perception of such treatment, and how it compared with expectations. Information was also obtained about temperamental variables, child rearing practices, and in particular, the amount of independence allowed to the child and the amount of anxiety shown about certain of the child's symptoms and behaviour. Rating scales were developed to code information obtained at the interviews, and the between-rater reliability of these has been established. The reliability of global ratings of disorder was assessed on transcripts by a rater, blind to the subject's status as a severe, mild, or control injury.

Information from the school. The child's class teacher was asked to complete a B2 version of the Rutter teachers' questionnaire (Rutter *et al.* 1970b; Rutter *et al.* 1975a) shortly after notification of the case. The teacher was asked to base replies on classroom behaviour during the 3 months before injury. This questionnaire was re-administered one year and 2–3 years after injury.

The class teachers of the children in the severe head injury group were interviewed briefly at the time of the final assessment 2–3 years after injury. This interview was designed to assess the child's school progress, residual physical handicaps, gross activity level, fatiguability, memory, ability to concentrate, peer relations and school adjustment.

Cognitive tests. Tests of cognitive functioning were chosen for their probable relevance to school performance and learning. The test battery included measures which other studies had shown to be sensitive to the effects of brain injury, and measures on which there was a substantial body of background knowledge in the form of data on reliability, validity, and correlation with educational progress. Administration of this latter type of test was considered essential, not least in providing a frame of reference for the psychologist to say something informative to the parents about their child's condition.

A six subtest version of the Wechsler Intelligence Scale for Children (1949) was used throughout to measure general intellectual ability. The verbal tests (similarities, vocabulary and digit span) were administered to all three groups at the initial assessment and the one year follow-up. Because these tests were no longer sensitive to the effects of head injury a year after injury, they were omitted from the test battery used at the final follow-up. The three performance subtests (block designs, object assembly and digit symbol) were used at the initial, one year and 2–3 year assessments. In addition, the digit span and coding subtests were included in the short test battery administered to the severe head injuries and controls four months after injury.

To provide a measure of scholastic attainment, the Neale Analysis of Reading Ability (1958) was given to children in all three groups at the initial assessment, and at the one year and 2–3 year follow-ups. To minimize practice effects, the A version of the test was used at the initial and final assessments and the B version was used one year after injury.

In order to provide finer detail on the types of cognitive impairment which may follow head injury, a variety of tests of specific cognitive abilities and sensori-motor functioning were administered to the children in the severe head injury group and their matched controls during the first year of follow-up. These tests are listed below:

Paired associate learning test. The child was required to learn and remember names to go with six photographs of children's faces. The general method of presentation and testing was essentially similar to that described by Meyer and Yates (1955). Delayed recall and speed of relearning were assessed at the end of the session.

Continuous performance task (Rosvold *et al*. 1956). An automated vigilance task in which the child had to maintain attention over a period of time and respond whenever an infrequent target stimulus was presented. The test was designed to examine sustained performance, attentiveness and reaction time.

Stroop colour-word test (Stroop 1935). A test of speed of colour naming and word reading speed which also provides a measure of proneness to distraction by irrelevant stimuli.

Matching familiar figures test (Kagan *et al*. 1964). A picture matching test designed to measure cognitive style on the reflective-impulsive continuum.

Object naming test (Oldfield and Wingfield 1964). A test of speed of picture naming, designed to quantify word finding difficulties.

Verbal fluency (Borkowski *et al*. 1967). Naming tasks which assess the child's ability to produce words of a particular semantic category, and also to name visible objects.

Manual dexterity (Annett 1970). The test measures the time required by the child to move ten pegs from one row of holes to another and involves both gross proximal-distal arm movements and fine motor control.

Repetitive finger movements (Denkla 1973). The number of time the child can press a switch in 20 seconds is measured on electrical counters.

Handedness inventory. The child was asked to perform a number of different activities to determine eye, hand, and foot preference.

By the time of the one year assessment, many of the tests listed above no longer showed significant deficits attributable to head injury. These were omitted from the test battery used at the final follow-up. In their place, new tasks were included to examine residual cognitive deficits in further detail and to explore some of the issues raised by earlier findings from the first year of follow-up. The new tests are listed below:

Reaction time task. Two- and four-choice visual reaction times were measured under 'symbolic' and 'non-symbolic' task conditions (cf. Gronwall and Sampson 1974).

Paced serial addition task (PASAT). A timed task which can be used to measure speed of cognitive functioning. Findings published shortly after the present study was started suggest that the test is sensitive to the effects of relatively mild head injuries (Gronwall and Wrightson 1974; Gronwall and Sampson 1974).

Arithmetic. The arithmetic subtest of the Wechsler Intelligence Scale for Children (revised edition, 1974) was included to provide a rough index of mathematical ability.

Translation task. This task was developed to examine the child's ability to work independently and maintain concentration in conditions approximating those encountered at school or in the course of doing homework. The child was allowed half an hour to translate a short story from Swedish into English with the aid of a simplified dictionary. The number of word units successfully translated was recorded every five minutes and the effects of various extraneous distractions was examined.

Behaviour ratings. At the end of each test session, ratings of various clinical aspects of the child's behaviour were made.

Neurological examination. At the final follow-up 2–3 years after injury, a systematic neurological examination of all children in the severe head injury group was carried out by a research neurologist. Standard methods were used to assess residual cranial nerve and sensory function; posture, gait and coordination; muscular power, tone and deep tendon reflexes.

Current status of the study (March, 1980)
Data collection and analysis have been completed and the results have been prepared for publication (Brown *et al*. 1980; Chadwick *et al*. 1980a, b; Rutter *et al*. 1980). The data are stored on punchcards. No further follow-up is planned.

Advantages of a longitudinal design

The primary advantage of this study lies in its contribution to understanding the *processes* which take place after injury, the natural history of sequelae, and their relation to injury characteristics. It should provide pointers toward identifying those children likely to be most at risk for post-injury difficulties, and toward predicting eventual outcome far more successfully than is currently the case. Such knowledge is clinically useful. Where dissatisfaction is expressed by parents concerning the hospital treatment of their children, lack of information about the chances, rate, and likely extent of recovery is frequently mentioned. Such lack, or felt lack, of adequate knowledge may create problems and uncertainties of many kinds, such as in making arrangements for future care and education.

Whilst recovery is usually the most striking process to be observed after head injury, there may be problems which develop over the course of time. Whereas measures of motor and specific cognitive functioning tend to show gradual improvement until a plateau is reached, there has been some suggestion that measures of behavioural abnormality may show a different pattern with significant problems emerging sometimes only at a relatively late stage (e.g. Black *et al*. 1971). A longitudinal study is essential in clarifying this problem and revealing possible causes operating.

To the extent that problems arise as a result of changes in the social and family response to the child and his injury, longitudinal studies may serve to throw light on the sorts of social changes which put the child at risk. A number of the severely injured children return to their schools only to find that neither they nor their schools can cope with each other. If the child is then moved to a special school there may be difficulties in adjustment for the child and his family. Alternatively, the family may take excessive steps to protect the handicapped child from either the physical or psychological dangers of his environment; or discord within the family may arise or be intensified as a result of anxieties raised by the accident. Again, more disturbance in the child may result. It is only by establishing the temporal sequence of such events that cause and effect can be disentangled, and this can only be done by following the child after his accident.

In addition to the research questions which longitudinal studies of head injury may serve to answer, they have a useful quasi-clinical role. A previous study of children with compound depressed fractures (Shaffer *et al*. 1975) showed that the hospital follow-up of such cases was often inadequate and inappropriate. Whilst longitudinal studies cannot be regarded as having an institutional role in dealing with problems such as those of head injured children, they can, through their duration, fulfil an important role in affecting a liaison between the child's family and the various treatment and social service agencies.

Limitations of prospective longitudinal studies

An essential feature of this type of prospective longitudinal research is the need for repeated measures. Such measures are decided upon, assembled, and then made at regular intervals on the sample under study. As those involved in the administration of tests, questionnaires, and interviews gain closer familiarity with the distinctive features of their population, the measures will come to be seen as only partially appropriate, and ways in which such measures could be improved will become apparent. In some cases innovative measures may be revealed as unreliable. In others, practice effects on the measures may appear and make interpretation of the data difficult. Either way, the longer the study progresses the more remote becomes the point at which a decision was reached about the appropriate measures to be included. When such studies end, the data which are analysed provide answers to questions which were formulated and put into operational terms a long time earlier. Longitudinal research in this respect is a somewhat cumbersome and inflexible tool, which allows only limited outlet for new ideas to be expressed in the form of new measures, and for these ideas to be examined empirically. Inevitably, such disadvantages have applied to the present study. However, they have been outweighed by the strengths in providing an adequate methodological framework for resolving the questions we set out to answer.

Administrative details

The study was funded from June 1974 to April 1977 by grants from the Mental Health Research Fund to Professor Michael Rutter and from H. S. Weavers and Co. to Dr D. Shaffer. Since May 1977 the study has been wholly supported by a grant from the Department of Health and Social Security to Dr D. Shaffer and Professor M. Rutter. Throughout the project the principal investigators have been Dr Oliver Chadwick (research psychologist) and Mrs Gillian Brown (research social worker).

57. Development among mentally defective children: a report on research in progress (France)

R. MISES and R. PERRON

Principles of the study

Until recently, mental deficiency states in childhood and adolescence were conventionally regarded as states of retardation. In the conventional model the term retardation has implied three conditions: a clear deficiency in intellectual capacity (usually demonstrated by means of intelligence tests); an organic origin of the deficiency, arising through mishap or heredity; and a prognosis of permanent intellectual deficiency ('incurability'), assumed as a result of the organic origin. The assumption has generally been that any treatment or educational measures undertaken, can only help the subject to utilize his capacities as best as he can, the limitations being insuperable.

This type of approach confuses diagnosis with prognosis, and has given rise to much controversy. Some longitudinal or semi-longitudinal studies have attempted to check the soundness of this conventional approach by focusing on the aspect of prognosis. The method used generally has involved measurement of IQs over a period of years to determine any changes. However, there were major methodological objections to this research, involving questions of universal validity and comparability of evaluations of children, adolescents, and adults, and problems which arose from the initial sampling and subsequent living conditions of the subjects. In addition, in many longitudinal studies, the thinning out of the sample group over a period of time introduces a gradual additional selection governed by criteria which are difficult to determine. Therefore, a different approach and a far different theoretical background must be adopted in carrying out such studies. This would include:

(1) Granting that there are widely differing nosographic pictures in the general field of mental deficiency, which means that greater importance must be attached than in the past to a simultaneous structural, functional, and genetic analysis of the pathological mental states responsible for a given condition, and hence that the criteria by which the initial sample is compiled must be listed in far greater detail;

(2) Carefully analysing the sociological and familial surroundings of children and adolescents sampled in the longitudinal study;

(3) Using a much more detailed system of periodic observation than the simple 'universal' intelligence tests which lead to the establishment of a uniform IQ.

These are the basic principles we have used in our research, described briefly in the present paper. We have, however, also been governed by a desire to initiate the study as early as possible in childhood.

Diagnosis and prognosis of deficiency states in childhood: some theoretical propositions

In any longitudinal study of defective structures, the sometimes decisive influence of neurobiological factors is worth bearing in mind, but at the same time the child's deficiency and disjointed development should not be equated with a direct expression of a dysfunction in the nervous system which ignores the gulf existing between the organic and the clinical. No more should any weight be attached to the exaggerations and simplifications uttered by the proponents of a pure psychogenesis for such conditions, though due credit should be given to the latter for pointing out certain important factors to be found in the relationship between the child and his family and society.

Many factors seem to be closely interwoven, and it may never be possible to measure exactly what stems from a dysfunction having

an organic causation and what results from distortions of a relational nature introduced at key phases in the establishment of the
personality. If proven organic damage is responsible for introducing relational disturbances, then conversely the psychogenetic factors least open to doubt have an impact on the way cognition and
instrumental function emerge and take shape. The crux is to be
found in the dialectic linking the two. In other words, there is no
'aetiology' of mental retardation but certain 'conditions' presiding
over its appearance, a fact which considerably diminishes the scope
of any classification devised from an aetiological basis. (A fuller
description of the implications derived from this theoretical stand is
available from the authors.)

Problems of method

From the point of view of method the work described in this paper is
significantly different from the pattern which ordinarily prevails in
longitudinal studies. In fact, we have taken an unusual risk which
we consider essential to justify, in dealing with the problem common to all such research, i.e. the need to choose between extensive
and intensive study. The pattern normally adopted consists in defining, in accordance with predetermined sampling rules, a group of
subjects termed 'cohort' who are studied over a period of time. A
number of technical problems must then be solved, which involves
the establishment of an initial sample that is as large in number as
possible, to ensure that it is representative, to offset diminution in
the numbers studied, and to be able to employ the statistical tools
considered essential, etc. In addition, only a limited amount of data
may be collected on each subject, for practical and financial
reasons. However, these procedures suffer from serious shortcomings as regards the study of mentally deficient children. At the
sampling stage the temptation exists for using a quite illusory
nosographic taxonomy; at the data collection and processing stage,
it is possible to lose sight of the multiple significance of each
symptom. We have therefore chosen to carry out a study primarily
based on a small number of cases and, by way of compensation,
investigating these cases in great detail so as to release a considerable amount of information on each of the subjects. The statistical
treatment of the data is consequently very different from that
generally used in extensive studies.

This type of intensive longitudinal investigation results in considerable importance being given to anamnestic and clinical procedures and to direct observation, and also to a strong background
of the requisite theory needed to govern the collection, collation,
and interpretation of such complex data. As regards the procedures, our research has primarily been conducted in an establishment where children and adolescents are treated on an in-
patient basis for a number of years, and is thereby carried out in
exceptionally favourable conditions. As regards the theoretical
background, our conceptual tools are drawn from a theory of child
psychopathology relying on psychoanalysis for a large proportion
of its references. This fact obviously raises difficult problems in
relation to the objectivity of the procedures involved in the collection, processing, and interpretation of the facts. Such problems are,
however, not peculiar to our approach and it is a well known fact
that the constantly necessary co-ordination between empirical
observation and the theory governing the latter are problems lying
at the very core of modern scientific epistemology. However, here
the general epistemological problem has a particular cast of its own
as regards intensive research into the psychopathology of children.
Moreover, the fact that longitudinal study of fairly extensive duration is involved creates additional difficulties resulting from 'time
drift' in terms of technique and theory which must be reckoned
with. Though it is not possible here to discuss the matter in any
greater detail, this type of problem should be noted.

We would also like to note that any study of this nature, irrespective of whether it is extensive or intensive, is bound to raise one
problem which is particularly delicate. Where a group of children
presenting with a certain type of problem is followed throughout
their development, the given study will obviously have the intention
of analysing their development in terms of the circumstances in
which they are placed. However, when, as is normally the rule, their
condition is being improved as much as possible by treatment and
education, one basic goal becomes an evaluation of the efficacy of
such intervention. The investigators are thereby faced with far
different conditions from those existing when the evaluation of a
development process unconnected with any research-linked intervention is involved, i.e. in 'natural' conditions (a term over which it
is important not to be misled, meaning simply that the researcher is
allowing 'normal' developmental conditions to come into play even
if he is taking account of them in his study plan as independent
variables). In work aiming at this type of evaluation of efficacy,
there is a temptation to resort to conventional 'control group'
techniques, made up of subjects as comparable as possible with
those of the experimental group but who are not undergoing any
intervention designed to improve their development conditions.
This obviously raises ethical objections of a serious kind; even if it
were possible to avoid this by finding a sufficient number of cases
for whom, for reasons unconnected with the researcher's will, no
treatment was possible, by all accounts the control sample which
resulted would no longer be comparable with the experimental
group. The elegant solution of a control group is therefore scarcely
possible, although differently constituted groups may be comparable as regards the nature of their initial problems or their
developmental conditions. This latter solution is the one that we
adopted.

Base-line studies

The research presented here has developed out of two previously
published studies. The first of these (Mises *et al*. 1971) was conducted on a group of 34 children in full-time care at the Fondation
Vallée, an institution for children displaying fairly serious mental
handicaps. The sample in the first study consisted of 34 girls whose
ages ranged between 8 and 11; their IQs, drawn up on the NEMI
scale, ranged between 31 and 80. Using an in-depth clinical
analysis, the children were divided up into three groups which
reflect our theoretical concerns:

Group A: Psychotic structure expressed as deficiency (10 children).
Cases in which a clear psychotic core was present, secondary processes were very precarious, and relational behaviour was quite
fragile.

Group B: Developmental disharmony with underlying psychosis (12
children). Representing cases where there is less evidence of a
psychotic core in the real symptoms displayed. In this group, secondary processes are less precarious than in Group A, and ensure both
better integration of the drives as well as of thought processes; the
way in which relational behaviour is managed is more successful,
the adaptive capacity is greater, and anxiety is less crushing. There
is a very noticeable difference in institutional life between children
in this group and those in the preceding category. The superstruc-
tures at the level of neurosis have succeeded in developing better
and more effectively than those in the first group. The psychotic
core is more difficult to reveal, even though it exists.

Group C: Disharmony deficiency in neurotic structures (12
children). Cases which can be distinguished from those in the
previous category by their greater skill in dominating upwellings of
primitive drives. In these cases we use the term neurotic structure
because in certain areas of behaviour the level of development
permits an opening up to sophisticated modes of investment and

identification. The degree of mental deficiency is consequently less marked than in the previous groups. (For a fuller description of these categories see Mises *et al.* 1971.)

Only those cases where a clear-cut structural diagnosis could be obtained, according to our theoretical criteria, were used for this study.

The cognitive functions of the 34 children were analysed using a battery of mental development test scales specially developed for the purposes of the present study. These scales are called Differential Scales of Mental Efficiency (Echelles Differentielles D'Efficience Intellectuelle: EDEI, Perron-Borelli 1974). The primary aim in designing the scales was to break with the illusions conjured up by the concept of a 'universal' mental level and with the way it is usually expressed in terms of one intelligence quotient. We chose to centre our evaluation method on processes related to the ability to symbolize and arrive at abstract concepts, which previous work had shown to be of key importance in intellectual development and which were understood to be selectively altered through disturbances or delay in such development. There are three scales related to mental activities of this type and for comparative analysis purposes 'practical adaptability' and 'social intelligence' tests were also introduced into the battery. The conventional distinction in intelligence testing between verbal and non-verbal tests was maintained, since a number of earlier studies suggested that decreased command of language was a very widespread feature of mental deficiency. The functional role of this selective deficiency in the genesis of mental retardation itself remains to be elucidated and was, in fact, one of the subjects of our study.

The results obtained by means of this type of analysis in the 34 cases in our sample made it possible for the double problem of structural diagnosis and prognosis to be restated in precisely the type of terms which led us to the present subject of study. The results revealed selective deficiency in the subjects examined, regardless of which group they belonged to, as regards their comprehension and abstraction abilities, in particular when it was a matter of establishing and making use of classes or categories of things. The results confirm and amplify earlier conclusions and can be considered as descriptors of a very general mode of deficiently functioning intelligence.

A second study utilizing the same methods but relating to 40 children aged between 8 and ten attending remedial classes in a school and at the level of what is conventionally termed 'mental deficiency', arrived at the same conclusion (Mises *et al.* 1974). In the following we refer to the subjects of the second study as Group D.

Significant differences among the four groups studied were found:

1. The gap between the two modes of mental operation under consideration was at its greatest for Group A (psychotic structure expressed as deficiency), less as regards Group B (disharmony with underlying psychosis), and still less for Groups C and D (disharmony in neurotic structures and retarded children from remedial classes). In the last two groups, the capacities to abstract and to symbolize (in relation to physical operations) were, relatively speaking, intact so long as language was not involved either as the substance of a test or as a vehicle for response;

2. The cases where deficiency psychosis was expressed (Group A) also displayed a very low level of social intelligence (skill in identifying relationships, social custom and convention, rules and roles, etc.) while conversely, such children succeeded in acquiring relatively sophisticated practical skills (given their very low mental capacity);

3. On the other hand, social intelligence appeared to be much better in cases with deficiency in neurotic structures (Group C)

and among those having 'slight or moderate mental disability' (Group D) but who remained within their families and were educated in special classes within ordinary educational establishments. These findings tended to confirm the theoretical expectations of the investigators.

Method used in the present study

Given the findings from these earlier studies, we have reformulated the links between diagnosis and prognosis as follows:

(1) Deficiency psychoses of childhood are displayed in seriously crippling mechanisms, in particular a critical shortcoming in the ability to produce abstract concepts or symbols. This fact leads to a rather pessimistic prognosis; the permanence of such overt disturbances, which are in turn fed by massive distress, persists in blocking mental development, and in levelling down mental ability to a very low standard;

(2) Developmental disharmony with underlying psychosis makes for a less pessimistic prognosis, in particular with regard to the use of language;

(3) Developmental disharmony in neurotic structures carries an even better prognosis. In this case, the structuring of the ego and adaptive capacity, the ability to produce symbols, and a broader grasp of language may set a process in motion leading to something like normalcy (where in some cases the subject may cease to be considered 'retarded' in the conventional meaning of the term).

Our present research is based on these hypotheses and is broken down into four activities:

(1) A re-examination after seven years of 20 out of the 34 cases studied under the research project summarized above, re-evaluating the way they have developed in the intervening period (consisting of 20 subjects still present in the Foundation, under observation for 10 to 12 years, and now between 15 and 18 years of age);

(2) A re-examination after between five and seven years, depending on the individual, of subjects forming the sample group used in the complementary study (1974) who were at that time pupils in special classes in the normal public education system (Group D);

(3) Extension of the study to very early screening, from the first year of life. This means checking and analysing 'warning signs' (initially in relation to the worries of those surrounding a child), by means of which note is taken of children who *could* develop deficient structures. The plan of work makes provision for a systematic comparison from this standpoint of cases which subsequently do develop defective structures and of those which do not.

(4) A re-examination of warning signs at the age of entry into primary school, in the 6–8 year age range. As part of this activity systematic analyses will be made of the reasons given by teachers who request admission of a given child to a remedial class; the analyses obtained will be compared, according to whether the child is or is not subsequently placed in such a class.

The four projects prove to lend themselves to varying degrees of implementation, for practical reasons. For the present, therefore, we will confine ourselves to a few comments on the first activity, which has so far registered the most progress. In this activity, the 20 subjects concerned are undergoing systematic case-by-case re-examination, including psychiatric reassessment, tests (the Differential Scales of Mental Efficiency or EDEI, overall intelligence tests, projective tests, etc.), and the collating of information contained in the file which has been used to 'follow up' the everyday life of the child throughout the seven years that have elapsed since the original study. At the moment of preparing the present interim paper, the material involved has still only been partially collected and processed. Nonetheless it is already possible to find in it a broad confirmation of the arguments put forward above as regards the links between diagnosis and prognosis. Cases of developmental disharmony in neurotic structures prove to have retained the most promise of development, though this is far from meaning that

normalcy in the development of intellectual capacity and good adaptation to the world surrounding them will always be obtained. On the contrary, the more obvious and the more active the psychotic core underlying the mental deficiency, the more serious will this deficiency remain and the more striking will be the relational disturbances and the psychopathy ruling them. Our present study, however, will doubtless make for better understanding of the 'retardation' processes in some cases of psychosis or disharmony with underlying psychosis.

58. Relapse of drunkenness (Sweden)

PER-ANDERS RYDELIUS

Introduction

The consumption of alcohol in Sweden has increased markedly since the Second World War, and in connection with changes in the political attitude towards alcohol. During the years 1946–50 3 litres of 100 per cent alcohol was consumed per inhabitant per year. In 1974 this figure was 6 litres, and by 1976 it had risen to 8 litres. The number of consumers of spirits, and also the number of offences committed under the influence of drink has increased and spread to even younger age groups. Despite this, and the fact that alcohol overconsumption comprises one of the larger social problems, drunken offences in children and adolescents have as a rule been considered as slight infringements. They have not led to further awareness or increased activity from child guidance or child welfare authorities.

Until 1 January 1977 in accordance with Swedish legislation, a drunken offence was considered a criminal act, and anyone found drunk by the police was routinely taken into custody at the police station. The subject was then allowed to sober up and later go home. At a later date, a magistrates court sentenced the offender to a fine. Registration of the drunken offence was recorded in both the local register as well as in a national register specially assigned for offences committed under the influence of alcohol. In reference to children and adolescents, notification was regularly made to the child welfare authority, when, usually after an investigation, the case was often dropped without procedural action.

Collett (1963) showed that the risk for relapse in drunkenness is greatest in the youngest age group, and that the earlier alcohol consumption was established the graver the prognosis for future alcohol addiction. Over half of the boys in the age group 15 to 17 years who were registered for first-time drunkenness relapsed at least once during an observation period. The risk for relapse increased with each new drunken offence so that the statistical risk for relapse into debauch after three drunken offences was more or less 100 per cent.

In order to obtain more knowledge of the risks of future alcohol addiction in children, a longitudinal prospective investigation was started in Stockholm in 1964 (Nylander and Rydelius 1973). The aim of the investigation was to detect clinically useable data for prognostic assessment when dealing with a case of first-time drunkenness.

Subjects and methods

All boys under 18 years of age, who were not previously known for asocial behaviour or addiction, and who came into custody for drunken offences in Stockholm, Sweden, during the period August – December 1964, were included in the investigation. The material consisted of 52 boys with a mean age of 16 years 3 months (range 14–17 years). Information was collected regarding the parents' situation, home relationship, the boys' previous social adjustment, previous alcohol habits, and circumstances surrounding the drunken episode which led to arrest. Supplementary information was obtained by a child psychiatric examination, which involved a case history obtained from the parents and a subsequent psychiatric assessment of the child. The boys' records, concerning relapses into drunkenness, were examined five years after the first drunken offence.

Results

All the boys came from Stockholm, the majority having grown up and living in a complete home. The majority also belonged to social group III and had 2 – 3 siblings. In a remarkably high proportion (in 31 per cent of cases), the father had a history of psychogenic disease or alcoholism. Psychogenic insufficiency in the mothers was less evident (in 21 per cent of cases).

Twenty-five per cent of the boys had symptoms of psychogenic insufficiency and similarly 25 per cent of the children had sought medical help for nervous troubles. Twelve of the children (23 per cent) drank alcohol regularly at the time of the first drunken offence, while the others had only sporadically tasted drinks containing alcohol. About half of the boys (44 per cent) showed a marked anxiety state when taken into custody by the police.

Relapse into drunkenness during a 5-year period

Twenty-three of the boys during the following 5-year period relapsed into drunkenness at least once. In eight cases this took the nature of one relapse of drunkenness, in seven cases two relapses of drunkenness, in two cases three relapses of drunkenness, and in one case each of four, six, eight, twelve, fourteen, and fifteen relapses of drunkenness.

Factors of prognostic significance

In order to determine factors of prognostic significance, eight boys who had been recorded for at least three relapses of drunkenness were compared with 29 boys who had not been registered for relapse. It was found that a mentally ill or alcoholic father, previously evident symptoms of psychogenic insufficiency, and disciplinary problems at school were significantly more common in the relapse group than in the non-relapse group. Apart from this, it was also demonstrated that the children in the non-relapse group significantly showed remorse and tension prior to the first drunken episode, as compared to the boys in the relapse group who did not react with anxiety when faced with arrest.

The experience and information obtained from this investigation led to the planning of the 'Umeå investigation' (Chapter 59), to determine whether early child psychiatric intervention and treatment could alter the prognosis in juvenile drunkenness.

59. The Umeå investigation: child psychiatric care of young alcoholics (Sweden)

PER-ANDERS RYDELIUS

Introduction

A prospective 5-year follow-up investigation of children up to and including 16 years of age was conducted. These children were treated at a child psychiatric clinic instead of being taken into custody by the police.

Until 1 January 1977 a drunken offence in Sweden was considered a criminal act. As a matter of routine, the police would take charge of the drunken individual and after transportation to the police station, the subject would sober up and be sent home. A trial investigation was started on 1 March 1967 at the Child Psychiatric Clinic at the University of Umeå to study whether it was possible, with the help of child psychiatric treatment, to prevent any relapse of drunkenness, and also to obtain further information of a predictive nature for use in the prognostic evaluation of drunken offences.

Umeå is a medium-sized university and magistrate town situated in the north of Sweden. It has no heavy industries. During the months November to April each year it has a winter climate with severe cold periods at times. At a meeting between representatives of the authorities concerned and the child psychiatric clinic, it was decided that the police should transport all arrested child and adolescent drunks, up to and including the age of 16 years, to the acute admissions department at the Umeå hospital, instead of the usual custody at the police station. (On those occasions when another criminal offence was suspected, the police were primarily involved in the custody of the youths.) Thus, instead of being jailed to sober up as was previously the case, and instead of waiting 2 to 3 months for the child welfare authorities to contact the child for investigation after the drunken offence, these procedures were replaced by hospital-organized child psychiatric care, with investigation in direct continuity to the drunken offence, and with possibilities to instigate treatment at an early stage. A room was arranged at the child psychiatric clinic where the children could sober up under hospital supervision, could eat, wash, receive their clothes (possibly laundered), and from where their parents could collect them at a later time.

When a child was admitted to the hospital, the case was seen by the physician on duty at the child psychiatric clinic, who took a case history from the child and the parents. The history was taken using a previously designed protocol which encompassed the parental situation, the home environment, the child's earlier social adaptation in the family and at school, previous alcohol habits, and the circumstances surrounding the drunken offence which led to police intervention. The investigation was completed with a physical examination, a psychiatric assessment, and an evaluation of the prognosis with regard to the relevant clinical data.

Depending upon the degree of intoxication, the child could either be admitted to the medical intensive care unit, a paediatric medical ward, or directly to the child psychiatric ward. After sobering up, the child could go home with the parents, start supportive therapy on an out-patient basis, or stay at the clinic for further investigation and treatment. In collaboration with the urban child welfare council, necessary supportive measures in accordance with the Swedish social legislation were also available for those cases where such measures were indicated.

Description of the sample

During the actual time period (1 March 1967 to 30 June 1972) of the investigation, 181 youths up to and including the age of 16 years were taken into custody in Umeå and its nearby surroundings. There were 130 boys and 51 girls with an average age of 15 years 5 months (range 10 years 0 months – 16 years 12 months). Thirty-two of the children taken into custody were Finnish youths on temporary visit to Umeå (the Finnish town of Vasa is the nearest town to Umeå). Since these children were not treated at the child psychiatric clinic in Umeå they were excluded from the investigation. Ninety-two (58 boys and 34 girls) of the remaining 149 children were admitted 99 times to the child psychiatric clinic, while 57 (40 boys and 17 girls) remained in the custody of the police. According to the police, these were kept in custody because of suspicion of a criminal offence, and in some cases because the subject refused to contact the clinic.

The 149 drunken youths did not comprise a randomized selection of the child population in Umeå, but in general came from insufficient or incomplete homes, with a single striving mother, an alcoholic father, or from economic misery. Several of the youths had previously shown disciplinary problems in school, asocial tendencies had been evident in the majority, while 20 per cent had been in receipt of child psychiatric contact before the first drunken offence. Thirty-one (14 boys and 17 girls) of the 92 youths admitted to the child psychiatric clinic lived under secure social circumstances, had previously been socially well adjusted, and exhibited no obvious symptoms suggestive of psychogenic insufficiency. In these cases, the drunken offence was judged to be an isolated event, and further treatment was not considered necessary. Fifteen boys and 6 girls stayed at the clinic for further investigation and treatment, while 29 boys and 11 girls commenced therapeutic out-patient contact subsequent to the first drunken episode.

Follow-up investigation

A 5-year follow-up investigation was conducted for all the children by collection of data from official registers in Sweden. Collection was directed with special reference to data concerning the total number of drunken offences, measures taken by the child welfare authorities, the amount of social assistance paid out, criminality, and sickness certification.

Results of the 5-year prospective follow-up investigation

Relapse of drunkenness. Fifty-two of the boys (53 per cent) and 13 of the girls (25 per cent) relapsed into drunkenness at least once. Advanced relapse, i.e. three or more drunken offences, occurred in 29 boys (30 per cent) and in 2 girls.

Criminality. Twenty-seven boys (28 per cent) and 2 girls (4 per cent) had been recorded in the Criminal Register for criminal acts (especially traffic offences, theft, robbery, and assault). In the majority of cases, the first record in the Criminal Register occurred 3–5 years after the first drunken offence, and at a somewhat shorter time for the children whom the police had retained in custody, as opposed to those children admitted to the child psychiatric clinic. This observation was not, however, unexpected since the majority of the youths were retained in custody by the police because of suspicion of some other criminal offence in connection with the drunken episode. A marked statistical correlation was evident between relapse of drunkenness and registration in the Criminal Register.

Social assistance. Social assistance in the form of economic support had been paid out to 34 boys (35 per cent) and to 13 girls (25 per cent). This support was paid out to 18 boys and to 10 girls on more than isolated occasions. No difference could be seen between the police cases and the hospital cases.

Sickness certification. Sixty-five boys (66 per cent) and 22 girls (43 per cent) were certified sick during the observation period. Absence because of sickness was in excess of 10 days per year in 33 boys (34 per cent) and in 13 girls (25 per cent) (in this age group the average sickness period throughout the country is 9·2 days per year). In the case of 12 boys and 4 girls, however, an absence because of sickness in excess of 30 days per year was recorded, and it must be noted that none of the girls were pregnant. The pattern of absence due to sickness was the same in both hospital and police cases.

Mortality. One boy and one girl died during the observation period, both from suicide. Both exhibited stigmata of severe alcohol problems, the boy having eleven drunken offences, the girl relapsing eight times into drunkenness.

Factors of prognostic significance

The 92 youths, 58 boys and 34 girls, who were admitted to the child and adolescent psychiatric clinic and who were examined by systematic child psychiatric investigation, were compared after division into two groups. One group consisted of children who, during the observation period, did not reappear in relapse of drunkenness (48 cases, 29 boys and 19 girls), and which was called the low risk group. The other group consisted of youths who relapsed at least three times in drunkenness during the observation time (18 cases, 16 boys and 2 girls), and is referred to as the high risk group. In these two groups, the data obtained upon examination in connection with the first drunken episode was compared in relation to records from the official registers during the observation period. Differences were demonstrated between the groups in the following respects:

(1) Boys were overrepresented in the high risk group;
(2) The frequency of children from insufficient home circumstances (psychogenic illness or alcoholism in the parents) or from incomplete homes was greater in the high risk group (72 per cent) as compared to the low risk group (25 per cent);
(3) The frequency of children jailed for drunkenness during week days was greater in the high risk group (61 per cent) in comparison with the low risk group (25 per cent);
(4) Only two children were found in the high risk group from the 31 children admitted to the child psychiatric clinic, who were assessed to live under such good conditions that continual supportive measures were not indicated.

Discussion

Eighteen (20 per cent) of the 92 youths admitted to the hospital developed alcohol addiction during the following 5-year period. This occurred despite early diagnostic identification, and access to both child psychiatric treatment and to other supportive measures. It seems probable that adolescents previously exposed to an insecure social environment with the resultant early development of symptoms of psychogenic insufficiency, have diminished resistance to the various damaging effects of alcohol.

This investigation has been published in detail in Swedish in 1978 in *Läkartidningen*, **75** (16), 1607–11.

60. Mortality rate and causes of death among male alcoholics (Iceland)

ALMA THORARINSSON and TÓMAS HELGASON

Introduction

This project was begun by the authors. The purpose of the study is a comparison of the observed numbers of deaths among 3000 male alcoholics who attended various treatment facilities for the first time during 1951–74, with the expected numbers based on the death rates of the male population in Iceland in the age groups 15 through 69.

Subjects and methods

The subjects have been selected from the psychiatric register by a computer. The registry collected its information from the records of all institutions in Iceland where alcoholics received treatment or rehabilitation during the above-mentioned period. The registry also obtained information about male alcoholics who had been treated by psychiatrists on an out-patient basis, in private practice or at the municipal out-patient clinic in Reykjavík. The mortality among in-patients and those who had only been out-patients, as well as causes of death in the two groups, will be investigated separately.

The following information has been obtained from the registry: the date of birth, date of the first admission to a hospital, or first psychiatric consultation, sex, occupation, residency (urban or town), marital status, primary and secondary diagnosis, as well as delirium tremens. Institutional records are searched for number of admissions.

A maximum follow-up is 24 years; a minimum is 4 years. The follow-up is carried out through the national register and institutional records.

Information pertaining to cause of death is obtained from the Statistical Bureau of Iceland. The date of death is recorded and the cause of death is coded using the Seventh Revision of the I.C.D. of the World Health Organization. Also, the basis for cause of death determination is mentioned. The death rates are standardized by age and sex and given by general and specific causes of death.

The overall relative risk for all age groups was calculated by summarizing the number of observed deaths and the number of expected deaths respectively and by calculating the ratio between these two. The calculation of man-years of exposure to the risk of death was performed by the same method as that of Schmidt and DeLint (1972).

vi. Children at risk

61. A longitudinal study of a risk group in Finland

GUNNEL WREDE, ROGER BYRING, STURE ENBERG, MATTI HUTTUNEN, SARNOFF A. MEDNICK, and CARL GUSTAF NILSSON

Introduction

In this paper we present a longitudinal study of a risk group composed of 212 children of mentally ill (mainly schizophrenic) mothers. The aims of this study are:

(1) To identify factors in the environment which are a threat to the mental health of the children;
(2) To find characteristics that distinguish the schizophrenics during premorbid periods of their lives.

In order to identify factors in the aetiology of schizophrenia we are conducting a follow-up study in Helsinki. The index group is composed of 183 children of schizophrenic mothers and 29 children of psychotic non-schizophrenic mothers. The control group comprises children of well mothers. The project was started in 1974 by Gunnel Wrede, Sarnoff A. Mednick, and Matti Huttunen as a study of the relation between obstetric complications and schizophrenia. Carl Gustaf Nilsson and Roger Byring later joined the project. The project is a risk group study, a special version of the prospective research method.

Risk factors and risk group research

Our assumption is that schizophrenia originates from the influence of a number of factors that may be called risk factors. These influence a person's life long before manifest schizophrenic traits can be observed. The risk factors may comprise everything from genetic dispositions to unfavourable environmental factors. The identification of these risk factors should be the logical basis for primary prevention, the ultimate goal of all research into the aetiology of schizophrenia.

The importance of a risk factor may be estimated by establishing the percentage of schizophrenic cases having been exposed to that factor in relation to the total number of cases (e.g. 10 per cent of the schizophrenics have a schizophrenic mother), or by establishing the percentage of cases of schizophrenia in a group exposed to that factor (e.g. 15 per cent of the children of schizophrenic mothers become schizophrenic themselves, 30–40 per cent of the children whose parents are both schizophrenic become ill themselves)

(Rosenthal 1970). However, all risk factors interact with the personality of the persons who are subject to them and with a large number of environmental factors. Thus, the predictive value of an isolated risk factor tends to be low. A more distinct notion of the role played by a certain risk factor in schizophrenic breakdown would be obtained if a cohort of children were followed up and the network of factors influencing the individuals observed; for example, among those children of schizophrenic mothers who had a schizophrenic breakdown 70 per cent were born with birth complications (Mednick 1970). The design is ambitious but may be realized if one focuses on a carefully selected group of individuals especially exposed to risk factors.

The results of such a study are in principle valid only for the investigated group. The right to generalize from this to other groups of cases depends on the representativeness of the investigated group. Our study does not pretend to give universal answers. Today the knowledge of the aetiology of schizophrenia is limited to a few separate risk factors. But methods have been developed to investigate constellations of risk factors. The next step would be to put these methods into use. The results of one study can only be validated by other studies. It is essential that many parallel studies are carried out with different groups and in different societies. In this way a basis for generalizations will be obtained.

The method by which constellations of factors can be investigated is the risk group method presented by Mednick and McNeil (1968). For our purpose it offers the following advantages:

(1) Control groups may be used—the pattern of factors that influence the growth of the schizophrenics-to-be can be distinguished from the pattern of factors that characterize the growth of well persons;
(2) The results may include effects of variables not foreseen in the hypotheses—the knowledge of relevant factors in the premorbid period is extended;
(3) Data collected during the growth of the children is not biased by an existing diagnosis—the investigation gains in objectivity;
(4) The time relation of the variables is known—the prerequisites for causal interpretations increase.

Schizophrenia and obstetric complications

The first risk factor to be examined here is the health of the mother during the pregnancy and the medical data concerning her delivery. It is generally assumed that an organ or a function is particularly sensitive to the influence of the environment during periods of rapid growth. The younger an individual is the more rapid is his general development. Influence during the foetal period and the delivery is therefore of special interest. Some hundred investigations have tried to establish the possible relation between birth complications and schizophrenia. Two questions stand out:

(1) Do schizophrenic women have more obstetric complications than women in general?

(2) Can the complications be considered a risk factor for schizophrenic breakdown among children of schizophrenic women?

In a survey McNeil and Kaij (1976) analyse a discussion about the aetiological influence of obstetric complications on schizophrenia. The paper presents 12 hypotheses including empirical findings related to each hypothesis. With a few exceptions the findings that elucidate the former question indicate that schizophrenic women do not have more complicated deliveries than others. The birth weight of the infant is dealt with separately. Nine different studies found no significant differences between infants of schizophrenic women and infants of control women. However, a couple of investigations found lower birth weights for the infants of schizophrenic women. The results thus seem inconsistent.

Regarding the second question the authors conclude:

. . . the weight of evidence at the present time might support the hypothesis that obstetric complications (OCs) in general increase risk for all types of schizophrenia (perhaps by default of further evidence), that OCs seem to interact with genetic influence toward schizophrenia, and that OCs occurring previous to schizophrenia in the offspring are independent, stressful factors and not a manifestation of 'schizophrenic' genes (McNeil and Kaij 1976; p. 39).

In our study of the relation between birth complications and schizophrenia we use a design in which we contrast the children of schizophrenic women ($N = 183$) with the children of well women ($N = 199$) and with the children of psychotic non-schizophrenic women ($N = 29$).

The 212 index children ($183 + 29$) form a cohort comprising all the children born in 1960–4 in Helsinki to all the female patients of the Helsinki mental hospital, 'Hesperia hospital', who at their admittance were diagnosed as schizophrenic or showing schizophreniform behaviour. We carefully checked that the cohort was complete. At Hesperia hospital we listed all female patients with the diagnosis mentioned who were born in 1916–48 ($N = 3243$). From the registers of residents of the city of Helsinki we listed each one of the patients who had given birth to children in Helsinki during the years 1960–4. We then checked the files at the birth clinics in Helsinki. The birth records of 199 children were found at the two big birth clinics. The other 13 children were either born at home (3) or at the small private clinics (10) where only poor records are kept. One matched control was chosen for each index child born at one of the two big clinics, i.e. the child who according to the patient number was born immediately before the index child.

A re-diagnosis of the illness of the mothers was made by a psychiatrist, Matti Huttunen. The categories that were used are presented in Table 61.1.

Status of data

The following data have been collected, coded, and punched:

1. The physical health of the mother during pregnancy (source: record from the Well Mother's Clinics);

2. The course of delivery (source: the birth record from the birth clinic);

3. The health of the child, aged 0–7 days (source: the birth record);

4. Social group of mother and father at the time of the index child's birth (source: the birth record);

5. Mother's admissions to mental hospitals in Finland (source: case records from different mental hospitals);

6. Mother's gynaecological history (source: mother's retrospective statements given at the birth clinic);

7. Mother's earlier pregnancies and deliveries (source: mother's retrospective statements given at the birth clinic at the time of birth of the index child).

Neurological examination

A follow-study of these children was conducted when they were aged 13–17 years. This follow-up included a neurological examination.

TABLE 61.1

Distribution of children according to the seriousness of mother's illness

Chronic schizophrenia with permanent social deficiency	58
Acute psychotic states, non-paranoid form, 3 or more admissions	46
Acute psychotic states, paranoid form, 3 or more admissions	31
Acute psychotic state, non-paranoid form, 1–2 admissions	28
Acute psychotic state, paranoid form, 1–2 admissions	20
Total	183
Definitely not schizophrenia	29

One of the reasons why birth complications may increase the risk of schizophrenia could be that a child delivered with complications may then develop neurological defects (see Cohler *et al.* 1975). The defects may retard the child's development (Whittam *et al.* 1966) and cause an increased vulnerability to maladjustment. A couple of risk group studies indicate that birth complications may have a special effect on children with psychotic parents (Gallant 1975; Mednick *et al.* 1971).

The study children now living in Helsinki and surroundings will be contacted to take the neurological examination. The aim of this part of the study is to compare the following four groups:

(1) Index children born with complications;
(2) Index children born without complications;
(3) Control children born with complications;
(4) Control children born without complications.

What is to be considered a birth complication has been defined by an obstetrician, Carl Gustaf Nilsson. He examined all the birth records and graded the deliveries according to the following criteria:

(1) No complications:
   birth weight at least 2500 g;
   duration of delivery no more than 24 h;
   foetal heart rate 160/min – 120/min;
   Apgar score 7–10.
(2) Moderate complications:
   birth weight at least 2500 g;
   duration of delivery 25–36 h;
   amniotic fluid meconium stained;
   foetal heart rate 180–160/min or 120–100/min;
   heavy analgesic medication during the course of delivery;
   Apgar score 4–6;
   abnormal presentation without acute distress;
   elective Caesarean section.

(3) Severe complications:
   birth weight under 2500 g;
   duration of delivery more than 36 h;
   foetal heart rate over 180/min or under 100/min;
   abnormal presentation;
   instrumental delivery;
   Apgar score 0–3;
   haemorrhaging during the I and II stage of delivery.

A case was assigned to group 3 if two or more of the criteria listed in group 2 occurred. Abnormal presentation refers mainly to breech presentation. Instrumental delivery includes also all but elective Caesarean sections (Barker 1966; Fairweather and Illsley 1960; Rauramo *et al.* 1961).

The neurological examination will be carried out by a physician, Roger Byring. In connection with the examination the children will be tested with some factor tests of intelligence (Heinonen 1963). A short standardized interview planned by a psychologist, Sture Enberg, is added. The parents are asked to give anamnestic data about the child. Roger Byring developed both the medical part of the examination and the questionnaire for the parents.

We have just started the neurological examination. As yet we have no guarantees that it will turn out well. There are very few neurological tests standardized for the age group in question (Peters *et al.* 1975; Spreen and Gaddes 1969). However, a pilot study indicates that our battery of tests discriminates among adolescents. We try two ways of data collection:

(1) to invite the children to a teenager polyclinic for the examination and
(2) to go to the children's school and do the examination during school time.

In both cases parents and teachers are informed that due to the time and place of birth the children belong to a study group that is being studied by the II Paediatric Clinic of Helsinki University and The Department of Psychology at Åbo Academy. We promise to inform the families about possible illnesses found and to suggest treatment.

Signs of vulnerability in adolescence

The schizophrenic breakdown is considered to occur at the earliest in adolescence. The teens may thus be considered a critical period from an aetiological point of view. Referring to their empirical research Strutt and Watt (1975) even suggest that the optimum time to identify children 'at risk' for schizophrenia is early adolescence.

We chose our index group so that it would be possible to collect data about the children's personalities and social adjustment in this critical period of life. The children's development from birth to adolescence can be followed only by means of medical and social registers and by retrospective information given by the parents.

It is possible that in some cases the schizophrenic breakdown occurs suddenly and without earlier signs of social maladjustment or personality problems. But it is probable that the breakdown, in at least some of the cases, is preceded by a primary process of illness. In the latter case the individuals are characterized by a certain stability and consistency in their personality development. It is reasonable to assume that such personality traits and patterns of behaviour may be found in them that may predict a future breakdown. We want to investigate if such signs may be identified among the teenagers in our study.

Personality development may be described by an interactional model of behaviour. According to this model, the individual's behaviour is 'characterized by consistency in terms of coherence, i.e. by idiographic reliable patterns of stable and changing behaviours across situations' (Magnusson 1976; p. 263). The model implies that there are fundamental traits in the personality that are modified by experience during the period of growth and that manifest themselves in different ways in different situations. Research into intelligence empirically supports the hypothesis that fundamental traits exist and that their manifestations in measurements may be constant if the measurements are done under highly standardized conditions. Analogously one can assume the existence of other fundamental personality traits, e.g. patterns of reactions which, with some variations, determine the behaviour of an individual in interpersonal situations.

The concept of vulnerability in psychopathology may be considered one such basic trait. The concept is a theoretical construct which refers to mediating processes not measurable as such. Like other psychic functions, vulnerability is assumed to vary in intensity among individuals. The more risk factors an individual is exposed to and the more experiences of threat against his mental health he has, the more severe his vulnerability is supposed to be. His stored information about his identity and his environment is loaded with negative experiences. These experiences may be limited to some particular social institutions in which he is involved (e.g. his home) or may include several (e.g. his home, school, and hobbies). This variation is likely to be reflected in the measurements of vulnerability. In the former case correct measurement of vulnerability will result in intersituational variance. In the latter case consistency over situations is expected.

Two different kinds of findings provide empirical support to the hypothesis that vulnerability is a fundamental personality trait. One kind of finding is based on a theory of schizophrenia proposed by Mednick (1962). The illness is described as a learned thought disorder reinforced by anxiety reduction. The fact that emotional states, among them anxiety, can be registered in several systems (verbal–cognitive, motoric, and physiological) is incorporated in the theory. Anxiety is registered as physiological arousal that is concomitant with the experienced state. In one theory, Mednick explains hypothetically how individuals with a certain physiological disposition develop schizophrenic traits by learning. Empirical results support the theory showing a relation between the physiological disposition and schizophrenic breakdown (Mednick 1970).

Another kind of finding seems to detect vulnerability from a purely empirical point of view. Retrospective *ex ante facto* studies deal with data based on direct observation of a phenomenon but collected for scientific purposes at a later point of time. These studies show a continuity of adjustment style over time that is 'much more impressive than the evidence of dramatic changes' (Watt 1978). The findings thus support the hypothesis of a basic personality trait. Furthermore, the findings show that 30–50 per cent of the children who at a later date develop schizophrenia are easily detected as deviant in school. School behaviour as a risk factor does not occur in aetiological theories which stress home conditions. It seems reasonable to assume that vulnerability tends to manifest itself in different connections and with some intersituational consistency.

Interestingly enough, the personality of pre-schizophrenic boys differs from that of girls. Negativistic, egocentric, and antisocial traits are characteristic of the boys, while the girls are introverted and silent though also egocentric. Both sexes are emotionally unstable and immature (Watt and Lubensky 1976). This corresponds well with the description of children with schizophrenic mothers obtained from prospective studies (Weintraub *et al.* 1975). Teachers rate these children higher than children with normal mothers on dimensions of classroom disturbance, disrespect–defiance, and inattentiveness–withdrawal. They are rated lower on comprehension, creative initiative, and relatedness to teachers.

The attributes mentioned may be considered concrete expressions of vulnerability. As such they have aetiological value.

They indicate indices of schizophrenia by stating that a certain percentage of schizophrenics show certain forms of behaviour. They will have prognostic value only when the percentage of schizophrenics is determined among individuals who behaved in the above-mentioned way. Finally they will have explanatory value when the behaviour traits are put into a model of measurement which indicates why vulnerability as a latent property is reflected in the behaviour variables in question.

The measurement of vulnerability among our risk group children

Our intention is to try to identify those children in the risk group who manifest signs of vulnerability. We seek primarily expressions that fill the practical requirements of measurement techniques, expressions that can be measured quickly and inexpensively in a group scattered over a wide area. Expression that fill these requirements of measurement will be of great value in the prophylactic work that aims at primary prevention of schizophrenia.

During this academic year (1977) we are collecting data on the school behaviour of our risk group. At a later point in time we hope to find out whether any of the index or control children have been admitted to a mental hospital. It will then be possible to estimate the prognostic value of the description we get this year of the pattern of behaviour of the teenagers.

As sources of information we use the study children's classmates and teachers of Finnish. We use self-ratings as well. For the stated aim the combination of these three means has been shown to be superior to other sources available in this study (Bower *et al.* 1961). Classmates and teachers have had numerous opportunities to become familiar with the study children's behaviour in school. They have also developed their own norms for rating normal teenage behaviour. In comparison with the study children's own parents these teachers are qualified to be more objective. Other studies testify that classmates and teachers possess an ability to identify children with emotional problems (see survey of literature in Strutt and Watt in press).

We constructed a peer rating scale which is based on the knowledge about premorbid traits that is available at present. The instrument comprises 44 personality attributes. The reliability of each item has been estimated separately. Items with low reliability were excluded. The teachers are required to answer two rating scales. One scale is a Finnish version of the Hahnemann High School Behaviour Rating Scale (Spivack and Swift 1972). The other scale uses the lay-out of Lambert and Hartsough's Pupil Behaviour Rating Scale (1973). The pupils are rated by the teachers on 11 scales. Detailed verbal descriptions of separate points of the scale aim at uniformity of the interpretation of the grades on the scale.

In order to protect the anonymity of the index children all the classmates of the same sex as the study child rate each other. Neither the pupils nor the teachers know which one of the children belongs to our study. Later the teacher will perform her rating of the study child as well as of a control child chosen at random from the class. To guarantee the teacher's co-operation with the project, we obtained a written recommendation for the project from the Central Board of Schools, and from the Trade Union of the Teachers. The teachers will get a fee for their contribution, the amount of which is stated by their trade union.

Special problems of the project

The project progresses at a rate restricted by its modest budget. Greater resources would not only have speeded up the work but would also have increased the possibilities of tracing those study children who, under prevailing circumstances, will apparently be lost. The size of the loss is still impossible to estimate.

Results

The analyses done until now show several tendencies for the index children to start their lives under slightly more unfavourable conditions than the controls. Briefly, though medical care is free of charge and offered all pregnant women, 9 per cent of those who later developed chronic schizophrenia had almost no predelivery medical care whatsoever; 1·6 per cent of the controls had almost no predelivery care. The index mothers who accepted medical care complained more than the controls about nausea, heartburn, and headache. At the mothers' arrival at the birth clinic, symptoms of illness (e.g. proteinuria, hypertension) were noted significantly more often among the index than among the control subjects. Of the foetuses of the chronic schizophrenics, 9 per cent had their heart sound affected, while the corresponding figure for the controls was 0·5 per cent. The manner of birth for the index subjects differed more often from what is considered normal (Caesarians, breech presentations, etc. . .). The index mothers gave birth to more prematures (11 per cent among the chronics; 3 per cent among the controls). The birth weight of the neonates was slightly lower among the index children. As a whole, 15–24 per cent of the index subjects (depending on the subgroups) were considered to have severe complications during the delivery; 9 per cent of the controls had severe complications. At last, nurses notes about the health of the neonates taken during their first day of life and during the six following days indicated that the control babies were in better health.

The follow-up of the index and control groups is proceeding. At this point it is clear that the index group begins life with a more difficult birth and a poorer state of health. The untangling of the relative importance of these perinatal conditions, the genetic background, and their interaction will be the future task of this project.

62. Schizophrenics' offspring reared in adoptive homes (Finland)

PEKKA TIENARI

Review of related studies

The rates of schizophrenia have been significantly higher for the sibs of schizophrenia index cases than for the general population. The median risk for second-degree relations has been lower than the median risk for the sibs. The median risk for third-degree relatives has been lower than the median rate for second degree relatives and higher than the median rate for the general population. The concordance rate for MZ twins has always been higher than that for DZ twins. Children who have one schizophrenic parent have about a 10 per cent median risk of developing schizophrenia themselves. When both parents are schizophrenic, the median risk in children increases to about 40 per cent. All these findings are consistent with the genetic hypothesis. On the other hand shared environments occur to lesser extents as the degree of blood relationship becomes further removed, thus possibly accounting for the observed correlations.

Family-dynamic studies have revealed both the frequent occurrence of disorders graver than the neuroses in the members of the families of schizophrenic patients, and the presence of certain typical disturbances in the interactional relationships between the family members. From the family-dynamic studies carried out, a number of useful experimental techniques for testing interactional relationships and communication models have also emerged.

In seeking to assess the effects of hereditary factors and those of family-dynamic factors separately, psychiatric research is faced with the difficulty that disordered parents, who have transmitted the genetic factors to their offspring, have also generally brought them up. In a study of adoptive children dealing with cases where the offspring of a schizophrenic parent has early enough been given away for adoption, discrimination between these two kinds of factors is possible. Yet the study of adoptive children has so far been rather limited and based on small samples. The newest but still provisional data from the Danish adoption studies (Rosenthal *et al*. 1974; Kety *et al*. 1975) have confirmed the findings of the earlier reports. That is, there were more schizophrenia and schizophrenia-related disorders in the biological relatives of schizophrenic adoptees and in the adopted-away children of schizophrenic parents than in their control groups.

A point open to criticism in these most recent and most careful studies is that the concept of schizophrenia has been replaced by a broader concept of a 'schizophrenia spectrum disorder', which has been made to cover also milder conditions quite different from schizophrenia and even conditions of the character disorder type.

(Wynne *et al*. 1976) were able to find the same type and amount of communication disturbances among adoptive parents of schizophrenic patients as among those parents who had themselves brought up their schizophrenic children. These disturbances did not exist in those adoptive parents whose children were either neurotic or normal.

The present study

In the present study, it has been possible to secure information on most of the women who were under treatment at the Finnish psychiatric hospitals on 1 January 1960, or were admitted in to those hospitals for treatment between 1 January 1960, and 30 April 1970, and were diagnosed as schizophrenics. When only those cases were taken into consideration in which the patients had been born in 1910–1954, a total of 9832 women meeting the criteria were found. The time and age limits were applied, because we believed the older case histories in hospitals to be unproperly filled and to have insufficient information for diagnosis. We also wished to avoid diagnostic difficulties with people over 60 years. Regarding these women, continued efforts have been made for years to find out which of them, after giving birth to a child, have later given the child away for adoption. To this end, the population registers of each locality in which any one of the women concerned had resided during her life had to be consulted, because when a mother moves to another locality, the population register authorities of the new locality are not informed about any of her children possibly adopted away.

A total of 121 children given away for adoption have been identified. Judging by the information thus far secured by us, 93 of them have been placed in adoptive homes in their first four years of life and 10 later than that, while 12 have been adopted abroad and 5

by relatives. The number of these cases is likely to increase, however, because we are still in the process of covering all the psychiatric hospitals in Finland.

The *subject series* consists of the adoptive families into which children born of schizophrenic mothers had been adopted and placed during the child's first four years of life.

A *control series* consists of a *double number* of adoptive families in which neither the adopted child's biological mother nor his father has been under psychiatric treatment. This group will be matched with the subject group as regards the following parameters: the child's age and sex and the age at which he or she was placed in the family, the adoptive family's social class, its urban/rural background and its structure (father and mother vs. only mother or father). *The families in the two series will be numbered at random in such a way that the psychiatrists who perform the personal examination will not know which of the two groups the adoptive family belongs to.*

In the field study we must in practice investigate families living in various parts of Finland. The examination of each family will require at least two days, since the following will be necessary:

1. A careful individual interview of both parents and the 'index child', including psychological tests (Rorschach test and an abridged version of the WAIS for all; MMPI only for children).
2. Examination of the parents' interactional relationship and communication disturbances by means of conjoint interviews and the Spouse Rorschach.
3. Examination of the whole family, particularly the interactional relationships between the children and their parents, with conjoint interviews and application of experimental family-dynamic examination techniques, the Family Rorschach (Loveland *et al*. 1963) and the Interpersonal Perception Method (Laing *et al*. 1966).

The interviews and the experimental parts of the study must be tape-recorded so that in scoring them, use can be made of blind comparative classifications.

Every effort will be made to identify and locate the biological parents in both groups. All the possible registered information is being collected about the children and their adoptive and biological parents.

Research questions

In the study an effort will be made to shed light particularly on the following:

1. The frequency and degree of disturbances in the children belonging to the subject series and the two control series. If disturbances are more frequent and/or more serious in children of the biological parents suffering from schizophrenia in both groups, this would lend support to the hereditary theories;
2. The extent to which the families of disturbed children differ from the families in which the children are not suffering from psychiatric disturbances. Would the health of the family and the absence of certain disturbances seem to prevent the development of disturbances in the so-called risk children? What kinds of disturbances in the family would seem to promote the manifestation of disturbances in the child?
3. By a prospective follow-up of the group of children who are at presently at puberty or younger, it will be possible to investigate the ability of family-dynamic methods to prognosticate the development of graver disturbances in the so-called risk children.

4. To what extent does the degree of severity of the biological mother's illness correlate with the disturbances observed in the adopted child? What is the contribution to the later disturbances in the children adopted to other families of the sick mother and the mother-child relationship that has possibly developed pathologically?

5. The conclusions concerning the prevention of mental health disturbances to be drawn from the results.

The study will be carried out by the Psychiatric Clinics of the Oulu and Turku Universities in co-operation with each other. The following research team was appointed for it in Spring, 1975: Professor Pekka Tienari (principal investigator), Professor Yrjö Alanen (expert in family research), Ilpo Lahti, Lic. Med. (Turku), Mikko Naarala, Lic. Med. (Oulu), and Anneli Sorri, Lic. Med. (Oulu).

63. A fifteen-year follow-up of children with schizophrenic mothers (Denmark)

SARNOFF A. MEDNICK, FINI SCHULSINGER, and PETER H. VENABLES

In the pages which follow we will consider the difficulties of investigating the origins of mental illness by traditional research designs. We will suggest that the prospective–longitudinal–interventive method holds some promise. We will then describe a research programme which may be considered an initial step in this direction.

Problems in traditional research methods in mental health which encourage the consideration of the prospective, longitudinal design

When we consider the prodigious efforts which have been made to understand the aetiology of the variety of psychiatric and social deviance that man exhibits it can prove depressing for a researcher to assess the yield. Some have responded to this apparent lack of progress by searching for mystical sources of understanding, or magical, often poetic treatments. Others have responded with nihilistic humour. One observer has characterized the growing mountain of writings on the aetiology of mental illness as having produced an 'independent problem of waste disposal'. J. N. Morris (1975), the English epidemiologist, has rather dryly commented on schizophrenia research, 'up to now, unhappily, this activity has yielded few new facts; a deficiency somewhat obscured by the communicativeness of psychiatrists and social scientists' (p. 218).

Perhaps, one reason for the impatience with research efforts in this field is the fact that the more 'physical' illnesses have yielded their secrets more readily. There is value in considering some of the reasons for this. Statements of aetiology are statements of causes. It is difficult to construct causal statements without the benefit of experimental manipulation. This is the method of choice in attempts to understand the causes of disease. We can inject a laboratory animal with a suspect virus and observe directly whether it develops a given illness. With proper controls and assuming that the animal succumbs to the illness, we can unequivocally conclude that we have established at least one partial cause of that illness. By analogy, to properly conduct experimental–manipulative research into the causes of psychoses or recidivistic delinquency, we would have to systematically inflict children with those suspect life circumstances (biochemical, physiological, social–environmental) which we hypothesize to be aetiologically important and observe the outcome. Of course we will not and cannot do this research; the experimental–manipulative method is not available to us in research into the causes of mental illness or social deviance. For the more physical illnesses, on the other hand, organ systems sufficiently similar to those of humans may be found in laboratory animals. These laboratory animals can be the subjects for experimental–manipulative research. The organ system under most seri-

ous suspicion in *mental* illness may not be sufficiently similar in man and other animals. (There is also uncertainty among most serious investigators that drug or situationally-induced deviance in laboratory animals or humans are in every way equivalent to a behavioural disturbance acquired by a human over a period of many years.) We are thus forced to ignore our most powerful methods for understanding the causes for human deviance. This is very likely a large part of the reason for our poor progress rather than greater stupidity, laziness, or scientific ineptitude. We are hampered simply because our subjects are human. Because their illnesses are peculiarly human, we are barred from using our most effective tools. Instead, we have struggled to elaborate empirical correlates of human deviance and on this basis to construct theories which we cannot test directly.

Primary prevention research–experimental-manipulative

But there is a way in which clinical research can exploit the efficiency and clarity of the experimental–manipulative method. The same humane code which inhibits us from experimentally manipulating the lives of children in order to attempt to cause them to become mentally ill would only encourage and support careful and well-founded attempts at experimental manipulations which are aimed at preventing mental illness. Let us hasten to make clear that even if such preventive attempts were effective, they would not point directly to aetiology; but let us not be discouraged by this fact. The history of medicine documents clearly that prevention of an affliction can precede full understanding of its cause. Second, the types of interventive manipulations which prove to help to prevent mental illness may suggest where we might most profitably search for causes. For these reasons, research on the primary prevention of human deviance suggests itself then as a method for consideration.

There are other reasons for a shifting emphasis towards research on prevention. Our progress and our capability of maintaining life has actually produced an *increase* in the population of the chronically ill. In a letter to *Lancet*, Gruenberg (1976) has called attention to this unforeseen consequence of the healing profession's increasingly sophisticated technology of treatment. This increase in the number of chronically ill has in turn produced a heightened level of desperate need for treatment in the population. Our response to this desperation has been an increase of treatment technology research. The devotion of an increasing portion of society's resources to research on prevention may help to reduce this accelerating level of human suffering and expenditure of society's resources.

It perhaps should be pointed out that no matter what the causes of mental illness might be, the emphasis on prevention research will very likely be appropriate. If the causes are biochemical or neurophysiological, these conditions may not prove to be readily reversible. It is even more likely that the learned reactions to such biological deficiencies or environmental inadequacies may become extremely difficult to change by the time the condition is recognized. Even if the original cause of a mental or social deviance is removed, the fixed habits of response to such deviance may be resistant to treatment. Primary prevention will cost less and reduce suffering.

Problems in cross-sectional research on deviance

Control groups. The launching of projects in primary prevention of human deviance may seem rather a giant step—perhaps more careful preparation is necessary; perhaps we should wait 100 years more. But we would suggest that it is precisely because of the immature nature of the field that long-term prospective research aimed at primary prevention is necessary. What are the alternatives? The most prevalent alternative is the comparison of the deviant with 'controls'. The researcher typically recognizes that his research design involves some biased selection of deviant cases. An attempt is often made to overcome this bias by observing control groups matched for 'relevant' factors. But do we really know what factors are relevant? We must begin to face the fact that almost any control group we select will be biased in some respects. For example, for valid generalization, the number of patients and controls in a study should be in proportion to their numbers in the population to which you wish to generalize. Otherwise, generalization is likely to be highly fallacious. This oft-repeated fallacy in research design is well known in epidemiological research; it has a name, Berkson's Fallacy. To quote Berkson,

If the sub-population. . . of a group X and its control not-X is not representative in the ratio of the marginal totals of X and not-X. . . in the general population, then association will appear even if it does not exist in the general population from which the study population is drawn. (Berkson 1955)

We might add that associations that do exist in the parent population may also be masked by control groups not representative of the not-X population. This also means that another investigator drawing a small sample from the same control population in the same manner is very likely to select a population biased in some other way. This problem is very likely at the root of most failures to replicate research results in the fields of mental illness and asocial behaviour.

The impossibility of the task of obtaining appropriate control subjects is most dramatically evident in the case of research in schizophrenia. The behaviour of schizophrenics is unquestionably markedly altered in response to the consequences of the illness. The schizophrenic experiences educational, economic, and social failure, pre-hospital, hospital, and post-hospital drug regimens, long-term institutionalization, chronic illness, and sheer misery. It is clear that appropriate control groups are not easily available. Consequently, in comparisons of controls and schizophrenics, it is often difficult to judge what portion of the reported differences have unique relevance to the aetiology of shizophrenia, and what portion is a function of the consequences of schizophrenia. For example, a study by Silverman (1964) demonstrated critical differences between acute and chronic schizophrenics on a perceptual task. Silverman *et al.* (1966) repeated the same tasks with long-term and short-term non-psychiatric prisoners. They found that the differences observed on these tasks among the normals and 'acute' and 'chronic' prison inmates were almost precisely the same as those observed among the normals and acute and chronic schizophrenics. The actual scores for the imprisoned and the hospitalized were highly similar at equal levels of institutionalization. The original differences observed were interpreted as due to institutionalization. Any differences found between schizophrenics and controls can as well be related to the consequences of the illness as to the causes. In effect, schizophrenics may be so contaminated by the consequences of their illness that they are usually not suitable subjects for research into the causes of their own illness. These same conclusions may be drawn at least to some degree with respect to conditions of social deviance and for less serious conditions of mental illness.

Studies of the families of schizophrenics have often been based on the aetiological assumption that disturbed family processes have a role in the development of schizophrenia. It is, however, just as reasonable to assume the obverse of this assumption: that the presence of a schizophrenic child or adolescent plays a role in the development of family disturbance. There is evidence for the latter assumption: studies of families with children with other severe physical illnesses found them to be similar to families with schizophrenic offspring. Note that this does not imply that family variables are not involved in the aetiology of schizophrenia. The study of families in which one member is already schizophrenic is simply not an excellent way to investigate this question.

All of these objections to the cross-sectional study of the correlates of mental illness or social deviance or the differences between deviants and controls are not to suggest that these methods are bankrupt and should be abandoned. The message is that, in addition to such research, carefully controlled, prospective studies of primary prevention of deviance seemed indicated.

But to proceed with this type of research we need:

1. Well-founded hypotheses;
2. Methods for the early detection of individuals in the population who have a very high probability of succumbing to deviance.

The latter need arises because our interventions may be psychologically intrusive. Therefore, we cannot use population-wide broadcasting of intervention such as in fluoridation of water or vaccines. We must restrict ourselves to high-risk groups. Hence the need for early detection.

Early detection of the schizophrenia-prone: fifteen-year follow-up of children at high risk for schizophrenia

This research programme was directed at the problem of the early detection of individuals with a very high likelihood of becoming schizophrenic. It was first formulated in 1960. At that point it was planned to

test and interview a group of normal children. . .from these tests and interviews we shall predict which of these children will become schizophrenic. . .we have decided to select a group in which the prevalence rates are considerably elevated. . . individuals who have one or two parents who have been schizophrenics. If our predictions prove to be supported, we are then in a position to do research which is aimed at the prevention of schizophrenia. We might observe a normal population with our tests, detect those individuals who are potential schizophrenics, and then explore the possibilities of intervention (Mednick 1960; p. 69).

In accordance with this overall plan, in 1962 we intensively examined a group of 207 children at high risk for schizophrenia. (They have schizophrenic mothers.) We also examined 104 control subjects. We followed this group until 1967 when 20 of them evidenced a variety of psychiatric breakdowns. In good agreement with the general theory guiding this research, an autonomic nervous system (ANS) variable, fast recovery rate, proved to be the best variable to discriminate the breakdown subjects from their carefully chosen high-risk and low-risk controls. We then took this 'best discriminator' to Mauritius where we examined the ANS functioning of all of the three-year old children in two communities (1800 children). In accordance with our theoretical position (Mednick 1958; Mednick and Schulsinger 1973) we selected out the 6 per cent of the 1800 (108 children) who evidenced the fastest recovery and greatest responsiveness in the population. Half of these individuals, along with controls, were then placed in specially established and organized nursery schools. The other 54 children were considered community controls, and were only identified in our files. (For the first description of this project see Schulsinger *et al*. 1975). In chapter 69 we shall pick up the thread of the prevention project in Mauritius and relate the promising outcomes observed.

The 20 breakdowns in 1967 ranged from schizophrenia and extreme schizoid states to antisocial behaviour. The follow-up of the Copenhagen high-risk subjects continued in order to see whether ANS recovery and/or other variables would predict specifically to later breakdown with *schizophrenia*. The results of these follow-up activities will form the basis of this paper.

The Copenhagen 1962 high risk project

Method of procedure

In 1962 we intensively examined 207 children at high risk (HR) for schizophrenia. They have schizophrenic mothers. We also assessed 104 children at low risk (LR) for schizophrenia. The identifying characteristics of these samples are given in Table 63.1. Table 63.2 presents the list of examination procedures. Some of the measures which will be critical for our later remarks stem from the interview made by a social worker with the individual responsible for the rearing of the child. From this interview we derived information on the social status and the intactness of the family and retrospective comments on the child's behaviour as an infant and small child.

TABLE 63.1

Characteristics of the experimental and control samples

	Control	Experimental
Number of cases	104	207
Number of boys	59	121
Number of girls	45	86
Mean age*	15·1	15·1
Mean social class**	2·3	2·2
Mean years of education	7·3	7·0
Per cent of group in children's homes (5 years or more)†	14	16
Mean number of years in children's homes (5 years or more)†	8·5	9·4
Per cent of group with rural residence††	22	26

* Defined as age to the nearest whole year.
** The scale runs from 0 (low) to 6 (high) and was adapted from Svalastoga (1959).
† We only considered experience in children's homes of 5 years or greater duration. Many of the experimental children had been to children's homes for brief periods while their mothers were hospitalized. These experiences were seen as quite different from the experience of children who actually had to make a children's home their home until they could go out and earn their own living.
†† A rural residence was defined as living in a town with a population of 2500 persons or fewer.

From the files of the Demographic Institute in Risskov and the mother's hospitalization record we extracted information relating to the form and seriousness of her illness. Danish midwives attended the birth of our subject population and prepared a written report on the pregnancy and delivery which we have coded. The psychophysiology examination yielded two important channels of information: heart rate and electrodermal responding. We shall centre our discussion on the electrodermal behaviour.

TABLE 63.2

List of experimental measures: 1962 high-risk assessment

1. Psychophysiology:
   A. Conditioning–extinction–generalization;
   B. Response to mild and loud sounds.
2. Wechsler Intelligence Scale for Children (Danish adaption).
3. Personality inventory.
4. Word association test.
5. Continuous association test:
   A. 30 words;
   B. 1 min. of associating to each word.
6. Adjective check list used by examiners to describe subjects.
7. Psychiatric interview.
8. Interview with parent or rearing agent.
9. School report from teacher.
10. Midwife's report on subject's pregnancy and delivery.

The first 20 psychiatric breakdowns. Following the intensive examination in 1962, an alarm network was established in Denmark so that most hospital and all psychiatric admissions for anyone in this sample would be reported to us. The number of reports of serious psychiatric or social breakdowns reached 20 in 1967. Very brief summaries of their case histories are given in Table 63·3. We then looked back to our data from 1962 to find characteristics that distinguished the schizophrenia breakdown individuals from carefully matched HR and LR controls. The most important characteristics distinguishing the Sick Group from the controls are given in Table 63.4. We shall call attention to a few of these characteristics.

TABLE 63.3

Descriptions of conditions of sick group

Male, born 16 March 1953; extremely withdrawn, no close contacts, 2 months' psychiatric admission following theft, currently in institution for boys with behaviour difficulties, still performing petty thieveries.

Female, born January 1943; married, one child, extremely withdrawn, nervous. Evidence of delusional thinking, pulls her hair out, has large bald area.

Female, born 29 March 1946; promiscuous, highly unstable in work, no close contacts, confused and unrealistic, psychiatric admission for diagnostic reasons, recent abortion, some evidence of thought disorder.

Male, born 1 July 1946; under minor provocation had had semipsychotic breakdown in Army, expresses strange distortions of his body image, thought processes vague, immature.

Male, born 2 May 1944; severe difficulties in concentrating; cannot complete tasks; marked schizoid character; marginally adjusted.

Male, born 3 June 1947; lonely in the extreme; spends all spare time at home; manages at home only by virtue of extremely compulsive routines; no heterosexual activity; marked schizoid character.

Male born 1 October 1953; no close contact with peers, attends class for retarded children, abuses younger children, recently took a little boy out in the forest, undressed him, urinated on him and his clothes, and sent him home.

Male, born 17 January 1954; has history of convulsions, constantly takes antiseizure drug (Dilanthin), nervous, confabulating, unhappy, sees frightening 'nightmares' during the day; afraid of going to sleep because of nightmares and fear that people are watching through the window, feels teacher punishes him unjustly.

Female, born 18 March 1944; nervous quick mood changes; body image distortions, passive, resigned; psychiatric admission, paranoid tendencies revealed, vague train of thought.

Male, born 14 March 1952; arrested for involvement in theft of motorbike; extremely withdrawn, difficulties in concentration; passive, disinterested, father objected to his being institutionalized; consequently he is now out under psychiatric supervision.

Male, born 10 October 1947; level of intellectual performance in apprenticeship decreasing, private life extremely disorderly; abreacts through alcoholism.

Male, born 20 January 1944; severe schizoid character, no heterosexual activity; lives an immature, shy, anhedonic life, thought disturbances revealed in TAT.

Female, born 25 May 1947; psychiatric admission, abortion, hospital report suspects pseudoneurotic or early schizophrenia; association tests betray thought disturbance, tense, guarded, ambivalent. Current difficulties somewhat precipitated by sudden death of boy friend.

Male, born 13 August 1950; sensitive, negativistic, unrealistic; recently stopped working and was referred to a youth guidance clinic for evaluation. Is now under regular supervision of a psychologist.

Male, born 28 May 1947; history of car stealing, unstable, drifting, unemployed, sensitive, easily hurt, one-year institutionalization in a reformatory for the worst delinquents in Denmark.

Female, born 1 June 1945; psychotic episode, one year of hospitalization; diagnoses from 2 hospitals: (1) schizophrenia; (2) manic psychosis.

Male, born 3 September 1946; severe schizoid character; psychotic breakdown in Army, preceded by arrest for car thievery. Now hospitalized.

Male, born 28 January 1953; perhaps border-line retarded; psychiatric admission for diagnostic reasons; spells of uncontrolled behaviour.

Male, born 23 June 1948; repeatedly apprehended for stealing; severe mood swings, sensitive, restless, unrealistic; fired from job because of financial irregularities.

Female, born 5 July 1941; highly intelligent girl with mystical interests. Very much afflicted by mother's schizophrenia. TAT reveals thought disorder. Receiving psychotherapy.

---

(1) The Sick Group suffered considerably more early separation from their parents than the two control groups;

(2) Rather than the classic textbook picture of the preschizophrenic child, the Sick Group subjects were disciplinary problems, domineering and aggressive in their classroom behaviour;

(3) While a number of psychophysiological variables predicted to their Sick Group status, the one which was the best discriminator was the rate of recovery from momentary states of autonomic imbalance;

(4) The Sick Group evidenced considerably more pregnancy and delivery complications.

TABLE 63.4

Distinguishing characteristics of the sick group

---

1. Lost mother to psychiatric hospitalization relatively early in life.
2. Teacher reports disturbing, aggressive behaviour in school.
3. Evidence of associative drift.
4. Psychophysiological anomalies.

   A. Markedly fast latency of response;
   B. Response latency evidence no signs of habituation;
   C. Resistance to experimental extinction of conditioned GSR;
   D. Remarkably fast rate of recovery following response peak.

5. 70 per cent of the Sick Group had suffered serious pregnancy and/or birth complications.

An interesting sidelight with respect to these perinatal events is the fact that the high risk group which had not suffered breakdown evidenced fewer perinatal difficulties than did the low risk control group. This suggested to us that perhaps there is a special interaction between the genetic predisposition for schizophrenia and pregnancy and delivery complications. It was almost as if in order for a high-risk subject to fare well, he needed a complication-free pregnancy and delivery. In the paper reporting the findings (Mednick 1970), mention was made of the fact that there was a marked correspondence between the pregnancy and birth complications and the deviant electrodermal behaviour. Almost all of the electrodermal differences between the groups could be explained by these perinatal difficulties in the Sick Group. The perinatal difficulties in the low-risk group were not as strongly associated with these

extreme electrodermal effects. This further suggested that the pregnancy and delivery complications trigger some characteristics that may be genetically predisposed.

The theory

A mini-theory has guided this longitudinal project but has not dominated it. The theory was first published in 1958 (Mednick 1958). It suggests that the syndrome of schizophrenia is an evasion of life, learned on the basis of physiological predispositions. It suggests that the combination of exposure to an unkind environment and possession of an autonomic nervous system that responds too often and too much *and* an abnormally fast rate of autonomic recovery provide an aptitude for learning evasive avoidance responses. If an individual is to become schizophrenic, he must possess both the ANS responsiveness *and* recovery characteristics. If an individual is rapidly, exaggeratedly, and untiringly emotionally reactive, he may become anxious or even psychotic, but will not tend to learn schizophrenia, unless his rate of recovery tends to be very fast. It also seems likely that an extraordinarily reactive ANS will only require moderately fast recovery, while an extraordinarily fast rate of recovery will only require moderate reactiveness. Both very high reactiveness and very fast recovery will result in a very heavy predisposition for avoidance learning and hence for schizophrenia.

Diagnostic assessment, 1972

The Reisby study (1967) gave us reason to expect that at the average age of 25 years, we should expect to be able to diagnose approximately one-half of the eventual schizophrenics in the high-risk group. Thus, we initiated an intensive assessment of the high and low-risk samples in 1972 when they reached an average age of 25·1 years. (They ranged between 20 and 30 years of age.) The central goal of this re-assessment was the establishment of a reliable diagnosis and an evaluation of their current life status.

Method of procedure

The 1972 assessment consisted of psychophysiological and cognitive tests, a social interview, and, most importantly, a battery of diagnostic devices. The diagnostic devices included a 3¼ hour clinical interview by an experienced diagnostician, (Hanne Schulsinger), a full MMPI, and the psychiatric hospitalization diagnoses and records where they existed. The diagnostic interviewer completed the Endicott and Spitzer (1972) Current and Past Psychopathology Scales (CAPPS) and the Present Status Examination, 9th edition (PSE) (Wing *et al.* 1974). The interview itself was structured as a clinical procedure and not as a questionnaire.

The coded PSE and CAPPS materials were sent to New York and London respectively. (We wish to thank the test authors for their helpful co-operation.) Computer diagnoses were returned. Table 63.5 presents information on the results of our follow-up contacts with the subjects. Ten of the high-risk subjects have died in the course of the follow-up, seven by suicide, two by accidental causes, and one by natural cause. None of the low-risk subjects have died. This is a dramatic difference which we shall explore further in future papers. Of the ten, six died before the assessment began; three of the other four took part in the assessment. Thus, of the 201 high-risk subjects available for the assessment, 91 per cent took some part in the interview (10 only had a home interview by the social worker). Of the low-risk subjects 91 took part in the full interview, and six took part in the home interview. Thus, 93 per cent of the low-risk group has taken some part in the interview. Subjects are still trickling in for the assessment.

Table 63.6 presents identifying information on those who completed the full interview. The groups seemed to be well matched with each other and with the total original sample with respect to age, sex, and social class.

TABLE 63.5

1972 Follow-up results with 1962 samples

	High risk (N = 207)	Low risk (N = 104)
Full assessment complete	173	91
Home interview only (social worker)	10	6
Not yet contacted (Parent objected or the subject could not be located)	6	2
Living abroad	6	0
Deceased	10	0
Subject refused	6	5

TABLE 63.6

Identifying characteristics of high- and low-risk subjects participating in full interview (1972)

	High risk	Low risk
Number—full interview	173	91
Mean age at 1962 assessment	14·9	15·1
Mean social class	2·1	2·4
Number of males	97	53
Number of females	76	38

Reliability of the diagnosis

The diagnosis of schizophrenia made by the interviewer is based on the presence of Bleuler's primary symptoms: thought disorder, autism, ambivalence, and emotional blunting, as well as Bleuler's secondary symptoms: delusions and hallucinations. For a diagnosis of schizophrenia it was not necessary that all of these symptoms were observed at the time of the interview; they might also be drawn from the case history. In two separate papers (Mednick *et al.* 1975b; Schulsinger 1976) detailed descriptions of the tests of the reliability of the diagnoses have been reported. For our purposes here, it is sufficient to say that across the two computer-derived diagnoses, the MMPI (analysed blindly by Professor Irving Gottesman) and the clinical diagnosis as well as an independent diagnosis arrived at by two Danish psychiatrists listening to the audiotape of the entire interview for ten subjects, rather excellent diagnostic agreement was achieved. (We wish to thank Drs Lise Hauge and Raben Rosenberg for their work on the reliability tests.)

The interview was, in part, coded in the form of a rather extensive series of questions. A very significant portion of these questions refer to symptoms of mental illness. It is interesting that one of the Danish psychiatrists listening to the audiotapes of these interviews has almost perfect agreement with the interviewer's codings of the CAPPS items. The codes for these items range from 1 to 6. In 91 per cent of the items his coding was no more than one unit different.

Another indication of the reliability of the coding and diagnoses may be found in the two important measures of severity of illness resulting from the interview. At the conclusion of the CAPPS interview form, the interviewer is required to rate the severity of illness on a scale from one to six. Ratings of five and six only occurred for those who were diagnosed schizophrenic. This rating correlated 0·70 with a rating of severity derived from the PSE.

Results of 1972 assessment

Distinguishing premorbid characteristics of those diagnosed schizophrenic

The interviewer diagnosed 13 schizophrenics in the high-risk group. (Of the interviewer's 13 schizophrenics, 6 were female and 7 were male.) In a previous publication we have compared these 13 schizophrenics with 29 borderline schizophrenics, 34 neurotics, and 23 high-risk subjects with no mental illness. This report (Mednick *et al.* 1975b) suggested that these high-risk subjects who became schizophrenic were characterized by the following factors:

1. All of the mothers of the high-risk subjects were seriously schizophrenic. The mothers of the children who became schizophrenic, developed their illness at a younger age;
2. Most of the 13 schizophrenics had been separated from their mother and father and many placed in children's homes quite early in their lives. This stands in sharp contrast to the patterns in the other diagnostic groups;
3. The birth of the schizophrenic group was relatively difficult. The period of labour was longer and characterized by more complications;
4. The rearing social class of the schizophrenic group was not noticeably different from that of the other groups;
5. The school teachers reported that the schizophrenics were extremely disturbing to the class, evidenced inappropriate behaviour, were easily angered, and violent and aggressive. They posed a disciplinary problem for the teacher;
6. ANS recovery rate (measured in 1962) was found to predict very well to later schizophrenia (Mednick 1978) and especially well to individuals suffering symptoms of hallucinations and delusions and thought disorder.

Sex differences in factors predisposing to schizophrenia

In considering these preliminary reports one factor seemed extremely striking. We were sensitized to this factor of sex differences in high-risk children by Dr Helen Orvaschel. Almost all of the findings we have listed above have been cited in the literature as being especially responsive to sex differences in schizophrenics. Gardner (1967) and Sobel (1961) have reported that the degree of mother's illness, for example, affects the level of schizophrenia in females, but not in males. Rosenthal (1962) has commented on the higher concordance for female monozygotic schizophrenics than for males. Male discordance in monozygotic twins with schizophrenia is twice as great as for females. While there are some sampling problems in these twin studies, such information might suggest that schizophrenia in females is more genetically determined, and that schizophrenia in males has a heavier environmental weight.

With respect to the pregnancy and delivery complications, in our more recent high-risk study especially studying perinatal factors (Mednick *et al.* 1971) we have found differential sex effects of perinatal complications. It is also well known that males are more vulnerable to pregnancy and delivery difficulties. Finally, aggressive school behaviour has been shown by Watt *et al.* (1970) to be associated with later schizophrenia in men, but not women.

In view of the fact that almost all of the findings reported in the two preliminary reports mentioned above are highly sex dependent, we determined to conduct separate analyses of these variables for males and females.

Hypotheses to be examined. The analysis of the factors potentially predispositional to schizophrenia were conducted separately for male and female HR individuals. It was hypothesized that:

1. The *seriousness of illness* of the mother (as indicated by early onset) would be of significance for both sexes, but would be more important for women;
2. *Separation from parents* during early life would be important for both sexes;
3. *Pregnancy and birth complications* would increase the probability of the development of schizophrenia in both sexes. Because of the male foetus' greater vulnerability to perinatal stress, we hypothesized greater effects for males than females;
4. *ANS recovery and responsiveness* would be involved in the development of schizophrenia.

In summary, we hypothesized that for female HR individuals the development of schizophrenia would be especially related to early onset of the schizophrenic mother's illness. In males we hypothesized that the perinatal variables would be especially predictive. In both sexes ANS factors and early separation were hypothesized as predispositional to schizophrenia.

Method of statistical analysis: path analysis

While a practical goal of this statistical analysis is to develop identifying characteristics of children who will later become schizophrenic, an underlying hope is progress toward an understanding of the aetiology of schizophrenia. The problem is one of causation. As mentioned above, we are barred in studies of the aetiology of schizophrenia from making use of the experimental–manipulative approach. Thus, it has been impossible for researchers in the field of schizophrenia to pretend to such causal statements. All we can ever note and interpret is co-variation. Certainly for research in a naturalistic setting (such as this longitudinal project) this point must remain unchallenged.

Methods have been developed, however, in the field of genetics and later used extensively in the field of economics which allow for hypothesized causal models to be stated in mathematical form in a way that allows their agreement with observed co-variances to be examined. So while we can never completely validate or prove a 'causal' statement, we can examine its expected consequences by examining the goodness-of-fit of hypothesized co-variances (i.e., generated under a hypothesized model) to observed co-variances.

In this analysis we are operating with variables which span the lifetimes of the individuals involved. We begin with the seriousness of the schizophrenia of the mother, examine perinatal factors, consider the intactness of their homes, see all this in the light of their socio-economic status during rearing, the functioning of their autonomic nervous system, and their sex. We know that many of these independent variables are intercorrelated. For example, the earlier the onset of illness of the mother, the more separation from the mother the child experiences. Other, less obvious, intercorrelations also exist in these data. Therefore, multiple analyses of individual independent variables in relationship to the dependent variable, schizophrenia, run the risk of repeatedly rediscovering a single or few common findings. Therefore, we chose a model in which all of the interrelationships are estimated simultaneously and all other intercorrelations are taken into consideration. We also foresaw the possible problems inherent in mediated effects. Thus, the seriousness of illness of the mother might not have any direct effects on her child's development of schizophrenia, but may have its effect mediated by the resulting disruption of the child's home life. For these and other reasons (See Chapter 4) we chose a statistical technique which could estimate both the direct and the mediated effects—the Jöreskog and Sörbom (1977) maximum likelihood estimation procedure for structural equations (LISREL). LISREL is a special case of Jöreskog's earlier analysis of co-variance structures (Jöreskog 1970) and is an advanced form of path analysis. It is a statistical tool which has great advantages for the analysis of data from longitudinal projects.

Definition of constructs

In the Jöreskog LISREL path analysis important factors are represented as constructs. The constructs are not directly measured, but are defined by indicators. These indicators of a construct go through a process which may be seen as roughly analogous to the development of communalities in factor analysis. (This analogy is presented for heuristic purposes only. The actual process is *not* mathematically related to factor analysis.) These 'communalities' then represent the construct. Rather than relate the individual, and relatively unreliable, indicators to one another, the constructs are interrelated. This serves to reduce some of the unreliability inherent in any individual indicator of a construct. For example, as indicators of the construct 'separation from parents' (separation) in the first five years of life, we used three indicators from the first five years of life:

(1) Amount of separation from the father;
(2) Amount of separation from the mother;
(3) Amount of time the child spent in children's homes.

For the construct 'age of onset of mothers's schizophrenia' (mother's onset) we used two indicators:

(1) Age of first appearance of symptoms;
(2) Age at first psychiatric hospitalization.

Thus, when we are interrelating separation and mother's onset we are interrelating two constructs rather than individual indicators.

The indicators of the constructs
Table 63.7 lists the constructs and their indicators. Certain of the constructs may require explanation.

TABLE 63.7

The 'early factors' constructs and their indicators

Construct name	Indicators
Mother's age of onset (of illness)	1. Age at first appearance of symptoms 2. Age at first hospitalization
Parental separation (first five years of life)	1. Amount of separation from father 2. Amount of separation from mother 3. Amount of time in children's homes
Pregnancy and birth complications (PBC)	1. Number of complications 2. Weighting for most severe complications 3. Total weighted score for all complications
ANS (responsiveness × recovery)	1. Per cent of electrodermal responses × recovery rate (Conditioning) 2. × recovery rate (Tests for conditioning) 3. × recovery rate (Extinction testing)
Socio-economic status	Caretaker's occupational title (see Svalastoga 1958)
Schizophrenia (in the high-risk child)	Factors: 1. Hallucinations and delusions 2. 'Hebephrenic' features 3. Thought disorder 4. Autistic features

Age of onset of mother's schizophrenia (mother's onset). Age of onset of schizophrenia is a rather good indicator of the seriousness of the condition. The mother's age at the beginning of symptoms was taken from her hospital case record. Her age at first hospital admission was taken from the Risskov Demographic Institute's Psychiatric Register.

Pregnancy and birth complications (PBCs). The scale has been described in previous publications (Mednick 1970; Mirdal *et al.* 1974). It is based on weights assigned by obstetricians and paediatricians to the various pregnancy and delivery complications noted by Danish midwives in their reports.

ANS (recovery × responsiveness). In the above discussions of the theory we have indicated that if an individual is relatively autonomically unresponsive, fast recovery will be that much less of an aptitude for avoidance learning. Conversely, a highly sensitive ANS will not lead to schizophrenia if not associated with fast recovery. Thus, the theory specifies an interaction effect which can be most simply expressed mathematically, in a single score, as a *product* of recovery rate and responsiveness. 'Responsiveness' was taken as the per cent of measurable responses in the entire 1962 electrodermal examination. Mean recovery rates were taken from conditioning, tests for conditioning, and extinction testing. The distribution of recovery rates in the high-risk group evidenced kurtosis. This was due to a small group of the *most* schizophrenic high-risk subjects who had the very fastest recovery rates. These outliers (who will be the subject of special study) resulted in highly exaggerated correlations between recovery rate and the outcome variables (such as hallucinations and delusions). Before producing the recovery–responsiveness products we transformed the recovery rates by a square root transformation which reduced kurtosis to an acceptable level. The intercorrelations of recovery rates and three product scores were 0·90, 0·86, and 0·92; the intercorrelations of the per cent responses with the three product scores were 0·73, 0·70, and 0·68.

Schizophrenia in the high-risk children. The diagnostic interview took about three-and-one-quarter hours and consisted of a rather extensive series of symptom descriptor items. These items were subjected to factor analyses which yielded (among others) four factors which described the schizophrenia symptoms of the high-risk children (see Table 63.8). The four factors were named:

(1) Hallucinations and delusions;
(2) 'Hebephrenic' features;
(3) Thought disorder;
(4) Autistic features.

TABLE 63.8

Indicators of the schizophrenia construct: symptoms defining the four factors

Hallucinations and delusions

1. Hears voices or sounds, sees, feels, smells, or tastes something with no apparent source outside of himself (CAPPS 227);
2. Auditory hallucinations (CAPPS 228);
3. Visual hallucinations (CAPPS 229);
4. Level of preoccupation with hallucinations and delusions (PSE 95);
5. Acts upon delusions and hallucinations or expresses them in public with strangers (PSE 96);
6. Systematization of hallucinations and delusions (PSE 93);
7. Concealment of hallucinations and delusions (PSE 94).

'Hebephrenic' features

1. Silliness—laughs or giggles in a foolish way (CAPPS 239);
2. Retardation—lack of emotional expression (CAPPS 240);
3. Speech disorganization—impairment in form of speech . . . aimless, no logical connection, irrelevant (CAPPS 248);

4. Denial of illness (CAPPS 251).

Thought disorder (items from diagnostic interview)

1. Tends to shift or drift spontaneously in train of thought;
2. Thought sequences are unrelated;
3. Quality of transition between ideas, themes, and topics is impaired.

Autistic features (items from diagnostic interview)

1. Emotionally impoverished;
2. Frankly psychotic defences;
3. Autistic, withdrawn. No eye contact, no emotional contact;
4. Autistic . . . only empathy regarding own affects.

Results of path analysis

We shall express the results of the path analysis in two ways. First by means of path diagrams we shall present the significant direct effects, then by means of bar graphs we shall consider the sum of the direct and indirect effects of the hypothesized predispositional variables on the outcome, schizophrenia.

Path diagrams

Figure 63.1 presents the path diagram for men. Significant path coefficients (and their probability levels) are indicated. Note that 'PBCs' have no direct effect on 'schizophrenia'; its effect is mediated by the ANS construct. Childhood separation and the ANS construct are directly related to later schizophrenia in high-risk men, as hypothesized. Also as hypothesized, the ANS factors are rather well predicted by PBCs. Childhood separation is predicted by an early age of onset of the mother's schizophrenia which does not evidence a direct relation to schizophrenia.

The LISREL computer program calculates a multiple *r* of 0·62 for the prediction of schizophrenia by these predispositional variables for the high-risk men. Figure 63.2 presents the path diagram for the women. In this path diagram the only construct which is

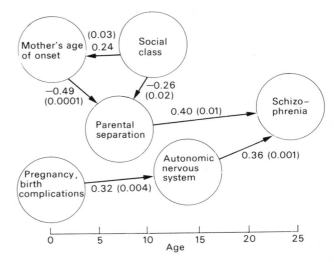

FIG. 63.1. Path diagram for men. Coefficients are indicated on the paths (arrows) along with their probability levels.

significantly directly related to the development of schizophrenia is the age of onset of the mother's schizophrenia. The pattern for the women is quite different from that seen in Figure 63.1 for men. The ANS construct (a reliable predictor for men) is not significantly related to schizophrenia in women, nor is childhood separation. Comparison of the path diagrams strongly suggests that some aspects of the aetiology of schizophrenia are quite different in high-risk men and women. The multiple *r* for the prediction of schizophrenia for women is 0·49.

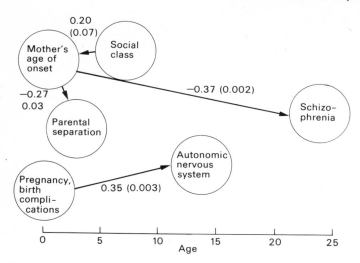

FIG. 63.2. Path diagram for women. Coefficients are indicated on the paths (arrows) along with their probability levels.

Direct and indirect effects. Before leaving the path diagrams, note that in these reported relationships socio-economic status (SES) is included and consequently held constant. SES has no direct, significant relationship with the construct schizophrenia. It does, however, influence schizophrenia via the mother's age of onset (in men and women), and amount of childhood separation (in the case of the men). The indirect effect of SES on schizophrenia via separation may be calculated by simply multiplying the two relevant path coefficients (0·26 × 0·40), yielding an indirect effect of 0·104. Note that we have earlier observed a similar interaction of social class and separation experience in relation to breakdown (Stern *et al*. 1974).

By adding the direct and indirect effects on to schizophrenia, the total effect of each construct in this path diagram can be calculated. Figure 63.3 presents a bar graph depicting the total direct and indirect effects of each of the constructs on the construct schizophrenia.

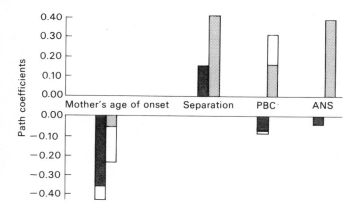

FIG. 63.3. Direct and indirect effects of childhood constructs on schizophrenia construct. Blank bars indicate indirect effects; cross-hatching indicates direct effects on females; and solid bars indicate direct effects on males.

Discussion of path analysis results

From the lives of our high-risk subjects we have chosen a small group of childhood variables to explore their relationship to the subject's current diagnosis of schizophrenia. These early factors seem to relate to the development of schizophrenia quite differently for men and women. We have presented the material in some detail so as to illustrate the path analysis method as discussed by Sörbom in Chapter 4.

In interpreting these results we must keep in mind the fact that for women, schizophrenia tends to have a later onset (greater incidence for women aged 35; Yolles and Kramer 1969). This assessment took place when the subjects ranged from 20–30 years of age; the results for the later-onset women may be different.

Aside from this age factor we cannot suggest other serious reservations regarding these findings. Perhaps, in some cases, the 1972 interviewer learned about the separation factor (and even something about the mother's age of onset) while talking to the subjects. It seems rather unlikely, however, that this would affect her coding of the schizophrenia symptoms listed in Table 63.7. It seems even more unlikely that her ratings would be influenced differently for men and women. At the time of the interview (and in fact to date) the interviewer was totally blind regarding the perinatal and psychophysiological data. It should perhaps also be pointed out that at the time these early variables were recorded, there was no information available regarding who, among the high-risk subjects, would become schizophrenic.

It does not seem overly imprudent to begin to accept the possibility that these four factors have some relationship to the development of schizophrenia in these high-risk individuals. The interpretation of the meaning of these results, some of which were rather unexpected, may be less straightforward.

Early detection

Our initial aim is the identification of factors which might be useful in the early detection of individuals in the general population who are at high risk for schizophrenia. With respect to this aim, these four early factors are worthy of some consideration and testing. However, it should be pointed out that we have only demonstrated that they predict reliably within a group of children born to schizophrenic women. The level of separation from the parents experienced by these children is unusually high. In a general population, this factor may not account for as high a proportion of the variance as it does for these high-risk families. The variable, age of onset of the mother's schizophrenia, is also not generally and directly applicable to population studies. Perhaps when we understand better what role the mother's early onset plays in her daughter's schizophrenia, some hypotheses regarding predictive measures may be suggested.

The ANS construct (the product of recovery and responsiveness) is an individual measure which is more promising for utilization in early detection in general populations. It has been a central variable in the theoretical framework of our research for the past 20 years. It predicted quite well the 1967 psychiatric breakdowns; almost all published studies with schizophrenics (with one exception, Maricq and Edelberg 1975) have supported the hypothesis of faster ANS recovery for schizophrenics (see Mednick 1978; Mednick *et al*. 1975b). Interestingly enough, almost all of these studies have been carried out on *male* schizophrenics. Our path analysis suggests that these reported results would not replicate with female schizophrenics. A senior member of our research group, Peter Venables, has repeatedly failed to find ANS differences between female controls and female schizophrenics. The ANS measures would seem to be a useful addition to an assessment of risk in a male general population.

These ANS results also support our reliance on fast ANS recovery and responsiveness for selection of the high-risk three-year olds in Mauritius. These sex-specific ANS results will now send us back to our Mauritius data to attempt to find analogous relationships.

Interpretation of findings

It is the fate of longitudinal researchers to continually be presenting interim results. Now we must await the next wave of schizophrenic breakdowns as we have indicated above. In addition to these inexorable developments and changes in our subjects over the years, we also face the problem of analysing literally lifetimes of data. In this case we are slowly and more or less systematically (but certainly slowly) analysing the individual and life-event factors related to the outcome, schizophrenia. This is an analysis which is very much in progress. Thus, this report must be understood as interim also for this reason. We now will attempt to transmit to you our reflections on the meaning of these results. These reflections will suggest our strategy for future data analyses. We present these reflections very tentatively for each of the early factors which were shown to relate to the construct, schizophrenia.

Mother's age of onset

Figure 63.3 depicts the direct and indirect effects of mother's age of onset on the construct of schizophrenia for both men and women. Note that while there is a strong tendency for 'onset' to relate to schizophrenia in the males, the relationship is almost completely mediated by 'separation'. Sons of 'early-onset' women have an especially heightened risk of themselves becoming schizophrenic. This relationship seems to be almost completely explained by the separation from parents which follows the mother's early onset of illness.

In the women, the 'onset' variable also has an important relationship to later schizophrenia. However, in the case of the women the indirect effects are negligible. This simply means that either the effect is actually only direct, or that the critical mediators were not included in this path analysis. We examined correlation matrices including some early childhood variables and 'onset' for the male and female high-risk children. Early onset of the mother's illness is associated mildly and significantly with the girls evidencing low verbal IQ, disturbed and peculiar word associations and continual associations, and adult thought disorder. Curiously enough, in males none of these relationships are observed. For the males, mother's early onset is better related to adult characteristics associated with a diagnosis of 'psychopathy'.

Some tentative reflections related to mother's age of onset

1. Perhaps the seriously ill mother is genetically transferring some language deviation to her daughters and not to her sons. This sex-linked transmission is, of course, a possibility which we must contrast with an identification-learning hypothesis. We must relate the seriousness of the daughter's illness to the amount of contact she had with her mother. The course of illness for the HR parents and their children is currently being compared by Ms Sharon Talovic.

2. The earlier development of language behaviour in girls than in boys, and the fact that girls tend more to identify with their mothers, may combine to differentially influence the associative and verbal responses of daughters of severely schizophrenic women. Maccoby and Jacklin (1974) suggest that this childhood advantage of girls in the acquisition of language behaviour probably exists only before the age of three. In future analyses this suggestion may help us to pinpoint possible critical periods of development for further intensive analysis. Careful analysis of our case files should enable us to estimate the amount and closeness of the contact between the mothers and their children at various age levels as well as the relation between the child's age at the time of mother's breakdown and the child's adult diagnostic status.

3. It is also possible that the more seriously schizophrenic mothers pass on some specific characteristic to *both* their daughters and their sons. But perhaps this characteristic predisposes to schizophrenia only in the daughter because of differences in the manner in which society deals with the two sexes. We shall return to this thought when we discuss the ANS construct.

4. In male, high-risk children, 'onset' is not directly related to schizophrenia. As mentioned, inspection of the case material for the boys indicates that for them, 'mother's early-onset' is significantly associated with adult symptoms of psychopathy. We know that the schizophrenic mothers (in this sample) tend to mate with criminal men (Kirkegaard-Sørensen and Mednick 1975; see also Lewis *et al.* 1976). We intend to examine the possibility that for the most early-onset schizophrenic women this tendency is even stronger. If this is true, it might explain the heightened psychopathy of the sons who have early-onset mothers (Schulsinger 1972; Hutchings and Mednick 1974). It might also suggest hypotheses regarding the mother–daughter findings.

Separation in childhood (0–5 years)

Early separation from parents is highly and significantly related to later schizophrenia for male, but not for female, high-risk children. The path coefficient for the females is in the same direction as for the males, but not statistically significant. Differences between the girls and boys in *amount* of separation are minimal and not statistically significant.

Some tentative reflections related to separation in childhood

1. The amount of separation experienced by the boys (but not the girls) is related negatively to their social class status. It is possible this social class factor may mean that the treatment of boys separated from their parents is of a different (poorer) quality than the treatment of girls. We shall attempt some modest examination of this possibility by interviewing individuals who worked in these children's homes in the 1940s and 1950s. We must also check to see whether reasons for selection of children to be placed in children's homes are different for the two sexes. We do have some suggestive evidence, for a subsample of the HR group, that children's home placement is partly dependent on pre-placement infant characteristics (Herrmann 1973).

2. Perhaps the reason early separation is a more important variable for boys than girls is that boys experience more 'separation anxiety'. While the research evidence on this issue is far from unequivocal, Maccoby and Jacklin (1974) suggest that where sex differences exist 'boys cry more when the mother or father leaves the room; and at the early age of 9–10 months they are more likely to crawl quickly after the mother if she moves into an adjacent room' (p. 196). Perhaps the boys in this study (because of their sex-linked immaturity) did suffer a stronger separation reaction than did the girls. This may have, in some way, been involved in the chain of events leading to their eventual schizophrenia. Unfortunately, our longitudinal project does not contain reliable data concerning the children's reactions to their separation from their parents. The high ANS reactiveness of the boys who eventually became schizophrenic could suggest that separation from their parents may have produced a relatively strong emotional reaction.

PBC factors

The high-risk boys suffered slightly more serious and a greater number of perinatal complications than the girls (not statistically significant). This direction of results is in keeping with our expectations. For boys there is a large significant relationship between PBCs and later schizophrenia (Fig. 63.3). The relationship for the girls is actually negative (not statistically significant). For the boys, most of the PBC-schizophrenia relationship is mediated by an ANS-schizophrenia relationship which is not found in the girls.

There is evidence that females' electrodermal responsiveness is related to their menstrual cycle (Bell *et al.* 1975a). One could suggest the hypothesis that the lack of a relationship between ANS factors and schizophrenia for the females is due to a menstrual-cycle-related lack of reliability of the ANS measures in the females. (We failed to note menstrual data in 1962.) Note, however, that the PBC–ANS relationship is at least as strong in the females as it is in the males. It is unlikely that this would be true, unless the females' ANS responsiveness were as reliable as the males'. ANS reactiveness and recovery are reliably related to PBCs in the girls, but this increased reactiveness is not associated with an increased risk of schizophrenia.

ANS factors

We have observed unexpected sex differences in the effect of the ANS factor on schizophrenia. These differences are puzzling; we offer some observations related to sex-differences in ANS-relevant emotional behaviour.

What is the nature of sex-differences-related emotional reactiveness?

Maccoby and Jacklin (1974) suggest that if there are sex differences in *amount* of emotionality, they are very small. The self-reported lower fearfulness of boys is almost certainly explained by their unwillingness to admit their fears and anxieties. Boys are much more defensive than girls. For a boy to admit emotionality, is to admit a weakness and to risk being called a 'sissy'. Girls 'are simply more willing than boys to admit that they feel anxious' (Maccoby and Jacklin 1974; page 186). It is not unfeminine to admit being afraid. Boys conceal and avoid such emotions more than girls do. Under some conditions and in some social circumstances, emotionality in women may be seen as a positive, feminine attribute. In males it is often regarded with considerable suspicion; it is not masculine.

Little girls are freer to express fear and to cry when disappointed without being judged a sex-role deviant. 'Parents show considerable more concern over a boy being a "sissy" than over a girl being a tomboy' (Maccoby and Jacklin 1974; page 362). Perhaps girls have less need than boys to avoid expressing fear or anxiety. In that case perhaps little girls need *not* learn deviant ways of thinking and behaving to avoid emotional expression.

Little boys tend to learn that they must avoid emotional expression. The little boy who has an extremely reactive ANS may often be pushed by parents, guardians, teachers, and peers to suppress this emotionality. Thus, any response (such as irrelevant thought or bizarre behaviour) which will avoid an encounter with a potentially emotion-provoking stimulus (such as an approaching person) will be reinforced and quickly learned. Fast ANS recovery will assure a relatively powerful reinforcement for such an avoidance response and will increase its probability of being elicited. The repetition of this learning sequence over the years could produce an effective screen of avoidance behaviour which will function to isolate the schizophrenic and support his withdrawal. What about the female schizophrenics? This discussion implies that (not being influenced by the ANS factors) the women should develop a less withdrawn form of schizophrenia. The clinical picture for the male schizophrenics is dominated by withdrawal, isolation, thought disorder, and hallucinations. The women evidence serious thought disorder, but are frequently quite promiscuous and socially 'active'. The fact that schizophrenic women become married three times as often as schizophrenic men (Forrest and Hay 1972) probably has many explanations, but in any case does testify to less avoidant, withdrawn behaviour than is the case for male schizophrenics. Forrest and Hay (1972) express some suspicion regarding early onset diagnoses of schizophrenia in women. They report that it has been their experience (over a specific two-year period) that 'almost every female patient first admitted under the age of 20 years with a presumptive diagnosis of schizophrenia later has this diagnosis revised to personality disorder or manic-depressive illness' (p. 55). This statement is probably too extreme for most clinicians to accept.

These reflections suggest two related notions which may repay some consideration by investigators. First, perhaps the condition we call schizophrenia takes a different form in men and women; second, perhaps the aetiology is, in part, different for men and women.

Most investigators (including ourselves) have until now neglected to consider the *possibility* of sex differences in the schizophrenics. Frequently, an area of research which has almost exclusively studied male schizophrenics is reviewed (with no mention of the sex variable) and the conclusions generalized to all schizophrenics. These analyses suggest that we may explain more variance if we consider the sexes separately.

Conclusions

The presence of schizophrenia in HR women is related negatively to the age of onset of their mothers' illness. The factors of early parental separation, ANS recovery and responsiveness, and perinatal complications did not relate significantly to the development of schizophrenia in these HR women.

In men the pattern is quite different. The age of onset of the mother's illness is related to schizophrenia in her son only because it produces parental separation. Parental separation relates directly to the development of schizophrenia in the HR boys. Perinatal complications in male HR children relate to their later development of schizophrenia. This apparently results in large part because the perinatal complications seem to produce ANS fast recovery-responsiveness effects in the HR children. In the HR boys the ANS deviance is reliably related to the later development of schizophrenia.

The discussion suggests that the form which schizophrenia takes in men and women may be different along the withdrawal-activity dimension (Depue 1976; Plovnick 1976). These differences may be related to the hypothesized role of ANS factors in the learning of avoidance–withdrawal.

Postscript

The project is continuing. We hope to conduct another clinical follow-up within five years. This will enable us to test our speculations regarding sex differences and schizophrenia.

Acknowledgement

The high-risk research is being supported by USPHS Grant No. MH 25325 and was supported earlier by the Foundation for Child Development. The perinatal study was supported by MH 19225. The Mauritius research was originally supported by grants to the Psykologisk Institut from the World Health Organization. We wish to express our gratitude to the Mauritian government for their continuing support during the entire project and to date. The assessment of the Mauritian children was supported by a grant from the British Medical Research Council to Peter Venables. The Danish Organization for Aid to Developing Nations (DANIDA) supported the nursery schools.

64. Children of alcoholic fathers: a longitudinal prospective study (Sweden)

PER-ANDERS RYDELIUS

Introduction

Children from alcoholic homes comprise a risk group. Since Jones *et al.* (1973) from the United States described the so-called alcohol-foetopathy syndrome, the number of scientific articles has increased rapidly, mostly being reports of children of alcoholic mothers. Similar reports have been published not only from France and the Soviet Union, but also from Sweden, which apart from describing the alcoholfoetopathy syndrome, demonstrate that intellectual handicap can result in the child of a mother with a high alcohol consumption during pregnancy. This has been well known from a historical point of view, as is apparent from the historical summary of the subject presented by Rebecca Warner and Henry Rosett in both American and British publications (Warner and Rosett 1975). The effects on the physical and mental health of children in a society where alcohol consumption increases in an uncontrolled spiral are presented in this article. The situation is considered to be frightening.

The number of scientific publications has also increased with respect to the mental development of adolescents growing up in alcoholic families, irrespective of alcoholism in the mother, the father, or in both parents. All authors emphasize the psychogenic risk group these children comprise (Aronsson 1963; Fine *et al.* 1976; Chafetz *et al.* 1971; Freiova 1966; Plante *et al.* 1973; Bourgeois 1975; Bosma 1973; Burk 1972; McCord 1972; Kammeyer 1971; Goodwin *et al.* 1973; Garcoia 1974).

The study

An investigation was started in Sweden at the end of the 1950s, the object of which was to reveal which symptoms were evident in children living in an emotionally stressful home environment. In child psychiatry and paediatric medical and surgical practice, the clinical impression was such that symptoms like headache, nausea, palpitations, diffuse abdominal pain, and tiredness were not always considered to have an organic aetiology. The clinical impression was that these symptoms were grounded in psychogenic tension in the child as a result of disharmonic home relationships, such as psychogenic disease or alcoholism in the parents, divorce situations, etc. (Ekstrom and Nylander 1959; Nylander 1959).

The subjects in the study were children from families where the father had a known severe alcohol overconsumption of several years duration, and had sought treatment by both hospital physicians and by the Council for Alcohol Addicts. The population consisted of 229 children between the ages 4 and 12 years, and coming from 141 male alcoholic families. A control group was selected, in accordance with the principle of social twins, from children matched with regard to age, sex, housing area, class group classification, and economic situation. In the case of school children, the control children were matched in the same class as the investigation group, and were assessed by the school teachers as having the same intellectual ability. Social twins were available to 163 children of alcoholics. The investigation was conducted using clinical child psychiatric methods, with interviews and assessment of parents, and with child psychiatric and paediatric ratings of the children. The first part of this investigation was published by Prof. Ingvar Nylander as a monograph (1960).

Results

Alcoholism in the paternal grandparent was present in 33 per cent of the investigation group as opposed to only 0·6 per cent in the control group.

Thirty-two per cent of the mothers in the investigation group were assessed as psychogenically insufficient compared to 10 per cent of the mothers in the control group (2 of the mothers in the investigation group were alcoholics). Fifty-two per cent of the mothers in the former group were working in civil life as opposed to 36 per cent of the mothers in the latter group. Children of alcoholics often had poor dental hygiene with severe caries in 39 per cent as compared to 21 per cent in the control group.

Twenty-nine per cent of the children of alcoholics were psychogenically insufficient, and a further 34 per cent experienced milder psychogenic symptoms. In this respect there was a marked difference in comparison with the control group.

Seventy-four per cent of the boys from alcoholic homes exhibited obvious difficulties at school, and as a general group, 48 per cent of the children of alcoholics were assessed as having school problems which were not of an intellectual nature.

Children of alcoholics experienced symptoms of a psychosomatic type more often; and while these children on the average exhibited three of the investigated symptoms, the children in the control group showed less than one symptom. All of the 24 symptoms investigated occurred more often in children of alcoholics, the following 10 so frequently, that the difference between the investigated group and the control material was statistically significant at the 0·01 level of significance. These ten frequently occurring symptoms were:

headache, abdominal pain, growing pains, tiredness, nausea and vomiting, sleep disturbances, emotional lability, anxiety, depression, aggressiveness, and difficulties in maintaining friendships.

An analysis of the material was performed with reference to the following background factors, in order to establish which factors could possibly influence the children of alcoholics in a positive manner. The background factors studied were:

1. Sex and age;
2. Social group;
3. Mental constitution and body build;
4. Possible head injury;
5. The nature of the father's alcoholism;
6. The father's contact with the Council for Alcohol Addiction;
7. The father's psychiatric profile;
8. The father's social adaptation;
9. The type of abstinence experienced by the father;
10. The mother's psychiatric profile;
11. The mother's profession and work;
12. The number of children in the family and the sibling order of the child;
13. Type of housing;
14. Presence of divorce conditions;
15. The psychiatric condition of the paternal grandfather;
16. The psychiatric profile of siblings.

This analysis showed that if the mother was in good psychogenic balance, the children felt better, especially the daughters. It was also shown that the children's situation was better if the father had contact with the Council for Alcohol Addicts and was under its care. The boys reacted with increased anxiety in connection with divorce, but in general none of the previously cited factors influenced the children's situation.

This investigation supported the hypothesis that children living under psychogenic stress as a consequence of serious emotional conflict at home reacted with non-organic somatic symptoms, and that children born to alcoholic families comprised a psychogenic risk group. A prospective longitudinal follow-up was planned as a continuation of this study, in order to determine how children of alcoholics establish their life as adults. This follow-up investigation was also designed to test the hypothesis that children from male alcoholic families have problems in their own social adaptation as adults, and that even as adults have a greater incidence of somatic and psychiatric disease, including a higher frequency of alcoholism. At the first examination in the investigation, the families were informed of the study and given advice regarding the children's situation at that time. However, since that occasion, the investigators have had no direct contact with the children. In those cases in which psychiatric or some other treatment has been given, it has been administered by other physicians.

By 1973, the children had attained adulthood, between 19 and 27 years of age, and the first follow-up investigation was started. This was conducted by collecting data from official registers in Sweden. Data was collected from the Social Register (containing details concerning social welfare measures, child care procedures, details from the Council for Alcoholic Addicts), the Criminal Register, the Income Tax Authority's special register of prosecutions involving drunkenness, the National Insurance Bureau's register over health and sickness certification, and finally from hospital registers regarding treatment of psychogenic and somatic disease.

All the children in both the investigation and the control group could be followed up. It was evident that children in the alcoholic group moved more often than children in the control group, since approximately 20 per cent of the children from alcoholic homes were still living in their original housing area as compared to the figure of 60 per cent for the control group children. Two girls from alcoholic homes had died as a result of accidents, while in the control goup one boy had died of a road accident, and one girl of autoimmune disease. Over 20 per cent of the children from alcoholic homes had been subject to child welfare measures during adolescence in accordance with Swedish Child Welfare Legislation, as opposed to 9 per cent of the children in the control group. Eleven per cent of the children in the alcoholic group as compared to 0·6 per cent in the control group were involved in more serious procedures as stipulated by the Swedish Welfare Legislation.

Fifteen per cent of the children born to alcoholic homes had come to attention through misdemeanours associated with their own drunkenness as opposed to 7 per cent in the control group. Four per cent of the children of alcoholics were considered to show signs of alcoholism themselves.

Twenty per cent of the children from alcoholic homes had been reported for varying types of crime in the Criminal Register, as compared to 8 per cent of the children from the control group.

It was found after collection of details of health and sickness certification, that children from alcoholic families had a greater number of days off work than children from the control group. The data regarding sickness certification is not yet collated.

This part of the study is to be presented as an academic thesis, but even the preliminary data which is presented above strongly suggests that children from male alcoholic homes experience as adolescents difficulties with social adaptation, and may also develop their own problems associated with alcohol consumption.

65. Longitudinal studies of institutional children and children of mentally ill parents (United Kingdom)

MICHAEL RUTTER and DAVID QUINTON

This chapter describes a programme of family studies begun in 1964. Because the unifying theme has been a concern to understand how family influences help shape children's development (and in particular how they may play a part in the genesis of psychiatric disorders), most, but not all, of the investigations followed some kind of longitudinal strategy. Each investigation has had a quite specific focus on a particular family variable or child-rearing pattern but, equally, in each case a rather broad range of detailed measures has been employed in order to better delineate the possible psychological mechanisms which might be involved. As a result, there has been a gradual shift of focus with the development of the programme, as new findings have emerged and as a better understanding of family processes became available. The first project started from the observation that the offspring of mentally ill parents had an increased rate of psychiatric disorder. A four-year prospective study was undertaken to investigate why and how this occurred. The results demonstrated the importance of family discord and disruption. It was then necessary to see whether this applied in a non-patient population, so an epidemiological investigation of the general population was carried out. It showed a similar pattern of associations confirming the impact of family disharmony on children's development. Both studies emphasized the many exceptions to these associations—many children reared in unhappy homes develop well in spite of the stresses. Both also showed the apparent greater vulnerability of boys and pointed to the need for a follow-through into adult life to see if girls showed their impairment in a different form later. Accordingly, a new project combining a retrospective enquiry with a longitudinal study was set up to examine possible links between childhood experiences and later functioning as adults and parents. This was designed in a way to allow a particular search for possible protective or ameliorating factors. The literature suggested the importance of early bonding and of the development of lasting personal relationships in this connection. Accordingly, the last two projects have focused on this issue by examining the consequences of atypical child-rearing experiences which have been thought to interfere with social development—namely an institutional upbringing, fostering, and adoption.

Family illness study

Numerous cross-sectional studies prior to the 1960s had noted significant associations between mental illness in parents and psychiatric disorder in their children (see Rutter 1966 for review). However, a detailed case note study of Maudsley Hospital patients showed that there was only a limited connection between the clinical form of disorders in parents and children. On the other hand, the psychiatric risk appeared to be particularly great when the parental condition directly impinged on the family, or was associated with marked family disturbance (Rutter 1966). Thus, the evidence suggested that parental mental illness might adversely influence the development of children through effects on family life and relationships. But findings came from retrospective studies and in order to adequately test the hypothesis there was a need for a longitudinal study with direct and detailed measurement of family functioning.

In 1964, one of us (M.R.) launched such a study. The aim was both to provide a more rigorous test of earlier findings and also to explore how and in what circumstances mental illness in one member influenced the health and social functioning of other members. Throughout the 8 years of the most active phase of the project, funding was provided by the Association for the Aid of Crippled Children (now called the Foundation for Child Development). From the start, the investigation was planned as a four-year longitudinal study preceded by a period for the development of new instruments to assess family functioning. Because the need for this kind of time scale was fully appreciated by the funding body there were no major problems in financing.

Development of measures

The earlier work had been limited at least as much by the inadequacy of the measures used as by the retrospective nature of many of the data. It was realized that the value of the longitudinal study would be heavily dependent on our ability to generate sensitive and robust measures of psychiatric state, of family life and functioning, and of the quality and patterning of relationships. These were also the requirements for the Isle of Wight studies (see Chapter 21) which began at about the same time. Resources were pooled in order to develop appropriate methods of assessments and then to go on to test their reliability and validity. Screening questionnaires for completion by teachers (Rutter 1967; Rutter *et al.* 1975a) and by parents (Rutter *et al.* 1970b) were devised to pick out behaviourally deviant children. A 'malaise inventory' was used to tap emotional disturbance in adolescents and adults (Rutter *et al.* 1970b). Standardized interviews with parents (Graham and Rutter 1968) and children (Rutter and Graham 1968) were utilized for a more detailed individual assessment of psychopathology in the child. We collaborated with Professor John Wing and his colleagues (1967) in the development of their structured appraisal of adults' present mental state; but went on to adapt the approach to make it more suitable for assessing depressive and neurotic symptomatology in non-patient populations (Rutter *et al.* 1975a). Finally, we created a style of interviewing which could both obtain factual information about family functioning and also elicit attitudes and feelings about family relationships, and a discriminating measure of these was devised. Its validity was shown, not only by the observation that independently obtained accounts from husband and wife agreed very well, but also by its good predictive correlation with marital breakdown over the next four years (Quinton *et al.* 1976). Of course, the longitudinal study itself was needed for this last test of validity.

These early methodological studies showed the value of interview measures, but also emphasized the need for further naturalistic and experimental study of interviewing techniques. This led to a research project designed specifically to evaluate the effects of different types of interview methods (see Rutter and Cox 1977).

Sampling

Because our objective was to study the *process* by which parental mental illness led (in some cases) to disorder in the children, we needed a sample of parents who had *recently* developed some kind of psychiatric condition. For the same reason it was essential to interview the parents as rapidly as possible after their disorder became manifest. In order to obtain an accurate picture of the nature and extent of the associations between illness in parents.

and children it was also necessary to have a representative sample of ill parents. This meant that a sample from a single hospital would not be satisfactory.

The Camberwell Psychiatric Register, established by the Medical Research Council Social Psychiatry Research Unit on a grant from the Department of Health and Social Security to Professor John Wing, provided the kind of sampling frame we needed (Wing and Hailey 1972). Camberwell was an inner London borough with a population of about 170 000 in which the Institute of Psychiatry was situated. (A reorganization of borough boundaries has meant that Camberwell no longer exists in this form.) The Register receives regular reports from all psychiatric facilities serving Camberwell (irrespective of whether the clinic is sited outside the area). In this way information is available on all persons (adult or child) living in the borough who make contact with psychiatric services in the National Health Service. This does not include private patients but in England these only constitute a small proportion of patients. Thus, the sample used in the longitudinal study included 20 per cent from the professional and managerial social classes, a similar proportion to that found in the general population.

The advantages of basing the study on the Camberwell Psychiatric Register were many, including:

(a) Ease of sampling;
(b) Possibility of contacting patients very soon after first clinic attendance (or hospital admission);
(c) Use of a sample from a known geographical area (and hence the possibility of calculating population rates from which realistic estimates of service requirements can be determined);
(d) The availability of data on the overall population from which the sample was drawn (so allowing a determination of how far a sample of patients who were parents differed from a sample of all adults);
(e) Reduction of the practical difficulties of following and interviewing families.

The specific criteria for our longitudinal sample were:

(i) The patient must be living in the Borough on the day of psychiatric contact;
(ii) No psychiatric contact for at least 1 year previously (76 per cent of cases had had *no* previous contact);
(iii) The main language spoken in the home must be colloquial English (in practice recent immigrants from Asia and the West Indies were excluded);
(iv) At least one child under the age of 15 years to whom the patient has been a parent either by being the biological father or mother or by taking a social parental role for a period of at least 6 months.

The sample which formed the basis of the project was collected during 1966–7 and consisted of all patients (fulfilling the above criteria) who came under psychiatric care during a period of 10 months, a total of 218 patients. From this total consecutive sample a 2 in 5 subgroup was randomly selected for more intensive interviewing (the remainder all had a briefer personal interview assessment). Analysis of the consecutive sample indicated that there were rather small numbers of men and of patients in certain diagnostic categories. In consequence, additional groups of male, psychotic, and alcoholic patients were collected consecutively from the Register in the same way. Altogether, the intensively interviewed group included 137 families with 292 children in the sample and the more briefly studied group, 118 families with 264 children in the sample.

Sample collection took place during the development of the Psychiatric Case Register. In order to ensure that no eligible cases were omitted, extensive checks of Register information were undertaken (these included comparisons with case notes). Our approach was to include all potential cases from the Register, and then to check their eligibility personally. This proved to have been a wise decision as results showed it would not have been satisfactory to rely on the Register as the sole source of information.

Some of the difficulties were simply a reflection of teething troubles of a new Register and we would not experience the same problems using the Register today. However, it is likely that other limitations would still be present. We had to know whether the patient was a parent and (because of our reliance on interview methods) whether colloquial English was spoken at home. Neither item was well recorded (on the Register and sometimes not in the case notes either, presumably because psychiatrists do not see them as very important clinically. It is not possible to design a sampling frame which adequately meets all purposes and however good the Register (and the Camberwell Register maintains a very high standard indeed) some degree of personal checking will almost always be necessary.

When a patient was selected as fulfilling the criterion, the responsible psychiatrist (and social worker where relevant) was contacted for permission to interview the family. Only one consultant refused permission for any of his cases to be seen (meaning that 17 were missed). In addition, one patient refused to be seen and a further 4 could not be traced. The remainder were all interviewed. Initial contact was by letter followed by a personal visit to describe the study and arrange an interview. We explained our purpose in terms of an interest in family and social problems with a view to improving knowledge and providing better services. The sample was not paid and the information was treated as entirely confidential (so that feedback to services or access by others to our data was given only with the express permission of subjects).

Controls

As our main interest concerned *within* sample comparisons we did not interview a non-patient control group at the time of the study of patients' families (however, we did so later for reasons outlined below). Nevertheless, we wished to obtain some measure of the extent to which the children of patients had a rate of disorder above that in the general population. Accordingly, we obtained behavioural questionnaires completed by teachers for all school age children in the patients' families. (As the study progressed and more children entered school, questionnaires were completed on them in the same way together with two controls.) For each study child, two control children were selected by us from the class register and teachers completed questionnaires on them in the same way. The method of selection was devised in such a way that no one at the school was aware of which children were in the study and which were controls. The teacher was simply given three names and asked to complete questionnaires on them. The head teacher was aware of our procedure and the reasons for it but was not told who the study children were.

The objects of this rather time-consuming exercise (we had to personally visit all schools in order to discuss the procedure and then to peruse the class registers) were two-fold:

(a) To retain the confidentiality of our information on families (if the school did not know the parent was ill it was not ethically acceptable for us to inform them of this);
(b) To ensure that the questionnaires were completed without bias resulting from knowledge of which children were under study.

Data collection

The initial study of intensively investigated families consisted of:

(1) An interview by one investigator with the patient to measure various aspects of his (or her) psychiatric disorder and to obtain systematic assessments of family life and relationships;
(2) An interview by a second investigator with the spouse to determine the impact of the illness on family life, the social context of the symptoms, attitudes towards the patient, the spouse's own mental state, and also to assess family life and relationships in the same manner as used with the patient;
(3) An interview by a third investigator with the patient and spouse together to assess their relationship with each other and to obtain information on family health and on medical and social service contacts.

The interview with the mother (wife), irrespective of which parent was the patient, was used to obtain detailed systematic information on the behaviour of two of the children (chosen randomly). The restriction of intensive information gathering to two children only was made because it proved impractical to do this for more than two. However, screening questionnaires were completed for all children in the family and interview information on certain indicators such as separation experiences and clinical contacts was also obtained for all. Another separate interview with the mother (wife), by a different investigator, was used to obtain standardized information on the temperamental attributes of children in the family aged 3 years 0 months to 7 years 11 months.

While it was slightly cumbersome having multiple investigators involved with each family, this was necessary to ensure that information gathering was not contaminated by knowledge obtained from another source. The arrangement was well accepted by families and it had the additional practical advantage that the husband and wife could be seen simultaneously (but separately), thus avoiding the possibility of one spouse overhearing the other's interview and perhaps listening to himself (or herself) being talked about. This was especially important when there were marital tensions.

Contact with families

Families were interviewed on 5 occasions over a period of 4 years. A full interview lasting between 2 and 3 hours (sometimes split between two interview sessions) was completed with both the husband and the wife (separately) on the initial assessment, at the 1-year follow-up and at the final follow-up after 4 years. In the initial assessment only there was also a conjoint interview with the husband and wife together. A more limited interview with one parent only, covering just demographic and psychiatric information on the families, was undertaken on the follow-ups at 2 years and at 3 years.

Co-operation from families was very good throughout. We failed to interview only 2·4 per cent of families at the time of first contact; and 8 per cent at both the 1-year and 4-year follow-ups. We made less vigorous attempts to obtain interviews in the interviewing second and third years so that data were lacking on 15 and 21 per cent for these occasions.

These refusal (or failure to contact) rates are very much lower than in most previous studies involving lengthy interviewing in the home. In view of the importance of keeping missing information to a minimum (see Cox *et al.* 1977), it is important to consider possible reasons for our success. We would lay emphasis on four main factors (although we lack systematic evidence on their relative importance). First, it is crucial to obtain personal contact, preferably in the home rather than on the doorstep. Once people can meet the interviewer personally and discuss the study, they rarely refuse. A prior letter of introduction helps but initial contact by telephone increases the refusal rate (see Robins 1966). Second, persistence is an essential quality for all interviewers. In some cases it was necessary to call back *dozens* of times before finding someone in and willing to answer the door. Moreover, people who did not refuse to be seen but who repeatedly said 'yes, but some other day', often willingly agreed to be interviewed if the investigator was sufficiently persistent. It should be added that we found some people very willing to be seen at the 4-year follow-up who had previously refused. A change of personal circumstances may alter people's attitudes. Third, the *flow* and balance of the interview seems to make a big difference to how people respond. The ordering of questions needs careful planning to avoid having an excess of either demographic enquiry (because that may be seen as boring and irrelevant) or of very personal questioning (because that may be felt as unduly intrusive) at the beginning. Once rapport is established, however, almost anything can be asked if it is done in the right way. The overall style is also vital so that the informant perceives the interview as a conversation with a relevant purpose rather than the reading of a questionnaire or interview protocol. Fourth, people tend to be more co-operative with the interviewer if the interviewer is helpful to them. This means being willing to discuss the purpose of the study and to answer questions (at the end of the interview as well as at the beginning), and to provide practical assistance in contacting services when this is wanted. Unsolicited advice is generally *not* welcome and we have always made it clear that we cannot offer services ourselves. Nevertheless, our willingness to put them in touch with services and to be available to discuss what they should do at times of crisis has been appreciated.

The fact that the parent was a newly referred patient was also probably a help at the time of our first contact. On the other hand it was sometimes a disadvantage later in cases where psychiatric care had not provided a remedy. We have found that the refusal rate can be kept below 10 per cent in all our other studies of non-patient samples, so that patient status cannot be a crucial factor.

Findings

The study has given rise to an immense body of findings (currently being written up in book form) and only a few key results with implications for research strategies will be given here. The findings confirmed that, compared with general population controls, the children of mentally ill parents had an increased risk of psychiatric disorder (Rutter 1970b). This was evident at the first (cross-sectional) assessment but longitudinal data were needed to bring out the true extent of the risk (Rutter 1977a). This was because behavioural deviance was more *persistent* in the children of patients than in the control children. Altogether, twice as many children in the patients' families sample showed persisting deviance, as assessed from the teachers' questionnaire.

The results also confirmed that the risk to the child was heavily dependent on psychosocial circumstances. *Within* the patient sample the children were most likely to show psychiatric disorder if there was serious marital discord. Indeed, this difference *within* the sample, according to the state of the parents' marriage, was greater than that between cases and controls. This suggested that the parental illness led to an increased psychiatric risk in large part through its association with family discord and disharmony. If this was so, it implied that similar associations with marital discord should be found in non-patient samples. This was one of the reasons for our decision to study a general population group in a closely comparable way (see below).

As in the earlier retrospective enquiries, the clinical diagnosis of the parents' illness was of little moment except that the children of parents who showed a lifelong personality disorder were particularly at psychiatric risk. In addition, the children were more likely to suffer if their parents' disorder directly involved them in some way.

Originally we had intended to use our longitudinal design to test how far these associations represented causal influences. The idea (along traditional lines) was to determine whether the children's problems ameliorated when parental marital relationships improved or when the parents ceased to be mentally ill. However, we were frustrated in these aims. One of the most striking findings of the study was the considerable persistence of both marital difficulties and mental health problems. Moreover, very few parental disorders consisted of illnesses with a clear beginning and end. Instead there was a close intermingling of psychiatric symptomatology, personality difficulties, and problems in interpersonal relationships. The time span was too short and marked changes in family circumstances too infrequent to study the temporal relationships between disorders in parents and children. This was unfortunate as the retrospective data from our study indicated that the risk to the child did diminish significantly when family relationships greatly improved (Rutter 1971a).

Previous studies had tended to focus on the traumata associated with children's separation experiences. Because we had detailed assessments of family life and relationships we were able to show that separations as such did *not* constitute the main danger to children. The damage more often came from longstanding discord and disharmony and, to a considerable extent, separations were associated with disorders in children simply because they often reflected family disturbance (Rutter 1971a). The finding has important public health implications but, in the present context, it is also important to note that it illustrates the research importance of having detailed and sensitive measures of family functioning.

Children's temperamental attributes proved to be strongly predictive of later psychiatric disorder (Graham *et al.* 1973; Rutter 1979a)—a finding which could only have come from a longitudinal analysis. It also emphasizes the importance of individual differences. This was evident, too, in our finding that boys were much more likely than girls to suffer from family discord (Rutter 1970b). However, this last finding raises the question of whether girls are truly less susceptible to psychosocial stresses or rather whether girls show their disability in different ways—perhaps later in terms of either adult psychiatric disorder or difficulties in parenting. This possibility emphasized the need for a longitudinal study to examine possible links between childhood experiences and adult functioning—a strategy we decided to follow on completion of the family illness study (see below).

The last issue to note here is the observation that even in the families associated with the greatest psychiatric risk, many (usually most) of the children did *not* succumb. This has been noted in all previous studies but it is a particularly striking finding in an investigation with such a wealth of detailed measures on a wide range of psychosocial risk factors. In retrospect, we have regretted that we did not gather more information on positive influences or protective factors. The question of why so many children are *not* damaged by chronic stress and disadvantage now seems more important than the usual question of why some *are* damaged (Rutter 1979a). In our current longitudinal study (see below), therefore, we are making special efforts to identify modifying factors which enable children to resist stress.

The existing literature is rather weak on what such factors might be. However, the evidence suggests that protection may be related in part to the development of stable personal relationships and the building up of self-esteem (Rutter 1979a). This consideration has led us to explore the influence of early patterns of child-rearing on both aspects of psychosocial development (see below).

Overview

There have been no particular problems in either following subjects or in gaining their co-operation. As a result, subject loss over time has been minimal. We have also been fortunate in maintaining considerable continuity of staffing throughout the study (M.R. has been director and D.Q. has been one of the principal investigators from the beginning). On the other hand, inevitably, there have been changes of staff and this has posed particular problems in a project which has relied heavily on highly skilled interviewing. Each new investigator has required two to three months full-time training and this has meant a considerable investment of time and energy from the experienced staff. We have now got more streamlined training techniques but in the earlier stages of the project these were not available.

We have also found that great effort is needed to maintain high motivation and good morale among interviewers in a longitudinal study of this kind. The stresses arise in part from the very demanding nature of intensive interviewing, especially when much of it has to be done in evenings and when one successful interview may require half a dozen fruitless journeys. In part, too, it is a consequence of the great strains of a longitudinal study in which there is the relentless pressure of interviews requiring to be done *now* just because the follow-up date has arrived. This lack of a breathing space makes it difficult to give adequate time to either concurrent data analysis or the planning of the next stage of the study. If this means (as it usually does) that results are slow in coming, the long delay in positive feedback to researchers may make it more difficult to keep drive and enthusiasm at a high level. In spite of these difficulties the study ran fairly smoothly most of the time but, in retrospect, it is clear that it would have been helpful to have left one year in the middle of the project free of data collection in order to give adequate time and energy to data analysis and strategic planning.

There have been three main difficulties in data analysis. The first has stemmed from the dilemma of whether the family or the individual child was the main focus. It seemed logical, as that was the way the sample was collected, to use the family as our base. We received statistical advice on the organization of the data to allow us also to sort the findings by child. In the event, the advice proved to be wrong, and we had considerable difficulties in analysing both by child and family. As a consequence, we needed to spend considerable time re-organizing our data into a child 'pack' of cards (then put onto tape) as well as a family 'pack'. The main difficulty arises from the fact that there is a variable number of children per family and, moreover, the number of eligible children for each family varies from year to year. Quite minor (but fundamental) changes in the way we dealt with the data at the outset could have avoided these difficulties.

The second problem has been the lack of an adequate statistical framework for handling longitudinal data and the need to derive special codings which can show the patterns of particular variables and associations over the follow-up period. Of course, this is a problem common to any longitudinal study with measurements at more than two points in time. It is not surprising that most longitudinal studies report their findings in terms of a cross-sectional style of analysis. However, this solution means that much of the value of a longitudinal approach is lost. There is little point in having data for several consecutive time periods unless you can determine whether the children who show X at point 1 are the same children who show X at point 2 and again at point 3. It is important to determine how the children who show a stable pattern of characteristics over time differ from those showing great temporal instability. Our attempts to deal with these problems have meant that data analysis has taken much longer than originally planned.

The third problem has come from our choosing to study a wide age range of children. This seemed necessary because data were lacking on which age group was most at risk. However, we have suffered from the difficulties of ensuring that all measures mean the same thing at all stages in development. How do you equate psychiatric disorder in a 3 year old with that in a 16 year old? It is not easy to see which is the correct solution but, given our time again, we would focus our most intensive measures on a narrower age range, while still maintaining screening measures over the very broad age group.

As already noted, the value of this study has depended in large part on the adequacy of its sampling and the quality of its measures.

With respect to both it has been a major advantage working in a research setting where we could collaborate with experienced colleagues. The study had its origins within the MRC Social Psychiatry Research Unit which established the Camberwell Psychiatric Register. The family measures were developed in collaboration with Professor George Brown and other sociologists, the adult psychiatric measures with Professor John Wing and other psychiatrists, and the children's measures together with Professor Jack Tizard and other colleagues on the Isle of Wight project (see Chapter 21). The teachers' questionnaire had its origin in the Aberdeen study (see Chapter 11) and was more fully developed in the Isle of Wight surveys. It would not have been possible to accomplish what we did if we had had to work in isolation.

Despite these difficulties, the bulk of the analysis on this family illness study is complete and a final report in book form is being prepared. The data are stored on both punchcards and tape and further analyses are being undertaken from time to time as new questions cause the data to be re-examined for a different purpose. The subjects could be identified for a further follow-up and the possibility of such an investigation is being considered with the aim of studying the adult psychiatric status of the children born to mentally ill parents.

London general population study

The Family Illness Study indicated that child psychiatric disorder was associated with various kinds of family discord and disharmony, as much as with parental mental illness. It was essential to determine if these associations held in a non-patient sample. For this purpose, it was necessary to take a general population sample from inner London (where the patients' families lived), but there was no need for a longitudinal design. For the reasons outlined above, it was decided to focus on one age group—namely 10 year olds and their families—and to use an epidemiological approach. This study was undertaken in 1970 and the results have been reported in a series of papers (Rutter *et al.* 1975a, b; Rutter and Quinton 1977). In brief, the findings showed that the factors associated with child psychiatric disorder in the patients' families sample were closely similar to those in the general population sample. We concluded that the longitudinal associations found in the Family Illness Study were likely to have general applicability and were not specific to families with a mentally ill parent.

Childhood experiences and parenting behaviour

This project began in 1975 by M.R. and D.Q. jointly with the London Borough of Southwark, and was funded on a contract with the Department of Health and Social Security and the Social Science Research Council. The study aims to investigate the links between childhood experiences and parenting behaviour, with special reference to children received into the care of the Local Authority. The investigation is being carried out in two stages, the first retrospective and the second prospective. In the first stage the families of children currently 'in care' were compared with a general population control group from the same socially disadvantaged area in inner London. Retrospective information was sought about the parents' childhood experiences, as well as concurrent data about their family situation and social circumstances. This study was needed to determine what proportion of currently malfunctioning families include parents with seriously adverse childhood experiences, and how this proportion compared with a randomly selected control sample. The retrospective study also provided the opportunity to obtain leads on the likely factors of importance in determining adult functioning, and it enabled a testing of the measures to be used in the longitudinal study.

The second stage consisted of a follow-up of persons, now adult, who were reared in institutions. Systematic comparisons are being made with a similarly aged control group also studied in childhood with the same measures (originally this was the control group for the Family Illness Study). Both groups are now being followed up when they are in their early 20s and hence likely to have begun families of their own. This part of the project is concerned with the mirror image of the question studied in the retrospective enquiry—that is it is asking what proportion of children with seriously adverse childhood experiences turn out to be malfunctioning adults. For obvious reasons this can only be satisfactorily answered through a longitudinal study. The design also has the important merit that, by comparing 'good' and 'bad' outcomes within the 'in care' sample, it can focus on protective factors or variables that enable individuals to develop normally in spite of early adversity.

Retrospective enquiry

Information on all children admitted into care by the Borough of Southwark is collected routinely and is collated in a central index. A sample of 48 families with a child recently admitted into care was chosen from this index according to the following criteria:

(1) Both parents born in the British Isles or mainland Europe;
(2) At least *two* separate admissions of children into care from that family (this specification was included to rule out families in which the admission into care is solely due to some temporary crisis);
(3) The recently admitted child was living with the biological mother at the time of admission;
(4) At least one child in the family aged between 5 and 8 years (to ensure comparability with the control group).

The control group was selected from two group general practices in the north of the Borough, contacted initially through the Health Visitors' Service in the Area Health District. Selection was made from the age/sex registers kept by each practice choosing families randomly from within those who met the same age and place of birth criteria as the 'in care' sample, and in which:

(1) *No* child in the family had ever been admitted into care;
(2) The child was living with the mother at the time we contacted the family;
(3) The family lived in the northern (more disadvantaged) half of the Borough.

General approval to contact families with children 'in care' was obtained, following discussions with Social Services departments and with Area Teams, through the normal process of local government decision-making. Permission to contact individual cases was negotiated with the social worker mainly responsible for the family. Initial contact was by letter followed by a personal visit to explain the project and to arrange an interview. The 'in care' sample was very mobile and considerable patience and the help of the health agencies and social workers was necessary in order to trace many of the families. Co-operation from families was generally good but in about one in six cases interviews were only obtained after repeated visits, sometimes extending over as long as 8 months during which a relationship with the families was established. Both the mothers and their co-habitees were interviewed with a failure rate of about 11 per cent for mothers and 29 per cent for fathers.

The initial contact with controls was through a letter from the general practitioner which provided an opportunity for refusal. If no refusal was received within two weeks the family was visited to explain the study and arrange an interview. Co-operation from control families was very good and only 8 per cent of mothers and 10 per cent of co-habitees were not interviewed. However,

arrangements for interviewing were complicated by the high proportion of working mothers.

The G.P. registers proved to be a most satisfactory means of obtaining a general population sample. However, naturally the register often did not include the information needed to determine whether the family met the selection criteria. As a result it was necessary to contact some two families for every one finally included. There was also a difficulty due to changes of address. G.P.s are often not told about moves of house and as a result a substantial number of families had to be traced through agencies or information from neighbours.

The main source of information was a standardized interview of about 2 to 3 hours in length, which utilized previously developed techniques of known reliability and validity (see section on family illness study). Retrospective information on the parents' childhood included details of periods 'in care', admissions to hospital, material circumstances, quality of relationships with parents and with sibs, marital discord and breakdown, parental discipline, parental deviance and psychiatric contacts, and school experiences and problems. Similar variables were covered for the teenage years with additional information on peer relationships, teenage deviance, early pregnancy, marital history, and housing experience.

The assessment of parenting skills concentrated on parental handling of peer relationships, disobedience/defiance, and fears/worrying. Systematic data were also collected on daily patterns of family life and on parent–child interaction.

The data are stored on punchcards and on tape. Identifying personal characteristics are not included on the data files but means are available to identify subjects for follow-up. The data have been analysed and the findings written up (Quinton and Rutter 1980a, b).

Follow-up study

Both the index sample and the control group were available because they were investigated in childhood as part of other studies. The index sample consists of 206 persons who, when first studied in 1964 by Professor Jack Tizard and his colleagues, were in the care of the local authority in two residential institutions for children. All were admitted from homes in inner London. Behavioural questionnaires completed by teachers are available on all but 19 children. Parental questionnaires completed by House parents are also available for 200 of the children (either a parent or teacher questionnaire is available for all 206 children). In addition, contemporary background family and personal data obtained during childhood are provided in the Social Services records which are open to us. Data on the two Children's Homes in which the children lived are also available through Professor Jack Tizard's original study. The people were all aged between 20 and 25 years inclusive on 1 January 1977.

The control group consists of 100 persons in the same age group who were studied in childhood because they constituted the control group for the family illness study. The sample all lived in inner London during their teens and behavioural questionnaires completed at that time by teachers are available for all the children. No contemporaneous family or social data exist.

The assessment at follow-up consists of two parts:

(1) Interviews with the subjects and their spouses (planned by D.Q. together with Christine Liddle);
(2) Observations in the home of parent–child interaction (planned by Linda Dowdney and David Mrazek).

The interview covers early experiences and the intervening life history in much the same way as that used in the retrospective study. Contemporary social work records provide a check on the reliability of some of the key data about family circumstances during childhood. In addition to the variables covered in the retrospective study, the intervening life history was expanded to provide a better coverage of compensatory 'positive' experiences and continuities in relationships. Current circumstances, relationships, and psychiatric states are systematically covered. In this stage the children studied are between the ages of two and three and a half. The parenting section of the interview have been adapted accordingly.

The observations of mother–child interaction in the home are based on time and event sampling techniques. Attention is paid to such items as reciprocal interaction, sensitivity to the child's needs and signals, emotional expression, control techniques, amount and type of play interaction, and verbal communication. New techniques for measuring *sequences* of mother–child interaction have been developed.

Data analysis will focus on delineation of the chains of circumstances which differentiate *within* the child care group and *within* the control group those individuals who do and who do not have family and parenting difficulties at follow-up. Attention will be paid to the extent to which this differentiation (concerning *dis*continuities in intergenerational cycles of disadvantage) depends on experiences in childhood, later experiences, the marriage partner, the current social situation, or the individual's psychiatric state.

This research design has several advantages. The longitudinal nature of the data is crucial to the linkage between childhood experiences and adult status or functioning. However, the possibility of using samples on whom information was previously collected in another investigation a decade ago greatly shortens the time span of the research (and incidentally immensely reduces its cost). It illustrates both the value of retaining basic data from completed studies and the potential implicit in collaboration between investigators. It is particularly important for the purpose of comparing the index and control groups that the *same* behavioural measures were obtained in both during childhood (in spite of the two studies being quite independent). There is considerable merit in different investigators including common measures whenever this is possible. The fact that information is available for both samples on psychiatric state (as reflected in questionnaire scores) during adolescence will be valuable when examining intervening variables and processes. The availability of a large sample of individuals with identified family problems during childhood not only allows a specific focus on relevant adverse experiences but also permits a *within* sample comparison between those who develop normally and those who do not. Finally, the combination of interview and observation measures should increase both the sensitivity and validity of the family assessments at follow-up.

Currently the study is at the stage of tracing, interviewing and observing families. The major problem has concerned the tracing. The high geographical mobility of the sample has meant that multiple diverse tracing methods, combined with persistence and ingenuity, have been essential. The major environmental and administrative changes in inner London over the last dozen years or so also complicate both tracing and the interpretation of findings.

Institution-reared and fostered children

The early studies on 'maternal deprivation' suggested that an institutional upbringing was particularly likely to interfere with personality development (see Rutter 1972b). It seemed that the damage probably came from having an ever-changing roster of caretakers none of whom remained long enough for personal bonds with the child to develop (Rutter 1978h). If this was indeed the explanation (rather than separation from parents or genetic influences), the social development of fostered children and institution-reared children should be different. Previous work has concentrated on the effects in infancy and little was known about any

effects persisting into middle childhood or later. Accordingly, it was decided to focus on the infant-school period (5 to 8 years) when children are first away from the home environment for a considerable part of the day and when peer relationships are beginning to be established. The project began in 1974 and was planned and undertaken throughout by Mrs Penny Dixon, supported by a Social Science Research Council Fellowship.

Sampling

The institutional children had to meet the following criteria:

(1) Admission to a residential nursery or Children's Home before the age of one year;
(2) Continuous care in one or more residential nurseries or Children's Homes since the first admission;
(3) No mental or physical handicap requiring special schooling.

The foster care children had to meet the criteria of:

(1) Admission to foster care before the age of one year;
(2) Continuous care in the *same* foster home since then;
(3) No mental or physical handicap requiring special schooling.

Both groups were individually matched in terms of age and sex with 'control' children attending the same school class. The control group had to be reared with their natural parents and not to have experienced admission into care; otherwise they were chosen simply on the basis of the next child of the right age and sex on the school register. The groups were also generally comparable in ethnic background.

If the findings were to be valid it was essential that the samples be truly representative and not biased in any way. Several checks were made to ensure the adequacy of sampling. Early on in the investigation it became clear that very few infants remained in institutions and not many remained in foster care (partly because of policies of early adoption in the case of abandoned babies). Accordingly, it was necessary to tap many sources for cases. Three-quarters of the 32 local authorities and 2 of the 3 voluntary societies which were approached agreed to participate and to make a detailed search of their records. Checks were available through a complete analysis of records in one authority and a personal search of all records in one local authority and one voluntary society. No additional cases were found through these extra enquiries. Foster children were identified in a similar way for 13 of the local authorities in London. In all cases permission was sought from house/foster parents before contacting the school. No Children's Home refused to participate and only one institution-reared child was lost through a refusal by the school. One foster child was excluded because the social worker refused permission (on the grounds that placement was breaking down); and one parent of a control child, although agreeing to other parts of the study, would not allow psychometric testing.

It was also necessary to check three other possible sources of bias. Because a requirement of the fostered group was that they should have remained with the same foster parents throughout, it was possible that the level of behavioural disturbances might be artificially low simply because the disturbed children had had to be removed from their first foster home. Enquiries are being made about who moves homes in order to check on this possibility. Second, it is possible that the institution children had remained in institutions just because they were handicapped in some way. The possibility is being examined by an investigation of the reasons for fostering or leaving children in Children's Homes. Third, any differences between the groups could be a result of genetic rather than experiential factors. While this possibility could not be excluded in the case of comparisons with the control groups, it could be checked with respect to differences between the institution-reared and fostered children. Case records were systematically searched to obtain all relevant data on the characteristics and background of the children's parents (as well as on the children's birth history and physical health). No differences in background between the institution–reared and family–fostered were found.

Measures

Prior to any interviews or observations (in order to avoid any possible influence stemming from discussions about the children's behaviour) the teachers completed 'B2' behavioural questionnaires (Rutter 1967; Rutter *et al.* 1970b; Rutter *et al.* 1975a), and the house/foster parents completed 'A2' questionnaires (a modified version of the 'A' scale described in Rutter *et al.* 1970b). B2 scales were completed for controls as well as cases but A2 scales are available only for the residential and foster children. The teachers also completed a further set of B2 scales (with additional items on social and attention-seeking behaviour) for residential children and controls one year after the initial assessment, in order to determine the temporal stability of any differences found.

Standardized interviews were conducted with teachers to obtain more detailed information on all children with respect to their friendship patterns, attachment, dependency and attention-seeking behaviour, lability of behaviour/mood, classroom behaviour, changes in behaviour over the last year, and contact with the home. Standardized interviews were also conducted with House parents and foster parents (but not with the natural parents of control children) on the children's behaviour (including patterns of attachment), and on family composition and characteristics.

The residential children and the foster children, together with the matched controls for the fostered group, were tested individually on the Wechsler Intelligence Scale for children and the Neale Analysis of Reading Ability. Children with very poor reading skills (i.e. at or below the floor of the Neal) were also tested on the Schonell reading test. Systematic ratings were made of the children's behaviour during testing.

Time-sampled observations in the school classroom were made for all children in a way which ensured that the children were unlikely to be aware which children were being observed at any one time. Task behaviours were observed during 5-second time samples and recorded during the succeeding 5 seconds (observation and recording periods were indicated to the observer through the use of a prerecorded cassette tape and earphone). The behaviours noted included measures of mobility, attention, on and off task activity, and a variety of miscellaneous behaviours. Social interactions were observed during 10-second time samples (with 10 seconds for recording) and the categories used included both the actions of the target children and those of children who approached or were approached by them. The measures included assessments of the nature of physical contact (positive, negative, or neutral), the frequency of approach and avoidance actions, socially disruptive behaviour, co-operative behaviour, reciprocal interaction, and conversation. Observations on residential children and controls extended over two days initially and over two half days at follow-up; the foster children and controls were observed for one day each.

Data analysis

All measures on the children have been obtained and record checks are complete. The questionnaire findings indicate marked differences between the groups in terms of restlessness and lack of concentration together with attention-seeking and socially disruptive behaviour; with the institution-reared children most deviant, the controls less so, and the foster children intermediate. The data from the interviews and observations have been prepared for data analysis, which is currently in progress.

Self-image, identity formation, and family ties of fostered and adopted children

The family studies which have been already completed clearly indicate the powerful impact of family discord and disharmony on children's behaviour. The preliminary findings of the investigation of institution-reared and fostered children also indicate that, quite apart from the damage done by disturbed personal relationships, children's social development may be influenced by the pattern of family ties experienced during the early years. Children reared in institutions with a large number of caretakers who keep changing seem to have particular difficulties in maintaining close stable friendships later. Because of these (and other) concerns, very few children in Britain today are reared in residential nurseries. Foster placement is generally preferred. However, the foster child has to share ties between his biological and foster parents, he has uncertainty about his future family placement, and he is likely to experience and feel less whole-hearted family commitment, if only because ties are partially dependent on the decisions of other people such as social workers and the biological parents. There are suggestions in the literature that the factors may influence self-image, identity formation, and the strength and nature of family ties, but systematic information is lacking. Mrs Daphne Holbrook, initially on a Central Council for Education and Training in Social Work Fellowship for Advanced Studies and later on a grant from the Hilden Trust, is currently undertaking a study to investigate these issues.

Twenty children aged 10 to 13 years who experienced long-term fostering with the same foster parents from before 18 months of age are being compared with a matched group of children adopted in infancy. Children fostered or adopted by relatives, handicapped children and children from ethnic minority groups were excluded in order to reduce the heterogeneity of the sample and the complexity of the issues. The foster sample was obtained through four London Social Services Departments and the adoptive sample through the Independent Adoption Society. Both groups are being compared with a control group of 20 children living with their biological parents; this group was obtained through a family doctor practice.

The main sources of data have been personal interviews with the children themselves and with their foster/adoptive/biological parents. Sensitive and detailed non-schedule standardized interviews, based on those used in the earlier family studies were employed. The interviews are complete and data analysis is currently in progress. This will involve both comparisons between the three groups and also an examination of the associations between self-image and the pattern of family relationships experienced.

Conclusion

This programme of family studies started with what seemed a quite circumscribed question about the impact on children of parental mental disorder. However, the initial cross-sectional study suggested that the mechanism partly lay in disturbed family relationships. A four-year prospective study was undertaken to examine the family processes involved. This broadly confirmed the initial hypothesis but also added knowledge on the relative importance of different features of family life. It seemed that, in large part, parental mental disorder was important because it intensified stresses and difficulties of a kind experienced by many families. Strains specific to mental illness appeared less important. A cross-sectional study of the general population confirmed this impression but re-emphasized the finding, first noted in the longitudinal study, that many children developed well in spite of chronic deprivation and disadvantage. The more recent family studies have focused on this observation and have sought to identify the relevant protective factors and ameliorating influences which facilitate normal development in children who experience long-standing family discord and disharmony. This issue highlighted the need to investigate normal social development and to identify how the nature of early family ties might serve to shape later social behaviour. The studies of institution-reared, fostered, and adopted children have been undertaken with this purpose in mind.

What started 16 years ago as a simple study of family illness patterns has grown into a series of investigations into the whole process of psychosocial development. The methods have extended from records to interviews to direct observations in the home; and the age period has also been extended to examine possible links between early childhood experiences and later functioning as a parent and as an adult. Perhaps most important of all the focus has shifted from an enquiry about why development sometimes goes wrong to a study of why so often it goes right in spite of stress and adversity. Because the emphasis has been on understanding the process of development, many of the studies necessarily have had to use a longitudinal strategy. Nevertheless, the benefits have often come from a *combination* of prospective, cross-sectional, and follow-up approaches. Moreover, what success has been achieved has depended at least as much on the development of reliable and sensitive measures as on the collection of longitudinal data. Knowledge on development requires detailed, appropriate, and valid measures as well as the collection of data at several points in time.

66. A re-examination of children who spent the first part of their lives in permanent nurseries in Zurich, Switzerland

NORA CHARITOS-FORSTER

First examination—re-examination

In the years 1958 to 1961 a medical and psychological examination of the babies and small children up to two years of age staying in permanent nurseries was started by M. Meierhofer, M.D., Ph.D. h.c. and her team at the Institute for Mental Health in the Child. By including all nurseries in the town of Zurich and two from the canton, the original population of examined children aged more than 3 months was 354.

At the time of re-examination, from 1971 to 1973, the age of the 143 children who could be re-examined varied between 14 and 15 years. The reasons for non-performance of the final re-examination are shown in Table 66.1. Twelve children were tested in the course of an earlier pilot study. Twenty-two children had to be eliminated from the data set of the evaluation due to suspicion of a minor brain dysfunction. Thus the final report deals with the remaining 122 cases. According to demographic criteria this population is representative of the original one.

TABLE 66.1

Reasons for non-performance of re-examination

Reasons	N
Address not found	82
Re-examination not allowed	64
No reaction	24
Too large distance from Zurich	13
Other reasons	10
Child dead	2

Measuring criteria and tests

The main interest of the project was to find out whether the children of this population, with early deprivation as the one common characteristic, are generally healthy at the age of 14 or 15. In order to answer this question a medical check-up was made. In addition, psychosomatic symptoms, emotional problems, and behavioural particularities were recorded and later systematized (in a manner shown below in the symptomatology section).

In order to reliably judge the actual state of development of every child, and to obtain the information on symptomatology, the following tests were used:

(a) WIP (intelligence);
(b) KAT (latent fear);
(c) Foto Hand Test (covert aggressivity);
(d) Rorschach test, for a quite differentiated personality description;
(e) The tree test, which provides information on certain projective interrelations between the characteristics of the drawn tree and the personality of the child.

The advantage of these tests lies in the intended complexity of the individual description derived from them. However, this complex information gathering, prompted by human interest in every child's development and fate, does not correspond well to the requirements of exact measurement methods. The disadvantages of this fairly qualitative method were thus found in the difficulty of constructing from it a quantitative evaluation which would have to abstract data about the traits of individuals in order to determine characteristic traits of certain subgroups of the population in question. Another more external disadvantage was the fact that regarding the psychological tests there were no results of any comparison group. Therefore, for the purposes of this report, these psychological tests will not be mentioned any further.

Social background of the population

(a) *Fixed, non-influenceable social parameters*. Most of the families who placed their babies in a permanent nursery after birth belong to the lower classes. Categories of salary, position, and educational standard, were each subdivided into three groups, forming a nine-point scale. This scale was coded as presented in Table 66.2, showing the frequency of the three final socioeconomic groups. Note that our socio-economic group III is at best to be considered as lower middle class.

TABLE 66.2

The socio-economic groups of the families whose children were re-tested

Socio-economic group	Per cent
I (3–4 points)	48
II (5–7 points)	40
III (8–9 points)	12

By the time of the re-examination, 10 per cent of the total population (Table 66.3) in the canton of Zurich were Italian guest-workers. (This percentage refers to the official 1970 statistics of the canton of Zurich.) It should be noted that this ethnic group is overrepresented in our population. In this specific population a highly significant intercorrelation was found between Swiss or Italian nationality and the socio-economic status of the families (Fig. 66.1). There are remarkably more Italian children whose father (or unmarried mother) is a non-qualified worker, has a low salary, and a low position.

TABLE 66.3

Distribution of the nationalities

Nationality	Per cent of total population of project	Total population in canton Zurich	
		Per cent	N
Swiss	48	81	897 684
Italian	37	10	109 104
Other	15	9	100 850

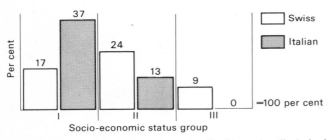

FIG. 66.1. Socio-economic status by nationality (the nationality 'other' was eliminated for this figure).

Our main concern was to show that in certain cases there might be a 'social risk' for children with a certain family background. If this could be documented by our re-examination we could then institute measures of prevention, including better planning, and psychological or even therapeutic help where needed. One of the primary risk criterion, for obvious reasons, is the illegitimacy of the child (Table 66.4). The importance of this probable risk criterion for other social and psychological handicaps will be discussed later.

Another non-influenceable risk for the development of the children is psychosocial affliction in the family, which includes criminality, deviant social behaviour, psychopathy, alcoholism, epilepsy, imbecility, and other deviations with uncertain diagnosis. Table 66.5 shows the frequency distribution of the occurrence of psychosocial affliction in the family.

(b) *Not fixed, influenceable social indicators.* This category includes the age at which the children joined families (their own or adopted or foster parents) and how many of these children are still resident in homes. Figure 66.2 shows that 64 children had been

placed in families by the age of 5; 35 children were placed between ages 6 and 14; and 23 children (19 per cent) are still resident in homes. The proportions of children distributed amongst the different family agencies are given in Table 66.6. These numbers present raw data about the characteristics of the social frame in which these children are now living. We realize that slightly more than 50 per cent of the children are living in their own families (or in substitutes). The rest of 35 children could definitely re-enter a family only later. A relative majority is accepted by their own complete family.

We present two other social indicators which relate to the quality of these children's life circumstances. The first of these indicators is

TABLE 66.4

Distribution of the civil status of the sample

Status	Per cent
Legitimate	51
Illegitimate	36
Legitimized	16

TABLE 66.5

Psychosocial affliction in the family

	Per cent
Mother	24
Father	21
Relatives	33
Single or multiple affliction	55

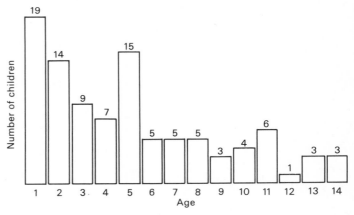

FIG. 66.2. Age of re-entry into a family.

TABLE 66.6

Families in which the children are actually living

Type of family	Per cent
In institutions	19
Complete own family	49
Family with added parent	13
Incomplete family	10
Adopted family	6
Foster family	3
Total	100

derived by counting the number of different placements in the first three years, the duration of living together with their own mother, and the occurrence of disturbances in the living milieu. From this we constructed the index for 'Early life quality' (Table 66.7).

TABLE 66.7

Index of early life quality

	Per cent
Rather favourable circumstances	15
Fairly unfavourable circumstances	45
Quite unfavourable circumstances	40

The second social indicator we formulated uses information about how stable the living milieu was during the years before re-examination. If the child joined his complete family right after his first nursery stage (even if he received additional care in day nurseries) we classified him as having a fairly stable milieu. If the child lived in 3 to 5 different situations (alternate homes or foster families) he was considered to have had a rather unstable milieu. Children with six and more different living changes (the absolute maximum was 15 stages) were counted as having had an extremely unstable milieu. The index of milieu stability (Table 66.8) relates to less qualitative characteristics than that of the early life quality. Nevertheless, the quantitative aspect of stability implies that the more unstable a milieu the more the family climate is apt to be disturbed. Table 66.8 shows this tendency quite clearly.

TABLE 66.8

Index of milieu stability

Milieu	Without disturbances (per cent)	With disturbances (per cent)	Total (per cent)
Fairly stable	19	4	23
Rather unstable	42	21	63
Extremely unstable	4	10	14

With regard to the above two social indices, we first investigated the social parameters and later the symptomatology with regard to various hypotheses. We found that neither ethnic context nor legitimacy give a significant bias to the latter index of stability (Fig. 66.3). We did find that there are comparatively more Italian children living finally in their own family. Only three Italians are still in homes whereas 14 children in all are still living there. With great probability this is a side-effect of the biased proportion between nationality and legitimacy. In this population there are 27 illegitimate Swiss children and only 5 illegitimate Italians. As a matter of fact, of the 13 illegitimate children still in homes, 7 are Swiss, 6 are foreigners, and from those there is only one Italian.

In Table 66.9, the early life quality index cross-tabulated by legitimacy shows the frequency relationship between these variables. Those Swiss children who re-entered their families did so earlier than their Italian mates. As background information for this statistical relation we should remember that the socio-economic status of the Italian families was remarkably lower, so that we might conclude that the Italian families or mothers who were late in taking their children back into the family were so because of a living standard which didn't permit them to do otherwise, rather than

because of negligence. The same could be said of the unmarried mothers as well. It has been shown that there are significantly fewer psychosocial disturbances in the Italian subgroup than amongst those of Swiss origin who brought their children at that time to the permanent nurseries. Psychosocial disturbances are considered to be of negative influence for normal family life.

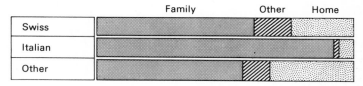

FIG. 66.3. Distribution of children among homes, families, and 'other' forms of accommodation for the various ethnic groups.

TABLE 66.9

Early life quality and legitimacy

Circumstances	N	Rather favourable (per cent)	Fairly unfavourable (per cent)	Quite unfavourable (per cent)
Legitimate	62	23	46	39
Illegitimate	44	4	39	57
Legitimized	16	12	44	44

We therefore might say that the Italian children dealt with in this particular research project are mostly socially disadvantaged but not so much psychologically disadvantaged, whereas the Swiss children not living in their own families are primarily disadvantaged by illegitimacy which, in the serious cases, is almost regularly combined with negligence and psychic problems such as nonacceptance by the mother. The institutional care, even if well-organized and functioning at its best, is not a substitute for a primary and an emotionally satisfying relationship with parents.

Due to the nature of the living circumstances brought about by illegitimacy, the age of return to the family and dwelling place both vary significantly with this parameter (illegitimacy) (Tables 66.10 and 66.11). Note that the significant differences lie in the numbers re-entering their families during the early years. The legitimized children are eliminated from Table 66.10; they have been distributed between the legitimate and illegitimate children for purposes of this particular analysis.

From Table 66.11 it is obvious that there are various placement solutions for the illegitimate child which do not imply any qualitative bias in themselves. In addition it can be seen that neither the

TABLE 66.10

Age of re-entry into a family for legitimate and illegitimate children by legitimacy

Re-entry into family	Per cent
Up to 6 years	
Legitimate	49
Illegitimate	22
From 7 to 14 years	
Legitimate	15
Illegitimate	14
Total	100

TABLE 66.11

Actual dwelling place as a function of legitimacy

Dwelling place	Legitimate (per cent)	Illegitimate (per cent)
Complete family	44	2
Completed family	4	10
Incomplete family	1	9
Adoptive family	1	6
Foster family	0	2
Home	8	12
Total	58	42

early nor the late changes rate higher for the illegitimate than for the legitimate children. A correlation matrix between all descriptive parameters and indicators showed sufficiently high coefficients only between single indicators used for the computation of the index 'stability' and this very index itself. We therefore conclude from this data that there are neither several single dominating parameters nor one multiple one which could be used as a causal factor for the life circumstances variables. Thus, in order to discuss whether social parameters or indicators can be declared as risk factors at all, we will have to consult the outcome of the symptomatology in combination with the above descriptive variables.

Symptomatology

The general view

The somatic status of the children was carefully examined. They can be considered as generally healthy within the range of a comparison group from Children's Growth Centre in Zurich which measures the children according to international standards coordinated at the Centre international de l'Enfance, Paris. Also, anamnestically the amount of sickness or the occurrence of accidents does not deviate from the values of the control group. Our main question about the health of these children concerns their psychic balance and their behaviour amongst the different reference groups.

All the information gathered in interviews with the adolescents themselves, their parents, or educators were later systematized into a schedule of symptoms (Table 66.12); this was then compared with the data from the Children's Growth Centre. The symptomatology system we used was originally elaborated by Jonsson and Kälvesten (1964). It enquires into psychosomatic and motoric disturbances as well as emotional and social particularities.

Amongst the psychosomatic symptoms we include: sleeping difficulties, nervous stomach, intestinal pain, and nervous headache. Psychosomatic disturbances may manifest as a restriction of activity (or, in the contrary, as hyperagility), as nail biting, or as stereotypic movements in the extremities where jactatio capitis is often a later development of another stereotypic movement. Speaking dysfunctions such as stuttering belong to this group as well; it has been shown that speaking a foreign tongue at home does not influence the statistical proportions of this symptom.

The following affective reactions were studied: sensibility, agitation or restriction of aggressive feelings, fear and anxiety, and the tendency to a depressive mood. Social retreat might also be one consequence of the early restrictions of social contacts at permanent nurseries.

From Table 66.12 it can be seen that some symptoms characteristically occur more frequently in our population than in the control group. According to the range of their frequency these are: sensitivity, biting nails, aggressive effects, depressive states, sleep-

ing difficulties, stereotypes and tics, speaking dysfunctions, stealing, and destructive behaviour.

In order to further validate this comparison we also compared our data with those of a longitudinal study of children at Birmingham (Shepherd *et al.* 1973) and an application from this study to the canton of Zug, Switzerland; the methodology was slightly different, but still comparable. In addition to the symptoms mentioned above, some further symptoms were found to have a higher frequency in our population than in the Children's Growth Centre; however, the frequencies in our population did not differ significantly from the other two comparison groups. These are: nervous stomach troubles, nervous headache, psychomotoric activity, difficulties in contact, and telling lies from time to time.

TABLE 66.12

Frequency comparison of the various symptoms

Sympton	Our population (per cent)	Control group† (per cent)
Sleeping difficulties	37	6
Eating troubles	15	16
Nervous stomach troubles	22	10
Nervous headache	29	3
Allergic complaints	16	13
Enuresis	5	1
Psychomotoric activity	18	4
Stereotypes and tics	19	9
Biting nails	46	25
Thumb sucking	6	1
Speaking dysfunctions	17	1
Negativism (overadjustment)	44	50
Aggressive affects (restr.)	45	6
Social behaviour	30	11
Depressive states	38	25
Sensitivity	57	8
Fear, anxiety	26	18
Truancy	2	1
Tramping around	11	18
Lying, fantasizing	34	7
Stealing	11	2
Destructive reactions (overcarefulness)	10	1

† Children's Growth Centre.

The frequencies of eating troubles, fears, allergic complaints, enuresis, thumb-sucking, playing truant, and restlessness are more or less the same in all control groups. These symptoms thus do not contribute to an understanding of the particularities of our population.

The affliction scale

In most cases we noted for each child more than one single symptom. Thus we computed an affliction scale demonstrating the degree of symptomatizing. This scale combines the amount of symptoms with the intensity of each. The scale became one of the quantitative indicators of health in its largest (not only medical) sense. For purposes of measuring with the criterion variables, the two extreme groups (slightly versus heavily afflicted) were made to be of equal size. The maximum affliction ranges from 15 to 28 symptoms. On the other end of the scale, there were two children who had no symptoms at all. Roughly speaking, each extreme group comprises a quarter of the population, with the remaining 50 per cent in the medium group.

The persistence of symptoms

We systematized the different symptom traits anamnestically for two earlier time periods (ages 2 to 7; 7 to 14). It was thus possible to attempt to describe the history of the actual state of symptoms. We found that if the persistence is noted from the first time it is observed at the permanent nurseries, those which are still found to be the most frequent are: nervous stomach troubles and psychomotoric activity (or passivity).

A relatively constant symptom persistence found from age 2 on is a complex of symptoms related to aggression-management. This complex is characterized by aggressive behaviour, including an extreme restriction of aggression, allergies, nail biting, and a general tendency to irritation as well as to depression. These particularities may be directly connected with early deprivation. In addition, there is another group of symptoms we have distinguished with high frequency at the age of $14\frac{1}{2}$. These latter symptoms often seem to be secondary reactions to early experiences or later uneasiness, such as many changes in educational climate or disturbed developmental processes. In this group of symptoms we include sleeping difficulties and negative social behaviour.

Trends of interrelationship of social background with symptomatology

A simple cross-tabulation as well as a regression analysis were performed using the general indicator 'affliction scale' as a variable. Both of these analyses showed the strongest statistical dependence to be between *stability* and *affliction*.

The ranks of condition variables resulting from the regressions equation support the original hypothesis that early life conditions at the permanent nurseries might influence the later development of the children. The home indicators, such as 'time spent with the child per day', range second (after stability); next rank are two other home indicators found to have relatively high intercorrelations.

The psychosomatic symptoms range the social parameters and indicators according to the height of the coefficients in different matter: stability (again first) is followed by the frequency of sicknesses in the anamnestic period II, then by legitimacy, and further on by two home indicators. Only then does the psychosocial affliction in the family have weight. The rest of the parameters have too small of a coefficient to explain a sufficient part of the variance.

With regard to the emotional symptoms we again have the stability factor in the first rank and even with a higher starting coefficient than above. Second of importance here is whether a child had many or few foster relations, which should actually be understood as a specification of the first-mentioned stability factor. The original maternal attitude toward pregnancy and the coming child ranged high in relation to emotional symptoms; it was third in rank. It should be noted that this maternal attitude factor was not ranked highly for any symptom group other than emotional. Age of re-entering the family and sex of child were next in rank.

The indicators which explain a part of the variance of the sensitivity syndrome are: number of home stages, development standard of the first permanent nursery, stability, nationality, the number of foster relations, and the frequency of having been ill from ages 7 to 14. The symptoms which depict the social characteristics range as follows: original maternal attitude towards pregnancy and child, number of foster relations, nationality and stability, the frequency of having been ill, the development standard of the first nursery, and legitimacy.

The amount of explained variance for social behaviour is lowest—it is fairly low in all other regression equations as well, which can be interpreted as a consequence of the primarily qualitative nature of the data. Thus, the importance of these regressions must not be overemphasized. However, the above-mentioned ranks of the path regression do give more information about the priorities in the network of the descriptive variables than a simple one-by-one cross-tabulation would provide.

In the final publication from this re-examination project we plan to present statistically demonstrated characteristics which will be illustrated by casuistic examples, so that the complex tendencies can be understood in a biographical frame of reference.

Schooling characteristics of the population

Although this population's IQ distribution does not deviate from the standard one, these children are obviously handicapped in their schooling career (Table 66.13). They are significantly more represented in lower level school types. The same could be said of course of lower class children in general. We were able to show some empirical background data which had previously been lacking in the official statistics. In our population 25 per cent of the children had not only one but two or three of the problems shown in Table 66.13.

TABLE 66.13

Frequencies of several schooling problems

Problem	Per cent
Later entrance into school	11
Repeating a class†	39
Special classes	16
Psychological examination	13

† The official statistics report that only 20 per cent of the pupils are repeating a class.

Our evaluation shows that the greatest portion of the children with school problems belong to the subgroup which experienced poor stability. When we say 'stability' we mean implicitly the emotional or psychosomatic difficulties connected with it. From what is known from the therapy of learning disability these very symptoms divert energy and concentration from school matters. In this context it has to be remembered that Italian children in general had better parental care than the Swiss subgroup, and consequently, in spite of being socially disadvantaged and having a different mother tongue, they showed less difficulties in concentration as well as fewer school problems.

Summary

1. The former babies in permanent nurseries who were re-examined at age $14\frac{1}{2}$ years, were physically normally developed and, excluding some psychosomatic symptoms, practically healthy.

2. Among these children we found more cases with behavioural problems and psychosomatic symptoms than are found in a control group. The observed symptoms indicate a tencency toward neurotic maladjustment, but there are no signs of social deviance or criminality. The large number of cases with sensitivity symptoms, which were observed even more often in girls, is striking. In addition, a tendency for over-adjustment combined with restriction of aggression was found, particularly in children who returned early to their families. Many of these youngsters are still in an infantile attitude of dependency. This latter attitude might be interpreted as a very strong need to be secure in the familiar reference group as a consequence of early frustration of that original drive.

3. The intelligence of the children is normal. However, even in cases of a relatively high intelligence, school success is difficult when environmental and psychological difficulties interfere.

4. A prognosis for these children is quite uncertain. According to their educational handicaps it seems that they will probably meet further difficulties before reaching an appropriate professional fulfilment or career.

B. Experimental–manipulative research

67. Preventive parent training (Switzerland)

J.-C. VUILLE and R. LÜTHI

Theoretical background

Preventive efforts in the field of mental health should start early in childhood, because the first years of life constitute the most sensitive period of emotional and social development. Though the links between childhood and adult psychopathology are not as tight as generally claimed, early intervention would appear to be able to attack at least one source of long-lasting mental disability. In modern industrial society intervention by experts appears to have become necessary because important bonds between the generations have been disrupted. Many of the behavioural rules which used to govern human interactions are no longer valid, leaving a vacuum and a sense of insecurity in young parents. It is one of the major hypotheses to be tested in the present project, that this vacuum can be filled to the benefit of the children with knowledge derived from the educational and medical sciences. In particular, learning theory is seen as one of the most important contributions to the knowledge and skills which are easily taught and readily applicable in everyday situations.

Experiences with *secondary* prevention, either in the form of an at-risk-strategy, by means of crisis intervention, or through systematic population screening, have shown that though such efforts may be worthwhile, their efficiency is as yet unsatisfactory. Attempts at *primary* prevention through parent education, on the other hand, have hitherto not been able to demonstrate a sufficient impact either, mainly because the participation rates were notoriously low. In order to overcome this difficulty, parent education should be integrated into the programme of those organizations which are already widely accepted as a support for families of young children. All industrialized countries provide some form of organized health care for mothers and infants. In many countries these MCH-services reach almost 100 per cent of all families with infants. This high acceptance rate is achieved by keeping the social distance between provider and user as small as possible without compromising the professional competence, by means of an active home-visiting policy, and through the provision of services which every family with young children needs, irrespective of social status.

The present project is an attempt to implement a well-defined preventive programme for mental health in an established Maternal and Child Health Service. The programme is built up as a combination of primary and secondary prevention. Its overall effectiveness will be assessed by comparing the outcome in the experimental and in two control groups. The goals of the programme are as follows:

1. To reach as many parents of 1 to 4 year olds as possible;
2. To make parent–child interactions more gratifying through better recognition of the child's true needs and through increased use of positive contact in adequate situations;
3. To enhance the subjective feeling of parental competence in mothers and fathers;
4. To provide parents with a simple language (derived from learning theory) in terms of which child-rearing problems can be discussed;
5. To improve the ability of parents to recognize signals of developmental disturbances in their child and to seek adequate help;
6. To promote parents' confidence in those who provide help and advice for problems in child-rearing, and to establish and maintain a close contact with the child health team;
7. To reduce the prevalence of behavioural troubles in the child.

Organization

The project is directed by Dr J.-C. Vuille, Asssociate Professor of Social Paediatrics and Deputy Director of the Institute of Social and Preventive Medicine, University of Bern. Dr R. Lüthi, Educational Psychologist, is the author of the training course; he is also responsible for individual counselling. Other collaborators are: 2 secretaries, 14 child health nurses, 10–20 'mediators' (mainly women trained as parent educators), and 20 interviewers.

The project is a joint enterprise of different organizational settings: University of Berne (Institute for Social and Preventive Medicine and Institute of Psychology), Bernese Association for Parent Education, and Maternal and Child Health Services of 14 districts in the Canton of Berne. The project is supported by grants from the Swiss National Science Foundation (Grant Nr. 3·823–0·76).

Selection of the sample

The three groups (one experimental and two control groups) were recruited from 4 or 5 child health districts each (one nurse per district). Each district was randomly assigned to one of the three groups. The criteria for inclusion of individual families were:

Living within the district;
First child of family born between 1 November 1975 and 30 April 1976;
Two contacts or more with child health nurse during the baby's first year (for nutritional counselling, etc.);
Sufficient comprehension of Swiss German dialect.

Each group thus includes approximately 200 families (participants and non-participants).

In the experimental group (group A) and in control group B the parents were invited to take part in the programme when the baby was between 9 and 12 months old. The personal invitation by the nurse was preceded by an informative letter. Two or more yearly personal contacts were scheduled for the participants in both groups; these contacts could be initiated either by the parents (preferably) or by the nurse. These contacts were essentially informal in character. In addition, the nurses of group B were free to organize course or group meetings of a traditional type. In control group C no special programme was offered to the parents. They were asked, however, whether they would participate in a programme of parent education if such a programme were available in their district. This question was necessary in order to allow a separation of potential participants and non-participants in group C.

The non-participants of all three groups were tracked again when the child was four years of age, and great efforts were made to include as many of them as possible in the final evaluation. Dropouts were followed by the responsible nurse only in so far as they stayed within the Canton of Berne. They will also be included in the final evaluation.

The programme of the experimental group (group A)

When the first child was 18 months old, the parents were invited to participate in basic training in small groups (12 persons) which consisted of six programmed sessions. The sessions were guided by 'mediators' who had previously been trained as 'parent educators' by the Bernese Association for Parent Education, and who had had an additional intensive course concerning the details of the six group sessions. Each session consisted of a complete package with precisely stated teaching goals, a written manual, all the necessary material (films, overhead-projections, working sheets, etc.), and planned exercises using video-recording. In spite of this rather rigid teaching method there was enough opportunity for free discussions. However, problems concerning individual children were not discussed in depth during this group work. A year later another series of 4 sessions was organized. This time the discussions focused on problem-solving strategies with material provided by the parents themselves.

During the 2½ years following the basic training, individual contacts between the parents and the consulting team (consisting of a child health nurse, one or more 'mediators', a consultant paediatrician, and a consultant psychologist) took place at irregular intervals. As a rule the team was represented by the nurse, but a wish for primary contacts with other persons was not refused. Experts were consulted whenever this appeared appropriate according to the kind or the severity of the problems. This procedure constituted the *secondary prevention* in our programme. In order to obtain high acceptance rates and reliable information also during this part, formal screening procedures were replaced by frequent personal contacts with one, and preferably the same, person.

Participation

Fifty per cent of the families in group A (selected according to the principles mentioned above and invited by letter and through personal contact) participated in the basic training. The percentage of later drop-outs for reasons other than moving out of the area was very low. While a participation rate of 50 per cent is high if compared with previous achievements in the same region using traditional methods of advertisement, it is still insufficient from the point of view of public health. The families with the most urgent need for help in child-rearing may experience the greatest difficulties to participate in discussion groups. Therefore, a home interview was conducted with 90 per cent of the non-participating mothers still resident in the area. The results of this interview are still being analysed, but the main conclusion is already clear: in the majority of nonparticipating families the situation of the child was good. These parents already applied most of the principles taught in our training and their judgment of not needing any parent training was probably correct. In a small percentage (5–10 per cent) however, we found evidence for child-rearing attitudes and practices implying a high risk for a distorted emotional and social

development. An effective preventive strategy will have to find ways of how to establish a continuous contact with these withdrawing high-risk families.

Methods of evaluation

Background information

For all participants in all three groups the following information was gathered initially:

Structure of the family;
Character of place of residence;
Type and size of dwelling;
For mother and father separately:
 Date of birth
 Profession
 Occupational situation
 Degree of employment
 Civil status
 Religion.
Concerning first child:
 Complications of pregnancy
 Complications of delivery
 State of health of newborn
 Psychomotor development (rough estimate whether normal or not)
 Severe and/or chronic disease or handicap.

Psychological examinations

Before the start of the training in group A and 2½ years later (when the first child was 4 years old), the following assessments were performed:

Test of social development;
Inventory of behavioural symptoms in the child;
Parents' knowledge of educational principles;
Parents' attitude towards certain educational situations;
Parents' rating of own competence as a parent;
Parents' educational style;
Parents' attitude towards medical and educational experts and institutions;
Parents' personality;
Direct observation and analysis of parent–child interaction (video);
Immediately after the basic training the parents' experiences and opinions concerning this course were also assessed.

Groups B and C are given the same tests at the end of the observation period. Certain tests were also administered initially, in order to assess the degree of comparability between the three groups. The greatest problem is with group C, which was intended to represent a true control with no intervention at all. Obviously, a thorough psychological examination with many intricate questions at the beginning might very well provide the incitement for a dialogue between the parents and/or the consultation of an expert, which would perhaps not have taken place without the interference of the evaluation process. Therefore, a 50 per cent random sample from group C was chosen and given the following tests: Vineland Social Maturity Scale, inventory of behavioral symptoms in the child, parent attitude towards certain educational situations, and attitude to parent training courses.

Data analysis

A vast amount of data has accumulated during a period of 3 years, and electronic data processing is therefore inevitable. In order to preserve the anonymity of the participants, the names and addresses are kept at the Child Health Centres. The documents used for the evaluation are identified by number only. Further follow-up of individuals would be possible by going back to the lists at the Child Health Centres.

Status of the project

As of March 1980, the interventions in group A have been completed and the final interview and testing in all three groups is in progress. The evaluation will be completed in about 2 months, but it will take at least another year before any quantitative results will be available. A preliminary analysis has been performed concerning the gain in theoretical and practical knowledge immediately after the basic training (Lüthi 1979). This analysis showed a significant increase in cognitive scores concerning basic principles of learning theory and their practical application in everyday situations. No significant increase was observed, however, in the problem-solving potential. Whether this capacity could be enhanced during the second training has not yet been studied.

Problems encountered

The most important problems encountered during the initial phase of the project relate to ethical issues and to questions of professional policy. The most rigorous critics maintain that any active strategy is unethical because it threatens the autonomy of the parents and is a mechanism of transfer of responsibility from the parents to the state. (In our view, the project aims rather at providing the parents with better opportunities to assume their responsibility.)

Another rather widespread criticism is concerned with the use of learning theory as the theoretical background of the basic training. Some people fear that the parents might be taught how to manipulate their children, and that this might eventually produce a generation of opportunists. (As a matter of fact the emphasis of the training is very much on the rights of children as individuals, on how to help them to reach independence and to assume responsibility for their own business.)

Finally, there has been some controversy concerning which profession, medical or educational, has the ultimate responsiblity for this preventive action with small children. Our concept relies on the fact that in infants and small children any disturbance of behaviour has important biological and medical aspects, and that parents generally address themselves to their physician or nurse for advice. The established Maternal and Child Health Organization appears therefore as the most natural framework for the implementation of an educational programme. On the other hand, it is recognized that the medical profession is not prepared well enough for this task, and therefore, educational and/or psychological experts have to join the health team. For the age groups of five to six years and older the professional roles might be reversed; when the school becomes the most important social setting outside the home, it appears logical that the educational profession should assume the responsibility for organizing preventive activities and invite medical experts to join their team.

68. Psychophysical crises observed in children living in complete families from birth up to the age of four years. Some results of the follow-up study to an experiment of early educational guidance in the town of Zurich (Switzerland)

LYDIA SCHEIER and MARIE MEIERHOFER

Introduction

In 1961 Mrs M. Meierhofer founded a medical-psychological consulting centre for mothers in a district of Zurich. This service was offered to all mothers of healthy first-born babies if the children could grow up in complete families (year of birth 1961–3). Almost all collaborated. Later on, they also brought along to the consulting centre their later born children (year of birth 1963–6). At the same time there were enquiries from mothers who had heard of this consulting possibility; most of these mothers were also given advice if their children were healthy at birth and if the families were complete (year of birth 1963–71).

Between 1961 and 1974, 51 children from birth up to four years of age were regularly examined, tested, and observed, while their mothers were advised in matters of child education. Some children were examined and tested again at the age of 7 and 11 years; parents as well as teachers had to answer a questionnaire.

This study is based on the data of twenty of these children (year of birth 1961–5). The data mainly consists of the written records from tapes of the consulting talks between physician and parents of the children and direct observations by the physician during examination. The aim of this longitudinal project was to collect data on psychophysical crises, to evaluate their severity, and to log their further development. Psychophysical crises can be observed in the following fields:

(1) Eating and digesting problems;
(2) Sleeping problems:
(3) Allergic reactions:
(4) Psychomotoric disturbances;
(5) Fears;
(6) Reactions of resistance and obstinancy;
(7) Aggressions;
(8) Mood disturbances.

The criteria used was the parents' feeling that this particular 'phenomenon' was a disturbance or at least a problem for them. The present study is not concerned with the influence of early educational guidance on the observed phenomena. The occurrences of psychophysical crises in 20 healthy children living in their families from birth up to four years of age were registered and related to circumstances and happenings in the near-surroundings of the children. Through this study paediatricians, infant nurses, children's educators, and also parents should become aware of all occurrences possible within the limits of a 'normal' development. Often such occurrences create serious worries and demand profound ability from the persons in charge.

Besides the present study which attempts to give a general view of the whole spectrum of observed psychophysical phenomena, several more specific studies of these same children have been carried out and partly published. These studies relate to such topics as: relations between siblings and rivalry between them (Savioz 1968); fears in children (Schäppi-Freuler 1976). A study about 'explicit and implicit sexual education in the family' is in preparation.

The data

For each child there are tapes of interview reports and a letter file containing copies of consulting reports, anamnestic sheets, regularly collected physical data (height and weight, tooth development, and test results), a developmental test up to two years, and an intelligence test for older children. For some of the 7-and 11-year-old children there is a test battery and an interview with a standardized questionnaire on file. There are also follow-up observation reports of nursery school children since the age of 3 years, and for some children observation reports in their families as well. For each child there is a series of photographs.

The group of 20 observed children is not representative of the whole group of their peers in Switzerland or in the town of Zurich (their number is too limited indeed). On the other hand, they are not 'special' children: the conditions under which they are growing up represent the usual conditions in this district of Zurich, which means, middle class, urban surroundings, no industry. These 20 children are 11 boys and 9 girls (birth year: 1961 to 1965); nine are first-born, nine second-born, and two are third-born children. Two are growing up as single children, 11 are in two children families, and 7 in three children families. These families are living in the traditional way—the father works away from home while the mother cares for the home and children full time.

Consultations and examinations

These took place as follows:

(a) With the infants between 0 and 10 months: once a month;
(b) Between 10 months and 4 years: once every three months;
(c) Between 4 and 6 years (according to special wishes of the parents): every three to six months;
(d) At the age of 7 and 11: a single examination.

If special problems emerged, the mothers could request a consulting talk in between testing dates. Dates missed because of illness, absence, etc. were made up for as soon as possible. The consultations have only been terminated if the families were moving too far out of the district.

It would be possible to again contact the families still living in Zurich, but the Institute for Psychohygiene is not able to carry out a new examination of the children who are now 15 and 16 years old.

Data analysis

The psychophysical crises reported by the mothers and recorded by the collaborators of the project during examinations have been quoted in a schedule distinguishing 8 main groups and showing the 8 half-year periods from ages 0 to 4. The registration list shows which phenomena appear most frequently (and at what age) and how early occurrences influence later development. Of course, a completion of the investigations which have been carried out after four years are of special interest. Such a completion for some of the 20 children is planned.

Background information

Such psychophysical crises in children are, as everybody knows, closely related to the reactions of the parents and near-

surroundings to the behaviour and special problems of the children. These have been registered during consulting talks, to the extent that the mothers spontaneously informed us; with the children observed directly at home, these reactions have been quoted systematically.

Information available about the parents includes age, professional position (former occupation of the mother), housing situation, moving during the follow-up period, contact with their own parents, and, where applicable, death of the grandparents. In addition, information about the development of the other children in the family and their education is available.

Problems encountered

Problems did not arise in receiving collaboration from the mothers (who benefited by free consultation), or from the children (who had to endure the whole procedure of being measured, examined, photographed, etc.), or in the regular examinations over the period of several years. The difficulties encountered consisted mainly in ensuring an objective comparability of the obtained data, due to the fact that in the 15 years of collecting data there were many changes in the educational practice of young parents as well as in the test methods used. In addition, the reports of the mothers are not in all cases equally complete and detailed. We noticed for instance that the mothers often reported in a much more detailed manner about their first child as compared to their later children; in many cases a mother who brought her second-born child for examination was constantly talking about difficulties caused by her first-born child.

A further problem is the large amount of data collected. In the 15 to 16 years since the start of this project a number of collaborators of the Institute of Psychohygiene in Early Childhood have participated in collecting, sorting out, and interpreting the data using individual 'systems'. The financial status of the Institute never allowed common work of several collaborators on the longitudinal material. At present we have, for each of the children examined, a big file of partly interpreted material, including pictures, drawings, and test results for 51 children. Each child's file could lead to a detailed case analysis. Presently we have to limit our work to those data which allow a comparative description of 20 cases. We are experimenting with a diagram-like description of material which can be completed by an analysis of a few cases, so in spite of the shortage in staff, it will be possible to complete a first report soon. The danger in such a longitudinal study is that by the time the test results are published, some of the data have already become 'out of date'.

Advantages

While in general in scientific literature more attention is paid to abnormal personal development than to so-called 'normal' development, we attempted here to register all psychophysical crises in the course of 'normal' development. Among them are also those which later on probably would have, without consultation, led to developmental disturbances (for example, severe eating problems or infant depression). Thus we must emphasize the necessity of *early* detection and treatment of children's disturbances. There is no other way of avoiding much pain to children and parents, self-reproaches of the parents, and also high costs for long treatment later on. In addition, the high number of mothers visiting the consulting centre shows that such an early consultation and examination meets the needs of the parents who are very often uncertain in educational matters.

69. The Mauritius project

SARNOFF A. MEDNICK, FINI SCHULSINGER, and PETER H. VENABLES

Introduction

Considerable ingenuity has been expended on devising relatively esoteric and technically sophisticated methods of treatment for the chronically ill (heart transplants, kidney machines, etc.), providing some form of therapy for the mentally disturbed and rehabilitation for the recidivistic criminal. In addition to *treatment* attempts, many of these patients and clients as well as welfare recipients must rely heavily on societal support for thier maintenance. These patients, clients, and welfare recipients are generally not made productive or happy by these ameliorative efforts. But at the present time these efforts are necessary, in fact, praiseworthy.

Paradoxically, from the point of view of society, these medical advances and care facilities and agencies serve only to aggravate the total treatment problem by radically increasing the number of chronically ill (Gruenberg 1977). This further taxes our treatment-technology research inventiveness. In the field of mental health, new psychotherapies with catchy names spring up like mushrooms; new drugs are sought to control the seriously disturbed behaviour of patients. But we would argue that if we are to reduce human suffering and the spiralling burden to the community, some appropriate proportion of society's resources should be devoted to finding ways to prevent the *initial* onset of mental illness.

As we foresee it, intervention programmes in the field of mental health will not take the form of blanket population treatments, such as water fluoridation. They are more likely to be somewhat more invasive or intrusive, both temporally and psychologically. As a consequence, the interventions will very likely have to be restricted to those at high risk of developing a mental disorder. A first step in mental health intervention research very likely must be to devise assessment procedures which will efficiently identify individuals (probably children) who are in great danger of some day becoming psychiatric patients. The longitudinal, prospective study design can make a contribution to the development of methods of early identification of such individuals. The high-risk design (Chapters 61–6) is especially devised for this purpose.

In the high-risk design subjects are identified (most often because of deviance in their parents) and intensively assessed (typically along with controls). They are then followed for an appropriate period of time until some level of decompensation is observed in some of the subjects. The life data and individual characteristics of the decompensated subjects are then examined to find characteristics which distinguish them from their more fortunate co-subjects. If these distinguishing characteristics can result in efficient and reliable discrimination, and generalization is feasible from high-risk subjects to the general population, then we will have devised an assessment battery which can be administered to an unselected population of children to identify a target group for intervention research. (For further elaboration see Mednick 1978; Mednick and Lanoil 1977.)

This strategy was first described in 1960 (Mednick 1960) and operationalized in 1962 in Copenhagen when we examined 207 children at high risk for schizophrenia (they have chronically, severely schizophrenic mothers) (Mednick *et al.* 1974). In 1967 when 20 high-risk individuals evidenced psychiatric breakdown, we discovered that certain autonomic nervous system variables (meas-

ured in 1962) discriminated the breakdown subjects from carefully chosen controls (Mednick and Schulsinger 1973). We then (1972) assessed a normal population of three-year olds in Mauritius with these same autonomic measures, detected those who resembled the breakdown subjects from Copenhagen, and began exploring the possibilities of intervention in specially established nursery schools (Schulsinger *et al.* 1975; Venables *et al.* 1978). This report describes the method and some results of the Mauritius intervention project.

The Mauritius intervention project

The results of the Copenhagen high-risk project suggested that certain autonomic measures could be useful in the early detection of children at risk for mental illness. Coincidentally, at that time one of us (SAM) was a member of a WHO Scientific Group of Neurophysiological Research which recommended that priority be given to 'longitudinal neurophysiological studies of high risk subjects'. WHO then invited the Psykologisk Institut in Copenhagen to undertake such research in Mauritius.

Despite the practical, logical, and methodological problems which we could foresee (only a fraction of those we encountered) we determined to follow the long-term plan (Mednick 1960) to use the high-risk study results to select individuals at risk from the general population and to begin research on primary prevention.

A visit to Mauritius indicated that local vaccination records would enable us to indentify a birth cohort which had survived to age three. Taking all three-year olds in two communities (Quatre Bornes and Vacoas) resulted in a population of about 1800 children. We combined forces with A. C. Raman, a Mauritian, English-trained psychiatrist, and established a laboratory in Quatre Bornes. As a result of the energetic efforts of Brian Bell, an English psychophysiologist who managed the project, the 1800 children were psychophysiologically assessed in the year beginning August 1972. In addition to the psychophysiological assessment we observed and coded play behaviour and examined cognitive development of the 1800 children. This aspect of the project was directed by Brian Sutton-Smith. Turan Itil and George Ulett taped EEGs for a part of the population. A family interview, a medical examination, and perinatal information were also recorded. The project owes a large debt to the Mauritian government. Sir Seewoosagur Ramgoolam, the prime minister (and a physician) and his cabinet ministers, particularly Sir Harold Walter (then his Minister of Health) offered intelligent criticisms, useful guidance, and practical support in the establishment and running of the project.

In undertaking this work we were aware that there were many potential pitfalls involved in the assumption that childhood autonomic deviance (assessed by peripheral measures) would predict to adult mental illness, especially when our expectations were based on preliminary results on adolescents in Copenhagen, and especially moving to a very different culture with different races and climatic conditions. However, a longitudinal study of a psychophysiologically-assessed, large, unselected population of children in Mauritius was deemed of sufficient importance in its own right to justify the project. In any case, were we to wait for evidence adequate enough to forestall criticism (Garmezy 1974) we would very likely not survive to write the grant application.

This report will concern itself only with data related to the skin conductance measures. (Details not appropriate for this brief presentation may be found in Schulsinger *et al.* 1975 and Venables *et al.* 1978.) These skin conductance measures were scored by hand in Mauritius, coded, and sent to Venables in England for analysis; 1796 usable records were obtained. Distributions of the skin conductance measures were plotted. Children evidencing deviant skin conductance behaviour, such as that evidenced by the Copenhagen breakdown group, were identified. (For more detail on the skin conductance variables see Mednick *et al.* 1974) Smaller groups with other deviance of special interest and controls with average skin conductance functioning were also identified. (For details see Venables *et al.* 1978) A total of 200 such children from the population of 1796 were isolated; 100 were placed in two specially established nursery schools. The remaining 100 were selected as matched controls and permitted to remain in the community (community controls).

The nursery schools were directed by Steen Møller and Bodil Birket-Smith, Danish experts who, as part of the project, also instituted the first nursery school teacher-training programme in Mauritius. Beyond the design of the nursery schools, no specific intervention programme was attempted in this first project. The nursery schools had several distinctive features, however, which should be mentioned:

1. The 100 children were almost completely from poor families. The children were bussed to and from school; the hours were 9.00 a.m. to 3.00 p.m. The nursery school children were given a hot lunch which almost certainly contained a higher protein content than the community controls received;
2. Because of the selection procedures, the nursery schools had a very high density of autonomically-sensitive children (about 50 per cent);
3. The directors and teachers were very highly motivated, well trained, and had a remarkable *esprit de corps*.

It should be stated that at no time was anyone in Mauritius informed regarding the autonomic status of the children. In addition to the intervention opportunity, the nursery schools provided us with a chance to systematically observe the behaviour of these children. The advantages of using nursery schools for interventive research are spelled out in Mednick and Lanoil (1977) and in Mednick *et al.* (1975a).

Results of nursery school experience

The autonomically deviant (Aut. High-Risk) and normal (Aut. Low-Risk) groups were first admitted to the nursery schools in 1973. They continued until 1976 when they all entered the primary school system. The community controls (matched for age, sex, race, and autonomic characteristics) remained undisturbed by us during this period except for some psychophysiological retesting in a laboratory in one of the nursery schools.

Just before the 100 community control and 100 nursery children began primary school in December 1976, they were invited in for a behavioural assessment session in order to compare them and estimate the effect of the nursery school. In order to bias the testing as little as possible, the play observation session did not take place at either of the nursery schools but at a third building. All children were dressed in new identical uniforms. Trained observers who had not previously met the children, provided standardized ratings of their behaviour using an adaptation of a system devised by Bell *et al.* (1971). New toys were provided for the play period. In other words, attempts were made to reduce the possibility of the identification of the nursery children by the observers or any advantage of the nursery children in familiarity with the setting, play materials, or observers.

The children were brought to the observation setting in buses in groups of four, one from each of the two nursery schools and one from each of the communities. (Thus none of the children knew each other.) The four children were brought together in a playroom; during the play period each child was observed for a period of eight minutes. Aspects of their behaviour were counted or timed. We will report on the timed behaviour which consisted of:

Watching. The observer timed periods when the child was passive and watching others.
Positive interaction. The observer timed periods when the child talked or played co-operatively with other children.
Constructive play alone. The observer timed the total number of seconds the child played constructively with toys by himself.

Since the total observation period for each child was eight minutes, the times spent in the three activities are not mutually independent. The data for the two nursery schools and communities were combined since previous analyses indicated that these were not significant variables.

Figure 69.1 compares the Aut. High-Risk and Aut. Low-Risk groups who experienced the nursery schools with the psycho-

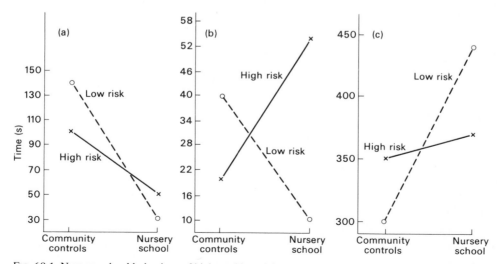

FIG. 69.1. Nursery school behaviour of high- and low-risk nursery and community control children: (A) watching; (B) positive interactions; (C) constructive play alone. (These three figures are presented together for ease of comparison. It should be emphasized that they are each drawn to a different scale. The reader is urged to note this and take these differences into account.)

physiologically-matched community controls who did not experience the nursery schools. The three figures were drawn together to make comparison easier. It should be emphasized that they are each drawn to a different scale. As might be expected, most of the children spent most of the eight minutes constructively playing with the new toys (Fig. 69.1(C)). In interpreting the results we assume that if the nursery children had not attended the nursery schools they would have been identical to their matched community controls at the time of this assessment.

Note that both Aut. High- and Aut. Low-Risk groups substantially decrease their inactive watching after having attended the nursery schools. The Low-Risk (Community) children are relatively high in positive interactions and watching. After the nursery experience they reduce both of these activities to the benefit of indulging in constructive play. The Aut. High-Risk (Community) children tend not to engage in positive interactions but are high in constructive play. It is gratifying that the greatest effect of the nursery school experience for the Aut. High-Risk children is their increase in positive interactions of a social nature (this, at the expense of time spent in isolated, inactive watching).

We offer the following interpretations of these results:

1. The psychophysiological selection criteria are correlated with specific characteristic behaviours before the influence of the nursery school.
2. The nursery school experience affects the social and play behaviour of the children.
3. The nursery school affects behaviour in the children differentially as a function of the psychophysiological characteristics used in selection.

What is most encouraging is the fact that the largest 'change' for the Aut. High-Risk group is an increase in positive social interactions. This increase is observed in a situation where they are thrown in with peers and adult observers who are unknown to them. In terms of the interventive goals of this project these results are rewarding. Perhaps most heartening is the fact that such a project could be completed.

Summary and conclusions

We began with the proposal that early detection is a useful first step in primary prevention research. The 1962 Copenhagen high-risk study suggested that specific autonomic variables might be useful in early detection. These were utilized in a population assessment of 1800 3-year-old, Mauritian children. Autonomically-defined high-risk children were identified and placed in specially established nursery schools. The chief effect of the nursery school on the autonomically-deviant children was to increase their engagement in positive social interactions. This result was in conformity with the aims of the intervention.

The high-risk selection criterion only made use of the autonomic characteristics of the children. A multidimensional selection device would doubtless do a better job. In this study, we concentrated on this single physiological channel because:

1. There were fewer problems in cross-cultural application;
2. It gave us the opportunity to conduct a longitudinal study of the long-term correlates of 3-year old autonomic status;
3. It reduced the complexity of the total experiment.

We are planning an assessment of the Mauritius cohort at age 10. This might be done in the context of summer camps (suggested by Richard Q. Bell) established for this purpose. This will enable us to observe the behaviour of the 1800 children as a function of their autonomic characteristics and to assess the possible long-term effects of the nursery school.

Acknowledgements

The high-risk research is being supported by USPHS Grant No. MH 31433 and was supported earlier by the Foundation for Child Development. The Mauritius research was originally supported by grants to the Psykologisk Institut from the World Health Organization. We wish to express our gratitude to the Mauritian government for their continuing support during the entire project and to date. The assessment of the Mauritian children was supported by a grant from the British Medical Research Council to Venables. The Danish Organization for Aid to Developing Nations (DANIDA) supported the nursery schools.

Part IV

Comments on methods and utility of longitudinal research

70. Reaction: the future of longitudinal studies

ERNEST M. GRUENBERG and LINDA LE RESCHE

Introduction

The European Region of the World Health Organization is to be congratulated for sponsoring this volume to call attention to an expanding set of activities conducted in the name of longitudinal research. This kind of an overview inevitably presents a mixed lot in terms of quality, scope, accomplishments, and promise. The thing which holds the set of proposals and reports together is the common feature of viewing time in a forward looking way, watching as one thing leads to another in the health situation of a defined population of people.

In this chapter we propose to put the development of longitudinal research projects in a historical context by describing the basic goals of epidemiology and by outlining the more common methods used to investigate the relationship between the causes of disease and their consequences. From this will emerge a recognition that the longitudinal study has developed out of a need to meet certain problems presented by studies which approached the issue of time in other ways. We hope that by classifying these other ways of relating investigations to time the special assets of longitudinal studies will emerge and highlight the appropriate place for longitudinal studies in epidemiological research. The special problems and weaknesses of longitudinal studies will also be mentioned.

Epidemiology

Epidemiology is the basic science of preventive medicine. It studies:

1. Who gets sick and who does not?
2. Why?
3. What can be done about it?

Epidemiology studies the patterns of occurrence of disease in populations. So epidemiology sometimes discovers preventable causes of disease; and whenever a programme seeks to lower the prevalence of a disease, epidemiology must be used to determine whether it succeeds. Therefore, epidemiology is the basic science of preventive medicine.

So epidemiology has two aspects. On the one hand, disease, disability, and death must be seen biologically as an inherent part of life, and the understanding of disease processes is as much a matter of scientific curiosity as is any other study of the nature of mankind. But there is also the practical aspect that when we understand how to modify certain circumstances so that fewer people become ill, we are on the path to prevention of disease and disability. Both the theoretical and the practical aspects will be given emphasis throughout this chapter. The distinction between the two can perhaps best be illustrated by a single example. It is well established that chronic poisoning with excessive alcohol leads to permanent damage to the brain and liver. On the surface, this knowledge would seem to provide a means for lowering the frequency of brain and liver damage from alcohol. But in the absence of any established socially organized method for reducing the frequency of self-poisoning with alcohol, this knowledge, even though correct, does not lead to a changed disease pattern.

When one considers the above description of what epidemiology is and does, it is obvious that many scientists and investigators have been doing epidemiology under many different rubrics. However, it is a mistake to think that epidemiology is simply a matter of common sense and intelligence. There is a technology which has been developed over the centuries, and it is not necessary for each new epidemiologist to repeat the mistakes of the past or to rediscover already established facts. The cumulative process by which knowledge has been gained has accelerated rapidly in the last hundred or so years, and a series of research techniques have accumulated which make it more likely that each decade will lead to fundamental advances in our knowledge and understanding. As a result of systematically applied empirical knowledge about the cause of disease, the whole pattern of disease experienced by mankind has been transformed in the last two centuries. It is of course true that there is still much disease and, in some respects, the way our knowledge has advanced has led to a rising prevalence of certain diseases (Gruenberg 1977). Nonetheless, the contributions have been enormous, and in particular, the life expectation at birth has risen fantastically. When looking at the potential of the longitudinal study, we should not begin by throwing away the methods which have led to such valuable insights in the past, but rather we should ask ourselves what new power longitudinal studies give us that the older methods did not.

Other epidemiological methods

Comparisons

The most elementary approach to understanding the factors which give rise to a disease is simply to compare a population in which a disease is common with another population in which it is not so common. Going back to the Hippocratic writings on epidemics, it had been observed by the ancients that malarial fevers were more common in some cities than in others, as were certain types of diarrhoea. This was recognized, not by careful counting, but by observant doctors noticing that each community had its own prevailing pattern of disease. Inferences were then drawn about what could produce these differences. Weather, wind, water, and social customs are all mentioned as probable causes of disease in these ancient writings with no statistical data whatever.

The purist might object that such crude observations can easily be erroneous, and he would be correct. However, it is wrong to think that all variations in occurrence of disease are too minute to be detected by thoughtful, systematic observation. All science starts by selecting out of the vast mass of observations key points that might be related to the phenomenon of interest. Something draws our attention to a particular event or sequence of events and we ask ourselves, 'What is this, how did it come about, and what can be done about it?' In epidemiology, the events which concern us are people becoming ill or disabled or unable to function as expected. The recognition that a problem exists starts with a complaint by someone to a clinician, who then formulates a diagnosis and gives a label to the problem. This cannot be emphasized too much, because it is very easy to develop the illusion that all such labels (e.g., autistic, delinquent, deviate) applied to people by such mechanisms have some inherent meaning. This is not to say that such labels cannot be used properly to group individuals as having something in common, but unless they are clearly defined and their sources clearly described, we can develop marvelous notions about what the labels mean without any baseline in reality.

So it is the clinician's observation that a group of people have something in common that is not desired that starts the problem on the way to definition and solution. For example, an ophthalmologist in Australia (Gregg 1941) noticed a sudden cluster in time of new-born infants brought to him with a cataract in the lens, an uncommon condition in that part of the world. He did not have to go back and count the cases he had seen in previous years to recognize that something new was going on. He connected this clustering of clouded lenses with an epidemic of German measles (rubella) which had occurred the previous year, and began to ask the mothers of the affected infants whether they had had German measles while they were pregnant. This led to more systematic investigations, to more careful counting, and ultimately to the very careful prospective studies of Hill *et al.* (1958) on German measles which showed not only that congenital cataracts, but also congenital malformations of the heart and mental retardation could be produced by German measles when experienced early in foetal development.

Pickles, the health officer and only practitioner for two villages, had made a habit of keeping systematic records and thinking about them in his attempts to understand the distribution of disease in his little population laboratory where he knew everyone personally. On this basis, he was able to elucidate the correlation between chicken-pox in children and shingles in adults and the nature of epidemic pleurodynia (Pickles 1948), both of which were fundamental, original observations.

Case-control studies

The case-control study begins with a straightforward observation that a condition is more common in one population than another. It then collects simultaneously a group of cases and a group of *comparable* controls and takes all information that is available or can be readily gathered on both groups to determine what characteristics the cases have in common that the controls do not have. Even if the factor which distinguishes the cases from the controls is not the actual cause of the disease, it may provide clues to the causal mechanism which might be involved (Lilienfeld 1976). Two recent examples of major progress using a case-control approach should be mentioned here.

At Massachusetts General Hospital, several cases of a vaginal carcinoma in young women (hardly ever recorded in the literature or in the case records of the hospital) appeared over a period of a few weeks. The epidemiologist and gynaecologists found a few more cases, picked matched controls of women born in the same hospital during the same time period, searched the medical records, and in a few weeks showed that what the cases had in common was that their mothers had been treated with stilbestrol while pregnant (Herbst *et al.* 1971). Here again, it was not necessary to do a lot of counting to know that something new had happened, since, from general knowledge of working in a stable situation, the gynaecologists knew that this was an extremely rare condition. Earlier, Ochsner and DeBakey (1939) had noticed that carcinoma of the lung was much more common among cigarette smokers than among non-smokers. The finding was largely ignored in the public health and medical literature until a series of case-control studies showed that the probability of a person with lung cancer having been a cigarette smoker was nearly 100 per cent, whereas the probability that a person without lung cancer had been a smoker was much less.

The case-control study is an enormously powerful tool, and is very often the sensible first stage of inquiry. But it has certain inherent weaknesses. In case-control studies, past events are used to make inferences about present health conditions. Information from the past obtained from medical records or from the self-reports of research subjects can be distorted. The problems of selective accumulation and selective survival, whether of case histories or patients' recollections, have been well documented.

A study without controls is like a compass without a needle; it can lead you anywhere you want to go and you will never know when you are off course. So controls are essential, but selecting them properly also presents fundamental problems. The most important of these can be termed the Berksonian bias (Lilienfeld 1976), which arises from picking a control population which is not comparable to the case population in every respect that may be relevant. For example, every medical service installation has built-in unknown biases regarding which examples of a given condition will come to its attention and be properly diagnosed. Selecting controls from the same medical facility does not ensure that their selection is biased in the same way as that of the cases. This can sometimes be avoided by taking neighbours of the cases from the same community for controls rather than using cases with some other medical condition in the same hospital. But the thoughtful investigator who looks over the literature will realize that in general this is not a totally soluble problem and that great judgement must be exercised in selecting controls.

A final problem with the case-control study is that although it can tell you that there is an increased risk associated with a suspected causal factor, e.g., cigarette-smoking and lung cancer, it cannot tell you the magnitude of the increased risk.

Prospective studies

In order to determine the magnitude of the risk, one must start with a population exposed to the risk factor and move forward in time to see how frequently the disease occurs (Lilienfeld 1976). Using such prospective investigations, it was possible to show that cigarette-smoking increases the risk of lung cancer many thousandfold, and that it doubles the risk of death from coronary heart disease (Sheps 1958; Levin 1953). The prospective study is a powerful tool and has made many contributions. However, it can be a costly and tedious process, particularly if there is a long interval between the time of exposure and the onset of disease. In this respect, it shares many of the limitations of longitudinal studies, as will be discussed later. Some investigators try to reduce the cost and complexity of the prospective study by searching for an existing source of earlier information on a defined population concerning the risk factors in which they are interested. They then try to find that population and to measure the frequency with which the disease has developed since the risk data were assembled. This approach is called a non-concurrent prospective design.

Preventive trials

A dramatic way to test a theory about the causes of disease in populations is to make a change in the situation. The preventive trial is the most powerful single tool for testing an aetiological hypothesis because it is the only method by which a single variable can be modified and the effects observed directly. The model preventive trial investigations are the Kingston–Newburgh studies (Ast *et al.* 1956) which showed that adding a trace of flouride to public water supplies reduces the frequency of dental decay. The most well known dramatic preventive trial was that of the Salk vaccine. Using double blind techniques on a national sample, the trial showed within a few months that the Salk vaccine was effective in preventing poliomyelitis (Francis *et al.* 1955). The preventive trial is also the most powerful single tool for theoretical purposes. As Brian MacMahon has said, (MacMahon and Pugh 1970), 'Epidemiology is the only science that proceeds on the principle of guilt by association'. If preventive trials were used as extensively as they should be, we would be able to exclude many innocent suspects from our theoretical presumptions of disease causation. But often, because they involve intervention in people's lives (even when the intervention is innocuous or positive), preventive trials raise social and ethical problems. They are sometimes thought to be too expensive, and are difficult to organize under the present research funding structure.

Ways of looking at time

Prevalence = incidence × average duration

Stop time for a moment, take a snapshot, and count who is sick and who is not. This produces what is called a point prevalence rate. It is simply the proportion of a defined population with a given condition at one moment in time, and it is the most direct measure of the importance of this particular condition to the people's health. In the end, it is the point prevalence rate which we seek to reduce with our disease control efforts. By measuring point prevalence rates at successive moments in time, e.g., 1910, 1920, . . ., 1980, we can tell whether a condition is becoming more or less common. The annual incidence rate is the number of new cases of a disease which begin each year, divided by the population at risk of developing that disease. It is the most fundamental measure of the force with which a disease is striking a given population.

Neither the point prevalence rate nor the annual incidence rate tells us anything about the duration of an illness episode. An illness may last a week or two like the common cold, or it may last for many years, like diabetes. The duration of all episodes of a condition beginning in the observed year divided by the number of episodes which began is the average duration. In a stable situation, the annual incidence rate multiplied by the average duration of cases is equal to the point prevalence rate.

From the above equation it is obvious that the prevalence rate can be reduced by reducing the annual incidence rate or shortening the average duration. With respect to disease control efforts, primary prevention reduces the prevalence rate by preventing a disease from starting, i.e., by reducing the incidence rate. Secondary prevention reduces the prevalence rate by shortening the duration of the average episode. An example of primary prevention is the Salk vaccine. It changed the prevalence rate of paralytic poliomyelitis radically by preventing new cases from occurring. Penicillin treatment for syphilis and desensitization treatments for hayfever are examples of secondary prevention. The incidence of these conditions has not been affected by these interventions, but because the duration of most cases has been cut dramatically, their prevalence rates have been reduced.

Accumulation

Any given individual's risk of developing a certain condition depends on a variety of factors, such as genetic make-up, medical history, and personal habits. Additionally, the person's risk may accumulate over time as he has lived under exposure to his life situation. There are life table techniques for summarizing these cumulative, or individual, risks with great accuracy, provided that good records are kept on movements into and out of the population.

The individual risk has played a major role in the study of genetic conditions and in the study of long-term consequences of chronic background states. For example, in genetic conditions, the assumption is made that the increased risk for the individual starts at the time of conception because of the genetic make-up of the individual organism. There are some conditions of this nature which manifest themselves shortly after birth, but others do not manifest themselves until the age of 20, 30, 40, or even later. There is then a concept of 'age of risk' involved, and what the investigator wishes to know is whether a person of a particular genetic background is more or less likely to develop a condition than people with a different genetic background. The Weinberg proband method has been developed specifically for calculating this kind of cumulative risk (1920). The method involves taking a cross-section picture of a total population for which histories exist as to who has had the condition in the past. People who have not lived through the full age of risk are regarded as having only partially demonstrated their freedom from the disease. By such methods, it is possible to make inferences about the increased risk of developing, e.g., schizophrenia or Huntington's chorea, among first degree relatives of cases as compared with the risk among first degree relatives of controls. But there are hazards to this kind of reasoning, and it is very difficult to separate social heritage from gene inheritance by these methods (Lilienfeld 1959).

Another use of the individual risk is actuarial. For example, the fact that a person has had a certain disease may be used as a basis for modifying life insurance rates. Whether or not the disease itself is a direct cause of death, it may be regarded as a contingency factor that increases a person's risk of dying at a younger age (Morris 1975).

Sequence of events

The developmentalists' point of view toward the sequence of events in the lives of individuals comes to be more and more important as we understand how diseases are produced. This is a rather new concept for epidemiologists, but the basic principle is a simple one: *we change as the result of experience*. These changes lead to changed responses to the same stimuli. A familiar example of this phenomenon is that of learning, but experience results in changes in other aspects of the organism besides the brain. The way tuberculosis develops as a disease was not understood until it became clear that the primary infection, which usually had no great effect on the health of the individual, modified the tissue responses to the next infection which might come many years later. The disease itself was an interaction between a new infection and a prior, changed state in the organism (Rich 1944). This process is also important in the immunity that results from prior exposure to a disease. For example, a single infection with poliomyelitis changes the organism in such a way that it becomes immune to all subsequent infection with the disease (e.g., Fox *et al*. 1957).

In part, it is this need for understanding sequence which makes the longitudinal study so attractive. We know that sequence can make a difference, but we usually lack exact hypotheses about how this occurs. So we feel that there will be an advantage in accumulating a data base with a good deal of information on a defined population which can later be inspected to bring out the effects of the sequences of events. Moreover, it is not the timing of the sequence that is important, but the fact that the sequence occurs. None of the other ways of looking at time can give us this information. Point prevalence rates, annual incidence rates, measures of duration, or measures of accumulated risk are of no help in understanding causal sequences.

Longitudinal studies

Sampling

It is unusual for a longitudinal study to be conducted using all the members of a community as subjects. In fact, the Lundby study is the only investigation reported in this volume which employed such a sample. Such a 100 per cent sample has the advantage that the subjects of the investigation are associated and in close touch with each other, so that each member of the study population can be used as a key informant about the other members of the population. However, in most communities where such close associations exist among people, there is no great variation in social class or living style. This is a disadvantage when such variation is thought to be important in the aetiology of disease.

Why do longitudinal studies?

Investigators who have used tables of routinely gathered information and more or less conventional research designs frequently feel dissatisfied. There is something a little dehumanizing about the whole process of what we like to call 'paper epidemiology'. The investigation lacks the vitality and concreteness of direct contact with research subjects and with the clinician's observations. The gathering of a limited amount of information on a focused topic always leaves the investigator feeling a little uneasy that some relevant issue could have been missed. Also, unanticipated events may occur that affect parts of the population and not others, and this may offer natural experiments once the data base has been established. A new exposure of one part of the population arising because of an industrial plant is a good example.

These are the motivations for fitting a data base on a defined population and moving forward in a longitudinal way. There has been a tendency to see a great advantage in registers of a particular condition (e.g., cancer registers), and a desire to create them as a basis for epidemiological investigations. These registers simply bring together all known examples of a condition in a defined population and make it possible for statistical and epidemiological studies to be made on data gathered in a routine fashion. They form a way of monitoring the frequency with which a condition or a group of conditions is occurring, and the effects that unanticipated events may have on the registered cases.

Like other epidemiological investigations, longitudinal studies require the assembly of information on many individuals to provide a perspective on disease which looks at what happens to a whole population rather than at what happens to each individual in it. This is the opposite of the current tendency towards reductionism—the tendency to look at smaller and smaller elements to infer the cause of what happens to the whole. Epidemiology is a population-based science, and epidemiological questions about the causes of disease in populations are questions about the whole population, not about each individual. The two lines of investigation run parallel historically. The field investigator of populations must be thoroughly familiar with the laboratory and clinical knowledge about the disease being studied, because it is at the clinical level that the questions arise. It is at the laboratory level that many of the scientific principles are elucidated and it is at the population level that consequences are felt and understood in human biological terms and in practical disease prevention.

Risks and limitations

The thalidomide scandal shook many public health workers thoroughly. Here was a new medication which produced devastating congenital abnormalities. It took an unconscionably long time to link the new epidemic of phakomelia to this new drug, and even when the link had been made, it took an unreasonable amount of time to ban the drug. Because of this failure, literally thousands of children were born without upper limbs, to live a lifetime of major disability. One inevitably asks whether this danger could have been anticipated. The answer is not clear. In contrast, the connection between diethylstilbestrol and vaginal carcinoma was discovered very quickly. Yet, no one could possibly suggest that this tragedy could have been avoided by any rational system of monitoring; the time interval between exposure during foetal life and the onset of the condition in early adulthood was too great. We could have been more cautious, we could have been more worried, and we could have been less excited about the possible usefulness of this poten-

tially dangerous treatment. But no conceivable system of monitoring would have revealed this problem any quicker. So our anxieties will not be rationally allayed by simply setting up rigid monitoring systems. The speed with which epidemiological responsiveness occurs in the presence of something new, the readiness of investigators to be deployed to confront a new situation, the intelligence and resourcefulness which attack the problem on an *ad hoc* basis all seem to be more important.

Before a longitudinal study is begun, its risks and limitations must be faced up to, and a cost–benefit analysis done. One of the great risks of longitudinal studies has to do with the way scientific knowledge accumulates. Each year more scientific events occur, more scientific findings are published, more scientists are working, and each scientist has more accumulated knowledge and a larger body of research skills to work with than the year before. The single crucial investigation that changes the whole scene is rare indeed, and it is not the usual way knowledge accumulates. Each question really does require several independent investigators approaching the same problem by somewhat different methods in order for us to be sure of the conclusions. Today, hardly anyone starts off as Charles Darwin did on his voyage on the Beagle with a general interest in biology, a loosely formulated set of ideas, and an opportunity to spend half a decade in service, wondering and speculating. But even then, Wallace was simultaneously developing the same insight. The investigator who undertakes to invest four years in a question and at the second year discovers that somebody else's findings have made his question irrelevant has lost two years of his life as a scientist. This is a gamble which every scientist must take. Hence, it is important to recognize that the quick study has its great advantages and has an ever growing place in scientific work in general. Nonetheless there are some questions that can only be investigated on a long-term basis. Yet one must expect that newly published researches can overtake the investigator's carefully laid plans.

In addition, those who deal with human populations on a longitudinal basis must always recognize the risk that the human population will disappear in front of their eyes, either through natural disaster or major social upheaval. The investment in a stable long-term investigative situation on a defined population is a serious gamble for the investigator and for those who provide the social underpinnings for the investigations. Both should recognize what is going on when such long-term investments are made.

Population losses can occur from many sources. In contrast to the stratified random sampling approach, longitudinal community population studies have the advantage of starting with a defined population so that when there are losses they are visible. But if continuing contact over a long period of time cannot be maintained in practice, many of the advantages of the longitudinal study are lost. It is often difficult to estimate the extent to which losses will occur. In many parts of the world, a longitudinal investigation is not practical because of the very high and rapidly increasing mobility of the population. In a few countries, particularly in Europe, where population registers have been maintained on a national basis, it becomes easier to follow a population, even as it migrates. But the planners must not minimize the cost of doing so. Withdrawal from participation is an additional problem and it is not easy to maintain continuing co-operation between the investigators and the research subjects. Careful estimates need to be made about this from the beginning and repeated throughout the study.

The scientific world is rapidly changing, and longitudinal studies take time. Because research workers must be able to pursue their careers, outside pressures for advancement and publications can divert attention away from the main purposes of the longitudinal study. Staff may move on to opportunities elsewhere, and the ideas of new personnel, not only about data-gathering, but also about research objectives, may differ from those of the principal investigators. Moreover, because it may take years before useful publications emerge from the longitudinal study, 'spin-offs' are a necessary part of any research project. Because of the high priority which publications represent for the developing team, these spin-offs can come to overwhelm the original goals of the study. Given the difficulties of mobilizing personnel and the pressures of publication, delay and procrastination are especially destructive for longitudinal studies.

Because the longitudinal study starts off with a new set of hypotheses and a desire to follow a population, it is important to realize that vast quantities of data will be gathered. Beginning investigators like to think that they will do a better job than their predecessors, that they will know what the data mean, and that they will see to it that the data are reported consistently and truthfully. This is a very healthy attitude, but it is very easy to denigrate the 'sloppy records' that you have inherited without facing up to the question of whether or not you will in fact be able to make better records. Consistency, diligence, and accuracy are extremely important, but very hard to maintain. A general law about routinely gathered data is that when it is not respected and used and interpreted on an ongoing basis, quality will tend to deteriorate because those making the records get little feedback of criticism or correction. Unless the investigators are close to the data gathering process, unanticipated problems will arise and those on the firing line will work out solutions to their own satisfaction. But when the investigator starts to use the data, he may find that those solutions do not satisfy him. There is also the added danger that he will never find out that new rules have been introduced on data-gathering that make the data appear to have a relevance that they do not actually have.

In addition, new personnel moving into the research situation may reinterpret old instructions and begin to gather data on a new basis, while using the same label. Maintenance of comparable language and symbol systems becomes a problem in itself, and an atmosphere of false consistency can readily emerge. Therefore, documentation of data-gathering procedures is extremely important and short lines of communication between senior research workers and the most junior data gatherers are essential.

The storage of records becomes an ever mounting problem and it is hardly ever possible to have enough well trained and well supervised personnel to keep them at a high level. The rapidly growing library of data needs meticulous attention constantly. It is very difficult to organize and deploy a sufficient staff for this purpose. Furthermore, data must be organized and reorganized as different issues emerging from spin-offs arise. If every event is dated and recorded properly, it is always possible to reconstruct the sequences, but unless these data-processing activities are planned for, it is very easy to lose track of these sequences. In fact, one of the biggest hazards illustrated in one of the chapters in this book is that the volume of data gathered can become so overwhelming that specialists in 'data reduction' must be brought in to reduce the data to manageable proportions. When these reductions produce a smaller data set that will satisfy some author and editor for publication the investigator may be pleased; but such pleasure does not guarantee that the reduction did not introduce misinterpretations of the data. This is throwing out the baby with the bath water and is a very serious danger when the volume of data gathered exceeds the capacity of the research team to investigate its meaning.

Recommendations

It is essential that sufficient attention be paid to ensuring a team structure that will incorporate the necessary multiple perspectives and develop rigidity of standards combined with flexibility of procedure in the light of new knowledge. The team must have a principal investigator, each topic for investigation must have a single scientist in charge, and the cross-fertilization of multiple disciplines is almost always necessary.

Built-in methods for cross-checking and maintaining rigidity of standards must be included and this is a high cost which should be budgeted. A data librarian is absolutely necessary. It is difficult to recruit and hold such a person, but if he is adequately paid, it is possible. The data handling mechanisms must be over-budgeted because data-processing equipment and technology keep changing and only those familiar with the content of the data can handle it properly. Stability is crucial.

It is desirable that any longitudinal study have an advisory group of consultants who are senior scientists and perhaps potential users and teachers. This Advisory Group should relate itself to the investigations in such a way that it shares the investigators' objectives and brings to the investigating team a set of different perspectives as to the meaning of the longitudinal study. It should meet at least once a year, preferably twice a year, at the locus of the longitudinal study. The advisers should participate as paid consultants; otherwise they will tend to pull the study toward their own private professional goals. They must be persuaded to see membership in the Advisory Group as a prestigious, useful scientific contribution. They should provide an audience which gives the staff an opportunity to present developing ideas, preliminary analyses of data, and preliminary suggestions of work to be undertaken. They must have no direct relationship to the funding agency or those providing administrative support because what the investigators need is an independent cadre of senior scientists who share their objectives, but can help the leaders and investigators see the implications of their work for the broader scientific community. The investigators can gain from time to time by inviting a representative of the funding agency to be present at the meetings but the meetings should not be decision-making activities but rather scientific colloquia to maintain stimulation and contact with the broader world. Simultaneously the scientific staff of the research group should have adequate budget for travel to visit colleagues working on related problems so that they stay in close contact with developing technology. They should have opportunities to go to scientific meetings, and there should be regular journal club and seminar meetings in the research group if it is to stay alive and vigorous. (An Advisory Group of distinguished senior professionals will also provide junior staff with personal contacts in their own professions, and a sense of access to the broader professional recruitment world which they may have to enter later in their careers.)

Since it is impossible for a longitudinal study to take full advantage of its data base even when it is well organized, arrangement should be made from the beginning to have space and resources for visiting scientists who wish to work in collaboration with one or more of the scientists in the research group making use of data and preparing joint publications. This is another way in which the isolation of the research team can be reduced and the maximum benefits of the longitudinal study realized.

Too great a burden usually falls on the leader of a longitudinal study to maintain relationships with the community and with the study subjects. Help is needed in this respect and it is really a full-time job, even for smaller-scale longitudinal studies. There are two aspects to external relations. First is contact with key informants and decision-makers of the community where the study is located, so that the relevant people of prestige, whose opinions are respected, are kept fully informed of the progress and purpose of the investigations. The sensibilities and sensitivities of the local community must always be kept in mind. The members of the community who are participating in the study or just know of its existence should be informed by various methods from time to time of its existence, its scientific reputability, its professional and governmental reputability, and the caution with which the privacy of the individuals and the reputation of the community are constantly being considered. Second, and even more important and more difficult, is the problem of personal relations with the research subjects over a long period of time. What is needed is someone who is empathic with the attitudes and feelings of the research subjects yet identifies with the research objectives of the investigators and can act as an intermediary, an interpreter and a molifier between these two groups. Although the qualifications of such a person are hard to spell out, he should be able to sense the research subjects' resentments and reluctance before they become a source of resistance to continued participation.

The most important and difficult recommendation to implement is that the organization, financing, and administrative structure of a longitudinal study must be given a combination of stability and supervision so that people can dedicate their professional lives to working on the team. An atmosphere of constant grant-hopping, job insecurity, and professional uncertainty is not one in which people can buckle down to the long pull. On the other hand those who finance and support the study are entitled to intermittent reviews to be sure that the study is productive and should continue in its current direction. The needed stability and supervision can probably be achieved by a mixture of the right institutional support and the appropriate Advisory Group, with productive interactions between the two. But as far as we know this problem has not been faced adequately in any ongoing longitudinal studies.

Many of the practical problems outlined above have been confronted successfully by three ongoing longitudinal projects: the Lundby studies, the Aberdeen studies, and the British National Child Development studies. Anyone undertaking to start a new longitudinal population study could profit by carefully scrutinizing these projects. For this reason, this chapter will conclude with a brief review of the accomplishments, potential, and problems of these three studies.

Three important longitudinal studies

The British national child development study

The results of the British National Child Development Study illustrate the advantages which can be gained from a well conceived longitudinal study carried out on a large population base. It should be noted at the outset that many of these advantages stem from the size (originally 16 000) and representative nature of the sample (originally a birth cohort, when immigrants were added and emigrants were dropped it became a national age cohort), and from the diversity of information collected in the surveys, rather than from the longitudinal nature of the study. The cross-sectional spin-offs from the main longitudinal study have been valuable enough to justify the programme's costs. For example, incidence rates of fairly common conditions, such as congenital defects (Alberman 1969) and speech problems (Butler et al. 1973; Sheridan 1973; Peckham 1973) were easily calculated from a sample of this size. In addition, numerous sociological variables (social class, family size, housing state) could be correlated with medical, behavioural, and educational measures taken at the same point in time (e.g., Goldstein 1971; Pearson and Peckham 1972; Ferri 1973).

Of much more interest are the data which exploit the *longitudinal* features of the cohort, looking at medical, social, psychological, and educational experience of the children in the NCDS sample to find predictors of future health and behaviour from prospective concurrent data. The longitudinal approach to time, coupled with the collection of a wide variety of data under a broadly stated set of research goals, has unmatched advantages. For example, the long-term effects of smoking during pregnancy (Fedrick et al. 1971; Goldstein 1976) have been assessed, as has the relationship between prepartum influenza and cancer in the child (Fedrick and Alberman 1972) (a finding which, we suspect, just 'turned up'); and the results of being in care outside the home at various ages have been evaluated (Essen et al. 1976).

A further advantage of the longitudinal approach which is illus-trated by this study is that the stability of educational and behavioural measures over time can be assessed. This has been done specifically for differences in educational attainment in relation to a number of social factors such as social class, social mobility, and family size (Fogelman and Goldstein 1976).

In addition to the findings already published and those expected from studies now in progress which have implications for policy in health care delivery (Sheridan and Peckham 1975), education (Davie 1971), child-rearing (Ferri and Robinson 1976), and health education (unpublished), the methodological contributions of the NCDS have been substantial (e.g., Goldstein 1968, 1975; Goldstein and Fogelman 1974; Healy and Goldstein 1976).

Yet the diverse and important results presented so far by the National Children's Bureau represent only a fraction of the information which could be gleaned from the data already collected. Furthermore, the next follow-up wave of the survey could enrich the data base along a whole new dimension by providing information on the children of the original cohort. These possibilities make the National Child Development Survey an invaluable resource for medicine and social science, a resource which can produce new information at relatively low unit costs; its maintenance costs, therefore, should be looked at in light of the speed with which questions can be answered if studies are based on this population.

Lundby

The nature of the population information, as well as the information collected in individual interviews in the Lundby study make it one of the most valuable longitudinal projects ever undertaken. The study was greatly facilitated by the Swedish population registration system, which allows complete enumeration, virtually total follow up, and knowledge of familial relationships. Furthermore, because the original investigators (Essen-Möller et al. 1956) were primarily interested in the familial clustering of personality variants in a *normal* population, every individual in the entire population was carefully and thoroughly interviewed in the 1947 survey wave, and this practice was repeated in subsequent surveys in 1957 (Hagnell 1966a, b) and 1972 (Hagnell and Öjesjö 1975). While the interviews were wide-ranging, a core of information was consistently obtained, making the interview protocols an especially rich source of data on personality, physical illness, mental health, and problems of living. In addition, information was obtained from official records of hospitals, police, temperance boards, etc., which, coupled with interview information, allows an analysis of how well services are meeting particular needs.

The specific advantages of obtaining information on every individual, and of obtaining a history of disorder over the interval between surveys, become apparent when the longitudinal aspects of the project are considered. For in addition to point prevalence rates, one can calculate the incidence and duration of particular conditions in the population. This makes it possible to look at trends in these measures over the twenty-five-year period, and to assess the impact of specific changes on the disease pattern of the population (Gruenberg and Hagnell in press; Gruenberg 1977). Furthermore, it becomes possible to discover precursors of undesirable conditions, and to calculate a relative risk for different subgroups of the population. Even such questions as the aetiology of mutual mental illness in husband–wife pairs (Hagnell and Kreitman 1974) can be addressed.

The rich and flexible data base of the Lundby study has already yielded one comparative study of mental illness (Leighton et al. 1971) and promises several more. It has provided the best base-line estimates of the incidence rates of mental disorders yet gathered through naturalistic observation of a human population. This information can be invaluable to investigators when planning studies in other populations.

The weakness of this laboratory is in its staffing and financing. It has not had full-time professional staff. The assistants are recruited without prior experience in record keeping and the laboratory lacks facilities for providing them with in-service training. Professor Hagnell has been generous in collaborating with other investigators who have recognized the value of the data base, but these excursions into the data still further deplete his time and energy, since he must carry a service and teaching load, most of which could be handled by an above average docent with no skills or interest in research.

The absence of full-time professional research staff is partially compensated for by the dedication of those involved and the continuing availability of Essen-Möller, Hagnell, and Öjesjö for case reviews, which provides rare continuity in standards.

The Lundby studies illustrate particularly well a general principle of all studies on human populations. Surveys are reported in the literature with varying degrees of detail about the population being studied. The people conducting the investigation are the 'investigators' who are recorded as 'authors'. In the text the way in which the 'investigators' learn the recorded facts about the 'subjects' is briefly mentioned under the heading 'methods'. There is merit in looking at each such survey as a *planned interaction between two populations*—the subjects and the investigators. Most of this information is unrecorded in the published literature and there is no scientific tradition for recording it. When the investigative team lives in close contiguity to the subject population, and has established a trusting relationship with the subject population through both formal and informal contacts, the sources of data are hard for an outsider to imagine! For example, while most of the 1947 cohort had moved away by 1972, the investigators did not have to travel to all the places they had moved for the 1972 interviews. Within 18 months most of them had paid a visit to relatives who had not migrated and these relatives telephoned the investigators and scheduled interviews while the subjects were in the neighbourhood. This is a level of collaboration between 'subjects' and 'researchers' which makes a crucial difference in evaluating the quality of the data.

Aberdeen

The Aberdeen longitudinal studies are unique because they are based on a virtually complete register of medical and developmental data (beginning with data on the obstetrical and gynaecological experience of the mother from early in pregnancy) in a defined, stable population over a 30-year period. The studies emerged from Sir Dugald Baird's interest in social obstetrics. The usual approach in longitudinal studies is to repeatedly survey a given population. In contrast, record-keeping, and hence data collection, in Aberdeen has been continuous throughout the period. This approach presents opportunities for some unusual and important analyses (e.g., time trends in medical problems and medical practices, seasonal influences), but carries with it immense difficulties in data management. It is therefore appropriate that the Aberdeen report in this volume (Chapter 11) deals extensively with problems of data access and their solution.

The numerous and various items of information gathered for each event in the life of each subject provide a rich data base which lends itself well to the study of broad questions which is characteristic of longitudinal work. Perhaps the main contributions of the Aberdeen neonatal project have been in the field of medical sociology, and have dealt with social factors influencing the birth process (e.g., Baird 1949, 1953; Baird and Illsley 1953; Illsley 1955, 1956; Billewicz and Thomson 1957; Fairweather and Illsley 1960). However, some spin-offs of the study have been purely clinical (Nelson 1955a, b; Stewart and Bernard 1954; MacGillivray 1961,

etc.); some have been purely sociological or demographic (e.g., Scott and Nisbett 1954; Illsley *et al.* 1963; Oldman and Illsley 1966); some have dealt with social problems (which may have medical aspects) such as illegitimacy and teen-age pregnancy (e.g., Illsley and Gill 1968a, b; Gill 1970; Gill *et al.* 1970); and many are best characterized as epidemiological studies of morbidity and mortality (e.g., Baird *et al.* 1954; Anderson 1956; Anderson *et al.* 1958; Herriot *et al.* 1962; Baird 1964). The rich data base has also been used in a comparative study of perinatal mortality in Aberdeen and Hong Kong (Thomson *et al.* 1963). Richardson's proposed follow-up study of individuals labelled retarded in their youth (Chapter 54) is an elegant example of how a specific hypothesis can be tested in conjunction with an ongoing longitudinal study.

The Aberdeen Child Development Study is a logical outgrowth of earlier investigations utilizing the maternity and neonatal data bank. Although many of the medical and sociological studies cited in the project report have historical components (e.g., Baird *et al.* 1968; MacNaughton 1961; Baird 1975), it is in the child development project that the potentialities for longitudinal studies embodied in the data base are most fully realized. The educational and behavioural parameters gathered at age 7, 9, and 11, meshed with child health histories during the school years and a wealth of data on children's experiences at birth provide a unique opportunity for analysis of the contributions of medical and social factors to school success. In addition, although the child development studies have not yet reached their full maturity, the possibilities for using this rigorously collected set of data in comparative studies are already becoming apparent.

A unique feature of the Aberdeen studies is their truly interdisciplinary nature. Begun under the auspices of a medical department of gynaecology and obstetrics, and inspired by a physician (Sir Dugald Baird), the studies are now carried out by the Institute of Medical Sociology in Aberdeen, which is headed by a sociologist, Professor Raymond Illsley.

Both the Child Development Study and studies based exclusively on the maternity data bank show that longitudinal investigations which are grounded on sound data collection procedures and a creative approach to the utilization of the collected information and which are carried out on a defined, stable population can contribute immeasurably to our understanding of diverse medical and social problems.

Conclusions

It seems clear after reviewing the present state of longitudinal research that there is a place for longitudinal community studies. There is a definite need that only they can meet. They act as a check on the findings from *ad hoc* miscellaneous hit-and-run studies (Gruenberg 1971). It is true that longitudinal work is fraught with difficulties and that most studies will probably yield few useful findings. Therefore, if the full potential of longitudinal studies is to be achieved, there must be some overinvestment in this type of research. At the same time, inadequately planned longitudinal studies are too costly to proliferate in large numbers. Scattering a lot of projects around a few continents is not going to do much good unless some of them are truly first rate. The three studies reviewed above are first rate. They have enormous potentialities that are untapped. These projects, and others of similar calibre, deserve continued attention and support.

71. Longitudinal studies: a psychiatric perspective

MICHAEL RUTTER

Longitudinal studies first came firmly into the psychological limelight with the group of major American investigations which began in the decade 1920–30 and which set out to chart the course of psychological development by following individuals from early life to maturity (see Kagan 1964; Stone and Onqué 1959; Bloom 1964). The enquiries were informative in indicating something of the extent of consistencies in development and in showing associations between various maternal measures and children's social–emotional development. However, conclusions were severely limited by vagaries in sampling, loss of contact with subjects, weak measures, and non-comparability of measures across studies and across time periods (Wall and Williams 1970).

Since those early pioneer projects, longitudinal research has made considerable progress. It has shared in the general improvement in methods of measurement, in sampling, in modes of statistical analysis, and in strategies of hypothesis-testing. But, also, as elegantly shown in Robins' (1978) comprehensive review, it has gained immensely from the appreciation that there are a variety of strategies which may be employed to link measures taken at two or more points in time. First, there is the 'real-time' prospective study in which a sample is selected and studied at time 1 and then re-examined after an interval at time 2. Second, there is the 'follow-back' study in which cases and controls are studied both contemporaneously and also in terms of some previously existing records. Thirdly, 'catch-up' prospective studies do the same thing the other way round. That is, the sample is identified as of time 1 on the basis of pre-existing records, but then followed up to the present. In this way, the sample will have already 'aged' before the research begins, thus eliminating any long waiting period. Fourthly, there is the use of a series of short-term longitudinal studies in an overlapping age-pattern so that a considerable age span can be studied within a much shorter time period (Bell 1953).

Samples may be large and nationally representative or they may be smaller and deliberately chosen to focus on some high-risk factor or some particular experience. Environmental change may be studied by capitalizing on some naturally occurring circumstance or through the introduction of some experimental intervention. Finally, it has been found that there are many ways of tracing individuals (see Laurence 1959; Robins 1966) and investigations have shown that it is possible to obtain 90 per cent contact even over periods as long as 30 years. (On the other hand, destruction of records and restrictions on access are making this increasingly difficult (Robins 1977).)

Most of these advances in methods of longitudinal study are represented in the accounts of European research provided in earlier chapters of this volume. The studies vary greatly in sophistication and complexity; also some are well advanced and have produced numerous reports of findings whereas others are still at the pilot stage. Accordingly, it would not be useful to attempt any kind of summary or review of the psychiatric implications of these studies as such. Rather, it seemed appropriate to consider longitudinal research more broadly in order to examine the ways in which this research method is making specific contributions to psychiatric knowledge which could not be obtained equally well in other ways. The advantages and disadvantages of different longitudinal strategies will be discussed both in relation to each other and to cross-sectional methods in connection with the various substantive issues considered.

Methodological issues

Sampling

Appropriate sampling is crucial to all research and in most cases it is necessary to ensure that the sample studied is truly representative of the population in question (Rutter 1977c). The population may be the general population, or all adopted persons, or all children with reading difficulties. But however defined there is the same requirement that the group studied should provide an unbiased sample. Robins (1970, 1978) has pointed out that longitudinal enquiries can often achieve a more complete sampling simply because it will be known how many have died, been incarcerated or hospitalized, or become vagrant. Cross-sectional studies tend to miss these people because the sampling usually has to be on the basis of school attenders or household enumerations.

On the other hand, the converse of this advantage is the major drawback that the longitudinal sample can only be representative of the population as it was constituted some years ago. This can lead to serious distortions if, for example, the general population has changed greatly through migration (as it has in Britain over the last 30 years). The in-migrants will be omitted from the longitudinal sample and as a result the findings will apply only to a group which no longer represents the population as it is now. The solution to this problem is to combine a longitudinal study with a new cross-sectional survey of all individuals of the appropriate age-group at follow-up. This procedure has been followed, for example, by both the National Child Development Study (Chapter 7) and the Isle of Wight study (Chapter 21). This combination of longitudinal and cross-sectional approaches gives the most comprehensive sampling frame possible.

Non-response bias

Almost all studies have a proportion of individuals for whom data are missing either through lack of co-operation or failure to contact. One of the grave disadvantages of most cross-sectional studies is that nothing is known about the people missed and hence it is not possible to determine how far or in what way the findings are biased. One asset of longitudinal enquiries is that information on missing cases is often available from an earlier stage of data collection.

The ways in which missing cases differ from those studied tend to vary according to both the type of investigation and the reasons for non-response. However, as Cox et al. (1977) showed using data from several studies, systematic differences are usually found. Often the missed cases are more deviant in some important respect. Thus, absentees from school tend to show more behavioural disturbance, to have lower levels of attainments, and are more likely to be heavy drug users (Cox et al. 1977; West and Farrington 1973; Baltes et al. 1971; Shepherd et al. 1971; Kandel 1975). Socially disadvantaged families are somewhat more likely to be missing from follow-up (see Chapters 7 and 6 on the National Child Development study and the 1946 birth cohort study) and antisocial individuals tend to be more difficult to locate because more of them lose contact with their relatives, change jobs frequently, and move about the country (Robins 1966). Often, the untraced individuals are more deviant than those who actually refuse to co-operate (Fogelman 1976).

Strength of measures

In all studies there has to be a concern to improve the strength of measures as far as possible. A common technique used for this purpose is the pooling of scales to produce some overall index. This method is equally applicable to cross-sectional and longitudinal studies but has been employed with great effect in several projects reported in this volume. For example, Farrington and West (Chapter 23) produced a global rating of 'poor parental behaviour' and Rutter and Quinton (Chapter 65) used summary measures of 'family adversity' (Rutter and Quinton 1977) and 'temperamental adversity' (Rutter 1978d).

However, the combination of measures over time can only be obtained from longitudinal data. Rutter and Quinton (Chapter 65) increased the strength of their measure of behavioural deviance by concentrating on children who showed deviant scores on a teachers' questionnaire on at least three occasions over a four-year period (Rutter 1977a). This approach increased the difference between the children of mentally ill parents and the controls because behavioural deviance was more *persistent* in the offspring of patients. Douglas *et al.* (1968) did much the same thing in the British National Survey (Chapter 6) by combining behavioural measures obtained at 13 and 15 years. Similarly, Farrington and West (Chapter 23) were able to differentiate isolated delinquent acts from persisting delinquency.

Testing the validity of measures

There are many ways to test the validity of psychosocial measures. None are entirely satisfactory (see Platt 1980), but one component of validity is the power to predict over time or situation. Cross-sectional data can be used for the latter purpose. Thus, Brown and Rutter (Brown and Rutter 1966; Rutter and Brown 1966) tested their measures of family relationships both by comparing the independent accounts obtained from husbands and wives and by comparing ratings based on single interviews with just one spouse with those based on conjoint interviews with both husband and wife together. However, a more stringent test is provided by predictors over time. Thus, Quinton *et al.* (1976) examined the validity of their measure of marital relationships by determining its power to predict marriage breakdown over the next four years in a longitudinal study of patients' families (Chapter 65). Obviously, longitudinal data are essential for this purpose.

The same approaches may be used with respect to behavioural deviance and psychiatric disorder. Again, comparisons between different measures obtained at much the same time are informative (e.g. Rutter *et al.* 1970b; Rutter *et al.* 1975a; Richman 1977a; Minde and Minde 1977), as are correlations over time (Rutter 1977a; Minde and Minde 1977; Richman 1977b). Low correlations over time do not indicate invalidity, as the measure may be a valid indicator of a transient behavioural feature. On the other hand, stability over time provides some support for validity.

Longitudinal data have also been crucial in demonstrating the validity of IQ measures in autistic children (see Chapter 55). It was once thought that the low IQ scores of autistic children represented social withdrawal, negativism, or poor motivation rather than cognitive capacity. However, longitudinal studies showed that IQ scores obtained in early childhood by autistic children showed the same stability over time as those obtained by other youngsters, and the IQ scores had a similar predictive relationship with later educational attainment and occupational level. Moreover, a low level of IQ was strongly associated with the development of epileptic fits dur-

ing adolescence (Bartak and Rutter 1976). As the same applied to children who were initially untestable, it was apparent that the children did not score on the IQ tests because their cognitive skills were at an extremely low level. In this way, follow-up findings were crucial in establishing the validity of IQ scores in autistic children.

Diagnostic validation by course of disorder

The one essential criterion for the scientific validity of psychiatric diagnostic categories is that the categories be shown to differ in terms of variables *other than the symptoms which define them* (Rutter (1965, 1978c). Since the time of Kraepelin, longitudinal studies have had a central role in this validation process through their value in differentiating conditions according to both response to treatment and long-term course. Kraepelin's follow-up of patients was chiefly of value in showing the differences between manic-depressive psychosis and schizophrenia in adult life. While the differentiation has since been validated in other ways (especially by genetic studies), a great deal has still to be learned about the longitudinal course of different psychiatric disorders. The Zurich study by Angst and his colleagues (Chapter 53), in which psychiatric patients first seen in 1959–63 have been followed up every five years, is a more sophisticated modern day equivalent of Kraepelin's approach to the study of psychoses. Angst has particularly focused on the differences between unipolar and bipolar affective disorders but also has compared both with schizo-affective conditions. Helgason's 6-year follow-up of psychiatric patients in Iceland (see Chapter 46) and the American 'Iowa 500' study (Tsuang and Winokur 1977), in which 500 schizophrenic and primary affective disorder patients have been followed up some 35 years after hospital admission, are other examples of this use of a longitudinal study.

Even less is known about the natural history of neurotic disorders and such few data as are available (Greer and Cawley 1966) provide little justification for sharp distinctions between discrete subcategories of neurosis (anxiety state, obsessional disorders, and the like). Slater's (1965) follow-up of so-called conversion hysteria also showed this to be a rather heterogeneous group chiefly distinguished by the frequency with which it was a *mis*diagnosis of some organic condition. Follow-up studies in childhood have shown much the same (Caplan 1970; Rivinus *et al.* 1975). Binder and Angst's prospective study of minor psychiatric disorders in young adults (see Chapter 27) should be of value in providing further evidence on how far distinctions between different types of neurotic disorder are justified by differences in long-term course.

In child psychiatry, longitudinal studies have been crucial in validating the broad differentiation between emotional disturbances and disorders of conduct (Rutter 1978c). Emotional disorders have been shown to differ in terms of a better short-term response to treatment (Cytryn *et al.* 1960), a better prognosis with respect to persistence of problems into adolescence (Graham and Rutter 1973—see also Chapter 21), a better long-term outcome (Robins 1966), and a linkage with different types of adult psychiatric disorder (Robins 1966; Pritchard and Graham 1966; Zeitlin 1972; Graham and Rutter 1973). Most children with emotional disturbance develop into normal healthy adults, but when disorders continue into adult life they usually take the form of depression or neurosis. In sharp contrast, youngsters with conduct disorders, if they show problems in adult life (as a high proportion do) tend to exhibit personality disorders with accompanying social difficulties as well as psychiatric impairment. While all studies have shown a substantial overlap between the groups, with many children showing a mixed clinical picture, longitudinal studies have shown the value of this important, but rather gross, diagnostic differentiation. The differences in natural history of the two diagnostic groups are paralleled by differences in sex ratio (see Isle of

Wight studies in Chapter 21), in associations with reading difficulties (also Chapter 22) and in links with family discord (Rutter 1971a; also Chapter 65).

Whether there are valid distinctions within the broad emotional disorder and conduct disorder groupings is more questionable (Rutter 1978c). The 12 year follow-up of institutionalized delinquents by Jenkins *et al.* (1977) showed that those with a 'socialized' disorder had a better prognosis in terms of adult convictions and imprisonment. However, it remains uncertain whether the finding reflects a distinction between *syndromes* or rather a differentiation according to *variables* present in all children to a greater or lesser degree. The latter possibility is suggested by the findings from other studies that both family characteristics (Power *et al.* 1974; Rutter 1977a) and quality of peer relationships (Roff *et al.* 1972; Sundby and Kreyberg 1968) predict outcome in delinquent and non-delinquent groups. It remains to be determined whether prognosis differs according to *type* of conduct disturbance or rather by *degrees* of personality disorder.

Clearly, additional follow-up studies of child psychiatric populations are needed to take the matter further. Curman and Nylander's (Chapter 48) 10- and 20-year follow-up of child guidance clinic patients should be informative in this connection. The Isle of Wight studies (Chapter 21) provide data on the course of disorders in a general population sample, and Rutter and Quinton's family study (Chapter 65) does the same for children in a high risk sample (parents with a mental disorder).

Autism is the other psychiatric condition in childhood for which longitudinal studies have provided vital evidence for diagnostic validity (see Chapter 55). Autism differs from the general run of child psychiatric disorders not only in terms of its relatively poor prognosis but also in terms of the high frequency with which epileptic fits develop in adolescence and the behavioural characteristics shown in adult life. Natural history studies of mostly untreated autistic children, studies of children in special educational units, and studies of children who were part of an intensive behaviourally oriented home treatment programme have all shown the great importance of levels of IQ and language as predictors of long-term social outcome. The findings emphasize the role of a cognitive deficit as a basic part of the syndrome—again a difference from most other psychiatric conditions in childhood.

Diagnostic differentiation by age of onset

A further diagnostic differentiation is by age of onset. When this is easily established by history-taking there is no need to use longitudinal data. Thus, the distinction between presenile and senile dementia is easily determined by routine enquiry, if it is not obvious from the age at which the patient comes to psychiatric notice. On the other hand, the determination of when behavioural problems began in early childhood is not so easy to establish by interview methods as parents so often misreport the timing (Chess *et al.* 1966). Longitudinal data are crucial for this purpose.

The importance of age of onset in relation to adolescent disorders was striking in the Isle of Wight study (Chapter 21). Psychiatric conditions present at age 14 years were subdivided according to whether behavioural deviance had or had not been evident when the same children had been previously studied at age 10 years. The disorders which had begun during the early adolescent years, rather than in earlier childhood, differed in three crucial respects:

(a) More occurred in girls;
(b) They were unassociated with educational retardation;
(c) They were less often associated with family discord, disruption, and disturbance.

It appeared that psychiatric conditions with an onset in adolescence were rather different from those beginning at an earlier stage of development.

Delinquency beginning in late adolescence or adult life also seems to differ somewhat from delinquency of earlier onset. Farrington and West (Chapter 23) found that, unlike juvenile delinquents, men first convicted as young adults were *not* particularly likely to have suffered poor parental behaviour (meaning marital disharmony, parental inconsistency, cruel or neglecting attitudes, etc). On the other hand they were just as likely to have come from large families with a criminal parent. Similar comparisons should be possible in the Aberdeen delinquency study (Chapter 11D) but have yet to be undertaken. Some years ago Robins and Hill (1966) found that delinquency beginning late was not particularly associated with school failure, although delinquency of earlier onset was. The matter requires further longitudinal study but it appears that the pattern of causation of disorders beginning in the teens and twenties may well be rather different from that for conditions arising in earlier childhood.

Overview

It is clear that longitudinal data have a crucial role to play in the study of methodological issues. A combination of longitudinal and cross-sectional methods probably provides the most effective sampling frame and longitudinal data are essential in the measurement of non-response bias. They are also valuable as a means of increasing the strength of measures (by pooling several assessments over time) and are very useful as one approach to the assessment of validity of both measures and diagnostic distinctions.

Course of psychological development

It might be thought that longitudinal studies would be most useful of all in the study of normal psychological development. Of course, they are indispensable for this purpose. Nevertheless, they have proved relatively disappointing in this connection and few studies in this volume address themselves to this issue. In part, this is a reflection of the fact that developmental psychology is much less well established in Europe than it is in the United States of America. However, it also reflects several basic difficulties.

First, there is the problem of measurement. The assessment of personality features is not nearly as advanced as that of cognitive functioning. On the other hand, worthwhile approaches have been found. For example, the Chess–Birch–Thomas approach to the study of temperament (Thomas *et al.* 1968) has stimulated some useful research. Thus, it has been found that temperamental differences in early childhood are significantly related to the later development of emotional and behavioural problems (see Rutter 1977d; Dunn 1980). In part, this is because a child's temperamental features help determine how other people will respond to him. Longitudinal data are essential to sort out sequences of parent–child interaction, but this type of analysis has proved remarkably difficult in practice (see Lewis and Rosenblum 1974).

Second, there is the uncertainty on how far measures at one age are comparable to those at other ages. This is especially a problem with assessments in infancy (Rutter 1970d). For example, Bell (1975) found that neonates who responded quickly and vigorously to interruptions of non-nutritive sucking were *less* emotionally responsive than other children when older. It appears that speculations about the meanings of neonatal behaviour are hazardous and potentially misleading. Empirical data on longitudinal connections are needed.

Third, there is the lack of any absolute scale. As a result it has not so far proved possible to develop any psychological equivalent of the growth curves which have been so informative in biological development (Tanner 1960). Concepts of 'immaturity' of personality are readily bandied about but no measures of psychological maturity have proved acceptable. There have been attempts to produce them (e.g. Sullivan *et al.* 1957), as well as endeavours to assess moral development (Kohlberg 1969). These provide useful leads for further research but there is a long way to go before psychological growth curves can be meaningfully compared. It is evident from the studies of temperamental development that children show quite varied patterns of change as they mature, but ways of analysing these have yet to be developed.

Fourth, although not a necessary feature of this type of research, in practice most studies utilizing the detailed individual measurement required for the assessment of personality development have suffered from either great selectivity in sampling or a high non-co-operation rate or both.

Fifth, the statistical handling of longitudinal data has given rise to innumerable headaches. There are difficulties in dealing with missing data but the linking of multiple assessments obtained at different time periods provides even greater difficulties. As a consequence of these problems, most reports of longitudinal studies have been confined either to cross-sectional analyses or to correlations between some initial indicator and various later outcomes. There are, at least partial, solutions available as shown by the various conceptual and methodological approaches described in the volume edited by Strauss *et al.* (1977) and the statistical techniques outlined by Sörbom (Chapter 4) and others. Both modern multivariate methods of analysis and the older techniques of life table analysis with standardization of rates have a place. Which is more appropriate needs to be decided in terms of both the type of data available and the type of questions being studied. However, whatever the statistic employed, a step-by-step conceptual approach will usually be more informative (see e.g. Robins *et al.* 1977, 1978) than putting everything into the computer and applying the latest statistical package.

With all these difficulties it is, perhaps, not surprising that the greatest gains have come from using longitudinal data to examine specific research questions which involve the *timing* of associations (the issue for which a longitudinal analysis is most essential). Thus, the National Child Development Study (Chapter 7) was able to show that *changes* in family social status (either up or down) were linked with comparable changes in the children's educational attainments. While this does not prove a causal relationship it certainly takes the argument a crucial stage beyond the crude social class-scholastic skills correlation. Or again, the National Survey (Chapter 6) was able to show that early puberty was associated with higher attainments both *before* and after pubescence. This clearly indicated that the intellectual superiority of early maturers was *not* due to any kind of cognitive growth spurt, although what the association does mean remains somewhat obscure. The parallel finding many years ago (see McCandless 1960) that early maturing boys had personality advantages over later maturers (whereas this was not so for girls) remains a fascinating observation which is waiting to be re-examined with the better methods of measurement and analysis now available. It may be that Kemper's longitudinal study of adolescence (Chapter 19) will provide some findings relevant to the issue. A closely parallel situation at the other end of the age span is the effect of the climacteric—being studied now by Hällström and Samuelsson (Chapter 26). Prospective data are crucial to the question of how far changes in psychiatric state are specifically connected with the onset of the menopause. Thomae's longitudinal study of ageing (Chapter 29) also emphasizes the value of a developmental approach to the investigation of personality and intellectual changes in later life.

Barbara Tizard's study (Tizard 1977; Tizard and Hodges 1978) which compares the social development of institution reared, home reared, and late adopted children is now throwing important new light on the development of social relationships. Her findings confirm that in many respects children's behaviour is greatly influenced by the *current* family situation. However, what is new and crucially

important is that certain aspects of the children's social functioning seems to be a consequence of experiences in the early years *even when experiences later have been very different.* Much has yet to be learned, and the children are still only 8 years of age, but the findings already open up new avenues in the understanding of social development. These could only have come from a longitudinal study.

Richardson's investigation of what it means to grow up as a mentally subnormal person (Chapter 54) emphasizes both the importance of examining the impact of various handicaps on development and, more especially, the need to study development in a social context. Both individual qualities and the social milieu within which the person grows are likely to be influential. Richardson stresses the formative influence of self-image and attitudes to handicap in this process.

Study of causal processes

Much psychiatric research has as its chief aim the identification of causal factors or causal processes which lead to disorder of one kind or another. Much the easiest approach to this issue is to use cross-sectional or retrospective data to determine the variables associated or correlated with the condition being studied. Patterns of associations are then examined in an attempt to find out the direction of relationships and in this way conclusions are drawn about possible causative influences. For most purposes this is quite an economical means of generating aetiological hypotheses and of determining variables where the likelihood of their having a causal effect is sufficiently great to warrant the considerable investment of time and resources needed to provide a proper test of the hypothesized causal mechanism. However, there are substantial hazards in using retrospective data to draw firm conclusions about causation.

In the first place, numerous studies have shown how often retrospective recall is distorted by systematic biases (Robbins 1963; Chess *et al.* 1966; Yarrow *et al.* 1970). In particular there is a tendency to distort accounts of the past to coincide more with current feelings and attitudes, with stereotypes of behaviour, or with prevailing views on child-rearing. On the whole, unpleasant experiences are less easily remembered than pleasant happenings (Lishman 1974), but when difficulties or disorder develop there may be a tendency to search the memory for stresses which could possibly have led to the problems. Alternatively the timing of events may be distorted so that, for example, problems are remembered as having begun *after* some stress when in fact they started *before* it (Chess *et al.* 1966). The possibility of wrong conclusions from misleading retrospective data is not just theoretical. An actual example is provided by the finding that Down's syndrome was associated with stresses during pregnancy and the suggestion that this might represent a causal relationship (Stott 1958), just before it became known that the syndrome was due to a chromosomal abnormality (Lejeune *et al.* 1959). Contemporaneous longitudinal data have the major advantage of not being subject to errors of recall.

Second, wrong conclusions may be drawn because a valid association between *A* and *B* is due to some prior variable *C* which could not be assessed retrospectively. For example, many surveys have shown enormous variation between secondary schools in delinquency rates (e.g. Power *et al.* 1967; Gath *et al.* 1976). This variation has been used to infer that some schools predispose children to commit delinquent acts. However, longitudinal data show that some of this variation is simply a function of some schools having a higher proportion of *already disturbed* pupils in their intake (see Chapter 23). On the other hand, longitudinal analyses also indicate that in addition there is also a significant secondary school effect on children's behaviour (see Chapter 21).

Third, retrospective data provide a most uncertain guide to prediction. Thus, it is well established that individuals with severe mental retardation are much more likely than other people to have had an abnormally low birth weight (McDonald 1967). The association certainly implies a causal link. On the other hand, the great majority of children of low birth weight are of normal intelligence. In the same way, cerebral palsy is strongly associated with reading difficulties (Rutter *et al.* 1970a) but reading difficulties are only rarely due to cerebral palsy (Rutter and Yule 1975). The apparent paradox is simply a function of markedly different base rates (low birth weight is very much more common than severe mental retardation) and these can be taken into account through the appropriate analysis of retrospective data (e.g. see Quinton and Rutter 1976). Even so, accurate predictive formulae can only be satisfactorily derived from longitudinal data.

Fourth, there is the related point that retrospective data are not easily utilized to study the phenomenon of 'escape'. With virtually all stresses numerous individuals survive unscathed (Rutter 1979a). Longitudinal data are needed to determine what was different about these apparently invulnerable people or what were the protective factors that enabled them to overcome deprivation or disadvantage.

Fifth, cross-sectional data generally cannot tell us the *direction* of relationships or *when* things developed. Thus, cross-sectional studies have shown that enuretic children tend to have a smaller functional bladder capacity than other children (e.g. Starfield 1967). But does a small capacity predispose to enuresis or rather is it that frequent wetting leads to a lower capacity because the bladder walls are less often fully stretched? Longitudinal data are needed to find out. Similarly, it is known that women with anorexia nervosa show various endocrine and metabolic abnormalities. However, return to normal with weight gain suggests that at least some of the abnormalities are a consequence of anorexia and not its cause (Halmi 1978).

For all these (and other) reasons longitudinal studies are frequently needed to study causal processes and many such investigations are reported in this volume.

Antecedent variables

The most common strategy has been to examine children's development or behaviour after some experience or happening which is thought to put them at risk. Thus, a variety of large general population longitudinal studies have shown the extent to which psychosocial disadvantage or deprivation is associated with educational difficulties, behavioural disturbance and delinquency (see for example chapters 6, 7, 9, 16, 17, 21, 23 and 25). It should be noticed, however, that many of the risk variables are ones which are easily and reliably studied through retrospective reports (e.g. social class, housing, working mothers, family size, admission into care, etc). In these cases, the longitudinal studies have done little more than confirm findings already well established by cross-sectional epidemiological enquiries (see e.g. Burt 1925, 1937; Rutter *et al.* 1970b; Birch *et al.* 1970). With variables of this kind it is striking how far longitudinal and retrospective analyses produce closely comparable findings. The demonstration that multiple hospital admissions are associated with an increased risk of later emotional or behavioural disturbance is a good example of this (Douglas 1975; Quinton and Rutter 1976).

Large-scale longitudinal studies have been particularly valuable when the variables have required contemporaneous measurement and when it was necessary to take into account intercorrelations with other risk factors. The British National Survey (Chapter 6), the Newcastle study (Neligan *et al.* 1976), and the National Child Development Study (Chapter 7) have been invaluable in this connection in showing that, compared with psychosocial variables, birth factors have a relatively weak effect on later psychological

development (apart from the causal links with cerebral palsy and severe mental retardation). On the other hand, they do have some effect and other longitudinal studies have been important in showing that biological and psychosocial effects cannot be regarded as independent (Sameroff and Chandler 1975). Perinatal hazards have their greatest adverse impact when *interacting* with psychosocial disadvantages. New insights come not just from having appropriate longitudinal data but also from the thoughtful application of suitable (often multivariate) statistical techniques.

How much more can be learned from the further longitudinal study of children who experience perinatal complications (such as in the various studies described in earlier chapters) remains to be seen. Perhaps the greatest need is to determine the consequences of new methods of obstetric care (e.g. see Chapter 45 for a study of the effects of induction) or of neonatal care (see Stewart 1977). It is most encouraging that the findings so far suggest that the prognosis not only for life but also for normal development in very low-birth-weight babies has improved considerably over the last 10 years.

Such studies need also to consider the possible inadvertent psychosocial *ill*-effects of improved techniques for dealing with physical disorder in early life. Recent longitudinal studies have pointed to the probability that denying mothers physical contact with their babies in the first day or so of life may sometimes impair later parenting (Klaus *et al.* 1972; Kennell *et al.* 1974; Leifer *et al.* 1972; Richards 1978). All these issues are dependent on longitudinal data for their effective study.

Longitudinal studies are also needed to determine the *mechanisms* involved in the development of different psychiatric conditions. The usual strategy here has been to take a high risk group of some kind. Thus, for schizophrenia the one well established risk factor is the presence of schizophrenia in a parent. However, until recent years it was not fully clear whether this was because the parental illness reflected a genetic predisposition or an environmental stress. Children adopted or fostered at birth provided a suitable group to test these two alternatives, and the availability of Scandinavian case registers made such studies possible (for example, Chapters 62 and 63). The very consistent finding from Heston (1966) onwards that schizophrenia in a parent is associated with a greatly increased rate of schizophrenia in the offspring even when the children have been adopted or fostered in infancy clearly points to a genetic effect—thus confirming the earlier twin findings (see Gottesman and Shields 1976). However, the mode of inheritance and exactly what is inherited remain to be determined. In Chapter 63, Mednick *et al.* describe how two longitudinal studies are being used to examine the possibility that psychophysiological variables constitute the crucial mediating variable. In Chapter 61 Wrede *et al.* outline their study to test the hypothesis that vulnerability is some kind of personality variable.

High-risk samples have been used in two rather different ways to study causal processes. First, groups may be defined in terms of some quite specific stress event to be studied. Thus, Judith Dunn and Claire Sturge in England both have short-term longitudinal studies to examine children's responses to the birth of a sib. Similarly, the Robertsons (1971) and others have used brief prospective studies to investigate children's reactions to hospital admission and various forms of residential care. Israeli workers (Lifshitz *et al.* 1977) have used a short-term follow-up design to investigate children's responses to bereavement according to the social system (kibbutz, moshav, or city) in which they were being brought up. Animal studies, too, have been most useful in delineating some of the possible mechanisms involved in acute and long-term responses to separation experiences (see Hinde and McGinnis 1977). As in humans, prospective strategies have been employed. In all these cases, the groups have been defined in terms of the specific stresses to be studied.

A second use of high-risk groups is to obtain a population in which there will be a high rate of the outcome variable to be studied. In these instances there is still an interest in the high-risk factor itself but the expectation is that many of the mechanisms involved will be non-specific. This approach was used for example by Farrington and West (see Chapter 23) in their prospective study of boys living in a high delinquency area; by Rutter and Quinton (see Chapter 65) in their 4-year follow-up study of children of adult psychiatric patients; by Wolkind and his colleagues (1976, 1977) in their longitudinal study of children born to mothers from a disrupted family of origin; by Rydelius (Chapter 64) in his investigations of the children of alcoholic fathers; and by Charitos-Forster (Chapter 66) in her follow-up of children who had started their life in residential nurseries. The expectation (confirmed by Rutter and Quinton in their parallel general population epidemiological studies) is that many of the causal processes studied will apply to the population generally and not be restricted to the high risk sample. The strategy has proved a powerful one and has emphasized the importance of family discord, parental criminality, parental mental illness, and poor supervision as factors predisposing to psychiatric disorder and delinquency.

Correlations over time

Cross-sectional data frequently give rise to correlations which suggest a *causal* relationship. Thus, significant associations have been found between styles of mother–child interaction and the child's intellectual development; or between watching violent television programmes and committing aggressive acts. But, almost always there is the problem of which way the causal process operates. In other words, does watching violence on television cause children to behave in a violent or aggressive fashion? Or, rather, is it that an interest in violence among aggressive boys causes them to watch more violent TV programmes? Or, yet again, are both TV viewing and aggressive behaviour due to some third variable (such as parental rejection)?

A variety of statistical techniques are available to disentangle the pattern of relationships. These help greatly in eliminating spurious associations but only the most indirect assessments of causality are possible if the data refer to only one point in time. However, as soon as there are *comparable* measures obtained at two or more different times, much more can be done to test causal hypotheses. Only the experimental method can do this decisively but the statistical analysis of appropriate longitudinal data can indicate with some power which causal hypotheses are more plausible.

The 'cross-lagged panel correlation' (Campbell and Stanley 1963) is a particularly useful technique in this connection. It requires two variables (X and Y) measured in the same way at two different points in time (T_1 and T_2), and deals with the problem of whether a significant correlation between X and Y is a result of X causing Y, or Y causing X. Put simply, the technique relies on comparing the two diagonal comparisons over time. Thus, if X causes Y, the correlation X_1Y_2 will exceed Y_1X_2; whereas if Y causes X the reverse will occur. In actuality, the situation is somewhat more complicated than that, both because it is necessary to take into account more than two rival hypotheses (Rozelle and Campbell 1969) and also because the findings will be influenced by varying reliabilities in measurement and by changes in the strength of causal relationships over time (Kenny 1975). However, statistical techniques are available to take these into account.

Several examples are available of the applications of this approach to substantive developmental problems in psychology. Thus, Eron *et al.* (1972) used it to determine the direction of the correlation between television violence and aggression. Their finding that watching violent TV in the third grade correlated 0·31 with aggression in the thirteenth grade, whereas aggression in the third grade correlated only 0·01 with watching TV violence in the thir-

teenth grade suggested that TV violence led to aggression rather than the other way round. (In fact, there are some problems in the analysis (see Kenny 1975) and alternative explanations are possible but the comparison was still valuable in indicating the relative plausability of two rival hypotheses.)

Clarke-Stewart (1973) used cross-lagged correlations to study the causes and consequences of mother–child interaction. The fact that the correlation between maternal attention at 11 months and the child's Bayley developmental quotient at 17 months was 0·60 whereas the reverse diagonal correlation was only – 0·04 suggested that the amount of maternal attention influenced the child's later intellectual competence (see Fig. 71.1). Interestingly, the existence of comparable measures at these ages (11, 14, and 17 months) indicated (through cross-lagged correlations) a changing reciprocal relationship over time with other aspects of mother–child interaction. At first, maternal attention increased infant attachment, but later, infant attachment led to more maternal attention.

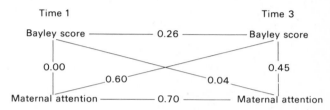

FIG. 71.1. Correlations between maternal attention and child's Bayley Developmental Quotient at ages 11 and 17 months (after Clarke-Stewart 1973).

In addition to the cross-lagged correlation method, there are a variety of other statistical approaches which are designed to use patterns of associations over time to sort out the direction of causal relationships. Thus, in addition to the more traditional methods (see Lazarsfeld 1972), multiple regression or partial correlation analyses may be used to delineate causal paths (Duncan 1976; Heise 1970) and factor analysis may also be employed to derive time-specific factors (Jöreskog 1969).

It is clear that the comparison of correlations over time (which require longitudinal data) can be very informative in the study of causal processes. Nevertheless, there are many statistical hazards to avoid and even the most sophisticated analyses are necessarily inconclusive. They do not 'prove' causation but they are most helpful in indicating which causal hypotheses are *likely* to be valid, and which are not.

Studies of process or change

Perhaps most of all longitudinal studies come into their own in the investigation of the results of psychosocial change or process. Some kind of longitudinal strategy is an essential component both because the interpretation of results is dependent upon a knowledge of what the individuals were like *prior* to the process under study, and because the measurement of an effect requires an assessment (and then a linking) of *change* in both the independent and dependent variables. Of course, causal relationships are most stringently tested by devising controlled situations in which randomly selected groups of subjects are experimentally exposed to contrasting environments or experiences and the consequences carefully measured. However, often it is not possible to introduce a genuinely experimental element into the social process—either because of politico–ethical difficulties or because the social events or circumstances cannot be accurately simulated in a planned experiment (Social Science Research Council 1975). It is in these circumstances that the natural experiment and evaluative longitudinal studies come into their own.

The natural experiment relies on the comparison of two situations similar in most respects but different in the one key variable under study. Often cross-sectional epidemiological studies are sufficient for this purpose (see Rutter 1977c) but in many instances longitudinal data provide the opportunity of a more critical test. These are crucial, for example, in educational studies because school performance is so strongly influenced by both family background and individual characteristics. In the inner London study of secondary schools (see Chapter 21) these variables were taken into account by following children from age 10 years (prior to secondary transfer) through the whole of their secondary schooling and to the end of their first year of employment. Measures of the children's family background, intelligence, scholastic attainments, and behaviour (together with primary school characteristics) at age 10 years were used to determine how far the variations between secondary schools in delinquency, exam success, attendance rates, and pupil behaviour were due to differences in intake, and how far to differences in the qualities of the schools as social institutions. The results showed that both were important. By studying in detail the features of schools associated with a good outcome it has been possible to identify which factors build up to constitute a successful social institution.

A similar research design was used to study the relative advantages of different types of educational unit in the treatment of autistic children (see Chapter 55). The improvements in children's behaviour and attainments over 3½ years were much influenced by which unit the children attended. It was possible to go on to show the features which characterized the most successful units.

It is useful to consider here the several steps needed to determine whether there is a true school (or other institutional) influence on children's development (and not just an artefactual association). First, it is necessary to show that schools vary in outcome measures of children's behaviour or attainments. Second, it has to be shown that this variation is not simply a consequence of differences in intake. This step requires longitudinal data and needs to take into account not only individual correlations over time (e.g. between the child's IQ or social class and later exam success) but also variations in the *balance* of intake. However, even this step is inconclusive in that all that it shows is that school variation still remains after controlling for all other specified variables. This may mean that there is a school influence or it may mean that other (non-school) variables which were not known or not taken into account led (artefactually) to school variation. A third step, which increases the likelihood that the school difference represents a *causal* influence, is to show that the school variation is systematically associated with differences in characteristics of the schools as social or pedagogic institutions. A fourth step is to check whether the school variations in outcome persist over time even when patterns of intake are altering. Nevertheless, a firm conclusion on a causal connection can only come from changing school practice and then following the children to see if the change in practice has led to the predicted change in behaviour or attainments. This kind of experimental intervention has only rarely been undertaken and as a consequence conclusions about psychosocial or educational experiences as causal influences on development usually have to be qualified or tentative. Such experimental studies are difficult to organize (and not always possible) but clearly there is a great need for more to be attempted.

In their absence, there has to be a reliance on psychosocial or educational variations which happen in an unplanned way. If properly undertaken, studies of such variations can be extremely informative and earlier chapters provide some nice illustrations of the many ways they can be used to provide relatively strong inferences of causation. For example, Farrington and West's longitudinal study of working class boys (see Chapter 23) has made excellent use of prospective data by focusing on the *timing* of associations. As a result the data have added greatly to our understanding of the origins of delinquency and crime. Because the data were prospective it was possible to be sure that the family adversities associated with delinquency had been present *before* delinquency occurred. The same data also showed that most of the family background factors related to violent delinquency were also significantly associated with aggressiveness at age 8–10 years. The strong implication is that the family variables were only related to violent delinquency because aggressive young boys tended to grow into delinquent teenagers. The existence of contemporaneously collected data at several points during the boys' development was also crucial in showing that convictions were *followed* by a worsening of delinquent behaviour which was not explicable in terms of any characteristics evident before conviction (Farrington 1977). None of these findings, all of which point to causal processes, could have come from a retrospective investigation.

There has been much speculation and theorizing by social scientists on the psychological effects of various kinds of social change—urbanization, industrialization, the introduction of universal schooling, changing roles of women, and rehousing schemes to mention but a few. But there have been remarkably few attempts to actually measure what happens in communities where such changes are occurring. A striking exception is the study by the Rosens (Chapter 32) in which they are attempting to determine the effects on mental health of rapid industrialization in the Shetland Isles, which is a consequence of the discovery of North Sea oil. The systematic comparison over time of two populations, only one of which is likely to be involved in the oil industrial complex, should provide invaluable knowledge on the psychiatric consequences of major social change. The design closely approximates a controlled experiment in that the two populations have been shown to be generally comparable at the outset and yet only one will experience the 'experimental treatment' (i.e. the industrialization). The comparison of changes over time in the two groups provides a good test, which is mainly limited by the fact that in real life both communities are likely to be influenced by the social change—albeit in rather differing ways. Nevertheless, the research design offers a good opportunity for examining causal processes—an opportunity all too rarely taken up.

Longitudinal data allow the timing of associations to be accurately measured, and knowledge on timing may be crucial in determining the meaning of associations. This is well illustrated in Plant's study of occupation and alcoholism (Chapter 31). The question is whether certain occupations attract alcoholics or rather whether particular jobs predispose to alcoholism. To answer that question it is crucial to know when heavy drinking and alcoholism developed—that is, before or after taking up a particular occupation. Plant's comparison of new recruits to the alcohol production industry and to other industries showed that the drink trade tended to attract heavy drinkers with a poor employment record. Follow-up interviews over the next two years should show whether, in addition to this selective intake, the job itself makes it more likely that alcohol consumption will increase or that dependency will develop.

The prospective study of children who experienced a head injury undertaken by Chadwick et al. (Chapter 56) demonstrates another use of longitudinal data to test causal relationships. In this instance the occurrence of intellectual *recovery* during the year after injury strongly suggests that the deficit noted immediately after the injury was *caused* by the injury (rather than being a prior characteristic of children who experience injuries). The findings were striking. Both children with mild and those with severe head injuries showed initially poor intellectual functioning compared with controls. But whereas the youngsters with severe injuries improved greatly over the next 12 months, those with mild injuries did not. The implication is that the relatively poor functioning of the children with mild injuries had nothing to do with the injury itself but rather was a reflection of what the child had been like before the injury. It is relevant in this connection that the circumstances in which the injuries occurred were rather different for mild and severe injuries, and that the children with mild injuries came from a more disadvantaged background. On the other hand, the demonstrated intellectual recovery of the individuals who experienced *severe* damage serves to confirm the causal nature of the relationship with the injury in that group.

One of the limitations of cross-sectional analyses is that the statistical associations generally refer to the same period of time, thus making it very difficult to disentangle the various stages of any causal process. Yet the same variable may have rather different effects at different points in the development of a disorder. This is well shown by Robins' study (Robins *et al.* 1977) of stages in the progression toward narcotic addiction in American men who served in Vietnam. It was found that young inner city blacks were the social group *most likely* to use narcotics (presumably because they come from a culture where drug taking is both common and socially accepted). In sharp contrast, however, these were the group of drug users *least likely* to become addicted on return. Drug dependence was most likely to develop in older white men from country areas (the fact that their drug usage was more deviant in their socio-cultural group suggested that this need for drugs was probably based more on individual compulsion than social convention). These two opposite associations served to cancel each other out in any overall association between demographic features and drug addiction. Longitudinal data were invaluable in indicating how different factors operated at different stages in the development of drug (or alcohol) dependence.

On the other hand, there is much evidence to indicate that most causal processes involve a *chain* of circumstances in which no single event or experience on its own can be considered 'the' cause (Rutter and Madge 1976). Cross-sectional data can do a great deal to delineate some of the steps involved. For example, epidemiological data were sufficient to show that inner city children had a higher rate of psychiatric disorder just because inner city families were more likely to experience all sorts of psychosocial adversity (Rutter *et al.* 1975b). The stresses of inner city life (whatever they may be) seem to operate on the parents rather than directly on the children. Inner city youngsters in homes *without* family adversity do *not* have any increased risk of disorder. Robins and her colleagues (1975) found the same with respect to black school boys in the United States. Longitudinal data, however, were important in their demonstration that the children's delinquency was linked more with their parents' adult criminality than with their delinquency as juveniles. They were also crucial in showing the connections between an individual's behaviour in childhood and his deviance in adult life (Robins 1972b; Robins *et al.* 1971).

Course of disorder

With respect to process, it is also relevant to note the importance of determining the factors which lead to a continuation or remission of psychiatric conditions once they have developed. It is an empirical question whether or not these are the same factors which led to the original genesis of the problem. Rutter and Quinton's longitudinal study (Chapter 65) showed that parental mental illness was not only a factor predisposing to psychiatric disorder in the children, but also tended to be associated with more persistent disorders. Power *et al.* (1974) found that family disharmony predicted both the development and persistence of delinquency. In infantile autism (see Chapter 55), cognitive/linguistic impairment is the most important variable in relation to both the development of autism and to its prognosis once it has developed. It is important that this has been found to be so in both treated and untreated cases—suggesting that it constitutes an essential part of the basic handicap. In all these cases the same factors predisposed to genesis and to perpetuation of

the condition. On the other hand, sometimes this is not the case. Both Robins' (1966) classical 10-year follow-up of child guidance clinic attenders and the Isle of Wight Study (Chapter 21) noted that the *type* or form of disorder in childhood was the most important predictor of outcome. Family variables were important in that they had different associations with different forms of child disorder, but once the disorder had developed they were of little importance in prognosis.

Prognostic studies are all illustrated in this volume by Rydelius' investigation of factors predicting relapse of drunkenness (Chapter 59), Ciompi *et al.*'s study of socio-psychiatric rehabilitation (Chapter 50), Ingham *et al.*'s longitudinal study of common psychological disorders (Chapter 49), and Stefánsson's follow-up of in-patients (Chapter 51). Prognostic studies are invaluable as a guide to the planning of treatment and advice to the patient; they also often shed light on the nature of the disorder being studied. For obvious reasons, findings on prognosis can only come from longitudinal studies.

Therapeutic intervention

Controlled trials of different forms of treatment are rarely considered in the context of longitudinal studies. To a considerable extent this is because most trials have been concerned with drug usage and assessments have been continued only for a matter of weeks, or at most months. Curiously, this has been so even when the therapeutic interventions have been applied to children with chronic handicapping disorders such as infantile autism, the hyperkinetic syndrome, or specific reading retardation. The lack of long-term evaluations of treatment is all the more regrettable because the criteria of successful outcome in these conditions must include the fostering of normal development, as well as the removal of symptoms or abnormal behaviours. As a result, our knowledge on the value of many of the methods of treatment used in psychiatry is rather limited.

Nevertheless, there have been important advances in the use of longitudinal studies to evaluate the long-term benefits and developmental gains consequent upon therapeutic interventions in childhood. First, as illustrated by Vuille and Lüthi's study of parent training (Chapter 67), researchers are beginning to attempt to evaluate preventive measures. Early work in the field was not encouraging. Several notable attempts to prevent delinquency through the provision of counsellors were singularly unsuccessful (e.g., Powers and Witmer 1951; Tait and Hodges 1962); compensatory education in the preschool years has only rarely been followed by lasting benefits (Bronfenbrenner 1974; Miller and Dyer 1975); and school programmes to aid mental health have not been very effective (Kellam *et al.* 1975). One attempt to increase community tolerance towards mental patients seemed actually to make things worse (Cummings and Cummings 1957).

The history of preventive psychiatry is a rather dispiriting one. Is there any reason to suppose that current attempts will prove any more effective? Time will tell, but two shifts of strategy offer some hope: preventive measures are tending to be more focused and systematic in approach, and increasingly the aim is to provide individuals with effective *coping* skills so that they may be better equipped to deal with new problems as they emerge. The work of Shure and Spivack (Spivack *et al.* 1976; Shure and Spivack 1978) in the United States in helping parents and children to learn social-problem-solving techniques has done much to break new ground in this area. Also Hemsley and her associates (see Chapter 55) have begun to develop ways of teaching and assessing parental coping skills relevant to the care of autistic children. Heber and Garber (1975) have shown that a great deal can be done to aid the development of socially disadvantaged black children born to mothers with an IQ below 80; Cullen's (1976) study of the counselling of parents of young children indicates that this may lead to a reduced rate of emotional disturbance; and school counselling also offers some promise (Rose and Marshall 1974). All these studies require replication before firm conclusions can be drawn, but they demonstrate both the possible potential of preventive measures and also the value of longitudinal methods in their evaluation.

A second development has been the appreciation that when services are in short supply (as they are in most parts of the world) the fact that, of necessity, only some individuals can receive treatment makes controlled trials of service delivery easy to arrange (and ethically acceptable). Thus, in the Isle of Wight studies (Chapter 21) controls were introduced into a naturally occurring situation in order to compare different methods of helping children with severe reading difficulties. Similarly, the opportunity was taken to examine the benefits to the children of giving their teachers in-service training on the skills of reading. In both cases, longitudinal data were used to assess the benefits a year or so later. In the study of a home-based approach to the treatment of autistic children (see Chapter 55), a long-term control group was obtained by using families living too far away to be involved in the intensive treatment programme but advised on an infrequent basis by the same therapists using the same therapeutic principles.

A third change has been to focus on children's behaviour in the ordinary environments of home and school and to include measures of normal development (in socialization, language, etc.) as well as of symptomatic features (fears, rituals, aggression, etc.). This shift has not only increased the scope of therapeutic evaluation but has also shed light on the nature of the disorders being treated. Thus, with autistic children (see Chapter 55) it has been striking that treatment has had a marked lasting benefit with respect to abnormal behaviours not specific to autism but has led to only marginal gains in language competence and no gains at all in intelligence. As language and cognition are also the most powerful prognostic features, the findings suggest that the basic handicap in autism involves a serious cognitive impairment which is relatively resistant to treatment. The follow-up of twin pairs (Folstein and Rutter 1977) indicates that the cognitive impairment is strongly influenced by genetic factors and that the development of autism is also associated with perinatal damage.

Fourthly, there has been a move from the global assessment of unspecified approaches encompassed under some general label such as casework or psychotherapy, to attempts to determine more precisely just which are the essential elements of successful treatment. Sometimes this has been done by comparing two alternative strategies, as in Reid and Shyne's (1969) study of focused and open-ended casework, or by comparing different therapist qualities, as in Truax and Carkhuff's (1967) investigations of Rogerian psychotherapy. In all cases it is desirable to have some measures of the process of therapy itself (in order to know better what is being evaluated). Such measures enable the researcher to use within-treatment comparisons to test whether the hypothesized therapeutic mechanism is indeed the operative factor. For example, if improved family communication is supposed to be the operative factor in family therapy, it would be helpful to determine whether (within cases all given the same treatment) changes in communication were linked with reductions in individual symptomatology. Alexander and Parsons (1973) made a start in this direction by applying the method to across-group comparisons, but so far little use has been made of the crucial within-group contrast.

Lastly, there has been the recognition that long-term assessments are needed to test the real value of therapeutic interventions, with chronic disorders. This is necessary not only because the benefits may prove transient but also because, with some treatments, time may be needed to consolidate the therapeutic gains. For example, Robins (1973) noted that this may be the case with group

psychotherapy methods. Either way it is clear that a longitudinal approach is required.

Longitudinal and cross-sectional methods

This overview of some of the ways in which longitudinal research is adding to psychiatric knowledge has emphasized the many strengths of this research approach. There are numerous scientific and policy questions which can *only* be answered effectively through the availability of longitudinal or follow-up data. In addition, there are others for which longitudinal data, although not essential, greatly improve the strength of hypothesis-testing. Nevertheless, it would be quite wrong to assume that longitudinal studies are necessarily the best means of answering psychiatric questions, or even developmental questions. All too often, longitudinal studies have been planned without any clear aims or hypotheses in mind, have involved a mindless collection of large amounts of data which are never adequately analysed, and which continue over so many years that by the end the original measures are hopelessly inappropriate for the purposes for which they are being used.

Some methodological issues in longitudinal research

Of course, most of these defects are a consequence of poor planning, and in any case the problems are by no means confined to longitudinal research. The crucial issues to be considered in planning a longitudinal study have been most thoughtfully and fully discussed by Robins (1978) and anyone undertaking longitudinal research would do well to consider carefully the issues she raises. Here, only a few key points will be mentioned. First, as already noted, most questions do *not* require that the same individuals be studied repeatedly over many years. For most purposes, 'follow-back' or 'catch-up' investigations or a series of short-term overlapping longitudinal studies will provide answers just as efficiently and very much more quickly. Furthermore, only certain sorts of issues require repeated assessments during the follow-up period.

Second, careful attention needs to be paid both to the size and characteristics of the index sample and also to the choice of control group. General population samples have the major advantage of avoiding misleading associations which stem from having unrepresentative or biased groups. As a consequence, they are often the first choice for the investigation of commonly occurring events and outcomes. On the other hand, for many purposes they are extremely wasteful of resources because so many normal children have to be studied in order to pick out the few who experience the stress or who develop the condition to be studied. For example, the huge American collaborative study had to examine 30 000 children in order to utilize longitudinal data to link pregnancy complications with the development of autism in just 14 children (Torrey *et al.* 1975)! In these circumstances there is much to be said for the use of stratified samples (in which there is oversampling from those portions of the population that are relatively rare but have important characteristics). Thus, Douglas (Chapter 6) and Robins (1972b) both oversampled school children of middle class background; and Rutter and his colleagues (Chapter 21) oversampled children with either deviant scores on a teachers' behavioural questionnaire or with reading difficulties. So long as the sampling fractions for each stratum are known, the unbiased total population can easily be reconstituted to produce representative prevalence estimates.

Another alternative is to use some kind of 'high risk' sample in order to inflate the proportion of individuals with the condition being studied. Thus, Rutter and Quinton (Chapter 65) studied the children of mentally ill parents; Mednick *et al.* (Chapter 63) followed the offspring of schizophrenic women; and Wolkind *et al.*

(1977) investigated children born to women who had themselves experienced disrupted childhoods. The strategy is powerful and legitimate but it is important to recognize that it inevitably involves distortions. Only a small minority of schizophrenics have schizophrenic mothers and it is possible that their psychiatric condition may arise from a different pattern of causes to those which operate in schizophrenia without a mentally ill parent. If the high risk strategy is followed prospectively it will almost always be necessary to combine it with some kind of 'follow-back' enquiry to check whether the high risk factor cases with the condition being investigated do or do not differ in important ways from individuals with the same condition but without the high-risk factor in this background.

A further issue in sampling is whether to take a national or local sample. Often it is argued that only the national sample is really representative. The argument, of course, is false because any such widespread sample is necessarily heterogeneous. A sample of all British children is quite unrepresentative of London or the Isle of Wight just because these areas are so different from each other, with neither similar to the nation as a whole (Rutter *et al.* 1975a, b). In the same way metropolitan Oslo and rural Norway are quite different (Lavik 1977). One value of epidemiological studies is the identification of just those ecological variables which do and those which do not influence the prevalence of psychiatric (or other) conditions. Large national samples may have enough cases to make appropriate regional comparisons (as for example in the National Child Development Study—see Chapter 7) but such large-scale surveys usually have to rely on questionnaire type data which may not give enough detail on the crucial environmental features. Whether an overall national sample or a series of more focused local samples (deliberately chosen to represent key variations in living conditions or socio-cultural context) is preferable will depend very much on the nature of the questions being asked. Of course, too, for some purposes international samples (e.g. the whole of Scandinavia, the EEC, or rural Africa) may be more suitable than either.

A longitudinal or cross-sectional approach?

The choice of whether to use a longitudinal or cross-sectional methodology involves many different issues. It is often argued that the main advantage of longitudinal studies is that they avoid the errors of retrospective recall. Unfortunately this is a rather misleading half-truth. Of course, they do diminish such errors insofar as their data gathering refers to contemporaneous events. But most longitudinal studies rely heavily on enquiries about past events. Thus, the 7-year-old sweep of the National Child Development study (Chapter 7) had to cover the whole 7 years from birth and the next sweep at 11 years had to gather information for the previous 4-year period. Necessarily, this means that many of the data are retrospective.

Even so, insofar as the data are contemporaneous and are gathered at two or more points in time, they do have the immense advantage of allowing an accurate determination of timing (of events or of changes in behaviour or of developmental modifications). It is this tremendous asset which gives the longitudinal enquiry its superiority over other methods for the study of development and for the investigation of causal processes. Only prospective data allow a proper assessment of predictive factors and of 'escape' from stressful experiences or happenings. It is for these reasons that the longitudinal strategy has proved itself such a powerful research tool in developmental psychiatry.

Longitudinal data are essential for the determination of developmental changes. Their strength in this connection is well illustrated by the issue of whether IQ scores declined with increasing age (Baltes 1968). Cross-sectional data on populations of varying ages had suggested that they did, but longitudinal analyses demonstrated that, to a considerable extent, this was an artefact of cohort or generation differences. Older people had a lower IQ, not so much because they were older, but because they were born in an earlier era and so were less well educated and less experienced in taking tests. The *combination* of longitudinal data and repeated cross-sectional data are essential to separate the effects of ageing, of generational differences, and of historical or cultural change (Schaie 1965; Schaie and Labouvie-Vief 1974). When the very substantial generational differences have been taken into account, it appears that there is some decline in IQ with age but not in all intellectual functions and probably not usually until either about age 60 years or the years leading up to death (Baltes and Schaie 1976; Horn and Donaldson 1976; Riegel and Riegel 1972).

What is sometimes less well appreciated is that repeated cross-sectional data are also crucial for this purpose. Changes over time in the same individual may reflect developmental alternatives or they may reflect secular changes in the population as a whole. Thus, delinquency rates have risen steadily throughout this century (Rutter and Madge 1976). Any increase in criminal behaviour between age X and age Y may have nothing to do with the maturation process. Rather it may be a consequence of secular changes in the population as a whole over the same time period. In short, both repeated cross-sectional and longitudinal data are needed to study development. Only in this way can developmental alterations and secular shifts be distinguished.

For many purposes it is necessary to differentiate the *incidence* of a condition from its *prevalence*. Longitudinal data are essential for this purpose. However, again, so are cross-sectional data. The point is that the population at risk may well have changed through immigration and this can only be checked through repeated cross-sectional surveys of the total population at that time (and not just those individuals who were present X years earlier).

The combination of cross-sectional and longitudinal data is also needed to take account of changing biological and social circumstances. For example, any prospective study linking birth weight with current adult intelligence is likely to be seriously misleading as a guide to the fate of babies born today because improved methods of neonatal care have greatly improved survival prospects (Stewart 1977). In the same way the National Survey data (Chapter 6) linking educational experiences with any other variable is of very limited relevance to the school child of today because the system of schooling in Britain now is very different from that operating when the 1946 cohort were being educated. Once more, a combination of longitudinal and cross-sectional methods are required. Because social circumstances and patterns of medical care change so rapidly, the cradle-to-coffin or even the infant-to-adult longitudinal enquiry has quite serious limitations. Really long-term prospective studies are needed for a few key research questions but for most purposes a series of shorter-term longitudinal studies (perhaps of overlapping age groups) is preferable.

A further problem of longitudinal studies, noted by Douglas in Chapter 6, is that biases may be created through repeated measurement. This may be checked by having a parallel sample studied only at infrequent intervals. Probably, the errors introduced in this way are quite trivial for most types of measures. Nevertheless, for some they may be larger and the possibility of repeated measurement bias needs to be checked.

Conclusion

There is not, and cannot be, any one most appropriate research strategy. Certainly the longitudinal approach (or rather the set of different longitudinal approaches) does not constitute such an all-purpose tool. Nevertheless, longitudinal studies represent a most important (and for some purposes indispensable) research technique. The variety of uses to which they may be put and the large number of research findings which could only have come from such a strategy have been illustrated in this review by reference to current investigations, most of which are represented in chapters

from this volume. They clearly indicate the great progress in longitudinal research which has taken place since the pioneer studies a half century ago. They also reflect some of the methodological and conceptual problems which continue to bedevil developmental research.

72. Developmental genetics and life-span ontogenetic psychology

I. I. GOTTESMAN

Overview

I have had the feeling, while contemplating some of the recent advances in developmental and molecular biology (e.g., Grouse *et al.* 1973; Hotta and Benzer 1972; Ohno 1972; Brown 1973; Brown and Goldstein 1976) that the longitudinal study of behaviour is more complex by an order of magnitude than is realized by the field. Valuable perspectives about the merits and problems of the longitudinal approach (e.g., Hindley 1972; Strauss *et al.* 1977) can only benefit by the fusion of parallel ideas and techniques from developmental genetics. We must start now to build a bridge between developmental genetics and ontogenetic psychology. My sentiments will be clearer if I paraphrase Paul E. Meehl's (1973) paraphrase of Albert Einstein and say that the trouble with the concept of development of behaviour over time is that it is too difficult for developmental psychologists, and further, it is too difficult for developmental biologists.

The potentials for genetic individuality and variability of our species are overwhelming (e.g., Brozek 1966; Harris 1975); there are some 3·8 billion human beings now alive but there are some seventy trillion potential human genotypes. Taking only twenty genetic markers for blood group systems we can calculate that the odds are one in two million that 2 people (excepting identical twins) would be matched; fortunately this degree of matching is not required for blood transfusions! It is estimated that our chromosome set contains three to five million genes, but a large number (perhaps 40–50 per cent) are redundant copies; the probable number of structural genes (see below) that code for an amino acid sequence in a protein is 60 000 to 100 000; the number of these that are polymorphic (a polymorphism is defined as the occurrence of two or more alleles at a given gene locus in a population, each allele having frequencies greater than 0·01) is 20 000 to 30 000 (but only some 50 have so far been discovered); and, the number of regulator genes (see below) is unknown and I can find no guesstimates. In the latest edition of McKusick's (1978) catalogue of Mendelian phenotypes identified in man are listed 1364 definites and 1447 probables for a total of 2811 gene loci of which 205 are on the X-chromosome. The extent of our ignorance about the structure and functions of the human genome is obvious; this in no way diminishes my awe at recent advances in molecular biology.

In a beautiful essay entitled 'Form, end and time' in his book *The strategy of the genes*, C. H. Waddington (1957) gave an overview of the conceptual framework I am grappling with in this paper. An adequate picture of any human can only be provided by considering the effects on him of three different types of temporal change, each being effective simultaneously and continuously.

The three time-elements in the biological picture differ in scale. On the largest scale is evolution; any living being must be thought of as the product of a long line of ancestors and itself the potential ancestor of a line of descendants. On the medium scale, an animal ... must be thought of as something which has a life history. It is not enough to see that horse pulling a

cart past the window as the good working horse it is today; the picture must also include the minute fertilized egg, the embryo in its mother's womb, and the broken-down old nag it will eventually become. Finally, on the shortest time-scale, a living thing keeps itself going only by a rapid turnover of energy or chemical change; it takes in and digests food, it breathes, and so on. In the biological picture toward which we are finding our way, the three time systems will have to be kept in mind together. That is the feat which common sense still finds difficult. Even in current biology, most of our theories are still only partly formed because they leave one or the other of the time scales out of account. (Waddington 1957; p. 6)

Therein lies one of the challenges to users of the longitudinal approach who have largely been working within the medium time scale: become aware of large-scale time (roughly equated with evolution and population genetics); remind yourselves of the importance of embryology and gerontology; and keep alert to the potential relevance of physiology and developmental genetics. Waddington went on to say:

One might compare an animal with a piece of music. Its short-scale physiology is like the vibrations of the individual notes, its medium-scale life-history is like the melodic phrases into which notes build themselves; and its long-scale evolution is like the structure of the whole musical composition, in which the melodies are repeated and varied. (Waddington 1957; p. 7).

Simultaneous contributions of genotype and environment to phenotypes

Throughout its young career behavioural genetics, following in the footsteps of agricultural and medical genetics, has been concerned with identifying the genotypes that correspond to certain behavioural phenotypes. This purpose was fairly well served by a conception of the genes as determiners of the structural end-states of an organism; the single-locus recessive disorder of PKU leading to mental retardation is a classical example of an inborn error of metabolism. The given trait (with implied structure) under investigation, be it intelligence of a rat in a maze, age at walking in infants, or predisposition to schizophrenia, was observed to be modified in many respects by environmental influences. (The identical twin concordance rate for onset of walking is 67 per cent while it is only 30 per cent in fraternals (Stern 1973; p. 717). Smiling and other indicators of sociability also appear to be under strong genetic control in infants (Freedman 1973).) It then became fairly standard practice, after appropriate experimental designs involving selection, or strain differences, or twins, to allocate proportions of the variance in individual differences observed to heredity, environment, and their interaction (cf., Fuller and Thompson 1978; Hirsch 1967; and McClearn and DeFries 1973). Such strategies will slowly give way to others suggested by the revolution in molecular biology ushered in by the eras of Watson and Crick (1953) and Jacob and Monod (1961), but they are an important starting point requiring understanding, before moving on to the more dynamic aspects of behavioural regulation and canalization (Wilson 1977; Denenberg 1979; Waddington 1957; Thiessen 1972).

One concept that I have found very useful for explaining the simultaneous contributions of genotype and environment to variations in phenotype, thus avoiding a number of pseudoquestions, is the reaction range (Gottesman 1963a, 1968; Gottesman and Heston 1972). It will serve to bridge the gap between static and dynamic aspects of structure and function. The explication may also serve to clarify the distinction I am trying to preserve between 'interaction' (cf., Erlenmeyer-Kimling 1972; Bouchard 1976) and simultaneous contribution or co-action. The fundamental points can be made by reference to Fig. 72.1 drawn from data collected by Krafka in 1919 on the effects on Drosophila eye facet number of

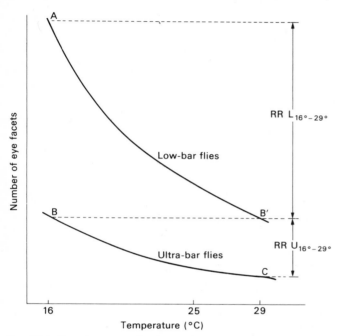

FIG. 72.1. Reaction ranges for *Drosophila* eye facet number as a function of larval-rearing temperatures. RR = reaction range.

rearing of their larvae at different temperatures (incidently a concrete example of *very* early experience). Samples of female flies of two genotypes, a low-bar and ultra-bar, were examined for eye facet number after the larvae from which they came had been subjected to seven different rearing temperatures (from 15°C to 29°C). Given these ideal circumstances of exquisite control over genotypic and environmental variability and these data, we can make a number of far-reaching statements that have potential application to behavioural phenotypes. Given uniformity of trait-relevant environment, almost all of the observed phenotypical variance in the trait must be attributable to genotypic differences: at 16° the difference is AB but it is only B'C at 29°, and in fact the genetic difference varies with the environment. Given uniformity in that part of the genome relevant to the trait, almost all of the phenotypical variance is attributable to environmental differences: the low-bar flies have A number of facets at 16° but the same flies have only B' facets at 29° while the other genotype, the ultra-bars have only B (= B') facets at the former temperature and C at the latter. The distances (or number of eye facets) AB' and BC are the Reaction Ranges (RR) of these two populations of flies over this particular range of environments; in other words, RR L and RR U are the two different environmental contributions to facet variability for these two genotypes under these conditions. The different sizes of RR suggest that there was differential buffering or environmental sensitivity of the developmental reactions of the

two genotypes to temperature changes; the differential response of two genotypes to a given environmental change is a 'clean' illustration of one of the meanings of genotype–environment interaction.

From this example we can conclude that the same genotype may have quite different phenotypes, and that similar phenotypes may have quite different genotypes. The latter is illustrated by the fact that the overlap in reaction ranges at the point B or B' would not allow you to distinguish between low-bar and ultra-bar flies from their number of eye facets, unless, of course, you had their complete developmental history. Given the usual state of affairs for human experimentation—genetic plus environmental heterogeneity—any observed trait variability must be attributed to some varying combination of genetic and environmental variances.

Fig. 72.2 illustrates the adaptation of the reaction range concept to variation in height for adolescent males and females based on some of the available morphological data (Greulich 1957; Meredith 1969; Mørch 1941). This trait is nearer to the interests of developmental psychologists and provides a shorter leaping distance to such behavioural traits as intelligence. The increased height in Japanese children born to Japanese parents in the United States compared to those born in Japan is well documented (Greulich 1957). It is a good example of (assuming no selective migration) a phenotypic change not associated with a genotypic one and is thus an example of the reaction range for height with the improved pre- and postnatal environment in the Japanese–Americans promoting a changed phenotype. The units for both X and Y-axes are only ordinal and not to scale.

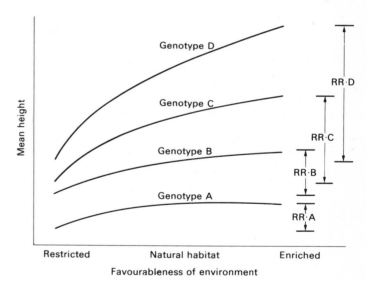

FIG. 72.2. The reaction range concept applied to adolescent height (units for both X- and Y-axes are only ordinal and not to scale). (See Gottesman 1963a; Bouchard 1976.)

Each curve in Fig. 72.2 can be construed as representing the phenotypic response of samples of individuals homogeneous for four different levels of genetic potential for height who have been reared in various trait-relevant environments (or niches) crudely characterized as restricted, natural habitat, and enriched. Curve Type A could represent a deviant mendelizing genotype, for example, the one associated with the dominant gene for classical achondroplastic dwarfism which has an incidence at birth of 1 in 10 000. (No connection has been demonstrated between this kind of 'growth failure' and that seen in pituitary dwarfs, a condition transmitted as one of a number of recessive loci.) The different environments to which such dwarfs have so far been exposed do not have much effect on their height; the mean height for 15-year-old cases (sexes combined) is only 120 cm. Curve Type B could represent samples of thirteen-year-old Japanese girls: in contemporary Japan they average 146·1 cm (= 'natural' habitat); thirteen-year-old girls measured in postwar Japan (1950) only averaged 139·9 cm. (= restricted environment nutritionally); thirteen-year-old Japanese girls born in the United States to Japanese parents averaged 150·5 cm. (= enriched environment). The Reaction Range (RR B) for the genotype represented by thirteen-year-old Japanese girls under the range of environments sampled would be the largest value minus the lowest or 10·6 cm. Curve Type C could represent the response of the genotypes of fifteen-year-old Japanese boys measured at the same time as the girls in B; we are dealing here with one more example of sexual dimorphism and a different genotype for height (cf., Tanner 1970). (The choice of 13- and 15-year-old girls and boys was dictated by the availability of data, but it does permit a rather close match for *maturity* with girls having a two- to three-year offset from boys in their velocity curves. 'Endocrinological age' is recommended as a criterion for matching sexes rather than chronological age throughout the behavioural sciences.) Post-war boys averaged 151·1 cm; contemporary boys in Japan, 158·2 cm; and, contemporary Japanese boys born in the United States, 164·5 cm for a reaction range of 13·4 cm, all attributable to environmental variations. The large difference in reaction ranges of 2·8 cm might suggest that an *XY* (again) is less buffered than an *XX* genome. Curve Type D could represent 15-year-old American white boys who average 168·7 cm. (13-year-old white girls average 155·4 cm.). Examples of the same phenotype with different genotypes are provided by some data on children of Japanese *X* United States white matings (fathers always white); the 15-year-old boys averaged 164·7 cm while the 13-year-old girls averaged 151·5. It appears that the hybrids matched the American-born Japanese and were about halfway between contemporary Japanese and white children (under natural habitat conditions). Other genotypes could have been added to Fig. 72.2 for such diverse groups as the Mbuti pygmies and Nuer of Sudan with adult mean heights of 144 cm and 184 cm, respectively. The thrust of the reaction range concept is that both heredity and environment are important in determining trait variation but in different ways, combinations, and degrees, some of which are amenable to dissection for some traits.

One of the major shortcomings of the reaction range concept is that it is not adequate for the task of encompassing changes observed over time intraindividually or interindividually. Fig. 72.3 presents the growth velocity curves of five boys followed with

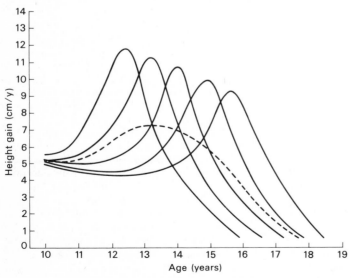

Fig. 72.3. Growth velocity curves (cm/year) of five British males during adolescent growth spurt with the dashed line representing the average for this sample. (After Tanner *et al.* 1966.)

repeated measurements over the period of their adolescent growth spurts (Tanner *et al.* 1966; Marshall 1971). Such a plotting of velocities (rate of growth cm/y) rather than distances (attained height at a point in time) has a number of important advantages:

(1) It maximizes the picture of individual differences in a dramatic fashion;
(2) It shows the gross kinds of distortion obtained from cross-sectional data compared to longitudinal observation and from averaging compared to individual observation (note that the dashed line represents the average velocity but characterizes no individual in the group);
(3) It forces to the forefront questions about the differential switching on of so-called maturational processes;
(4) It pinpoints the possibilities for critical or vulnerable periods in ontogeny for dramatically different tissue requirements (cf., Dobbing 1971; Winick 1976).

If we are to approach an understanding of the phenomena such as those on growth in Fig. 72.3 from a genetic point of view, we must extend the concepts so that genetic regulation and gene function are included.

Regulator genes and epigenetic landscapes

Many attractive albeit tentative hypotheses about the processes of development in mammals have been stimulated by the growing understanding of the switching on and off of metabolic processes in the cell of a bacterium. Only a rough and ready sketch of the principles involved and their possible extensions to gene expression in mammalian cells (Britten and Davidson 1969; Tomkins *et al.* 1969) can be provided here and the reader is referred to other sources (e.g., Darnell *et al.* 1973; Thiessen 1972; Bodmer and Cavalli-Sforza 1976) for details. (Protein synthesis and structure is more complex than implied by this abbreviated description. See Bodmer and Cavalli-Sforza (1976) and Harris (1975) for more details.) As Thiessen (p. 87) says,

Gene influence on behaviour is always indirect. Hence, the regulatory processes of a behaviour can be assigned to structural and physiological consequences of gene action and developmental canalization. The blueprint for behaviour may be a heritable characteristic of DNA, but its ultimate architecture is a problem for biochemistry and physiology.

Large, some would say radical, changes in the mechanisms involved in gene regulation are required conceptually before the bacterial model can be extrapolated to mammalian cells, but the important message for developmental psychologists is the same. That is, exquisite, precise systems have evolved that provide for qualitative differences in proteins and for quantitative variations in rates of synthesis that are cybernetically related to the needs of the organism. In one extension (Britten and Davidson 1969) *batteries* of structural genes are regulated by 'integrator and receptor' genes with the former under the control of 'sensor genes'; this model would permit responses to an external signal, production of a second signal which is transmitted to receptors unresponsive to the original signal, reception of the second signal, and a response to it in the form of structural gene transcription. Other points at which mammalian cells may be regulated with 'fine tuning' are suggested by the terms *post-transcriptional regulation* and *translational modulation* (cf. Darnell *et al.* 1973). The thorny problem of what switches on the switches that switch on the switches is tackled by Ohno (1972) who also argues that mammalian regulation involves simplification rather than complication of the bacterial model via changes in the power of regulatory genes vs. the acquisition of new structural genes. One of his pertinent and bold conjectures is that maleness and femaleness represent the switched on and switched off state of one and the same regulatory system!

A different but related concept from developmental genetics that should prove an important addition to the armamentarium of longitudinal researchers is Waddington's three-dimensional model for handling phenotypic changes in the states of organs (or organisms) as they develop toward some adult end state. The top surface of his 'epigenetic landscape' together with a peek at what is underneath it—all schematic of course—is given in Fig. 72.4. It allows for the conceptualization of the simultaneous and sequential effects of many genes and many external stimuli influencing the structure and function of an organism. The contour of the landscape is determined by the person's genotype; the surface is tilted so that time of fertilization is in the back plane and end states are at the bottom of the canals. The location of the ball represents the state of differentiation or development of some part of the fertilized egg, for example, that part destined to become the brain. The trajectory of the ball as it rolls toward you analogously represents the developmental history of an egg part. Don't destroy the artistry in the landscape by demanding too much explanatory power from it. You can see though that if, while the system is moving along, environmental or genetic forces push the ball slightly off course, it will return to its original path with some exceptions. One exception is the 'critical period' when the ball is at a fork in the path (T_2); even here individual differences in the depth of the canalization and the steepness of the walls determine the susceptibility to the forces (differential buffering). Underneath the epigenetic landscape you can see pegs representing a sample of structural genes while the wires connecting them to the surface are subject to variable tension as a function of gene expression (the regulation of the genes is not shown but see the discussion above).

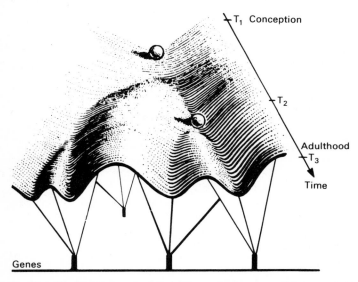

FIG. 72.4. Waddington's epigenetic landscape for conceptualizing genetic and environmental roles in ontogeny of an organ or organism.

A developmental psychology that incorporates developmental genetics is appropriately complex. The phenotype at any point in time is in a state of dynamic flux with its momentary value determined by all three time elements (p. 338). Since only a small portion of the genome (perhaps 5 to 20 per cent) is activated at any one time (cf., Grouse et al. 1973), the effective genotype upon which environmental forces are acting is constantly changing. As I shall show below, this phenomenon goes a long way towards accounting for the different developmental trajectories of monozygotic (identical) twins with respect to both states and outcomes.

Developmental behavioural genetics and psychopathology

We are still very much on the frontiers of applying a developmental behavioural genetic point of view to the area of psychopathology, but it has commenced (Gottesman 1960, 1965, 1966; Gottesman and Shields 1972; Shields et al. 1975; Hanson et al. 1977). Genetic disorders of behaviour with a variable age of onset and /or remissions and exacerbations provide the most fertile ground for a joining of developmental psychology and biology. Huntington disease (HD), caused by a dominant gene, and schizophrenia, a disorder with a well established genetic component, can be used to illustrate the ontogeny of psychopathology. In a paradigmatic application of the high-risk method (Pearson and Kley 1957; Mednick 1970), Lyle and Gottesman (1977) followed up 88 offspring of Huntington patients some 15 to 20 years after they had been tested with a battery of psychometrics. All 88 were free of clinical signs of HD when they were first tested; 44 would be expected to develop the disease eventually; 28 were found on follow-up to be affected. The results for the offspring at the time of initial testing on just the Wechsler Performance Scales as a function of their status on follow-up are given in Fig. 72.5. Up to this time the use of psychological or other tests to detect the presymptomatic carriers of the dominant gene has not been encouraging. Recently a group of investigators (Klawans et al. 1972) have reported promising results with a provocative test that elicited choreaform movements in 10/28 offspring of HD patients (but in none of the controls) after loading with the chemical levodopa; it will take a long-term follow-up to determine whether there is a one-to-one correspondence with overt disease.

Affected when tested	Early-onset carriers	Late-onset carriers	Normative 'average' adult	Still normal 'controls'
85.7	87.8	94.4	100	106.2

91.9

Premorbids

Critical contrast

FIG. 72.5. Mean Performance IQ scores at initial testing of Huntington disease offspring as a function of follow-up status 15–20 years later. (After Lyle and Gottesman 1977.)

Our analyses of the data from the Wechsler and other cognitive tests (but not the MMPI) can be interpreted to mean that the gene for HD has been having an effect on neural functioning before clear symptoms appear and that the nearer to overt disease, the greater the malfunctioning. The age of onset for HD ranges from under 5 to over 75 and appears from parent–child and MZ twin correlations to be under strong genetic control. The variability across families in symptoms and onset ages implicates regulatory genes and their triggers. The practical application of changes in psychometric status over time combined with a loading test to genetic counselling is some way off but appears to be promising at this point in time (Mednick 1978). Note that performance IQs of 94 or 88 would not ordinarily suggest pathology and it is only in contrast to the 58 offspring who remained unaffected that suspicions are aroused.

The premorbid detection of schizophrenia has so far met with little success (Shields et al. 1975). The application of high-risk methods (cf., Garmezy 1974) continues to hold promise, but most investigators (see Schulsinger 1976) do not yet have enough affected (with schizophrenia) children of schizophrenics to give definitive findings (Hanson *et al.* 1977). A diathesis-stressor model (to be explicated below) for understanding schizophrenia's aetiology appears to hold the most heuristic promise (Rosenthal 1963; Gottesman and Shields 1972) where the genes are necessary but not sufficient (Meehl 1972a, b). While we are waiting for the longitudinal studies of high-risk children to 'pay off', we can learn a great deal about some of the ontogenetic aspects of schizophrenia by looking at the course of the disorder once it has made its appearance.

Fig. 72.6 shows the MMPI profiles of a pair of female identical twins (MZ 22) age 28 from the Maudsley Schizophrenic Twin Study (Gottesman and Shields 1972); they both have had repeated admissions since they were first hospitalized at age 19. Both twins were tested in remission (A_1 and B profiles) showing the kinds of personality resemblance we have come to expect with identical twins (Gottesman 1963b) but the profiles do not indicate the presence of the kinds of schizophrenic psychoses both had experienced on five previous occasions. The very elevated and typically psychotic profile A_2 in Fig. 72.6 is from Twin A just eight weeks later; she had responded to an accumulation of environmental stressors with another decompensation and was admitted to a Day Hospital. Twin B was not tested in a psychotic state since she did not have her next breakdown for another two years, but our data on other MZ pairs tested when both were decompensated suggest their profiles would be very similar (see MZ 13 and MZ 21 in Gottesman and Shields 1972, p. 274). Despite their identical genotypes and identical predispositions or liabilities to developing schizophrenia, they were capable of showing quite different states because of the differences in their effective genotypes i.e., differences in which genes were activated or inactivated at one point in time.

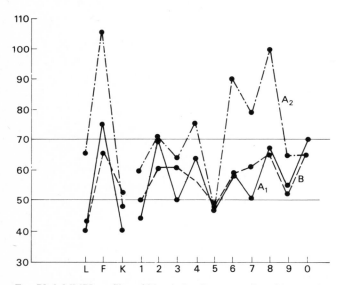

FIG. 72.6. MMPI profiles of identical twins concordant for recurring schizophrenia: in remission (A_1 and B) and after A decompensated (A_2) 8 weeks later. (After Gottesman and Shields 1972.)

This phenomenon of environmental determination of effective genotype was ubiquitous, as can be seen in Fig. 72.7. The in and out of hospital periods are shown for all ten pairs of identical twins and three pairs of fraternal twins who were concordant for schizophrenia in the Maudsley study using the consensus diagnoses of 6 judges. It should now be obvious how much information about psychodynamics and about gene regulation may be hidden by the all embracing term 'concordant'. Ages at first hospitalization are given to the left while elapsed time since then are indicated by a

time line in years at the top and bottom of Fig. 72.7. The longitudinal view of the course of schizophrenia after its onset (cf., Bleuler 1972) permits the reconciliation of views about the aetiology of schizophrenia that lean too heavily in either a genetic or an environmental direction.

The contribution of specific genetic factors to the genetic liability to schizophrenia suggested by the data from twin, family, and adoptee studies forms only a part of this epigenetic landscape. Comprehension of the *total* liability to schizophrenia requires the concepts schematized in Figs. 72.8 and 72.9. Fig. 72.8 portrays the various genetic and environmental contributors that combine in some fashion (additively and/or more complexly) to yield a net value on the dimension of combined liability; the concepts are cross-sectional or frozen in time. In addition to specific genetic liability, there are general genetic and general environmental contributions that serve as modifiers or potentiators. Additional axes are shown that provide for genetic and environmental *assets*; they have negative values to illustrate the role of factors that may decrease the total liability to schizophrenia, permitting a person to stay compensated or to go into a remission despite high values of genetic and/or environmental liability. The five dimensions in Fig. 72.8 are marked off in liability units of varying length to imply differential weighting effects (Gottesman and Shields 1972). The curve in the figure depicts the distribution of combined liability units in the general population together with the point defining the threshold value where a diagnosis of schizophrenia is highly probable. If the three liability values plus the two asset values sum to a suprathreshold value for an individual at a point in time, he has reached a schizophrenic state in his epigenetic landscape or in his ontogeny. Of course, the concepts are oversimplified and overschematic. There may well turn out to be specific environmental liability to schizophrenia (e.g., ingestion of LSD) in addition to the general one we have shown, but so far the candidates proposed have been found wanting (Schofield and Balian 1959; Kind 1966; Scharfetter 1970; Schuham 1967; Kohn 1973; Gottesman and Shields 1976).

The dimension of time must be added to Fig. 72.8 in order to increase the semblance to reality; an effort to represent a more dynamic view of a person's trajectory across the epigenetic landscape and thus do justice to the concept of a genetic diathesis being influenced by the environment so as to produce a schizophrenic phenotype is given in two-dimensional form in Fig. 72.9. The intention is to incorporate the concepts of changes in effective genotype by gene regulation, critical periods, and environmental inputs to a dynamic system. The time axis starts with the moment of fertilization so that prenatal factors can show their influence on states of combined liability towards schizophrenia. Both chance and ontogenetic constitutional changes will influence the path of the trajectories, leading to both upward and downward inflections. Environmental or genetic contributors to liability coming close together in time would be expected to have a cascade effect and be more influential than the same forces spread out in time (think about the ball and the modelling of the landscape).

G_1 is intended to indicate the trajectory of a person with a low (for schizophrenics generally) combined *genetic* liability to schizophrenia; over time environmental contributors to liability, say first the death of a spouse and then the onset of deafness, cause upward deflections of his trajectory to the threshold (T), culminating in a late-onset paraphrenia. The dashed line at the bottom of the zone of the so-called schizophrenic spectrum disorders (Kety *et al.* 1968, 1975; Rosenthal *et al.* 1968), is intended to convey the idea of a possible need for a second threshold in our model; Wright (1934) invoked a second threshold to account for the imperfectly formed fourth digit seen in crosses between a high and a moderate line of guinea pigs with liabilities to polydactyly.

G_2 could be the divergent trajectories of a pair of MZ twins, only the A-twin encounters the sufficient factors over time leading to schizophrenia for a person with his genotype. The B-twin at the time of observation is discordant for schizophrenia, but close to the threshold of schizophrenic spectrum disorders. Subthreshold values of combined liability make it clear why so many first degree relatives can have normal MMPIs (Gottesman and Shields 1972)

and why two phenotypically normal parents are typical for the vast majority of schizophrenics. The A-twin is shown to have an acute onset with an indistinguishable premorbid personality, and then a remission from schizophrenia into a chronic schizoid state.

G_3 is the posited trajectory of a person with a high genetic loading needing very little in the way of environmental contributors to

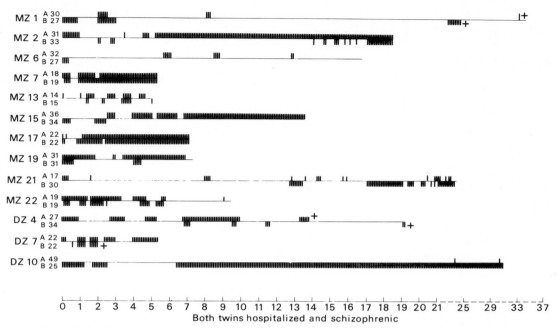

FIG. 72.7. Possible evidence of gene regulation form plotted hospitalization periods for concordant schizophrenic twins; fact of death indicated by a crown; years since first hospitalization of first ill twin on X-axis. (After Gottesman and Shields 1972.)

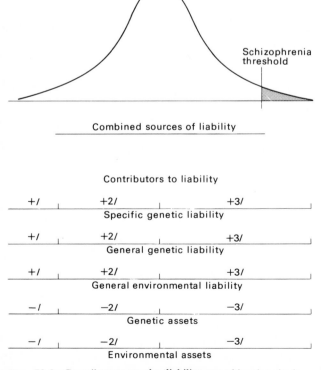

FIG. 72.8. Contributors to the liability to schizophrenia in a diathesis-stressor multifactorial threshold model. (After Gottesman and Shields 1972.)

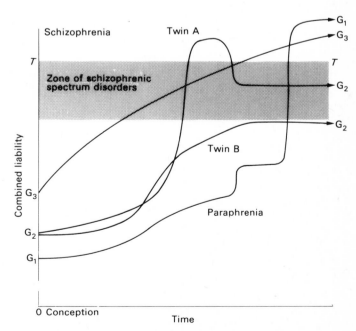

FIG. 72.9. Trajectories over the epigenetic landscape showing the schematic ontogenesis of schizophrenia for 3 different genotypes. T = threshold point of Fig. 72.8. (After Gottesman and Shields 1972.)

make him schizoid; he is shown as having a poor premorbid personality, an insidious onset, and a deteriorating course. Many other life trajectories could have been drawn to illustrate the unfolding of schizophrenia. It is easy to see how the hospitalization data in pairs of twins (Fig. 72.7) and the fascinating life-span histories of the Genain quadruplets (Rosenthal 1963) would augment the total perspective about the pathogenesis and ontogeny of schizophrenia.

Concluding remarks

I hope that the diverse subject matter of this chapter ranging from drosophila eye facet number, to height, to Huntington disease and schizophrenia will be seen to be appropriate for the apperceptive mass of life-span developmental psychology rather than aimless wandering about the landscape. Heuristic integration of the knowledge for longitudinal studies of behaviour is an enormous task and will require teams of scientists who appreciate the contributions each can make to the enterprise of understanding the development of our species.

This paper is an updated revision of 'Developmental genetics and ontogenetic psychology: overdue detente and propositions from a matchmaker', in *Minnesota Symposia on Child Psychology* (ed. A. Pick) Vol. 8. University of Minnesota Press, Minneapolis, 1974.

I am indebted to D. R. Hanson, L. L. Heston, and D. J. Merrell for their constructive comments on an earlier draft of this paper. A great deal of my thinking about the aetiology of schizophrenia has evolved from my long collaboration with the late James Shields.

References

ABDELLAH, F. G. and LEVINE, E. (1970). *Better patient care through nursing research.* New York: Macmillan.

ABELL, L. L., LEVY, B. B., BRODIE, B. B. and KENDALL, F. E. (1952). Simplified method for the estimation of total cholesterol in serum and demonstration of its specificity. *J. Biol. Chem.,* **195**, 357–66.

ADAMS, E. M. and FINLAYSON, A. (1961). Familial aspects of pre-eclampsia and hypertension in pregnancy. *Lancet,* **ii**, 1373.

ADELSTEIN, A. M., DOWNHAM, D. Y., STEIN, Z. and SUSSER, M. W. (1968). The epidemiology of mental illness in an English city. *Soc. Psychiat.,* **3**, 47–59.

AGUÉ, C., CIOMPI, L. and DAUWALDER, J. P. (1977a). La réadaptation socio-professionnelle des malades mentaux: la recherche en Angleterre et ses implications pratiques. *Soc. Psychiat.,* **12**, 95–106.

——, and —— (1977b). La rehabilitaciòn del enferme mental y estrategias de investigaciòn socio-psiquiatrica: I. Antecedentes y generalidades. *Psicologia Medica,* **3**(2), 179–203.

——, and —— (1977c). La rehabilitaciòn del enferme mental y estrategias de investigaciòn socio-psiquiatrica: II. Projectos, instrumentos y metodologia. *Psicologia Medica,* **3**, 265–81.

AHRLÉ, F. (1965). Die Entwicklung von Kindern berufstätiger Mütter in der Oberstufe. Unpublished Dipl. Thesis, Bonn.

AITKEN-SWAN, J. (1977). *Fertility control and the medical profession.* London: Croom Helm.

ÅKESSON, H. O. (1961). *Epidemiology and genetics of mental deficiency in a Southern Swedish population.* Uppsala: The Institute for Medical Genetics of the University of Uppsala.

ALBEE, G. W. (1951). The prognostic importance of delusions in schizophrenia. *J. abnormal soc. Psychol.,* **46**, 208–12.

ALBERMAN, E. D. (1969). The prevalence of congenital defects in the children of the 1958 cohort. *Concern,* **3**, 29–33.

ALEXANDER, J. F. and PARSONS, B. V. (1973). Short-term behavioural intervention with delinquent families: impact on family process and recidivism. *J. abnormal Psychol.,* **81**, 219–25.

AMARK, C. (1970). A study in alcoholism. *Acta Psychiat. Neurolog. Scand.,* Suppl. 70, 237–43.

AMIEL-TISON, C. (1969). Cerebral damage in full-term new-borns: aetiological factors, neonatal factors and long term follow-up. *Biologica Neonatorum,* **14**, 234–50.

AMNELL, G. (1966). The mentally subnormal in Finland and their need for care 1962, Medical part. *Official Statistics of Finland* (X32: 26). Helsinki.

—— (1974). Mortalitet och kronisk morbiditet i barnaåldern, En kohortundersokning av ar 1955 födda Helsingforsbarn. *Samfundet Folkhälsan.* Helsinki.

ANDERSON, E. (1973). *The disabled schoolchild.* London: Methuen.

ANDERSON, W. J. R. (1956). Stillbirth and neonatal mortality in twin pregnancy. *J. Obstet. Gynaecol. Brit. Empire,* **63**, 205–15.

——, BAIRD, D. and THOMSON, A. M. (1958). Epidemiology of stillbirths and infants deaths due to congenital malformation. *Lancet,* **1**, 1304–6.

ANGLEITNER, A. (1976). Changes in personality observed in questionnaire data from the Riegel Questionnaire on rigidity, dogmatism, and attitude toward life. In *Contributions to human development,* vol. 3, (ed. H. Thomae), pp. 68–80. Basel: S. Karger AG.

ANGST, J. (1966). *Zue aetiologie und nosologie endogener depressiver psychosen. Eine gentische, soziologische und klinische studie.* Monographie aus dem Gesamtgebiet der Neurologie und Psychiatrie. Heft 112. Berlin: Springer.

—— (1978). The course of affective disorders. II. Typology of bipolar manic-depressive illness. *Arch. Psychiat. Nervenkrankheiten,* **226**, 65–73.

—— (1980). Verlauf unipolar depressiver, bipolar manisch-depressiver und schizo-affektiver Erkrankungen und Psychosen. Ergebnisse einer prospektiven Studie. *Fortschr. Neurol. Psychiat.,* **48**, 3–30.

—— and FREY, R. (1978). The course of affective disorders. I. Change of diagnosis of monopolar, unipolar and bipolar affective illness. *Arch. Psychiat. Nervenkrankheiten,* **226**, 57–64.

—— and WEIS, P. (1967). Periodicity of depressive psychoses. *Proceedings of the Fifth International Congress of Collegium Internationale Neuropsychopharmacologicum,* pp. 703–10. Washington, D.C. March 1966. Excerpta Medica Foundation, International Congress Series No. 129. Amsterdam: Elsevier.

ANNETT, M. (1970). The growth of manual preference and speed. *Brit. J. Psychiat.,* **61**, 545–58.

Annual Reports Registrar General Scotland (1963–75), Part 1—Mortality Statistics. Her Majesty's Stationery Office. Edinburgh, Scotland.

APPLETON, T., CLIFTON, R., and GOLDBERG, S. (1975). The development of behavioural competence in infancy. In *Review of Child Development Research 4* (ed. F. D. Horowitz). Chicago: The University of Chicago Press.

ARAJÄRVI, T., HUTTUNEN, M. O., and TALVINKO, S. (1977). Family counselling in the prevention of children's psychiatric disorders. A preliminary report. Accepted for publication in *Psychiatria Fennica.*

ARONSSON, G. (1963). The adolescent sons of male alcoholics. *Arch. gen. Psychiat.,* **3**, 235–41.

AST, D. B., SMITH, D. J., WACHS, B. and CANTWELL, K. T. (1956). Newburgh-Kingston cariesfluoride study, XIV: combined clinical and roentgenographic dental findings after 10 years of fluoride experience. *J. Amer. dent. Assoc.,* **52**, 314–25.

ASTRUP, C. and NOREIK, K. (1966). *Functional psychoses: diagnostic and prognostic models.* Springfield, Illinois: Charles C. Thomas.

AVERIL, J. R. (1973). Personal control over aversive stimuli and its relation to stress. *Psychol. Bull.,* **80**, 286–303.

BACKETT, E. M. and JOHNSTON, A. M. (1959). Social patterns of road accidents to children: some characteristics of vulnerable families. *Brit. med. J.,* **i**, 409–13.

BAHNA, S. L. and BJERKEDAL, T. (1972). The course and outcome of pregnancy in women with bronchial asthma. *Acta Allerg.,* **27**, 397–406.

—— and —— (1974). The course and outcome of pregnancy in women with neuroses. *Acta Obstet. Gynecol. Scand.,* **53**, 129–33.

BAIRD, D. (1949). Social factors in obstetrics. *Lancet,* **1**, 1079–83.

—— (1953). Health and physique of mothers in various social groups. *The Eugenics Review,* **45**, 151–4.

—— (1964). The epidemiology of prematurity. *J. Pediat.,* **65**, 909–24.

—— (1974). Birth control pioneer. *New Scientist.*

—— (1975). Interplay of changes in society, reproductive habits and obstetric practice in Scotland between 1922 and 1972. *Brit. J. prevent. soc. Med.,* **29**, 135–46.

——, ANDERSON, A. R. M. and TURNBULL, A. C. (1968). Influence of induction of labour on caesarean section rates, duration of labour and perinatal mortality in Aberdeen primigravidae 1938–66. *J. Obstet. Gynaecol. Brit. Commonwth.,* **75**, 800–11.

—— and ILLSLEY, R. (1953). Environment and childbearing. *Proc. Roy. Soc. Med.,* **46**, 53–9.

—— and THOMSON, A. M. (1969). The effects of obstetric and environmental factors on perinatal mortality by clinico-pathological causes. In *Perinatal problems* (ed. N. R. Butler and E. D. Alberman), pp. 211–26. Edinburgh: Livingstone.

——, WALKER, J. and THOMSON, A. M. (1954). A classification of deaths by clinical cause: the effect of age, parity and length of gestation on death rates by cause. *J. Obstet. Gynaecol. Brit. Empire,* **61**, 433–48.

BAKWIN, H. (1968). Delayed speech: developmental mutism. *Pediat. Clinics North America,* **15**, 627–38.

BALDWIN, J. W. and EVANS, J. H. (1971). The (North East Scottish) Psychiatric Case Register. In *Aspects of the epidemiology of mental illness: studies in record linkage* (ed. J. A. Baldwin), pp. 17–38. Boston: Little, Brown and Co.

BALLOW, B., ANDERSEN, J. A., REYNOLDS, M. and RUBIN, R. A. (1969). *Educational and behavioural sequelae of prenatal and perinatal conditions* (Interim Report No. 3). U.S. Department of Health, Education, and Welfare.

BALTES, P. B. (1968). Longitudinal and cross-sectional sequences in the study of age and generation effects. *Human Develop.*, **11**, 145–71.

—— and SCHAIE, K. W. (1976). On the plasticity of intelligence in adulthood and old age: Where Horn and Donaldson fail. *Amer. Psychol.*, **31**, 720–5.

——, —— and NARDI, A. H. (1971). Age and experimental mortality in a seven-year longitudinal study of cognitive behaviour. *Develop. Psychol.*, **5**, 18–26.

BANHAM, K. (1964). *Manual for the ring and peg tests of behavioural development for infants and pre-school children. Ages: birth to six years.* Munster: Psychometric Affiliates.

BARKER, D. J. P. (1966). Low intelligence and obstetric complications. *Brit. J. prev. soc. Med.*, **20**, 15–21.

BARTAK, L. and RUTTER, M. (1971). Educational treatment of autistic children. In *Infantile autism: concepts, characteristics and treatment* (ed. M. Rutter). Edinburgh: Churchill Livingstone.

—— and —— (1973). Special educational treatment of autistic children: a comparative study. I. Design of study and characteristics of units. *J. child Psychol. Psychiat.*, **14**, 161–79.

—— and —— (1975). The measurement of staff–child interaction in three units for autistic children. In *Varieties of residential experience* (ed. J. Tizard, I. Sinclair and R. V. E. Clarke). London: Routledge and Kegan Paul.

—— and —— (1976). Differences between mentally retarded and normally intelligent autistic children. *J. Autism childhood Schizophrenia*, **6**, 109–20.

BAUMANN, U., MEYER, B. and SUTER, U. (1974). Formale und inhaltliche Ueberprufung der PND-Skalen. *Diagnostica*, **20**, 3–21.

BAUMRIND, D. (1966). Effects of authoritative parental control on child behaviour. *Child Develop.*, **37**, 887–907.

BAX, M. and WHITMORE, K. (1973). Neurodevelopmental screening in the school entrant medical examination. *Lancet*, **ii**, 368–71.

BAYER, M. L. and BAYLEY, N. (1959). *Growth diagnosis.* Chicago: The University of Chicago Press.

BAYLEY, N. (1955). On the growth of intelligence. *Amer. Psychol.*, **10**, 805–18.

—— (1964). Consistency of maternal and 'child behaviours' in the Berkeley Growth Study. *Vita Humana*, **7**, 73–95.

—— (1969a). *Bayley scales of infant development.* Berkeley: Institute of Human Development.

—— (1969b). *Manual for the Bayley scales of infant development.* New York: The Psychological Corporation.

BEAGELEHOLE, E. (1949). Cultural complexity and psychological problems. In *A study of interpersonal relations* (ed. P. Mullahy), pp. 256–68. New York: Hermitage Press.

BEEK, A., ZONNEVELD, R. J., FRENKEL-TISTZ, M. G. and MOES-SWAAB, G. P. J. (1968). Longitudinaal onderzoek naar de gezondheidstoestand in een Bejaardeninrichting. *Tijdschrift voor Sociale Geneeskunde*, **46**, 854.

BEHAR, L. and STRINGFIELD, S. (1974). A behaviour rating scale for the preschool child. *Develop. Psychol.*, **10**, 601–10.

BELL, B., CHRISTIE, M. J. and VENABLES, P. H. (1975a). Psychophysiology of the menstrual cycle. In *Research in psychophysiology* (ed. P. H. Venables and M. J. Christie). London: Wiley.

——, MEDNICK, S. A., RAMAN, A. C., SCHULSINGER, F., SUTTON-SMITH, B. and VENABLES, P. (1975b). A longitudinal psychophysiological study of three-year-old Mauritian children: The Joint Child Health Project. *Develop. Med. child Neurol.*, **17**, 320–4.

BELL, R. Q. (1953). Convergence: an accelerated longitudinal approach. *Child Devel.*, **24**, 145–52.

—— (1975). The Bethesda longitudinal study: the overall study and some specific findings. In *Life history research in psychopathology*, Vol. 4 (ed. R. D. Wirt, G. Winokur and M. Roff). Minneapolis: University of Minnesota Press.

——, WELLER, S. M. and WALDROP, M. F. (1971). Newborn and preschooler: organization and behaviour and relations between periods. *Monographs Soc. Res. child Develop.*, **86**, 1–145.

BENARON, H. B., TUCKER, B. E., ANDREWS, J. P., BOSHES, B., COHEN, J., FROMM, E. and YACORZYNSKY, G. K. (1960). Effect of anoxia during labour and immediately after birth on subsequent development of the child. *Amer. J. Obstet. Gynecol.*, **80**, 1129–42.

BENDER, L. (1949). Psychological problems of children with organic brain disease. *Amer. J. Orthopsychiat.*, **19**, 404–15.

BENNHOLDT-THOMSEN, C. (1942). Die Entwicklungsbeschleunigung. *Ergebnisse der inneren Medizin und Kinderheilkunde*, **62**, 1153–237.

BERGMAN, L. R. (1971). Some univariate models in studying change. *Reports from the Psychological Laboratories*, Suppl. 10. University of Stockholm.

—— (1972a). Change as the dependent variable. *Reports from the Psychological Laboratories*, Supplement 14. University of Stockholm.

—— (1972b). Inferential aspects of longitudinal data in studying developmental problems. *Human Develop.*, **15**, 287–93.

—— (1972c). Linear transformations and the study of change. *Reports from the Psychological Laboratories*, No. 352. University of Stockholm.

—— (1973a). Parents' education and mean change in intelligence. *Scand. J. Psychol.*, **14**, 273–81.

—— (1973b). Bloom's developmental formula: a methodological note. *Human Develop.*, **16**, 395–6.

—— (1974). Is intellectual performance more vulnerable in boys than in girls? *Reports from the Psychological Laboratories*, No. 417. University of Stockholm.

—— and MAGNUSSON, D. (1979). Overachievement and catecholamine output in an achievement-demanding situation. *Psychosom. Med.* (in press).

BERGSVEINSSON, J. (1974) Brug og misbrug af alkohol i Reykjavík (Use and abuse of alcohol in Reykjavík). *Nord. Psykiat. Tidsskr.*, **28**, 513–21.

BERTELSEN. A., HARVALD, B. and HAUGE, M. (1977). A Danish twin study of manic-depressive disorders. *Brit. J. Psychiat.*, **130**, 330–51.

BILLEWICZ, W. Z. and THOMSON, A. M. (1957). The effect of maternal social class and stature upon the incidence of prematurity. *Proc. Nutrit. Soc.*, **16**, v.

BINDER, J., SIEBER, M., and ANGST, J. (1979). Verzerrungen bei postalischen Befragungen: das Problem der Nichtantworter. *Z. für exper. und angewandte Psychol.*, **26** (1), 53–71.

BIRCH, H. G. (1964). The problem of brain damage. In *Brain damage in children* (ed. H. G. Birch). Baltimore: Williams and Wilkins.

——, RICHARDSON, S. A., BAIRD, Sir D., HOROBIN, G. and ILLSLEY, R. (1970). *Mental subnormality in the community: a clinical and epidemiologic study.* Baltimore: Williams and Wilkins.

BIRREN, J., BOTWINICK, J., WEISS, A. and MORRISON, F. F. (1963a). Interrelations of mental and perceptual tests given to healthy elderly men. In *Human aging: a biological and behavioural study* (ed. J. E. Birren, R. N. Butler, S. W. Greenhouse, L. Sokoloff, and M. R. Yarrow), pp. 143–56. Bethesda, Maryland: National Institute of Mental Health.

——, BUTLER, R. N., GREENHOUSE, S. W., SOKOLOFF, L. and YARROW, M. R. (eds.) (1963b). *Human aging: a biological and behavioral study.* Bethesda, Maryland: National Institute of Mental Health.

—— and MORRISON, D. F. (1961). Analysis of the WAIS subtests in relation to age and education. *J. Geront.*, **16**, 363–9.

——, WOODRUFF, D. R. and BERGMAN, S. (1972). Research, demonstration, and training: issues and methodology in social gerontology. *Gerontol.*, **12**, 49–83.

BJARNAR, E., MELSOM, R., REPPESGAARD, H. and ASTRUP, C. (1975a). A social psychiatric investigation of a rural district in Northern Norway. *Acta Psychiat. Scand.*, **51**, 19–27.

——, REPPESGAARD, H. and ASTRUP, C. (1975b). Psychiatric morbidity in Berlevåg. *Acta Psychiat. Scand. Suppl.*, **263**, 60–7.

BJERKEDAL, T. and BAHNA, S. L. (1973). The course and outcome of pregnancy in women with epilepsy. *Acta Obstet. Gynecol. Scand.*, **52**, 245–8.

——, —— and LEHMANN, E. H. (1975). Course and outcome of pregnancy in women with pulmonary tuberculosis. *Scand. J. Resp. Dis.*, **56**, 245–50.

—— and BAKKETEIG, L. (1972). *Medical registration of births in Norway, 1967–68: some descriptive and analytical aspects.* Bergen, Norway: University of Bergen, Institute of Hygiene and Social Medicine, Medical Birth Registry of Norway.

—— and —— (1975a). *Medical registration of births in Norway during the 5-year period 1967–71.* Bergen, Norway: University of Bergen, Institute of Hygiene and Social Medicine.

—— and —— (1975b). Surveillance of congenital malformations and other conditions of the newborn. *Int. J. Epidem.*, **4**, 31–6.

——, —— and BERGSJØ, P. (1975). *Maternity institutions in Norway per 1st July 1974. Personnel, equipment and care facilities. Changes since 1st January 1972.* Bergen, Norway: University of Bergen, Institute of Hygiene and Social Medicine.

BJÖRNSSON, S. (1973). Enuresis in childhood. *Scand. J. educ. Res.*, **17**, 63–82.

—— (1974). Epidemiological investigation of mental disorders of children in

Reykjavík, Iceland. *Scand. J. Psychol.*, **15**, 244–54.

—— Constellations of psychological symptoms in childhood and their association with cognitive, educational and socioeconomic variables (in preparation).

——, EDELSTEIN, W. and KREPPNER, K. (1977). *Explorations in social inequality. Stratification dynamics in Iceland.* Max-Planck Institut für Bildungsforschung.

BLACK, P., BLUMER, D., WELLNER, A. M. and WALKER, A. E. (1971). The head-injured child: time-course of recovery with implications for rehabilitation. In *Head injuries*. Proceedings of an International Symposium, 131–7. Edinburgh and London: Churchill Livingstone.

——, JEFFRIES, J. J., BLUMER, D., WELLNER, A. and WALKER, A. (1969). The post-traumatic syndrome in children. In *The late effects of head injury* (ed. A. E. Walker, W. F. Caveness and M. Critchley), pp. 142–9. Springfield, Illinois: Charles C. Thomas.

BLEULER, M. (1972). *Die schizophrenen geistesstorungen im lichte langjahriger krankenund familiengeschichten.* Stuttgart: Thieme.

BLOMFIELD, J. M. and DOUGLAS, J. W. B. (1956). Bed-wetting: prevalence among children ages 4–7 years. *Lancet*, **1**, 850.

BLOMQUIST, J. (1957). Some social factors and school factors. *Int. Rev. Educ.*, **3**, 165–73.

BLOOM, B. S. (1964). *Stability and change in human characteristics.* London: Wiley.

BLUM, G. S. and MILLER, D. R. (1952). Exploring the psychoanalytical theory of the 'oral character'. *J. Personal.*, **20**, 287–304.

BLUM, R. H. (1962). Case identification in psychiatric epidemiology: methods and problems. *Milbank Mem. Quart.*, **15**, 253–75.

BODMER, W. and CAVALLI-SFORZA, L. L. (1970). Intelligence and race. *Sci. Amer.*, **233**, 19–29.

—— and —— (1976). *Genetics, evolution, and man.* San Francisco: W. H. Freeman.

BOHMAN M. (1973). *Adoptivbarn och deras familjer: en undersökning av adoptivbarn, deras bakgrund, miljö och anpassning* (in Swedish). Stockholm: Almquist and Wiksell.

BOND, M. (1975). Assessment of the psychosocial outcome after severe head injury. In *Outcome of severe damage to the central nervous system* (ed. R. Porter and D. W. FitzSimons), pp. 141–7. Amsterdam: CIBA Foundation Symposium No. 34.

BORKOWSKI, J. G., BENTON, A. L. and SPREEN, O. (1967). Word fluency and brain damage. *Neuropsychol.*, **5**, 135–40.

BOSMA, W. G. A. (1973). Alcoholism and the family: a neglected problem (in Yugoslavian). *Alkoholizm*, **13**(3–4), 43–7.

BOUCHARD, T. J. (1976). Genetic factors in intelligence. In *Human behaviour genetics* (ed. A. R. Kaplan), pp. 164–97. Springfield: C. C. Thomas.

BOURGEOIS, L. (1975). Les enfants d'alcooliques. Une enquête sur 66 enfants d'alcooliques d'un service pédopsychiatrique. *Ann. Médicopsychol. (Paris)*, **2**(3), 592–609.

BOWER, E. M., SHELLHAMER, T. A. and DAILY, J. M. (1961). School characteristics of male adolescents who later became schizophrenic. *Amer. J. Orthopsychiat.*, **30**, 4.

BRADLEY, D. (1955). Organic factors in the psychopathology of childhood. In *Psychopathology of childhood* (ed. P. H. Hoch and J. Zubin). New York: Grune and Stratton.

BRANDT, U. (1964). Flüchtlingskinder. Eine Untersuchung zu ihrer psychischen Situation (A study on the psychological situation of children from displaced families). *Wissenschaftliche Jugendkunde*, vol. 6. Munich: J. A. Barth.

BREMER, J. (1951). A social psychiatric investigation of a small community in Northern Norway. *Acta Psychiat. (Kobenhavn) Suppl.*, **62**.

BRITTEN, R. J. and DAVIDSON, E. H. (1969). Gene regulation for higher cells: a theory. *Science*, **165**, 349–57.

BRONFENBRENNER, U. (1974). *Is early intervention effective? A report on the longitudinal evaluations of pre-school programmes.* Bethesda: Office of Child Development, U.S. Department of Health, Education, and Welfare.

BRONSON, W. C. (1966). Central orientations: a study of behaviour organization from childhood to adolescence. *Child Develop.*, **37**, 125–55.

—— (1967). Adult derivates of emotional expressiveness and reactivity-control: developmental continuities from childhood to adulthood. *Child Develop.*, **38**, 801–17.

BROOKS, D. N. (1976). Wechsler memory scale performance and its relationship to brain damage after severe closed head injury. *J. Neurol. Neurosurg. Psychiat.*, **39**, 593–601.

BROWN, D. D. (1973). The isolation of genes. *Sci. Amer.*, **229**, 20–9.

BROWN, G. W. (1974). Meaning, measurement, and stress of life events. In *Stressful life events* (ed. B. S. Dohrenwend and B. P. Dohrenwend), pp. 217–43. New York: John Wiley.

—— and BIRLEY, J. L. T. (1968). Crises and life changes and the onset of schizophrenia. *J. Hlth Soc. Behav.*, **9**, 203–14.

——, BONE, M., DALISON, B. and WING, J. K. (1966). *Schizophrenia and social care.* London: Oxford University Press.

——, CHADWICK, O., SHAFFER, D., RUTTER, M., and TRAUB, M. (1980). A prospective study of children with head injuries. III. Psychiatric sequelae (submitted for publication).

——, MONCK, E. M., CARSTAIRS, G. M. and WING, J. K. (1962). The influence of family life on the course of schizophrenic illness. *Brit. J. prev. soc. Med.*, **16**, 55.

—— and RUTTER, M. (1966). The measurement of family activities and relationships: a methodological study. *Human Relat.*, **19**, 241–63.

——, SKLAIR, F., HARRIS, T. A. and BIRLEY, J. L. T. (1973). Life events and psychiatric disorders. I: Some methodological issues. *Psychol. Med.*, **3**, 74–87.

BROWN, M. S. and GOLDSTEIN, J. L. (1976). Receptor-mediated control of cholesterol metabolism. *Science*, **191**, 150–4.

BROZEK J. (ed.) (1966). *The biology of human variation.* New York: New York Academy of Science.

BRUN-GULBRANDSEN, S. and IRGENS-JENSEN, O. (1967). Abuse of alcohol amongst seamen. *Brit. J. Addict.*, **62**, 19–27.

BRUUN, K. *et al.* (1977). *Alcohol control policies in public health perspective.* Helsinki: Finnish Foundation for Alcohol Studies (vol. 25).

BÜCKING, H., VAN EGMOND, J., ELSENGA, S. and HAAUSTRA, F. (1975). De konstruktie van een jeugdversie van de Nederlandse Persoonlijkheidsvragenlijst (de NPV-J) Heymans Bulletins, pp. 75–190. Psychologische Instituten R.U. Groningen, H.B.

BÜHLER, C. and HETZER, H. (1953). *Kleinkindertests.* Munich: Johann Ambrosius Barth.

BULLOCK, A. (1975). *Bullock report.* London: H.M.S.O.

BURK, D. (1972). Some contemporary issues in child development and the children of alcoholic parents. *Ann. N. Y. Acad. Sci.*, **197**, 189–97.

BURT, C. (1925). *The young delinquent.* London: University of London Press.

—— (1937). *The backward child.* London: University of London Press.

BUSS, A. H. and PLOMIN, R. (1975). *A temperament theory of personality development.* New York: John Wiley.

BUTLER, N. R. and ALBERMAN, E. D. (1969). *Perinatal problems.* Edinburgh: Livingstone.

—— and BONHAM, D. G. (1963). *Perinatal mortality.* Edinburgh: Livingstone.

——, PECKHAM, C. S. and SHERIDAN, M. D. (1973). Speech defects in children aged seven years. *Brit. Med. J.*, **5848**, 253–7.

BUTLER, S. and WALSH, D. (1976). *The St. Loman's case register 1971–1975.* Dublin: Medico-Social Research Board.

CALNAN, M., DOUGLAS, J. W. B. and GOLDSTEIN, M. (1978). Tonsillectomy and circumcision—a comparison of two cohorts. *Int. J. Epidemiol.*, **7**, 79–85.

CAMPBELL, D. T. and STANLEY, J. C. (1963). Experimental and quasi-experimental designs for research and teaching. In *Handbook of research on teaching* (ed. N. L. Gage). Chicago: Rand McNally.

CANTWELL, D., HOWLIN, P. and RUTTER, M. (1977). The analysis of language level and language function: a methodological study. *Brit. J. Disord. Commun.*, **12**, 119–35.

CAPLAN, G. (1974). *An approach to community mental health.* London: Tavistock.

CAPLAN, H. L. (1970). Hysterical 'conversion' symptoms in childhood. M. Phil dissertation, University of London.

CAREY, W. B. (1970). A simplified method for measuring infant temperament. *J. Pediat.*, **77**, 108.

CARLESTAM, G. and LEVI, L. (1971). *Urban conglomerates as psychosocial human stressors.* (A contribution to the United Nations conference on the human environment). Stockholm: Royal Ministry for Foreign Affairs.

CARNEY, M. W. P. and LAWES, T. G. C. (1967). The etiology of alcoholism in the English upper classes. *Quart. J. Stud. Alc.*, **28**, 59–69.

CARPENTER, W. T., SACKS, M. H., STRAUSS, J. S., BARTKO, J. J. and RAYNER, J. (1976). Evaluating signs and symptoms: comparison of structured interview and clinical approaches. *Brit. J. Psychiat.*, **128**, 397–403.

CASSEL, J. and TYROLER, H. A. (1961). Epidemiological studies of culture change. I. Health status and recency of industrialization. *Arch. Environ. Hlth.*, **3**, 25–33.

CATTELL, R. B. (1950). *Personality. A systematic theoretical and factual study.* New York: McGraw-Hill.

CEDERLÖF, R., FRIBERG, L., JONSSON, E. and KAIJ, L. (1961). Studies on similarity diagnosis in twins with the aid of mailed questionnaires. *Acta Genet. (Basel)*, **11**, 338–62.

—— (1966). The twin method in epidemiological studies on chronic disease. Thesis. Stockholm.

—— (1971). Twin registries in the study of chronic disease with particular reference to the relation of smoking to cardiovascular and pulmonary diseases. *Acta Med. Scand.* (Suppl.), **523**, 3–40.

Census, 1961, 1966 (Special Census Report) and 1971, Scotland, County Report, Zetland. (1962, 1967, 1972). General Register Office, Her Majesty's Stationery Office, Edinburgh, Scotland.

CHADWICK, O., RUTTER, M., BROWN, G., SHAFFER, D. and TRAUB, M. (1980a). A prospective study of children with head injuries. II. Cognitive sequelae (submitted for publication).

——, —— and SHAFFER, D. (1980b). A prospective study of children with head injuries. IV. Possible specific cognitive deficits (submitted for publication).

CHAFETZ, M., BLANE, H. and HILL, M. (1971). Children of alcoholics. Observations in a child guidance clinic. *Quart. J. Stud. Alc.*, **32**, 687–98.

CHERRY, N. (1974). Components of occupational interest. *Brit. J. educ. Psychol.*, **44**, 22–30.

—— (1976). Persistent job changing—is it a problem? *J. occup. Psychol.*, **49**, 203–21.

—— and KIERNAN, K. (1976). Personality scores and smoking behaviour. *Brit. J. prevent. soc. Med.*, **30**, 123–31.

CHESS, S., THOMAS, A. and BIRCH, H. G. (1966). Distortions in developmental reporting made by parents of behaviourally disturbed children. *J. Amer. Acad. Child Psychiat.*, **5**, 226–34.

——, —— and —— (1973). *Your child is a person.* New York: Viking Press.

CHRISTIANSEN, K. O. (1968). Threshold of tolerance in various population groups illustrated by results from a Danish criminological twin study. In *The mentally abnormal offender* (ed. A. V. S. de Reuck). Boston: Little, Brown and Co.

CICOUREL, A. V. (1968). *The social organisation of juvenile justice.* New York: John Wiley.

CIOMPI, L., AGUÉ, C. and DAUWALDER, J. P. (1977). Ein Forschungsprogramm über die Rehabilitation psychisch Kranker I. Konzepte und metodologische Probleme. *Nervenarzt*, **48**, 12–18.

——, —— and —— (1978a). Mise en evidence de changements psychodynamiques. *L'Evolution psychiatrique.* **43**, 369–77.

——, —— and —— (1978b). Ein Forschungsprogramm über die Rehabilitation psychisch Kranker II. Querschnittsuntersuchungen chronischer Spitalpatienten in einem modernen psychiatrischen Sektor. *Nervenarzt*, **49**, 332–8.

CLARK, I. R. (1975). Shetland—The oil boom and the future. *The Shetland Times*, July 18 1975, p. 10. (Special suppl.)

CLARKE, R. B. (1949). The relationship of alcoholic psychoses commitment rates to occupational income and occupational prestige. *Amer. Soc. Rev.*, **14**, 539–43.

CLARKE-STEWART, K. A. (1973). Interactions between mothers and their young children: characteristics and consequences. *Monographs Soc. Res. Child Develop.*, **38**, (6–7) (Serial no. 153).

COBB, H. V. (1966). *The predictive assessment of the adult retarded for social and vocational adjustment: a review of research. Part I.* Department of Psychology, University of South Dakota.

COBB, S. (1974). A model for life events and their consequences. In *Stressful life events* (ed. B. S Dohrenwend and B. P. Dohrenwend), pp. 151–6. New York: John Wiley.

COELHO, G. V., HAMBURG, D. A. and ADAMS, J. E. (1974). *Coping and adaptation.* New York: Basic Books.

COERPER, C., HAGEN, W. and THOMAE, H. (1954). *Deutsche nachkriegskinder.* Stuttgart: Thieme, 1954.

COHLER, B. J., GALLANT, D. H. GRUNEBAUM, H. U., WEISS, J. L. and GAMER, E. (1975). Pregnancy and birth complications among mentally ill and well mothers and their children. *Soc. Biol.*, **22**, 269–78.

COLEMAN, J. S., CAMPBELL, E. Q., HOBSON, C. J., McPARTLAND, J., MOOD, A. M., WEINFELD, F. D. and YORK, R. L. (1966). *Equality of educational opportunity.* Washington, D.C.: Office of Education, HEW.

COLLETT, J. (1963). Om risken for aterfall i fylleri. *Alkoholfragan*, **57**, 210.

COMMISSION OF THE EUROPEAN COMMUNITIES (1978). *Report on the joint EEC/WHO workshop on physical activity in primary prevention of ischaemic heart disease.* Luxembourg, 22–4 February, 1977, CEC.

COOLS, A. T. M. and HERMANNS, J. M. A. (1976). DOS-handleiding. *Denver Ontwikkeling Screeningtest.* Amsterdam: Swets and Zeitlinger.

COOPER, B. (1973). Epidemiological psychiatry (editorial). *Psychol. Med.*, 401–4.

COOPER, J. E. (1965). Epilepsy in a longitudinal survey of 5000 children. *Brit. med. J.*, **1**, 1020–2.

COPELAND, J. R. M., COOPER, J. E., KENDELL, R. E. and GOURLAY, A. J. (1971). Differences in usage of diagnostic labels amongst psychiatrists in the British Isles. *Brit. J. Psychiat.*, **118**, 629–40.

COURT, D. (1976). *Court report to the Department of Health and Social Security.* London: H.M.S.O.

COX, A., RUTTER, M., YULE, B. and QUINTON, D. (1977). Bias resulting from missing information: some epidemiological findings. *Brit. J. prevent. soc. Med.*, **31**, 131–6.

CRAFT, A. W., SHAW, D. A. and CARTLIDGE, N. E. (1972). Head injuries in children. *Brit. med. J.*, **3**, 200–3.

CRAIG, W. S. (1950). Intercranial irritation in the newborn: immediate and long-term prognosis. *Arch. Dis. Childhood*, **25**, 325–50.

—— (1960). Convulsive movements occurring in the first 10 days of life. *Arch. Dis. Childhood*, **35**, 336–44.

CRELLIN, E., PRINGLE, M. L. and WEST, P. (1971). *Born illegitimate.* Slough: National Foundation for Educational Research.

CULLEN, K. J. (1976). A six-year controlled trial of prevention of children's behaviour disorders. *J. Pediat.*, **88**, 662–6.

CUMMINGS, E. and CUMMINGS, J. (1957).

Closed ranks. Cambridge, Mass.: Harvard University Press.

CURMAN, H. and NYLANDER, I. (1976). A 10-year prospective follow-up study of 2268 cases at the child guidance clinics in Stockholm. *Acta Paediat. Scand. Suppl.*, **260**.

CYTRYN, L., GILBERT, A. and EISENBERG, L. (1960). The effectiveness of tranquillizing drugs plus supportive psychotherapy in treating behaviour disorders of children: a double-blind study of eighty outpatients. *Amer. J. Orthopsychiat.*, **30**, 113–29.

DALÉN, P. (1975). *Season of birth: a study of schizophrenia and other mental disorders.* Amsterdam: North-Holland Publishing Co.

DARNELL, J. E., JELINEK, W. R. and MOLLOY, G. R. (1973). Biogenesis of messenger RNA: genetic regulation in mammalian cells. *Science*, **181**, 1215–21.

DAVIE, R. (1971). Size of class, educational attainment and adjustment. *Concern*, **7**, 8–14.

——, BUTLER, N. and GOLDSTEIN, H. (1972). *From birth to seven. A report of the National Child Development Study.* London: Longman.

DE COSTER, W., DE ZUTTER, M., VANDIERENDONCK, A., THIERY, M. and DEROM, R. Psychomotor and cognitive development of twins from birth to six years. In press.

——, GOETHALS, A., VANDIERENDONCK, A., THIERY, M. and DEROM, R. (1976). Labor induction with prostaglandin F2α. Influence on psychomotor evolution of the child in the first 30 months. *Prostaglandins*, **12**(4), 559–64.

——, LEROU, J., DUTOIT, C., DE ZUTTER, M., DEROM, R., THIERY, M. and VANDIERENDONCK, A. (1977). Psychological follow-up study of twins from birth to 5 years. *Acta Genet. Med. Gemellolog.*, **25**, 198–212.

DEFARES, P. B., KEMA, G. N., VAN PRAAG, E. and VAN DER WERFF, J. J. (1970). *Syracuse–Amsterdam Groningen sociometrische schaal.* Uitgave voor Research doeleinden.

DENENBERG, V. H. (1979). Paradigms and paradoxes in the study of behavioural development. In *The origins of the infant's social responsiveness* (ed. E. B. Thoman). Hillsdale, N.J.: L. Erlbaum Assoc. (in press).

DENKLA, M. B. (1973). Development of speed in repetitive and successive finger movements in normal children. *Develop. Med. child Neurol.*, **15**, 635–45.

DEPARTMENT OF HEALTH AND SOCIAL SECURITY (1977). *Report on hospital in-patient enquiry for the year 1973.* H.M.S.O.

DEPARTMENT OF INDUSTRY. National survey of smoke and sulphur dioxide (1975). *The investigation of air pollution.* Warren Springs Laboratory, Stevenage, England, 1966–75.

DEPARTMENT OF TRADE (1975a). *Report of the working group on discipline in the fishing industry.* H.M.S.O. November 1975, pp. 10–4.

DEPARTMENT OF TRADE (1975b). *Report of the working group on discipline in the Merchant Navy.* H.M.S.O. November 1975, 16.

DEPUE, R. A. (1976). An activity-withdrawal distinction in schizophrenia: behavioural, clinical, brain damage and neurophysiological correlate. *J. abnorm. Psychol.*, **85**, 174–85.

DEROGATIS, L. R. (1974). The Hopkins Symptom Checklist. In *Psychological measurements in psycho-pharmacology. Modern problems of pharmaco-psychiatry* (ed. P. Pichot), vol. 7, pp. 70–110. Basel: Karger.

DEUTSCHER, I. (1962). Some relevant directions for research in juvenile delinquency. In *Human behaviour and social processes—an interactionist approach* (ed. A. M. Rose). London: Routledge and Kegan Paul.

DIGHT, S. E. (1976). *Scottish drinking habits.* Office of Population Censuses and Surveys.

DISTLER, G. (1959). *Längsschnittkinder mit geringer Differenziertheit im Grundschulalter.* Dipl. Thes., Erlangen.

DOBBING, J. (1971). Undernutrition and the developing brain: the use of animal models to elucidate the human problem. In *Normal and abnormal development of brain and behaviour* (ed. G. B. A. Stoelinga and J. J. Van der Werfften Bosch), pp. 20–30. Leiden: Leiden University Press.

DOHRENWEND, B. S. and DOHRENWEND, B. P. (eds.) (1974a). *Stressful life events: their nature and effects.* New York: John Wiley.

—— and —— (1974b). Overview and prospects for research on stressful life events. In *Stressful life events* (ed. B. S. Dohrenwend and B. P. Dohrenwend), pp. 313–31. New York: John Wiley.

—— and —— (1974c). A brief historical introduction to research on stressful life events. In *Stressful life events* (ed. B. S. Dohrenwend and B. P. Dohrenwend), pp. 1–15. New York: John Wiley.

—— and —— (1974d). Psychiatric disorders in urban settings. In *The American handbook of psychiatry* (ed. G. Caplan), pp. 424–47. New York: Basic Books.

—— and —— (1974e). Social and cultural influences on psychopathology. *Ann. Rev. Psychol.,* **25**, 417–52.

DOLL, E. A. (1953). *Vineland Social Maturity Scale.* New York: Psychological Corp.

DONNISON, D. V. D. and SOTO, P. (in press). *The Good City: a study of urban development and policy in Britain.* London: Heinemann.

DOUGLAS, J. W. B. (1964a). *The home and the school.* London: MacGibbon and Kee.

—— (1964b). Ability and adjustment of children who have had measles. *Brit. med. J.,* **2**, 1301.

—— (1970). Broken families and child behaviour. *J. roy. Coll. Physicians,* **4**, 203.

—— (1973). Early disturbing events and later enuresis. In *Bladder control and enuresis* (ed. I. Kolvin, R. C. MacKeith and S. R. Meadow), pp. 109–17. Spastics International Medical Publishers.

—— (1975). Early hospital admissions and later disturbances of behaviour and learning. *Develop. Med. Child Neurol.,* **17**, 456–80.

—— (1976). The use and abuse of national cohorts. In *The organization and impact of social research* (ed. M. Shipman). London: Routledge and Kegan Paul.

—— and GEAR, R. (1976). Children of low birthweight in the 1946 national cohort. *Arch. Dis. Childhood,* **51**, 820–7.

——, LAWSON, A., COOPER, J. E. and COOPER, E. (1968a). Family interaction and the activities of young children. *J. Child Psychol. Psychiat.,* **9**, 157–71.

——, ROSS, J. M. and SIMPSON, M. R. (1968b). *All our future.* London: Peter Davies.

DRILLIEN, C. M. (1964). *The growth and development of the prematurely born infant.* Edinburgh: Livingstone.

—— (1972). Abnormal neurological signs in the first year of life in low-birthweight infants. Possible psychiatric significance. *Develop. Med. Child Neurol.,* **14**, 575–84.

DUNCAN, O. D. (1976). Some linear models for two-wave two-variable panel analysis with one-way causation and measurement error. In *Quantitative sociology* (ed. H. M. Blalock *et al.*). New York: Academic Press.

DUNÉR, A. (1978). Problems and designs in research on educational and vocational career. In *Research into personal development: educational and vocational choice* (ed. A. Dunér). Report of the European Contact Workshop held in Saltsjöbaden, Sweden, in September, 1977. Amsterdam: Swets and Zeitlinger.

DUNN, J. (1980). Individual differences in temperament. In *Scientific foundations of developmental psychiatry* (ed. M. Rutter). London: Heinemann Medical.

DUPONT, A., VIDEBECH, T. and WEEKE, A. (1974). A cumulative national psychiatric register: its structure and application. *Acta Psychiat. Scand.,* **50**, 161–73.

EDGERTON, R. (1967). *The cloak of competence.* Berkeley: University of California Press.

EDWARDS, G., CHANDLER, J. and HENSMAN, C. (1972). Drinking in a London suburb. 1. correlates of normal drinking. *Quart. J. Stud. Alc.,* (Suppl. 6) 69–93.

EKEHAMMAR, B. (1977a). Test of a psychological cost-benefit model for career choice. *J. voc. Behav.,* **10**, 245–60.

—— (1977b). Intelligence and social background as related to psychological cost–benefit in career choice. *Psychol. Rep.,* **40**, 963–70.

—— (1978a). Toward a psychological cost–benefit model for educational and vocational choice. *Scand. J. Psychol.,* **19**, 15–27.

—— (1978b). Psychological cost-benefit as an intervening construct in career choice models *J. voc. Behav.,* **12**, 279–89.

EKSTROM, G. and NYLANDER, I. (1959). Neuroser—appendektomerade barn. *Nord. Med.,* **62**, 1759.

ELDRED, C. A., ROSENTHAL, D., WENDER, P. H., KETY, S. S., SCHULSINGER, F., WELNER, J. and JACOBSEN, B. (1976). Some aspects of adoption in selected samples of adult adoptees. *Amer. J. Orthopsychiat.,* **46**(2), 279–90.

ELKIND, D. (1967). Cognition in infancy and early childhood. In *Infancy and early childhood* (ed. Y. Brackbill), pp. 361–94. New York: Free Press.

EMANUELSSON, I. (1974). *Utbildningshandikapp i långtidsperspektiv.* (With an English summary.) Stockholm: Lärarhögskolan i Stockholm, pedagogiska institutionen.

—— and FÄGERLIND, I. (1968). *Uppföljningsundersökning 1938–1965 av en årskurs elever i Malmö skolor. Datainsamling.* (With an English summary.) Report No. 28. Pedagogiska institutionen, Lärarhögskolan i Stockholm.

——, —— and HARTMAN, S. (1973). *Vuxenutbildning och arbetsförhållanden. En enkätstudie inom malmöundersökningen av 1938 års tioåringar i 45-årsåldern.* (With an English summary.) Report No. 96. Pedagogiska institutionen, Lärarhögskolan i Stockholm.

ENDICOTT, J. and SPITZER, R. (1972). Current and past psychopathology scales (CAPPS). *Arch. gen. Psychiat.,* **27**, 678–87.

ENGELS, H. and THOMAE, H. (1950). Schuld und Sühne im Urteil jugendlicher Arbeiter der Gegenwart. *Unsere Jugend,* **2**, 288–96.

ERIKSON, H. E. (1951). *Childhood and society.* New York: W. W. Norton.

ERLENMEYER-KIMLING, L. (1972). Gene–environment interactions and the variability of behaviour. In *Genetics, environment, and behaviour* (ed. L. Ehrman, G. S. Omenn and E. Caspari), pp. 181–208. New York: Academic Press.

ERNHART, C. B., GRAHAM, F. K., EICHMAN, P. L., MARSHALL, I. M. and THURSTONE, D. (1963). Brain injury in the preschool child: some developmental considerations. *Psychol. Monog.,* **77**(11, Whole No. 574).

ERON, L. D., HUESMANN, L. R., LEFKOWITZ, M. M. and WALDER, L. O. (1972). Does television violence cause aggression? *Amer. Psychol.,* **27**, 253–63.

ESQUIROL, J. E. D. (1830). Remarques sur la statistique des aliens et sur le rapport du nombre d'aliéns à la population: analyse de la statistique des aliéns de la Norvège. *Ann. Hyg. publ. Med. leg.,* **4**, 332–59.

ESSEN, J. (1978). Living in one-parent families: income and expenditure. *Poverty,* **40**, 23–8.

—— and FOGELMAN, K. (1979). Childhood housing experiences. *Concern,* **31**.

——, —— and GHODSIAN, M. (1978b). Long-term changes in the school attainment of a national sample of children. *Ed. Res.,* **20**, 2.

——, —— and HEAD, J. (1978a). Childhood housing experiences and school attainment. *Child: Care, Hlth. Dev.,* **4**, 1.

——, —— and —— (1978b). Children's housing and their physical development. *Child: Care, Hlth. Dev.,* **14**.

——, —— and TIBBENHAM, A. (1979). Non-academic correlates of ability-grouping in the secondary school. *Educ. Studies,* **5**, 1.

—— and GHODSIAN, M. (1977). Sixteen-year-olds in households in receipt of Supplementary Benefits and Family Income Supplement. Appendix to *Supplementary Benefits Commission Annual Report 1976.* London: H.M.S.O.

—— and LAMBERT, L. (1977). Living in one-parent families: relationships and attitude of sixteen-year-olds. *Child: Care, Hlth. Dev.,* **3**, 301–18.

——, —— and HEAD, J. (1976). School attainment of children who have been in care. *Child: Care, Hlth. Dev.,* **2**(6), 339–51.

—— and PECKHAM, C. (1976). Nocturnal enuresis in childhood. *Develop. Med. Child Neurol.,* **18**(5), 577–89.

ESSEN-MØLLER, E. (1956). Individual traits and morbidity in a Swedish rural population. *Acta Psychiat. Scand. Suppl.,* **100**.

—— (1957). Individual traits and morbidity in a Swedish rural population. *Jap. J. human Genet.* (Suppl. 2), 44–7. Proceedings of the Symposium on Twin Research and Population Genetics in Tokyo, 1956.

——, LARSSON, H., UDDENBERG, C.-E. and WHITE, G. (1956). Individual traits and morbidity in a Swedish rural population. *Acta Psychiat, Neurol. Scand.* (Suppl. 100).

ESSING, W. (1964). *Faktorenanalytische Untersuchung des 'Psychologischen Gesamteindrucks' nach Thomae.* (Unpublished).

—— (1966). Untersuchungen zu einem Burteilungssystem der Persönlichkeit. *Arch. gesam. Psychol.,* **118**, 73–85.

EYSENCK, H. J. (1970). A dimensional system of psychodiagnostics. In *New approaches to personality classification* (ed. A. R. Mahrer). New York: Columbia University Press.

FÄGERLIND, I. (1975). *Formal education and adult earnings. A longitudinal study on the economic benefits of education.* Stockholm: Almqvist and Wiksell.

FAHRENBERG, J. and SELG, H. (1970). *Freiburger Persönlichkeitsinventar (FPI).* Göttingen: Hogrefe.

FAIRWEATHER, D. V. I. and ILLSLEY, R. (1960). Obstetric and social orgins of mentally handicapped children. *Brit. J. prev. soc. Med.,* **14**, 149–59.

FALKNER, F. (1958). Some international comparisons of physical growth in the first two years of life. *Courrier,* **8**(1), 1–11.

FALMAGNE, J. (1959). Etude comparative du développement psychomoteur. *Acad. roy. Sci. Outre-Mer,* Mémoires, 13.

The family study—a code book (1975). *Project Metropolitan Research Report Series,* No. 4.

FARIS, R. E. L. and DUNHAM, H. W. (1939). *Mental disorders in urban areas.* Chicago: University of Chicago Press.

—— (1947). Ecological factors in human behaviour. In *Personality and the behavior disorders* (ed J. M. Hunt). New York: Ronalds Press.

FARRINGTON, D. P. (1977). The effects of public labelling. *Brit. J. Criminal.,* **17**, 112–25.

FEDRICK, J., ALBERMAN, E. D., and GOLDSTEIN, H. (1971). Possible teratogenic effects of cigarette smoking. *Nature,* **231**, 529–30.

—— and —— (1972). Reported influenza in pregnancy and subsequent cancer in the child. *Brit. med. J.,* **2**, 485–8.

FEFFER, M. H. (1959). The cognitive implication of roletaking behaviour. *J. Personal.,* **27**(2), 152–68.

FENTON, G. W., FENWICK, P. B. C., DOLLIMORE, J., RUTTER, M., and YULE, W. (1973a). The EEG in adolescence: an epidemiological investigation. *Electroencephalog. clin. Neurophysiol.,* **34**, 719.

——, ——, RUTTER, M., and YULE, W. (1973b). The EEG in 14-year-old boys: some normative data obtained by visual inspection of records taken from a random sample of Isle of Wight boys. *Electroencephalog. clin. Neurophysiol.,* **35**, 416.

——, ——, DOLLIMORE, J., RUTTER, M., and YULE, W. (1974). An introduction to the Isle of Wight EEG study. *Electroencephalog. clin. Neurophysiol.,* **37**, 325.

FENWICK, P. B. C., DOLLIMORE, J., FENTON, G. W., RUTTER, M., and YULE, W. (1973). EEG autospectral data from a random sample of healthy 14-year-old Isle of Wight boys. stress. In *Stress and anxiety,* vol. 2 (ed. I. G. Sarason and C. D. Spielberger). New

FENZ, W. D. (1975). Strategies for coping with stress. In *Stress and anxiety,* (vol. 2) (ed. I. G. Sarason and C. D. Spielberger). New York: Wiley.

FERGUSON, T. (1952). *The young delinquent in his social setting.* London: Oxford University Press.

FERREL, E. and KARLBERG, P. (1960). The practical problems of recording and analyzing the data in the research. Child development: an international method of study. In *Modern problems in pediatrics,* vol. V (ed. F. Falkner). Basel: S. Karger.

FERRI, E. (1973). Characteristics of motherless families. *Brit. J. Soc. Work,* **3**, 91–100.

—— (1976). *Growing up in a one parent family.* Slough: NFER Publishing Co.

—— and ROBINSON, H. (1976). *Coping alone.* Slough: NFER Publishing Co.

FIELD, J. H. (1976). *Epidemiology of head injury in England and Wales.* H.M.S.O.

FIELD, M. J. (1960). *Search for security: an ethnopsychiatric study of rural Ghana.* Evanston, Illinois: Northwestern University Press.

FINE, E., YUDEN, L., HOLMES, J., and HEINEMANN, S. (1976). Behavioral disorders in children with parental alcoholism. *Ann. N.Y. Acad. Sci.,* **273**, 507–17.

FISCHER, M., HARVALD, B., and HAUGE, M. (1969). A Danish twin study of schizophrenia. *Brit. J. Psychol.,* **115**, 981–90.

—— (1971). Psychoses in the offspring of schizophrenic monozygotic twins and their normal co-twins. *Brit. J. Psychol.,* **118**, 43–52.

—— (1973). *Genetic and environmental factors in schizophrenia.* Copenhagen: Munksgaard.

FISSENI, H.-J. (1976). Perceived life space: patterns of consistency and change. In *Contributions to human development* (ed. K. F. Riegel and H. Thomae), vol. 3, pp. 93–112. Basel: Karger.

FOGELMAN, K. R. (1975). Developmental correlates of family size. *Brit. J. Soc. Work,* **5**(1), 43–57.

—— (ed.) (1976). *Britain's sixteen-year-olds.* London: National Children's Bureau.

—— (1978a). The effectiveness of schooling—some recent results from the National Child Development Study. In *Perimeters of social repair* (ed. W. H. G. Armytage and J. Peel). London: Academic Press.

—— (1978b). School attendance, attainment and behaviour. *Brit. J. ed. Psychol.,* **68**, 2.

—— (1978c). Drinking among sixteen-year-olds. *Concern,* 29.

—— (1979). Educational and career aspirations—findings from a national sample of sixteen-year-olds. *Brit. J. Guidance Counselling,* **7**, 1.

—— ESSEN, J., and TIBBENHAM, A. (1978). Ability-grouping in secondary schools and attainment. *Ed. Studies,* **4**, 3.

—— and GOLDSTEIN, H. (1976). Social factors associated with changes in educational attainment between 7 and 11 years of age. *Educ. Stud.,* **2** (2), 95–109.

——, ——, ESSEN, J., and GHODSIAN, M. (1978). Pattern of attainment. *Educat. Studies,* **4**, 2.

—— and GORBACH, P. (1978). Age of starting school and attainment at eleven. *Educ. Res.,* **21**(1), 65–6.

FOLSTEIN, S. and RUTTER, M. (1977). Infantile autism: a genetic study of 21 twin pairs. *J. Child Psychol. Psychiat.,* **18**, 297–321.

FORREST, A. D. and HAY, A. J. (1972). The influence of sex on schizophrenia. *Acta Psychiat. Scand.,* **48**, 49–58.

FOULDS, G. A. (1976). *The hierarchical nature of personal illness.* London: Academic Press.

FOX, J. P., GELFAND, H. M., LeBLANC, D. R., and CONWELL, D. P. (1957). Studies on the development of natural immunity to poliomyelitis in Louisianna. I. Overall plan, methods and observations as to seroimmunity in the study group. *Amer. J. Hyg.,* **65**, 344–66.

FRANCIS, T. J., KORNS, R. F., VOIGHT, R. B., BOISEN, M., HEMPHILL, F. M., NAPIER, J. A., and TOLCHINSKY, E. (1955). An evaluation of the 1954 poliomyelitis vaccine trials. *Amer. J. Publ. Hlth,* **45** (part 2), i–xiv, 1–63.

FRÄNDÉN, O. (1977). Who were the Leftists? Personality and sociopsychological antecedents. *Project Metropolitan Research Report Series,* No. 8.

FRANK, H., HEIL, W., and LEADOLTER, I. (1967). The liver and beer consumption. *Münch. Med. Wochenschr.,* **109**, 892–7.

FRANKENBERG, W. and DODD, J. B. (1967). The Denver developmental screening test. *J. Pediat.,* **71**, 181–91.

FREEDMAN, D. G. (1973). *Human infancy: an evolutionary perspective.* New York: Basic Books.

FREEMAN, H. E. and SIMMONS, O. (1963). *The mental patient comes home.* New York: John Wiley.

FREIOVA, E. (1966). [Alcoholism in parents and the moral impairment of school age juveniles.] (in Czech) *Ceskoslov. Psychiat.,* **62**, 188–92.

FREMMING, K. H. (1947). *Morbid risks of mental disease in an average Danish population.* Copenhagen: Munksgaard.

FREW, R. (1972). The prevalence of mental retardation in children. *Concern* (10), 27–31.

—— and PECKHAM, C. S. (1972). Mental retardation: a national study. *Brit. Hosp. J. Soc. Serv. Rev.,* **82** (4300), 2070–2.

FROSTIG, M. (1963). Visual perception in the brain injured child. *Amer. J. Orthopsychiat.,* **33**, 665–71.

FULLER, J. L. and THOMPSON, W. R. (1978). *Foundations of behaviour genetics.* St. Louis: C. V. Mosby.

GALLANT, D. H. (1975). Children of mentally ill mothers. In *Mentally ill mothers and their children* (ed. H. Grunebaum, J. Weiss, B. Cohler, and A. Cohler). Chicago: University of Chicago Press.

GARCOIA, C. (1974). [Childhood psychiatric pathology in children of alcoholics.] (In Spanish). *Actas Luso-Españolas Neurol., Psiquiat. Cienc. Afines,* **2**(6), 507–16.

GARDNER, G. G. (1967). Role of maternal psychopathology in male and female schizophrenics. *J. Consult. Psychol.,* **31**, 411–3.

GARFIELD, J. C. (1964). Motor impersistence in normal and brain damaged children. *Neurol. (Minneapolis),* **14**, 623.

GARMEZY, N. (1974). Children at risk: the search for the antecedents of schizophrenia. *Schizophren. Bull.,* **1**, 13–90. (With the assistance of S. Streitman.)

GATH, D., COOPER, B., GATTONI, F., and ROCKETT, D. (1976). *Child guidance and delinquency in a London borough.* London: Oxford University Press.

GERARD, H. B., JACKSON, T. D., and CONOLLEY, E. S. (1975). Social contact in the desegregated classroom. In *School desegregation* (ed. H. B. Gerard and N. Miller). New York: Plenum Press.

—— and MILLER N. (1975). *School desegregation*. New York: Plenum Press.

GESSEL, A. and AMATRUDA, C. (1954). *Developmental diagnosis*. New York: Paul B. Hoeber.

GHODSIAN, M. and CALNAN, M. (1977). A comparative, longitudinal analysis of special educational treatment groups. *Brit. J. ed. Psych.*, **47**, 162–74.

—— and LAMBERT, L. (1978). Mum and dad are not so bad. *J. Ass. ed. Psychol.*, **4**, 7.

GILL, D. (1970). Changing trends in illegitimacy and changing modes of explanation. *Roy. Soc. Hlth J.*, **90**, 154–9.

——, ILLSLEY, R., and KOPLIK, L. H. (1970). Pregnancy in teenage girls. *Soc. Sci. Med.*, **3**, 549–74.

GINSBURG, H. and KOSLOWSKI, B. (1976). Cognitive development. *Ann. Rev. Psychol.*, **27**, 29–61.

GLATT, M. M. (1967). Complications of alcoholism in the social sphere. *Brit. J. Addict.*, **62**, 35–44.

—— (1972). *The alcoholic and the help he needs*. London: Priory.

GLÖCKEL, H. (1960). Eine Vergleichsuntersuchung zur Frage des jugendlichen Idealerlebens. *Psychol. Rundschau*, **11**, 1–20.

GOFFMAN, E. (1963). *Stigma: notes on the management of spoiled identity*. Englewood Cliffs, N. J.: Prentice-Hall.

GOLDBERG, D. P. (1972). *The detection of psychiatric illness by questionnaire*. Institute of Psychiatry, Maudsley Monograph No. 21. London: Oxford University Press.

GOLDBERG, I. D., CHOI, N. W., KURLAND, L. T., and KURTZKE, J. F. (1973). Cerebral palsy, In *Epidemiology of neurologic and sense organ disorders* (ed. L. T. Kurland, J. F. Kurtzke, and I. D. Goldberg), pp. 232–45. Cambridge, Massachusetts: Harvard University Press.

GOLDMAN, F. (1950). Breastfeeding and character formation. II. The etiology of the oral character in psychoanalytic theory. *J. Personal.*, **19**(189), 196.

GOLDSTEIN, H. (1968). Longitudinal studies and the measurement of change. *The Statistician*, **18**, 93–117.

—— (1971). Factors influencing the height of seven-year-old children. Results from the National Child Development Study (1958 cohort). *Human Biol.*, **43**, 92–111.

—— (1975). A mathematical model for population disease screening. *Bull. Inst. Maths Appl.*, **11**, 64–6.

—— (1976). Smoking in pregnancy: the statistical controversy and its resolution. In *Proceedings of 3rd World Conference on Smoking and Health*. Washington, D.C: U.S. Department of Health, Education, and Welfare.

—— and FOGELMAN, K. R. (1974). Age standardization and seasonal effects in mental testing. *Brit. J. educ. Psychol.*, **44**, 109–15.

GOODENOUGH, F. (1926). *Measurement of intelligence by drawings*. New York: World Book Co.

GOODWIN, D., SCHULSINGER, F., HERMANSEN, L., GUZE, S. B., and WINOKUR, G. (1973).

Alcohol problems in adoptees raised apart from alcoholic biological parents. *Arch. gen. Psychiat.*, **28**, 238–43.

——, ——, ——, ——, and —— (1974a). Alcohol problems in adoptees raised apart from alcoholic biological parents. In *Genetics, environment and psychopathology* (ed. S. A. Mednick, F. Schulsinger, J. Higgins, and B. Bell). Amsterdam: North-Holland/American Elsevier.

——, ——, MØLLER, N., HERMANSEN, L., WINOKUR, G. A., and GUZE, S. B. (1974b). Drinking problems in adopted and non-adopted sons of alcoholics. *Arch. Gen. Psychiat.*, **31**, 164–9.

——, ——, Knop, J., Mednick, S., and Guze, S. B. (1977). Alcoholism and depression in adopted-out daughters of alcoholics. *Arch. gen. Psychiat.*, **34**, 751–5.

GORDON, D. A. (1976). Alcohol and work. Paper presented at Second Scottish School on Alcoholism, Ayr, April 2, 1976.

GORDON, G. H. (ed.) (1972). *Renton and Brown's criminal procedure according to the law of Scotland* (4th edn.). Edinburgh: W. Green.

GOTLIEB JENSEN, K. (1972). *Peptic ulcer. Genetic and epidemiological aspects based on twin studies*. Copenhagen: Munksgaard.

GOTTESMAN, I. I. (1960). The psychogenetics of personality. Unpublished doctoral dissertation. University of Minnesota.

—— (1963a). Genetic aspects of intelligent behavior. In *The handbook of mental deficiency: psychological theory and research* (ed. N. Ellis), pp. 253–96. New York: McGraw-Hill.

—— (1963b). Heritability of personality: a demonstration. *Psychol. Monog.*, **77** (9, Whole No. 572), 1–21.

—— (1965). Personality and natural selection. In *Method and goals in human behavior genetics* (ed. S. Vanderberg), pp. 63–80. New York: Academic Press.

—— (1966). Genetic variance in adaptive personality traits. *J. Child Psychol. Psychiat.*, **7**, 199–208.

—— (1968). Biogenetics of race and class. In *Social class, race, and psychological development* (ed. M. Deutsch, I. Katz, and A. Jensen), pp. 11–51. New York: Holt, Rinehart, and Winston.

—— and HESTON, L. L. (1972). Human behavioral adaptions: speculations on their genesis. In *Genetics, environment, and behavior* (ed. L. Ehrman, G. S. Omenn, and E. Caspari), pp. 106–22. New York: Academic Press.

—— and SHIELDS, J. (1972). *Schizophrenia and genetics: a twin study vantage point*. New York: Academic Press.

—— and —— (1976). A critical review of recent adoption, twin, and family studies of schizophrenia: behavioral genetics perspectives. *Schizophren. Bull.*, **2**, 360–401, 447–453.

GRAFFAR, M. (1956). Une méthode de classification sociale d'échantillons de population. *Courrier*, **VI**, 445–9.

GRAHAM, F. K., ERNHART, C. B., THURSTONE, D., and CRAFFT, M. (1962). Development three years after perinatal anoxia and after potentially damaging newborn experiences. *Psychol. Monog.*, **76**(522).

—— and KENDALL, B. S. (1960). *Memory for Designs Test*. Missoula, Montana: Psychological Test Specialists.

GRAHAM, P. and RUTTER, M. (1968). The reliability and validity of the psychiatric assessment of the child. II. Interview with the parent. *Brit. J. Psychiat.*, **114**, 581–92.

—— and —— (1973). Psychiatric disorder in the young adolescent: a follow-up study. *Proc. roy. Soc. Med.*, **66**, 1226–9.

——, ——, and GEORGE, S. (1973). Temperamental characteristics as predictors of behaviour disorders in children. *Amer. J. Orthopsychiat.*, **43**, 328–39.

GRANICK, S. and FRIEDMAN, A. S. (1967). The effect of education in the decline of test performance with age. *J. Gerontol.*, **22**, 191–5.

—— and —— (1973). Educational experience and the maintenance of intellectual functioning by the aged: an overview. In *Intellectual functioning in adults: psychological and biological influences* (ed. T. Jarvik, C. Eisdorfer, and J. E. Blum). New York: Springer.

GRAY, G., SMITH, A., and RUTTER, M. (1980). School attendance and the first year of employment. In *Out of school: modern perspectives in truancy and school refusal* (ed. L. Hersov and I. Berg). London: Wiley.

GREEN, R. F. (1969). Age–intelligence relationships between age sixteen and sixty-four: a rising trend. *Develop. Psychol.*, **1**, 618–27.

GREER, H. S. and CAWLEY, R. H. (1966). *Some observations on the natural history of neurotic illness*. Mervyn Archdall Medical Monograph No. 3, Sydney, N.S.W.: Australian Medical Association.

GREGG, N. M. (1941). Congenital cataract following German measles in the mother. *Trans. Ophthalmol. Soc. Austral.*, **3**, 35–46.

GREULICH, W. W. (1957). A comparison of the physical growth and development of American-born and native Japanese children. *Amer. J. Phys. Anthropol.*, **15**, 489–515.

GRIFFITHS, R. (1970). *The abilities of babies*. London: University of London Press.

GRÍMSSON, Ó. (1977) Delirium tremens á Íslandi. [Delirium tremens in Iceland.] *Laeknablaoio*, **63**, 135–44.

GROMBACH, H. H. (1976). Consistency and change of personality variables in late life. In *Contributions to human development* (ed. K. F. Riegel and H. Thomae), vol. 3, pp. 51–67. Basel: Karger.

GRONWALL, D. and SAMPSON, H. (1974). *The psychological effects of concussion*. Auckland: University of Auckland Press.

—— and WRIGHTSON, P. (1974). Delayed recovery of intellectual function after minor head injury. *Lancet*, **2**, 605–9.

GROUSE, L., OMENN, G. S., and McCARTHY, B. J. (1973). Studies by DNA-RNA hybridization of the transcriptional diversity of the human brain. *J. Neurochem.*, **20**, 1063–73.

GRUENBERG, E. M. (1961). *New York State Mental Health Commission: a mental health survey of older people, by the staff of the mental health research unit, New York State Department of Mental Hygiene*. Utica, N. Y.: State Hospital Press.

—— (1963). Epidemiology. In *Mental retardation* (ed. Am. Ass. Ment. Deficiency). Chicago.

—— (1964). Epidemiology. In *Mental*

retardation: a review of research (ed. H. A. Stevens and R. Heber). Chicago: University of Chicago Press.

—— (1971). Two research strategies, review of: Kessler, I. I. and Levin, M. L. (eds.), *The community as an epidemiologic laboratory. Science*, **172**, 251–2.

—— (1976). The future of community medicine. *The Lancet*, **2**, 262.

—— (1977). The failures of success. *Hlth Soc.*, **55**, 3–24.

—— and HAGNELL, O. (In press). The rising prevalence of chronic brain syndrome in the elderly. In *Society, stress, and disease*, vol. 5 (ed. L. Levi and A. R. Kagan). Oxford: Oxford University Press.

GUNDERSON, E. K. E. and RAHE, R. H. (eds.) (1974). *Life stress and illness*. Springfield, Illinois: Thomas.

GUOMUNDSDÓTTIR, B., KARLSDÓTTIR, E. and THORDARDÓTTIR, E. (1975). Námsferill Reykvískra Ungmenna. [Educational attainment of youth in Reykjavík]. Unpublished B. A. thesis. University of Iceland: Psychological Department.

HAGEN, W. (1954). Das Problem der kinderbeurteilung. In *Deutsche Nachkriegskinder* (ed. C. Coerper, W. Hagen, and H. Thomae), pp. 3–18. Stuttgart: Thieme.

—— (1964). *Wachstum und Entwicklung von Schulkindern*. Munich: J. A. Barth.

—— and PASCHLAU, G. U. R. (1961). *Wachstum und Gestalt* [Growth and form]. Stuttgart: Thieme.

—— and THOMAE, H. (1962). *Deutsche Nachkriegskinder*. Munich: Barth.

——, ——, MANSFELD, L. and MATHEY, F. J. (1958). *Jugendliche in der Berufsbewährung* [Occupation development of adolescents]. Stuttgart: Thieme.

HAGNELL, O. (1959). Neuroses and other nervous disturbances in a population living in a rural area of southern Sweden, investigated in 1947 and 1957. *Acta Psychiat. Scand.* (Suppl. 136).

—— (1966a). *A prospective study of the incidence of mental disorders in a Swedish population together with an evaluation of aetiological significance of medical, social and personality factors*. (Dissertation.) Stockholm: University Books.

—— (1966b). *A prospective study of the incidence of mental disorder*. Lund: Scandinavian University Books.

—— (1969). A prospective study of mental disorders in a total population. *Soc. Psychiat. Res. Publ. A.R.N.M.D.*, **47**, 22–46.

—— and KREITMAN, N. (1974). Mental illness in married pairs in a total population. *Brit. J. Psychiat.*, **125**, 293.

—— and ÖJESJÖ, L. (1977). Alcoholism among men in the Lundby population 1947–1972. Report from a prospective longitudinal study of a total population. To be published.

HAKOSALO, J. K. (1973). Cumulative detection rates of congenital malformations in a ten-year follow-up study. *Acta Patholog. Microbiol. Scand.*, Sect. A (Suppl. 242).

HALL, D. J., ROBERTSON, N. C., DORRICOTT, N., OLLEY, P. C., and MILLAR, W. M. (1973). The northeast Scottish psychiatric case register—the second phase. *J. chron. Dis.*, **26**, 375–82.

HALLGREN, S. (1939). Intelligens och miljö. En experimentell undersökning av barn i tredje

skolåret vid Malmö folkskolor och privata skolor, I–II. Unpublished lic.-thesis, University of Lund.

HALMI, K. A. (1978). Anorexia nervosa: recent investigations. *Ann. Rev. Med.*, **29**, 137–48.

HAMMOND, W. H. and CHAYEN, E. (1963). *Persistent criminals*. London:, H.M.S.O.

HANSON, D. R., GOTTESMAN, I. I., and MEEHL, P. E. (1977). Genetic theories and the validation of psychiatric diagnoses: implications for the study of children of schizophrenics. *J. abnormal Psychol.*, **86**, 575–88.

HANVIK, L. J., NELSON, L. E., HANSON, H. B., ANDERSEN, A. S., DRESSLER, W. H., and ZARLING, V. R. (1961). Diagnosis of cerebral dysfunction in children as made in a child guidance clinic. *Amer. J. Dis. Children*, **101**, 364–75.

HARRIS, H. (1975). *Principles of human biochemical genetics* (2nd edn.). Amsterdam: North-Holland.

HARTIKAINEN, A-L. (1973). Tutkimus Pohjois-Suomen synnyttäjistä. *Acta Universitatis Ouluensis*. Series D Medica Nr 4. Obstetrica et Gynecologica Nr 1, Oulu.

HAUGE, M., HARVALD, B., FISCHER, M., GOTLIEB JENSEN, K., JUEL-NIELSEN, N., RAEBILD, I., SHAPIRO, R., and VIDEBECH, T. (1968). The Danish Twin Register. *Acta genet. med. gemellolog.*, **17**, 315–32.

——, ——, and REID, D. D. (1970). A twin study of the influence of smoking on morbidity and mortality. *Acta genet. med. gemellolog.*, **19**, 335–7.

HAVIGHURST, R. J. (1975). Life style transitions related to personality after age fifty. Unpublished.

—— and DEVRIES, A. (1969). Life styles and free time activities of retirement. *Human Develop.*, **12**, 34–54.

HAVLÍNOVÁ, M. (1975). I.Q. trends in the same subjects at the age of 3 to 11 years. English summary. *Psychol. Patopsychol. Dietaťa*, **5**, 457–63.

——, NOVOTNÁ, M., and PROKOPEC, M. (1975). Report from the Institute of Hygiene and Epidemiology: 'Longitudinal follow-up of physical and mental development of children', p. 210 *IHE*, Praha.

HAWELL, W. (1963). *Factor analysis of longitudinal rating data*. Unpublished research report.

HEALY, J. J. R. and GOLDSTEIN, H. (1976). An approach to the scaling of categorized attributes. *Biometrika*, **63**, 219–29.

HEBER, R. and GARBER, H. (1975). Progress report III: an experiment in the prevention of cultural–familial retardation. *Proceedings of the Third International Congress, International Association for the Scientific Study of Mental Deficiency*. Warsaw: Polish Medical.

HEINONEN, V. (1963) *Alykkyystesteja lahjakkuuden eraiden alkeistekijain tutkimista varten*. Reports from the Institute for Educational Research, University of Jyvaskyla.

HEISE, D. (1970). Causal analysis of data from panel data. *Sociological methodology* (ed. D. F. Borgatta and G. Bohrnstedt). San Francisco: Jossey-Bass.

HELGASON, L. (1977). Psychiatric services and mental illness in Iceland. Incidence study (1966–1967) with 6–7 year follow-up. *Acta Psychiat. Scand.* Suppl. 268.

HELGASON, T. (1954). *Talning geó- og taugasjúklinga 15. marz 1953*. [*Prevalence of nervous and mental disorder in Iceland. March 15, 1953.*] (Mimeographed).

—— (1964). Epidemiology of mental disorder in Iceland. A psychiatric and demographic investigation of 5395 Icelanders. *Acta Psychiat. Scand.* Suppl. 173.

—— (1973). Epidemiology of mental disorder in Iceland: a geriatric follow-up (preliminary report). *Excerpta Med. Int. Cong.* (274), 350–7.

—— (1975). Studies on prevalence and incidence of mental disorders in Iceland with a health questionnaire and a psychiatric case register. *Social, somatic and psychiatric studies of geographically defined population*. Tromsö Seminar in Medicine, pp. 172–83.

—— (1976). Studies of psychiatric morbidity through record linkage. (Paper read at the XVIII Nordic Psychiatric Congress, Turku, June 1976). *Acta Psychiat. Scand.* Suppl. 265, 39.

——, ÁSMUNDSSON, G., BRODDASON, TH., ÓLAFSSON, H., HANNESDOTTIR, H., and STEFANSSON, J. G. (1977). Havfiskere og deres familier. [Deepsea fishermen and their families.] *Tidsskr. Nor. laegeforen.*, **97**, 1389–91.

HELLMAN, L. M. and PRITCHARD (1971). *Obstetrics*. London: Butterworths.

HEMSLEY, R., HOWLIN, P., BERGER, M., HERSOV, L., HOLBROOK, D., RUTTER, M., and YULE, W. (1978). Treating autistic children in a family context. In *Autism: a reappraisal of concepts and treatment* (ed. M. Rutter and E. Schopler). New York: Plenum.

HENRIKSON, M. (1973). Tonåringar och normer: en undersökning av tonåringars norm-klimat. (Investigation of teenage norms and norm-climate.) Educational research, sö-rapport, FoU4. Stockholm: Utbildningsförlaget.

HERBST, A. L., ULFELDER, H., and POSKANZER, D. C. (1971). Adenocarcinoma of the vagina: association of maternal stilbestrol therapy with tumor appearance in young women. *New Eng. J. Med.*, **284**, 878–81.

HERMANS, H. J. M. (1971). *Prestatiemotief en fallangst in gezin en onderwijs*. Amsterdam: Swetz en Zeitlinger.

HERRIOT, A., BILLEWICZ, W. Z., and HYTTEN, F. E. (1962). Cigarette smoking in pregnancy. *Lancet*, **1**, 771–3.

HERRMANN, E. (1973). Long range effects of early parental separation experiences in children with high and low risk for schizophrenia. Doctoral dissertation. New York: Graduate Faculty, New School for Social Research.

HESTON, L. L. (1966). Psychiatric disorders in foster home reared children of schizophrenic mothers. *Brit. J. Psychiat.*, **112**, 819–25.

—— and DUNNEY, D. (1968). Interactions between early life experience and biological factors in schizophrenia. In *The transmission of schizophrenia* (ed. D. Rosenthal and S. S. Kety). Oxford: Pergamon Press.

HETZER, H. (1937). *Kindheit und Armut*. Leipzig: Hirzel.

HEWETT, F. M. (1973). Conceptual models for viewing minimal brain dysfunction: developmental psychology and behavioral modification. *Ann. N.Y. Acad. Sci.*, **205**, 38–45.

HILL, A. B., DOLL, R., GALLOWAY, T. McL., and HUGHES, J. P. W. (1958). Virus diseases in pregnancy and congenital defects. *Brit. J. prev. soc. Med.*, **12**, 1–7.

HIMMELWEIT, H. (1955). Socio-economic background and personality. *Int. soc. Sci. Bull.*, **7**, 29–35.

—— and OPPENHEIM, A. N. (1958). *Television and the child*. London: Oxford University Press.

HINDE, R. A. and McGINNIS, L. (1977). Some factors influencing the effects of temporary mother–infant separation: some experiments with rhesus monkeys. *Psychol. Med.*, **7**, 197–212.

HINDLEY, C. B. (1972). The place of longitudinal methods in the study of development. In *Determinants of behavioral development* (ed. F. J. Mönks, W. W. Hartup, and J. de Wit), pp. 23–50. New York: Academic Press.

HINKLE, L. E. JR. (1974). The effect of exposure to culture change, social change, and changes in interpersonal relationships on health. In *Stressful life events: their nature and effects* (ed. B. S. Dohrenwend and B. P. Dohrenwend), pp. 9–44. New York: John Wiley.

HIRSCH, J. (1967). *Behavior–genetic analysis*. New York: McGraw-Hill.

HIRSCHI, T. and SELVIN, H. (1967). *Delinquency research—an appraisal of analytic methods*. New York: Free Press.

HITCHFIELD, E. (1974). *In search of promise*. London: Longman in association with National Children's Bureau.

HITZ, D. (1973). Drunken sailors and others: drinking problems in specific occupations. *Quart. J. Stud. Alc.*, **34**, 496–505.

HØGH, E. (1976). *Random numbers, probabilities, algorithms, and intuition*. Project Metropolitan, Copenhagen.

HOLLINGSHEAD, A. B. and REDLICH, F. C. (1958). *Social class and mental illness*. New York: John Wiley.

HOLM, N., HAUGE, M., and HARVALD, B. (1980). Etiological factors of breast cancer elucidated by a study of unselected twins. *J. Natl. Cancer Inst.*, **64**.

HOLMES, T. H. and RAHE, R. H. (1967). The social adjustment rating scale. *J. psychosom. Res.*, **11**, 213–8.

HOMANS, G. C. (1950). *The human group*. New York: Harcourt, Brace and World.

—— (1961). *Social behaviour, its elementary forms*. New York: Harcourt, Brace and World.

HONZIK, M. P. (1967). Environmental correlates of mental growth: prediction from the family setting at 21 months. *Child Develop.*, **38**, 337–64.

——, HUTCHINGS, J. J., and BURNIP, S. R. (1965). Birth record assessment and test performance at eight months. *Amer. J. Dis. Children*, **109**, 416–26.

HORN, I. (1959). Das Problem der Unehelichkeit. Erfahrungen aus einer Längsschnittuntersuchung. Medical doctoral dissertation, Bonn.

HORN, J. L. and DONALDSON, G. (1976). On the myth of intellectual decline in adulthood. *Amer. Psychol.*, **31**, 701–19.

HOROBIN, G. W. (ed.) (1973). *Experience with abortion: a case study of N. E. Scotland*. Cambridge University Press.

HOROWITZ, M. H., SCHAEFER, C., and COONEY, P. (1974). Life event scaling for recency of experience. In *Life stress and illness*

(ed. E. K. E. Gurderson and R. H. Rahe), pp. 125–33. Springfield, Illinois: Thomas.

HORSKÝ, J. and ZNAMENÁČEK, K. (1956). [Clinical research of causes of hypoxia and of origin of bleeding into the fetal CNS and of their prevention.] (In Czech.) Sb. věd. Prací: Fetal traumatism during labour, Prague.

HORWITZ, A. and WASSERMAN, M. S. (1978). Formal rationality, substantive justice, and discrimination: a study of a juvenile court. (Stencil)

HOTTA, Y. and BENZER, S. (1972). Mapping of behaviour in *drosophila* mosaics. *Nature*, **240**, 527–35.

HOTYAT, F. (1956). Le poids du social sur l'éducation. *Socialisme*, **16**.

HOWLIN, P., MARCHANT, R., RUTTER, M., BERGER, M., HERSOV, L., and YULE, W. (1973a). A home-based approach to the treatment of autistic children. *J. Autism Childh. Schizophren.*, **3**, 308–36.

——, CANTWELL, D., MARCHANT, R., BERGER, M., and RUTTER, M. (1973b). Analyzing mothers' speech to young autistic children: a methodological study. *J. Abnorm. Child. Psychol.*, **1**, 317–39.

HUGHES, C. C., TREMBLAY, M., RAPPORT, R. N., and LEIGHTON, A. H. (1960). *People of cove and woodlot*. The Stirling county study of psychiatric disorder and socio-cultural environment (vol. II) New York: Basic Books.

HULKKO, S., IKONEN, R. S., and KAUPPILA, O. (1973). Tampereen perinataalikuolleisuus 1955–69. *Duodecim*, **89**, 240–6.

HULTIN, H. (1973). Infant health services at child health centres in Finland in 1960. *Health services research of the national board of health in Finland II*. Helsinki.

—— and PAAVILAINEN, S. (1967). Health service of first graders in primary schools in Finland 1963/64. *Health services research of the national board of health in Finland 4*. Helsinki.

HUNT, K. W. (1970). Syntactic maturity in school children and adults. *Monogr. Soc. Res. Child Develop.*, **35**(1), 67.

HUSÉN, T. (1950). *Testresultatens prognosvärde*. (With an English summary). Stockholm: Almqvist and Wiksell.

——, EMANUELSSON, I., FÄGERLIND, I., and LILJEFORS, R. (1969). *Talent, opportunity and career. A twenty-six year follow-up of 1,500 individuals*. Stockholm: Almqvist and Wiksell.

HUTCHINGS, B. and MEDNICK, S. A. (1974). Registered criminality in the adoptive and biological parents of registered male adoptees. In *Genetics, environment and psychopathology* (ed. S. A. Mednick, F. Schulsinger, J. Higgins, and B. Bell). Amsterdam: North-Holland/American Elsevier.

HUTCHISON, D., PROSSER, H., and WEDGE, P. J. (1979). Prediction of educational failure. *Ed. Studies*, **5**, 1.

HUTTUNEN, M. O. (1971). Persistent alteration of turnover of brain noradrenaline in the offspring of rats subjected to stress during pregnancy. *Nature*, **230**, 53–5.

—— and NISKANEN, P. (1977). Psychiatric disorders among persons with prenatal death of their father. Submitted for publication in *Arch. gen. Psychiat*.

——, VARONEN, L., NYMAN, G., and ARAJÄRVI, T. (1977). A survey of the temperament of Finnish infants with a simplified

questionnaire. Submitted for publication in *Acta Paedopsychiat*.

ILLSLEY, R. (1955). Social class selection and class differences in relation to stillbirths and infant deaths. *Brit. med. J.*, **2**, 1520–4.

—— (1956). The social context of childbirth. *Nurs. Mirror*, Sept. 14 and 21.

—— (1966). Perinatal mortality: social aspects. *Proceedings of the 52nd Annual Conference of the National Association for Maternal and Child Welfare*, pp. 23–7.

—— (1967a). The sociological study of reproduction and its outcome. In *Childbearing—its social and psychological aspects* (ed. S. a Richardson and A. F. Guttmacher). Baltimore: Williams and Wilkins.

—— (1967b). Family growth and its effect on the relationship between obstetric factors and child functioning. In *Social and genetic influences on life and death* (ed. R. Platt and A. S. Parks). Edinburgh: Oliver and Boyd.

——, FINLAYSON, A., and THOMPSON, B. (1963). The motivation and characteristics of internal migrants. *Milbank Mem. Fund Quart.*, **41**, 217–48.

—— and GILL, D. (1968a). Changing trends in illegitimacy. *Soc. Sci. Med.*, **2**, 415–33.

—— and —— (1968b). New fashions in illegitimacy. *New Society*, November 14, 1968, pp. 709–11.

INGHAM, J. G. and MILLER, P. McC. (1976). The concept of prevalence applied to psychiatric disorders and symptoms. *Psychol. Med.*, **6**, 217–55.

——, RAWNSLEY, K., and HUGHES, D. (1972). Psychological disorder and its declaration in contrasting areas of South Wales. *Psychol. Med.*, **3**, 281–92.

INKELES, A. and SMITH, D. H. (1974). *Becoming modern: individual change in six developing countries*. Cambridge, Mass.: Harvard University Press.

J. I. F. (1947). Alcoholism: an occupational disease of seamen. *Quart. J. Stud. Alc.*, **8**, 498–505.

JACOB, F. and MONOD, J. (1961). Genetic regulatory mechanisms in the synthesis of proteins. *J. mol. Biol.*, **3**, 318–56.

JANSON, C.-G. (1965). Project Metropolitan, *Acta Sociol.*, **9**, 110–15.

—— (1971). A preliminary report on Swedish urban spatial structure. In *Comparative factorial ecology* (ed. B. J. L. Berry). Special issue of *Econ. Geogr.*, **47**, 249–57. See also Swedish urban spatial structure: 1965. *Bulletin from SIB*, **5**(1976).

—— (1975). Project Metropolitan—a presentation. *Project Metropolitan research report series*, No. 1.

—— (1977). The handling of juvenile delinquency cases. *Project Metropolitan research report series*, No. 7.

JENKINS, R. L., HENN, F., and BARDWELL, R. (1977). Outcome study of three diagnoses of boy delinquents. (Paper read at World Psychiatric Association Meeting, Honolulu.)

JENNETT, B. (1975). Scale, scope and philosophy of the clinical problem. In *Outcome of severe damage to the central nervous system* (ed. R. Porter and D. W. FitzSimons), pp. 3–9. Amsterdam: CIBA Foundation Symposium No. 34.

—— (1976). Assessment of severity of head

injury. *J. Neurol. Neurosurg. Psychiat.*, **39**, 647–55.

——, TEASDALE, G., GALBRAITH, S., PICKARD, J., GRANT, H., BRAAKMAN, R., AVEZAAT, C., MAAS, A., MINDERHOUD, J., VECHT, C. J., HEIDEN, J., SMALL, R., CATON, W., and KURZE, T. (1977). Severe head injuries in three countries. *J. Neurol. Neurosurg. Psychiat.*, **40**, 291–8.

JOFFE, J. M. (1969). *Prenatal determinants of behavior*. London: Pergamon Press.

JOHANSSON, G., FRANKENHAEUSER, M., and MAGNUSSON, D. (1973). Catecholamine output in schoolchildren as related to performance and adjustment. *Scand. J. Psychol.*, **14**, 20–8.

JOHN, E. R., KARMEL, B. Z., CORNING, W. C., EASTON, P., BROWN, D., AHN, H., JOHN, M., HARMONY, T., PRICHEP, L., TORO, A., GERSON, I., BARTLETT, F., THATCHER, R., KAYE, H., VALES, P., and SCHWARTZ, E. (1977). Neurometrics. *Science*, **196**, 1393–410.

JONES, H. E. (1958). Consistency and change in early maturity. *Vita Humana*, **1**, 43–51.

JONES, K. L., SMITH, D. W., ULELAND, C. N., and STREISSGUTH, A. P. (1973). Pattern of male formation in offspring of chronic alcoholic mothers. *Lancet*, **1**, 1267–71.

JONSSON, G. and KÄLVESTEN, A. (1964). *222 Stockholms pojkar: en socialpsychiatrisk undersökning av pojkar i skolaldern*. Stockholm.

JÖRESKOG, K. G. (1969). Factoring the multitest–multioccasion correlation matrix. *Educ. Testing Serv. Res. Bull.*, *RB-69-62*.

—— (1970). A general method for estimating a linear structural equation system. *Research Bulletin 70–54*, Princeton, New Jersey: Educational Testing Service.

—— and SÖRBOM, D. (1976a). Statistical models and methods for test-retest situations. In *Advances in psychological and educational measurement* (ed. D. N. M. de Gruijter, L. J. Th van der Kamp, and J. F. Crombag). London: Wiley.

—— and —— (1976b). *LISREL-III: estimation of linear structural equation system by maximum likelihood methods*. A FORTRAN IV Program. Chicago: International Educational Services.

—— and —— (1977). Statistical models and methods for analysis of longitudinal data. In *Latent variables in socioeconomic models* (ed. D. J. Aigner and A. S. Goldberger). Amsterdam: North Holland.

—— and VAN THELLO, M. (1972). LISREL—a general computer program for estimating a linear standard equation system involving multiple indicators of unmeasured variables. *Research Bulletin*, 72–56, Princeton, New Jersey: Educational Testing Service.

JUEL-NIELSEN, N. (1965). Individual and environment. *Acta Psychiat. Scand. Suppl.* 183.

KAGAN, J. (1964). American psychological research in psychological development. *Child Develop.*, **35**, 1–32.

—— and Moss, H. A. (1962). *Birth to maturity: a study in psychological development*. New York: Wiley.

——, ROSMAN, B. L., DAY, D. ALBERT, J., and PHILLIPS, W. (1964). Information processing in the child: significance of analytic and reflective attitudes. *Psychol. Monogr.*, **78**, 1–37.

KALVERBOER, A. F. (1973). Vroege ontwikkelingsdiagnostiek: enige feiten en

KAPALÍN, V., KOLANDOVÁ, J., NOVOTNÁ, M., and TESAŘOVÁ, M. (1970). Relations between

——, KOTÁSKOVÁ, J., and PROKOPEC, M. (1969). Groningen: Tjeenk Willing.

KAMMEYER, SR. M. L. (1971). Adolescents from families with and without alcohol problems. *Quart. J. Stud. Alc.*, **32**, 364–72.

KANDEL, D. (1975). Reaching the hard-to-reach: illicit drug use among high school absentees. *Addict. Dis.*, **1**, 465–80.

KAPALÍN, V., KOLANDOVÁ, J., NOVOTNÁ, M., and TESAŘOVÁ, M. (1970). Relations between growth values of children in longitudinally and semilongitudinally studied groups and some genetic and social factors of their families. *CIE*, Davos, 1970 tom *2*, 53–60.

——, KOTÁSKOVÁ, J., and PROKOPEC, M. (1969). *Physical and mental development of present generation of our children* (Czech with English summary). Praha: Academia.

KAPRIO, J., KOSKENVOU, M., ARTIMO, M., SARNA, S., and RANTASALO, I. (1979). *Baseline characteristics of the Finnish Twin Registry. Section I: Materials, methods, representativeness and results for variables special to twin studies*. Publication of the Department of Public Health Science M47, Helsinki.

——, SARNA, S., SISTONEN, P., and KOSKENVUO, M. (1977). Determination of zygosity in the Finnish Twin Registry. Unpublished.

——, KOSKENVUO, M., and RANTASALO, I. (1978a). *Baseline characteristics of the Finnish Twin Registry. Section II: History of symptoms and illnesses, use of drugs, physical characteristics, smoking, alcohol and physical activity*. Publications of the Department of Public Health Science M37, Helsinki.

——, ——, ——, and ——. (1978b). The Finnish Twin Registry: formation and compilation, questionnaire study, zygosity determination procedures and research program. In *Twin research: biology and epidemiology* (ed. W. Nance), pp. 179–84. New York: Alan R. Liss.

KATZ, M. M. (1968). A phenomenological typology of schizophrenia. In *The role and methodology of classification in psychiatry and psychopathology* (ed. M. M. Katz, J. O. Cole, and W. E. Barton). Public Health Service Publ. No. 1584. Washington D.C.: U.S. Government Printing Office.

KAUPPINEN, M. (1967). Maternal heart volume correlated to perinatal mortality, birth weight as well as to maternal weight and height. *Acta Paediat. Scand.*, Suppl. 159., 166–7.

KELLAM, S. G., BRANCH, J. D., AGRAWAL, K. C., and ENSMINGER, M. E. (1975). *Mental health and going to school: the Woodlawn program of assessment, early intervention and evaluation*. London: University of Chicago Press.

KEMPER, H. C. G. (1973). The influence of extra lessons in physical education on physical and mental development of 12- and 13-year old boys. *Proceedings of the Stallite Symposium of the XXV International Congress of Physiological Sciences: Physical Fitness*, pp. 212–6. Prague: De Vrieseborch.

——, BINKHORST, R. A., VERSCHUUR, R., and VISSERS, A. C. A. (1976a). Reliability of the Ergo-analyzer—a method for continuous determination of oxygen uptake. *J. cardiovasc. pulmon. Technol.*, **4**, 27–30.

——, POULUS, A. J., and VAN DER HELM, N. (1971). Circuit Training und Körpererziehung: Uber den Einfluss einer Kreistrainings beim Schulsport auf einige morphologische und funktionelle Merkale bei 12- und 13- jährige Jungen. *Med. Sport*, **6**, 179–84.

—— and VAN'T HOF (1978). Design of a multiple longitudinal study of growth and health in teenagers. *Eur. J. Pediat.*, **129**, 147–55.

——, VERSCHUUR, R., RAS, J. G. A., SUEL, T. SPLINTER, P. G. and TAVECCHIO, L. W. C. (1976b). Effects of 5 versus 3 lessons a week physical education program upon the physical development of 12- and 13- year old schoolboys. *J. Sports, Med. Phys. Fitness*, **16**(4), 319–26.

—— and —— (1977a). *Motor performance (MOPER) Fitness Test*. Thomas 3, 75–102.

—— and —— (1977b). Validity and reliability of pedometers in habitual activity research. *Eur. J. appl. Physiol.*, **37**, 71–82.

KENDALL, M. G. (1962). *Rank correlation methods*. London: Wiley.

KENNEDY, P., KREITMAN, N., and OVENSTONE, I. (1974). The prevalence of suicide and parasuicide (attempted suicide) in Edinburgh. *Brit. J. Psychol.*, **124**(578), 36–41.

KENNELL, J. H., JERAULD, R., WOLFE, H., CHESLER, D., KREGER, N. C., MCALPINE, W., STEFFA, M., and KLAUS, M. H. (1974). Maternal behavior one year after early and extended post-partum contact. *Develop. Med. Child Neurol.*, **16**, 172–9.

KENNY, D. A. (1975). Cross-lagged panel correlation: a test for spuriousness. *Psychol. Bull.*, **82**, 887–903.

KEPPEL, G. (1973). *Design and analysis. A researcher's handbook*. Englewood Cliffs, N. J.: Prentice-Hall.

KERN, H. (1959). Verlaufsformen der Entwicklung bei antriebsarmen und antriebsgehemmten Kindern. Dipl. Thesis, Erlangen.

KESSEL, N. and WALTON, H. (1971). *Alcoholism*. Harmondsworth: Penguin.

KETY, S. S. (1959). Biochemical theories of schizophrenia. *Science*, **129**, 1528–32, 1590–6.

——, ROSENTHAL, D., WENDER, P. H. and SCHULSINGER, F. (1968). The types and prevalence of mental illness in the biological and adoptive families of adopted schizophrenics. In *The transmission of schizophrenia* (ed. D. Rosenthal and S. S. Kety), pp. 345–62. Oxford: Pergamon.

——, ——, ——, and JACOBSEN, B. (1975). Mental illness in the biological and adopted individuals who have become schizophrenic: a preliminary report based on interviews with the relatives. In *Genetic research in psychiatry* (ed. R. R. Fieve, D. Rosenthal and H. Brill), pp. 147–65. Baltimore: Johns Hopkins Press.

KIERNAN, K. E., COLLEY, J. R. T., DOUGLAS, J. W. B., and REID, D. D. (1976). Chronic cough in young adults in relation to smoking habits, childhood environment and chest illness. *Respiration*, **33**, 236–44.

KIEV, A. (1972). *Transcultural psychiatry*. Harmondsworth, England: Penguin Books.

KILBRIDE, J. E. (1969). *The motor development of rural Baganda infants*. Pennsylvania State University.

KIND, H. (1966). The psychogenesis of schizophrenia: a review of the literature. *Brit. J. Psychiat.*, **112**, 333–49.

KINNEY, D. and JACOBSEN, B. (1978). Environmental factors in schizophrenia: new adoption study evidence. In *The nature of schizophrenia, new approaches to research and treatment* (ed. L. C. Wynne, R. L. Cromwell, and S. Mathysse), pp. 38–51. New York: Wiley.

KINSBOURNE, M. (1973). Minimal brain dysfunction as a neurodevelopmental lag. *Ann. N. Y. Acad. Sci.*, **205**, 268–73.

KIRK, S. A., McCARTHY, J. J. and KIRK, W. D. (1968). *The Illinois Test of Psycholinguistic Abilities. Examiners manual.* Urbana: University of Illinois Press.

KIRKEGAARD-SØRENSEN, L. and MEDNICK, S. A. (1975). Registered criminality in families with children at high risk for schizophrenia. *J. abnorm. Psychol.*, **84**, 197–204.

KLAUS, M., JERAULD, R., KREGER, N., McALPINE, W., STEFFA, M., and KENNELL, J. (1972). Maternal attachment—importance of the first post-partum days. *New Engl. J. Med.*, **286**, 460–3.

KLAWANS, H. L., PAULSON, G. W., RINGEL, S. P., and BARBEAU, A. (1972). Use of 1-DOPA in the detection of presymptomatic Huntington's Chorea. *New Engl. J. Med.*, **286**, 1332–4.

KLEIN, G. (1965). *Persönlichkeitsentwicklung in der Schule.* Heidelberg: Quelle and Meyer.

KLEMETTI, A. (1966). Relationship of selected environmental factors to pregnancy outcome and congenital malformations. *Ann. Paediatr. Fenn.*, **12**, (Suppl. 26).

KLONOFF, H. (1971). Head injuries in children: predisposing factors, accident conditions, accident proneness and sequelae. *Amer. J. Publ. Health*, **61**, 2405–17.

—, Low, M. D. and CLARK, C. (1977). Head injuries in children: a prospective five year follow-up. *J. Neurol. Neurosurg. Psychiat.*, **40**, 1211–19.

— and PARIS, R. (1974). Immediate, short term and residual effects of acute head injuries in children: neuropsychological and neurological correlates. In *Clinical neuropsychology: current status and applications* (ed. R. M. Reitan and L. A. Davison), pp. 179–210. Washington: Winston.

KNOBLOCH, H. and PASAMANICK, B. (1962). The developmental behaviour approach to the neurologic examination in infancy. *Child Develop.*, **33**, 181–98.

KNÖPFLER-v. MANN, H. (1964). Schulische Entwicklung und Berufsbewährung in psychischer, somatischer und sozialer Sicht. [Development in school and occupational training.] Phil.Diss., Bonn.

KNOPS, L. (1967). *Handleiding bij de analytische intelligentietest voor kleuters van vijf en zes jaar. Leuvense aanpassing van Thurstone's PMA (5–7).* Leuven: Leuvense Universitaire Uitgaven.

KOCH, H. L. (1966). *Twins and twin relation.* Chicago: University of Chicago Press.

KOHLBERG, L. (1969). Stage and sequence: the cognitive-developmental approach to socialization. In *Handbook of socialization theory and research* (ed. D. A. Goslin). Chicago: Rand McNally.

KOHN, M. L. (1973). Social class and schizophrenia: a critical review and reformulation. *Schizophren. Bull.*, **1**, 60–79.

KOSKENVUO, M., SARNA, S., KAPRIO, J., and RANTASALO, I. (1976). *Methodology and structure of the Finnish Twin Registry.* Department of Public Health Science, University of Helsinki.

——, LANGINVAINIO, H., KAPRIO, J., RANTASALO, I., and SARNA, S. (1979). *Baseline characteristics of the Finnish Twin registry. Section III: Occupational and psychosocial factors.* Publication of the Department of Public Health Science M49, Helsinki.

KOWALSKI, C. J. (1972). A commentary on the use of multivariate statistical methods in anthropometric research. *Amer. J. Phys. Anthropol.*, **36**, 119.

— and GUIRE, K. E. (1974). Longitudinal data analysis. *Growth*, **38**, 131.

KRAEPELIN, E. (1909). *Psychiatrie*, vol. I. Barth.

KRAFKA, J. (1919). The effect of temperature upon facet number in the bar-eyed mutant of drosophila. Part I. *J. gen. Physiol.*, **2**, 409–32.

KRAPF, E. E. (1964). Social change in the genesis of mental disorder and health. In *Population and mental health* (ed. H. P. David). Berne: Hans Huber.

KREITMAN, N. (1972). Suicide in Scotland in comparison with England and Wales. *Brit. J. Psychiat.*, **121** (560), 83–7.

KRINGLEN, E. (1970). Natural history of obsessional neurosis. *Seminars Psychiat.*, **2**, 403–19.

LAING, R. D., PHILIPSON, H., and LEE, A. R. (1966). *Interpersonal perception. A theory and a method of research.* London: Tavistock publications.

LAMBERT, L. (1977a). Sex and parenthood: sources of information for teenagers. *Hlth soc. Serv. J.*, **77**, 4536.

— (1977b). Measuring the gaps in teenagers' knowledge of sex and parenthood. *Hlth soc. Serv. J.*, April issue.

— (1978a). Careers guidance and choosing a job. *Brit. J. Guidance Counselling*, **6**, 2.

— (1978b). Living in one-parent families: leaving school and future plans for work. *Concern*, 29.

—, ESSEN, J., and HEAD, J. (1977). Variations in behaviour ratings of children who have been in care. *J. Child Psychol. Psychiat.*, **18**, 335–46.

— and PEARSON, R. (1977). Sex education in schools. *J. Inst. Hlth Educ.*, **15**, 4.

LAMBERT, N. M. and HARTSOUGH, C. S. (1973). Scaling behavioral attributes of children using multiple teacher judgments of pupil characteristics. *Educ. psychol. Measure.*, **33**, 859–74.

LAMBO, T. A. (1965). Developing countries and industrialization. In *Industrialization and mental health*, pp. 104–14. Geneva: World Federation for Mental Health.

LANDAU, S. F. (1978a). Discrimination in the handling of juvenile offenders by the police. (Stencil).

— (1978b). Do legal variables predict police decisions? (Stencil).

LANGNER, T. S., and MICHAEL, S. T. (1963). *Life stress and mental health—the midtown Manhattan study* (vol. II). London: Collier-MacMillan Ltd.

LAURENCE, K. M. (1959). Tracing patients. *Lancet*, **2**, 208–12.

LAVIK, N. (1977). Urban–rural differences in rates of disorder. In *Epidemiological approaches in child psychiatry* (ed. P. Graham). London: Academic Press.

LAZARSFELD, P. F. (1972). Mutual relations over time of two attributes: a review and integration of various approaches. In *Psychopathology* (ed. M. Hammer, K. Salzinger, and S. Sutton). New York: Wiley.

LEHR, U. (1959). Berichte über den Stand des Accelerationsproblems. I. *Vita Humana*, **2**, 191–212.

— (1960). Berichte über den Stand des Accelerationsproblems. II. *Vita Humana*, **3**, 32–60; 143–72.

— (1964). Die ersten sechs Lebensjahre in der Erinnerung Erwachsener und Jugendlicher. *Proceedings of the 24th Congress Deutsche Gesellschaft für Psychologie.* Vienna.

— (1969). *Frau im Beruf, Eine Psychologische Analyse der Weiblichen Berufsrolle.* Frankfurt: Athenäum.

— (1977). *Psychologie des Alterns* (3rd edn.). Heidelberg: Quelle Meyer.

——, SCHMITZ-SCHERZER, R. and THOMAE, H. (1972). Psychologischer status, subjektiver Gesundheitszustand und internistischer Befund. *Ärzt. Prax.*, **90**, 4393–401.

— and — (1976). Survivors and non-survivors: two fundamental patterns of aging. In *Contributions to human development* (ed. H. Thomae), vol. 3. Basel: S. Karger.

— and THOMAE, H. (1958). Eine Laengsschnittuntersuchung bei 30–40 jaehrigen Angestellten. *Vita Humana*, **1**, 100–10.

— and — (1965). Konflikt, seelische Belastung und Lebensalter. Opladen: Westdeutscher Verlag.

LEIFER, A. D., LEIDERMAN, P. H., BARNETT, C. R., and WILLIAMS, J. A. (1972). Effects of mother–infant separation on maternal attachment behaviour. *Child Develop.*, **43**, 1203–5.

LEIGHTON, A. H. (1959). *My name is Legion. The Stirling County study of psychiatric disorder and sociocultural environment* (vol. I). New York: Basic Books.

——, LAMBO, T. A., HUGHES, C. D., LEIGHTON, D. C., MURPHY, J. M. and MACKLIN, D. G. (1963). *Psychiatric disorder among the Yoruba.* Ithaca, New York: Cornell University Press.

— and LEIGHTON, D. C. (1964). Handbook for the psychiatric evaluation of personal data as developed in the Stirling County Study and the Cornell Program in Social Psychiatry. Mimeographed edn. Ithaca, N.Y.

LEIGHTON, D. C., HAGNELL, O., LEIGHTON, A. H., HARDING, J. S., KELLERT, S. R., and DANLEY, R. A. (1971). Psychiatric disorders in a Swedish and a Canadian community: an exploratory study. *Soc. Sci. Med.*, **5**, 189–210.

——, HARDING, J. S., MACKLIN, D. B., MACMILLAN, A. M., and LEIGHTON, A. H. (1963). *The character of danger.* New York: Basic Books.

LEJEUNE, J., GAUTIER, M., and TURPIN, R. (1959). Etudes des chromosomes somatiques de neuf enfants mongoliens. *Comptes Rendus Hebdomadaires des Seances de l'Academie des Sciences (Paris)*, **248**, 1721–2.

LEVI, L. (1974). Psychosocial stress and disease: a conceptual model. In *Life stress and illness* (ed. E. K. E. Gunderson and R. H. Rahe), pp. 8–33. Springfield, Illinois: Thomas.

LEVIN, M. L. (1953). The occurrence of lung cancer in man. *Acta Unio Internationalis Contra Cancrum*, **9**, 531–41.

——, BRIGHTMAN, I. J. and BURTT, E. J. (1949). The problem of cerebral palsy. *N.Y. State J. Med.*, **49**, 2793–9.

LEWIS, D. O., BALLA, D., SHANOK, S., and SNELL, L., (1976). Delinquency, parental psychopathology and parental criminality. *J. Child Psychiat.*, **15**, 665–78.

LEWIS, M. and ROSENBLUM, L. A. (eds.) (1974). *The effect of the infant on its caregiver*. New York: Wiley.

LIETZ, A. (1960). *Verlaufsformen niederer Anregbarkeitsvarianten*. Dipl. Thesis, Erlangen.

LIFSHITZ, M., BERMAN, D., GALIDI, A., and GILAD, D. (1977). Bereaved children: the effect of mother's perception and social-system organisation on their short-term range adjustment. *J. Amer. Acad. Child Psychiat.*, **16**, 272–84.

LILIENFELD, A. M. (1959). A methodological problem in testing a recessive genetic hypothesis in human disease. *Amer. J. publ. Hlth*, **49**, 199–204.

—— (1976). *Foundations of epidemiology*. Oxford: Oxford University Press.

——, PASAMANICK, B., and ROGERS, M. (1955). The relationship between pregnancy experience and the development of neuropsychiatric disorders in childhood. *Amer. J. publ. Hlth*, **45**, 637–43.

LILJEFORS, R. (1967). *Vilka blir straffade? En undersökning av de brottsliga i en population som följts upp under 26 år*. (With an English summary). Stockholm: Lärarhögskolan i Stockholm, pedagogiska institutionen.

LIN, T.-Y. and STANDLEY, C. C. (1962). *The scope of epidemiology in psychiatry*. Geneva: World Health Organization. (Public Health Papers No. 16).

LISHMAN, W. A. (1974). The speed of recall of pleasant and unpleasant experiences. *Psychol. Med.*, **4**, 212–8.

LOCKHART, R. and LIEBERMAN, W. (1976). Factor structure of the electrodermal response. Paper presented at the Society for Psychophysiological Research, San Diego.

LOCKYER, L. and RUTTER, M. (1969). A five to fifteen year follow-up study of infantile psychosis. III. Psychological aspects. *Brit. J. Psychiat.*, **115**, 865–82.

—— and —— (1970). A five to fifteen year follow-up study of infantile psychosis. IV. Patterns of cognitive ability. *Brit. J. soc. clin. Psychol.*, **9**, 152–63.

LORR, M. and KLETT, C. J. (1966). *Inpatient Multidimensional Psychiatric Scale*. Palo Alto, California: Consulting Psychology Press.

LOTTER, V. (1978). Follow-up studies. In *Autism: a reappraisal of concepts and treatment* (ed. M. Rutter and E. Schopler). New York: Plenum.

LOVELAND, N., WYNNE, L. C., and SINGER, M. T. (1963). The Family Rorschach: a new method for studying family interaction. *Fam. Proc.*, **2**, 187–215.

LOWMAN, J. (1975). *The inventory of family feelings: manual for research uses*. Department of Psychology, University of North Carolina at Chapel Hill.

LUBORSKY, L. (1962). Clinicians' judgements of mental health. *Arch. Gen. Psychiat.*, **7**, 407–17.

LÜTHI, R. (1979). Präventives elterntraining. Dissertation, Bern.

LYLE, O. E. and GOTTESMAN, I. I. (1977). Premorbid psychometric indicators of the gene for Huntington's Disease. *J. consult. clin. Psychol.*, **45**, 1011–22.

MAAS, H. S. and KUYPERS, J. A. (1974). *From thirty to seventy. A forty year longitudinal study of adult life styles and personality*. San Francisco: Jossey-Bass.

MACCOBY, E. E. and JACKLIN, C. N. (1974). *The psychology of sex differences*. Stanford: Stanford University Press.

MACGILLIVRAY, I. (1961). Hypertension in pregnancy and its consequences. *J. Obstet. Gynaecol. Brit. Commonwlth*, **68**, 557–69.

MACINTYRE, S. (1977). *Single and pregnant*. London: Croom Helm.

MACMAHON, B. and PUGH, T. F. (1970). *Epidemiology: principles and methods*. Boston: Little Brown and Co.

MACNAUGHTON, M. C. (1961). Pregnancy following abortion. *J. Obstet. Gynaecol. Brit. Commonwlth*, **68**, 789–92.

MAGNUSSON, D. (1976). The person and the situation in an interactional model of behavior. *Scand. J. Psychol.*, **17**, 253–71.

—— (1977). Overachievement as a person characteristic and its relation to physiological reactions. *Reports from the Department of Psychology*, University of Stockholm, No. 493. (To appear in proceedings from a symposium, organized by the Society for Life History Research in Psychopathology, Fort Worth, October, 1976).

—— (1978). A longitudinal problem oriented investigation of development and adjustment. In *Research into personal development: educational and vocational choice* (ed. A. Dunér). Amsterdam: Swets and Zeitlinger.

—— (1979). Methodology and strategy problems in longitudinal research. In *Proceedings from a seminar in longitudinal research in Aarhus* (ed. F. Schulsinger and S. Mednick).

—— and BACKTEMAN, G. (1978). Londitudinal stability of person characteristics: intelligence and creativity. *Appl. Psychol. Measurement*, **2**, 481–90.

——, DUNÉR, A., and ZETTERBLOM, G. (1975). *Adjustment—a longitudinal study*. Stockholm: Almqvist and Wiksell. (New York: Wiley).

MANSFELD, E. (1958). *Reifeentwicklung und Berufsbewährung bei Jugendlichen*. Schriftenreihe aus dem Gebiet des öffentlichen Gesundheitswesens, vol. 7, pp. 10–103. Stuttgart: Thieme.

—— and STRICKMANN, R. (1965). Accelerierte und retardierte Kinder im Längsschnittvergleich [Longitudinal studies on early and late maturing boys and girls]. Unpublished research report, Bonn, 1965.

MANSFELD, G. and LANG, K. (1962). Die Kreislaufregulation im Wachstumsalter. In *Wissenschaftliche Jugendkunde* (ed. W. Hagen and H. Thomae), vol. 3. Munich: J. A. Barth.

MAPSTONE, E. (1969). Children in care. *Concern*, **3**, 23–8.

MARICQ, H. R. and EDELBERG, R. (1975). Electrodermal recovery rate in a schizophrenic population. *Psychophysiol.*, **12**, 630–3.

MARKOWE, M., TONGE, W. L., and BARBER, L. E. D. (1955). Psychiatric disability and employment. I. A survey of 222 registered disabled persons. *Brit. J. prev. soc. Med.*, **9**, 39–45.

MARKUSH, R. E. and FAVERO, R. V. (1974). Epidemiologic assessment of stressful life events, depressed mood, and psychophysiological symptoms—a preliminary report. In *Stressful life events* (ed. B. S. Dohrenwend and B. P. Dohrenwend), pp. 171–90. New York: Wiley.

MARSHALL, W. A. (1971). Somatic development and the study of the central nervous system. In *Normal and abnormal development of brain and behavior* (ed. G. B. A. Stoelinga and J. J. Van der Werff ten Bosch), pp. 1–15. Leiden: Leiden University Press.

MARTENS, P. (1975). Project Metropolitan—a description of its data archives, as of March, 1975. *Project Metropolitan Research Report Series*, No. 2.

—— (1976). Patterns of child rearing ideology. *Project Metropolitan Research Report Series*, No. 5.

MARWICK, E. W. (1975). *The folklore of Orkney and Shetland*. London: B. T. Batsford Ltd.

MATHEY, F. J. (1956). Psychologische Längsschnittergebnisse zur Frage der seelischen Entwicklung des Grundschulkindes. *Psychol. Rundschau*, **7**, 163–76.

—— (1968). Reaktionen auf eine Belastungssituation im höheren Alter. *Berichte der Deutschen Gesellschaft für Gerontologie* (ed. R. Schubert), vol. 1, pp. 223–7. Darmstadt.

—— (1976). Psychomotor performance and reaction speed in old age. In *Contributions to human development* (ed. H. Thomae), vol. 3, pp. 36–50. Basel: S. Karger.

MAXWELL, A. E., FENWICK, P. B. C., FENTON, G. W., and DOLLIMORE, J. (1974). Reading ability and brain function: a simple statistical model. *Psychol. Med.*, **4**, 274–80.

MAY, A. R. (1976). *Mental health services in Europe. A review of data collected in response to a WHO questionnaire*. (WHO Offset Publication No. 23), Geneva: World Health Organization.

MAY, D. R. (1973). Illegitimacy and juvenile court involvement. *Int. J. Criminol Penol.*, **1**, 227–52.

—— (1975a). Juvenile offenders and the organisation of juvenile justice: an examination of juvenile delinquency in Aberdeen, 1959–67. Unpublished Ph.D. Thesis, University of Aberdeen.

—— (1975b). Truancy, school absenteeism and delinquency. *Scottish educ. Stud.*, **7**, 97–107.

—— (1977). Delinquent girls before the courts. *Med. Sci. Law*, **17** (3), 203–12.

MAY, P. R. A. (1968). *Treatment of schizophrenia: a comparative study of five treatment methods*. New York: Science House.

MAZER, M. (1976). *People and predicaments*. Cambridge, Mass.: Harvard University Press.

MCCABE, M. S., FOWLER, R. C., CADORET, R. J., and WINOKUR, G. (1972). Psychiatric illness among paternal and maternal relatives of poor prognosis schizophrenics. *Brit. J. Psychiat.*, **120** (554), 91–4.

McCANDLESS, B. R. (1960). Rate of development, baby build and personality. *Psychiat. Res. Rep.*, **13**, 42–57.

McCLEARN, G. E. and DeFRIES, J. C. (1973). *Introduction to behavioral genetics*. San Francisco: W. H. Freeman.

McCORD, J. (1972). Some differences in backgrounds of alcoholics and criminals. *Ann. N.Y. Acad. Sci.*, **197**, 183–9.

McDONALD, A. (1967). *Children of very low birth-weight*. Medical Education and Information Research Unit Monograph No. 1. London: SIMP/Heinemann.

McFARLANE, J. W. (1938). Studies in child guidance I. Methodology of data collection and organization. *Monogr. Soc. Res. Child Develop.*, **3**, 1–254.

McGARVEY, W. E. (1977). Longitudinal factors in school desegregation. Unpublished doctoral dissertation, University of Southern California.

McKINLAY, J. (1970). The new late comers for antenatal care. *Brit. J. prev. soc. Med.*, **24** (1), 52–7.

McKUSICK, V. A. (1978). *Mendelian inheritance in man* (5th edn.). Baltimore: Johns Hopkins Press.

McLOY-LAYMAN, E. (1974). Psychological effects of physical activity. In *Exercise and sport sciences reviews* (ed. J. H. Wilmore), vol. 2. New York: Academic Press.

McNEIL, T. and KAIJ, L. (1976). *Obstetric factors in the development of schizophrenia. Complications in the births of preschizophrenics and in reproductions by schizophrenic parents*. Second Rochester International Conference on Schizophrenia. May 2–5, 1976.

—— and WIEGERINK, R. (1971). Behavioral patterns and pregnancy and birth complication histories in psychologically disturbed children. *J. nerv. ment. Dis.*, **152**, 315–24.

——, ——, and DOZIER, J. E. (1970). Pregnancy and birth complications in the births of seriously, moderately and mildly behaviorally disturbed children. *J. Nerv. ment. Dis.*, **151**, 24–34.

MEAD, M. (1947a). The implications of culture change for personality development. *Amer. J. Orthopsychiat.*, **17**, 633–47.

—— (1947b). The concept of cultural change and the psychosomatic approach. *Psychiat.*, **10**, 57–76.

Measurement of morbidity (1954). A report of the Statistics Sub-committee of the Registrar General's Advisory Committee on Medical Nomenclature and Statistics. London:H.M.S.O.

MECHANIC, C. (1974). Social structure and personal adaptation: some neglected dimensions. In *Coping and adaptation* (ed. G. V. Coelho, D. A. Hamburg, and J. E. Adams), pp. 32–44. New York: Basic Books.

MEDICO-SOCIAL RESEARCH BOARD. *Annual Reports 1970–1976.*

MEDNICK, B. (1977). Intellectual and behavioral functioning of ten to twelve year old children who showed certain transient symptoms in the neonatal period. *Child Develop.*, **48**, 844–53.

—— and MICHELSEN, N. M. (1977).

Neurological and motor functioning of 10–12 year old children who showed mild transient neurological symptoms in the first five days of life. *Acta Neurol. Scand.*, **56**, 70–8.

MEDNICK, S. A. (1958). A learning theory approach to research in schizophrenia. *Psychol. Bull.*, **55**, 316–27.

—— (1960). The early and advanced schizophrenic. In *Current research in schizophrenia* (ed. S. A. Mednick and J. Higgins). Ann Arbor, Michigan: Edwards.

—— (1962a). Schizophrenia: a learned thought disorder. In *Clinical psychology* (ed. G. Nielsen). Proceedings of XIV International Congress of Applied Psychology. Copenhagen: Munksgaard.

—— (1962b). The associative bases of the creative process. *Psychol. Rev.*

—— (1970). Breakdown in individuals at high risk for schizophrenia: possible predispositional perinatal factors. *Ment. Hyg.*, **54**, 50–63.

—— (1976). *Undersogelser af high-risk born. Trin pa vejen mod en skizofreniteori.* Copenhagen: FADL's forlag.

—— (1978). Berkson's fallacy and high-risk research in schizophrenia. In *The nature of schizophrenia* (ed. L. C. Wynne, R. L. Cromwell, and S. Matthysse). New York: Wiley.

—— and HUTCHINGS, B. (1977). Some considerations in the interpretation of the Danish adoption studies in relation to asocial behavior. In *The bio-social bases of criminal behavior* (ed. S. A. Mednick and K. O. Christiansen). New York: Gardner Press.

—— and LANOIL, G. (1977). Intervention in children at high risk for schizophrenia. In *Primary prevention in psychopathology* (ed. G. W. Albee and J. M. Joffe), pp. 153–63. Hanover, N.H.: University Press of New England.

—— and McNEIL, T. F. (1968). Current methodology in research on the etiology of schizophrenia: serious difficulties which suggest the use of the high-risk group method. *Psychol. Bull.*, **70**, 681–93.

——, MURA, E., SCHULSINGER, F., and MEDNICK, B. (1971). Perinatal conditions and infant development in children with schizophrenic parents. *Soc. Biol.*, **18**, 103–13.

—— and SCHULSINGER, F. (1973). Studies of children at high-risk for schizophrenia. In *Schizophrenia: the first ten Dean Award lectures* (ed. S. R. Dean), pp. 245–93. New York: MSS Information Corporation.

——, ——, and GARFINKEL, R. (1975a). Children at high risk for schizophrenia: predisposing factors and intervention. In *Experimental approaches to psychopathology* (ed. W. Kietzman). San Francisco: Academic Press.

——, ——, HIGGINS, J., and BELL, B. (eds.) (1974). *Genetics, environment and psychopathology*. Amsterdam: Elsevier.

——, ——, TEASDALE, T. W., SCHULSINGER, H., VENABLES, P. H., and ROCK, D. R. (1978). Schizophrenia in high-risk children: sex differences in predisposing factors. In *Cognitive defects in the development of mental illness* (ed. G. Serban), pp. 169–97. New York: Brunner/Mazel.

——, ——, and SCHULSINGER, F. (1975b). Schizophrenia in children of schizophrenic mothers. In *Childhood personality and*

psychopathology: current topics, 2 (ed. A. Davids.), pp. 221–52. New York: Wiley.

MEEHL, P. E. (1972a). A critical afterword. In *Schizophrenia and genetics: a twin study vantage point* (ed. I. I. Gottesman and J. Shields), pp. 367–415. New York: Academic Press.

—— (1972b). Specific genetic etiology, psychodynamics, and therapeutic nihilism. *Int. J. ment. Hlth*, **1**, 10–27.

—— (1973). Why I do not attend case conferences. In *Psycho-diagnosis: selected papers* (ed. P. E. Meehl), pp. 225–302. Minneapolis: University of Minnesota Press.

MELLBYE, F. (1967). Medisinsk registrering av fødsel. *Tidsskr. Norske Laegefor.*, **87**, 1085–6.

MELLOR, C. S. (1967). The epidemiology of alcoholism. *Hosp. Med.*, 284–94.

MERCER, J. R. (1970). Sociological perspectives on mild mental retardation. In *Social–cultural aspects of mental retardation* (ed. H. C. Haywood), pp. 378–91. New York: Appleton-Century-Crofts.

MEREDITH, H. V. (1969). Body size of contemporary youth in different parts of the world. *Monogr. Soc. Res. Child Develop.*, **34**, (7, Ser. No. 131).

MEYER, V. and YATES, A. (1955). Intellectual changes following temporal lobectomy for psychomotor epilepsy. *J. Neurol. Neurosurg. Psychiat.*, **18**, 44–52.

MILLER, L. B. and DYER, J. L. (1975). Four preschool programs: their dimensions and effects. *Monogr. Soc. Res. Child Develop.*, **40** (5–6), (Serial no. 162).

MILLER, P. McC and INGHAM, J. G. (1976). Friends, confidants and symptoms. *Soc. Psychiat.*, **11**, 51–8.

MINDE, K. and MINDE, R. (1977). Behavioral screening of pre-school children—a new approach to mental health? In *Epidemiological approaches in child psychiatry* (ed. P. J. Graham). London: Academic Press.

MIRDAL, G., MEDNICK, S. A., SCHULSINGER, F. and FUCHS, F. (1974). Perinatal complications in children of schizophrenic mothers. *Acta Psychiat. Scand.*, **50**, 553–68.

MISES, R., BREON, S., and FUCHS, F. (1974). Etude d'enfants de classes de perfectionnement. Mise en question de la débilité mentale. *Rev. Neuropsychiat. Infant. Hyg. Ment. Enfance*, **22** (7–8), 457–502.

——, PERRON-BORELLI, M., and BREON, S. (1971). Essai d'approche psychopathologique de la déficience intellectuelle. Les déficits dysharmoniques. *Psychiat. l'Enfant*, **14** (2), 341–464. (Summarized in Mises, R. (1975). *L'enfant deficient mental*. Paris: PUF.)

MONCK, E. M. (1963). Employment experiences of 127 discharged schizophrenic men in London. *Brit. J. prev. soc. Med.*, **17**, 101–10.

MÖNKS, F. J., MUNCKHOF, H. C. P. VAN DEN, WELS, P. M. A., and KOWALSKI, C. J. (1975). Application of Schaie's most efficient design in a study of the development of Dutch children. *Human Develop.*, **18** (6), 466–75.

——, ROST, H., and COFFIE, N. H. (1969). *Nijmeegse schoolbekwaamheidstest (NST), monografie en handleiding*. Nijmegen: Berkhout.

MONTAGU, A. (1971). Sociogenetic brain damage. *Develop. Med. Child Neurol.*, **13**, 597–605.

Mørch, E. T. (1941). Chondrodystrophic dwarfs in Denmark. *Opera Ex Domo Biologiae Hereditarie Humanae Universitatis Hafniensis*, **3**, whole.

Moreno, J. L. (1934). *Who shall survive? A new approach to the problem of human interrelations*. Washington, D.C.: Mental Disease Publishing Co.

Morris, J. N. (1966). *Standards and progress in reading*. Slough: National Foundation for Educational Research.

—— (1975). *Uses of epidemiology*. London: Churchill Livingstone.

Moss, M. A. and Kagan, J. (1964). Report on personality consistency and change from the Fels longitudinal study. *Vita Humana*, **7**, 127–38.

Mowrer, O. H. (1960). *Learning theory and behavior*. New York: Wiley.

Myers, J. K. and Bean, L. L., (1968). *A decade later*. New York: Wiley.

Myrhed, M. (1974). Alcohol consumption in relation to factors associated with ischemic heart disease. *Acta Med. Scand.* (Suppl.), 367.

Neale, M. D. (1958). *Neale analysis of reading ability (manual)*. London: Macmillan.

Neligan, G. A., Kolvin, I., Scott, D. M., and Garside, R. F. (1976). *Born too soon or born too small: a follow-up study to seven years of age*. Clinics in Developmental Medicine No. 61. London: Heinemann Medical.

Nelson, T. R. (1955a). A clinical study of pre-eclampsia. Part I. *J. Obstet. Gynaecol. Brit. Emp.*, **62**, 48–57.

—— (1955b). A clinical study of pre-eclampsia. Part II. *J. Obstet. Gynaecol. Brit. Emp.*, **62**, 58–66.

Nichols, P. C. and Bilbro, W. C. (1966). The diagnosis of twin zygosity. *Acta Genet. (Basel)*, **16**, 265–75.

Nicolson, J. R. (1972). *Shetland*. Devon: David and Charles.

Nie, N. H., Hadlaihull, C., Jenkins, J. G., Steinbrenner, K., and Bent, D. H. (1975). *Statistical package for the social sciences*. New York: McGraw-Hill.

Nielsen, J. (1976). The Samsø project from 1957 to 1974. *Acta Psychiat. Scand.*, **54**, 198–222.

Nilsson, L. and Smith, G. (1962). Dimensions of overt behavior as represented in EEG and adaptive test patterns. *Acta Psychiat. Scand.*, **38**, 277–301.

Nixon, W. L. B. and Slater, E. (1957). Second investigation into the children of cousins. *Acta Genet. Statist. Med.*, **7**, 513–32.

Noreik, K. (1970). A follow-up examination of neuroses. *Acta Psychiat. Scand.*, **46**, 81–95.

Northern Constabulary Chief Constable's (Annual) Report (1969–74). Wick, Scotland, 1969–74 and Inverness, Scotland, 1975.

Novotná, M. (1971). The growth level of school. Beginners in the relation to the sequence of their birth, number of children and monthly income per head. *Českoslov. Hyg.*, **16**, 9–10.

—— (1973). The effect of family and kindergarten care on development level of preschool children. *Českoslov. Hyg.*, **18**, 2.

—— (1974). Einige ergebnisse der longitudinal forschung. *Z. gesamte Hyg. Grenzgeb.*, **12**, 20.

Nunnally, J. (1967). *Psychometric theory*. New York: McGraw-Hill.

Nye, F. I. (1959). Employment status and adjustment of adolescent children. *Marr. Fam. Liv.*, **6**, 260–7.

Nylander, I. (1959). Physical symptoms and psychogenic etiology. *Acta Paediat.* (Suppl. 117), **48**, 69.

—— (1960). Children of alcoholic fathers. *Acta Paediat.* (Suppl. 121), **49**.

—— (1979). A 20-year prospective follow-up study of 2164 cases at the child guidance clinics in Stockholm. *Acta Paediat. Scand. (suppl.)*. (To be published).

—— and Rydelius, P.-A. (1973). The relapse of drunkenness in non-social teenage boys. *Acta Psychiat. Scand.*, **49**, 435–43.

Nyman, G. E. (1952). Electroencefalografi och psykiatri. *Nord. Med.*, **48**, 1348–9.

Ochsner, A. and DeBakey, M. (1939). Preliminary pulmonary malignancy. Treatment by total pneumonectomy: analyses of 79 collected cases and presentation of 7 personal cases. *Surg. Gynecol. Obstet.*, **68**, 435–51.

Ödegård, Ö. and Herlofsen, H. (1955). A study of psychotic patients of consanguineous parentage. *Acta Genet. Statist. Med.*, **5**, 391.

Office of Population Censuses and Surveys (1978). *1970—2 occupational mortality, decennial supplement*. London: H.M.S.O.

O'Hare, A. and Walsh, D. (1975). *The Irish Psychiatric Hospital Census, 1971*. Dublin: The Medico-Social Research Board.

—— and —— (1977). *Activities of Irish psychiatric hospitals and units 1973 and 1974*. Dublin: The Medico-Social Research Board.

Ohno, S. (1972). Gene duplication, mutation load, and mammalian genetic regulatory systems. *J. med. Genet.*, **9**, 254–63.

Ojesjo, L. and Hagnell, O. (1980) Prevalence of male alcoholism in a cohort observed for 25 years. *Scand. J. Soc. Med.*, in press.

Olbrich, E. (1977). *Health, ecology and aging*. Paper presented at Institute de la Vie: World Conference on Aging: A challenge to science and policy. Vichy, France.

—— and Lehr, U. (1976). Social roles and contacts in old age: consistency and patterns of change. In *Contributions to human development* (ed. H. Thomae), vol. 3, pp. 113–37. Basel: S. Karger.

Oldfield, R. C. and Wingfield, A. (1964). The time it takes to name an object. *Nature*, **202**, 1031–2.

Oldman, D., Bytheway, W. and Horobin, G. (1971). Family structure and educational achievement. *J. Biosoc. Sci.*, **3**, 81–91.

—— and Illsley, R. (1966). Measuring the status of occupations. *Sociol. Rev.*, **14**, 53–72.

Olofsson, B. (1971) *Vad var det vi sa! Om kriminellt och konformt beteerde bland skolpajkar*. (Or delinquency and conformity among schoolboys). Stockholm: Utbildningsförlaget.

Olsson, U. and Bergman, L. R. (1973). *A structural model for testing the age-differentiation hypothesis*. Örebroprojektet, Delstudie 21.

—— and —— (1977). A longitudinal factor model for studying change in ability structure. *Multivar. behav. Res.*, **12**, 221–42.

Opler, M. K. (1956). *Culture, psychiatry and human values*. Springfield, Illinois: Thomas.

Orvaschel, H. (1976). An examination of children at risk for schizophrenia as a function of the sex of the sick parent and the sex of the child. Doctoral dissertation, New School for Social Research, New York.

Oster, H. (1963). Ergebnisse einer Schulreifeuntersuchung. *Öffentl. Gesundheits.*, **25**, 550–9.

Owens, W. A. (1966). Age and mental abilities: a second adult follow-up. *J. educ. Psychol.*, **57**, 311–25.

Paine, R. S. and Oppé, T. E. (1966). Neurological examination of children. *Clin. Develop. Med.*, No. 20/21.

Palmore, E. (1969). Predicting longevity: a follow-up controlling for age. *Gerontol.*, **9**, 247.

—— (ed.) (1970). *Normal aging*. Durham, North Carolina: Duke University Press.

—— (ed.) (1974a). *Normal aging II*. Durham, North Carolina: Duke University Press.

—— (1974b). Predicting longevity: a new method. In *Normal aging II* (ed. E. Palmore). Durham, North Carolina: Duke University Press.

Parkin, J. M. and Warren, N. A. (1969). *Comparative study of neonatal behavior and development*. Proceedings, University Social Science Conference. University of East Africa, Nairobi.

Partington, M. W. (1960). The importance of accident-proneness in the aetiology of head injuries in childhood. *Arch. Dis. Child.*, **35**, 215–23.

Pasamanick, B. 1954). *Epidemiology of behavior disorders: neurology and psychiatry in childhood*. New York: Williams and Wilkins.

—— and Knobloch, H. (1960). Brain damage and reproductive casualty. *Amer. J. Orthopsychiat.*, **30**, 298–305.

Pattie, F. A. and Cornett, S. (1952). Unpleasantness of early memories and maladjustment of children. *J. Personal.*, **20**, 315–21.

Pearson, J. S. and Kley, I. B. (1957). On the application of genetic expectancies as age specific base rates in the study of human behavior disorders. *Psychol. Bull.*, **54**, 406–20.

Pearson, R. and Lambert, L. (1977). Sex education, preparation for parenthood and the adolescent. *Community Hlth*, **9**, 84.

—— and Peckham, C. S. (1972). Preliminary findings at the age of eleven years on children in the National Child Development Study (1958 cohort). *Commun. Med.*, **27** (3318), 113–6.

—— and Richardson, K. (1978). Smoking habits of 16-year-olds in the National Child Development Study. *Publ. Hlth*, **92**, 3.

Peckham, C. S. (1973). Speech defects in a national sample of children aged seven years. *Brit. J. Disord. Commun.*, **8**(1), 1–8.

—— and Butler, N. R. (1978). A national study of asthma in childhood. *J. Epidemiol. Comm. Hlth*, **32**, 79–85.

—— and Pearson, R. (1977). Handicapped children in secondary schools. *Publ. Hlth*, **91**, 296–304.

——, Sheridan, M. D., and Butler, N. R. (1972). School attainment of seven-year-old children with hearing difficulties. *Develop. Med. Child Neurol.*, **14**(5), 592–602.

——, MARSHALL, W., and DUDGEON, J. A. (1977). Rubella vaccination in school girls: factors affecting vaccine uptake. *Brit. med. J.*, **1**, 760–1.

PEKKARINEN, M. (1970). Methodology in the collection of food consumption data. *World Rev. Nutr. Dietet.*, **2**, 145.

PERNANEN, K. (1974). Validity of survey data on alcohol use. In *Alcohol and drug problems* (ed. R. J. Gibbins, Y. Israel, M. Kalant, R. E. Popham, W. Schmidt, and R. G. Smart, pp. 355–74. New York: Wiley.

PERRON–BORELLI, M. (1974). *Echelles Differentielles d'Efficience Intellectuelle: EDEI*. Paris: Centre de Psychologie Appliqué.

PETERS, J. E., ROMINE, J. S., and DYKMAN, R. A. (1975). A special neurological examination of children with learning disabilities. *Develop. Med. Child Neurol.*, **17**, 63–78.

PHILLIPS, D. L. and CLANCY, K. L. (1970). Response biases in field studies of mental illness. *Amer. Sociol. Rev.*, **35**, 503–15.

PHILLIPS, L. (1953). Case history data and prognosis in schizophrenia. *J. nerv. ment. Dis.*, **117**, 515–25.

PIAGET, J. (1950). *The psychology of intelligence*. New York: Harcourt, Brace.

PICKLES, W. N. (1948). Epidemiology in country practice. *New Engl. J. Med.*, **239**, 420–7.

PILLING, D. (1973). The handicapped child. *Research Review*, vol. III. London: Longman.

PLANT, M. A. (1975a). Alcoholism in Scotland. *New Psychiat.*, **2** (25), 12–13.

—— (1975b) *Drugtakers in an English town*. London: Tavistock.

—— (1977). Alcoholism and occupation: a review. *Brit. J. Addict.*, **72** (4), 309–16.

—— (1978). Occupation and alcoholism: cause or effect? A controlled study of recruits to the drink trade. *Int. J. Addict.*, **13**(4), 605–26. New York: Marcel Dekker, Inc.

—— (1979a). *Drinking careers: occupations, drinking habits and drinking problems*. London: Tavistock.

—— (1979b). Occupations, drinking patterns and alcohol-related problems: conclusions from a follow-up study. *Brit. J. Addict.*, **74**, 267–73.

PLANTE, G., COTE, H., and PILIC, I. (1973). [Study on a group of inhibited children from a deprived urban area.] (In Fench). *Can. Psychiat. Assoc. J.*, **18**, 321–5.

PLATT, S. (1980). On establishing the validity of 'objective' data: can we rely on across-interview agreement? *Psychol. Med.* (in press).

PLOVNICK, N. (1976). Autonomic nervous system functioning as a predisposing influence on personality, psychopathy and schizophrenia. Doctoral dissertation, Graduate faculty, New School for Social Research, New York.

POLLACK, M. and WOERNER, M. (1966). Pre- and postnatal complications and 'childhood schizophrenia': a comparison of five controlled studies. *J. Child Psychol. Psychiat.*, **7**, 235–42.

POLLIN, W. and STABENAU, J. (1968). Biological, psychological and historical differences in a series of monozygotic twins discordant for schizophrenia. In *The transmission of schizophrenia* (ed. D. Rosenthal and S. Kety), pp. 317–32. New York: Pergamon Press.

POND, D. A., BIDWELL, B. H., and STEIN, L. (1960). A survey of epilepsy in fourteen general practices. Demographic and medical data. *Psychiat. Neurol. Neurochir.*, **63**, 217–36.

POPULATION INVESTIGATION COMMITTEE (1948). *Maternity in Great Britain*. London: Oxford University Press.

POWER, M. J., ALDERSON, M. R., PHILLIPSON, C. M., SCHOENBERG, E., and MORRIS, J. N. (1967). Delinquent schools? *New Society*, **10**, 542–3.

——, ASH, P. M., SCHOENBERG, E., and SOREY, E. C. (1974). Delinquency and the family. *Brit. J. Soc. Work*, **4**, 13–38.

POWERS, E. and WITMER, H. (1951). *An experiment in the prevention of delinquency: the Cambridge–Somerville youth study*. New York: Columbia University Press.

PRAHL-ANDERSEN, B. and KOWALSKI, C. J. (1973). A mixed longitudinal, interdisciplinary study of the growth and development of Dutch children. *Growth*, **37**, 281–95.

——, ——, and HEYDENDAEL, P. (1979). *A mixed longitudinal interdisciplinary study of growth and development*. New York: Academic Press.

PRECHTL, H. F. R. (1965). Prognostic value of neurological signs in the newborn infant. *Proc. roy. Soc. Med.*, **58**, 3–4.

—— (1967). Neurological sequelae of prenatal and perinatal complications. *Brit. med. J.*, **4**, 763–7.

—— and BEINTEMA, D. (1964). *The neurological examination of the full-term newborn infant*. London: Heinemann Medical Books.

The President's Panel on Mental Retardation (1962). *Report to the president. A proposed program for national action to combat mental retardation*. Washington, D.C.: U.S. Government Printing Office.

PRINGLE, M. L. (1967). Follow-up of adopted children. *J. med. Women's Fed.*, **43** (3), 146–8.

——, BUTLER, N. R., and DAVIE, R. (1966). *11 000 seven-year-olds*. London: Longman in association with National Children's Bureau.

PRITCHARD, M. and GRAHAM, P. (1966). An investigation of a group of patients who have attended both the child and adult departments of the same psychiatric hospital. *Brit. J. Psychiat.*, **112**, 603–12.

PROKOPEC, M. (1960). Report on the longitudinal follow-up of Prague children. *VI. Congrès International des Sciences Anthropologiques et Ethnologiques*, Tome 1, Paris, 519–27.

—— (1962). Harmonický vývoj dětí do 3 let. *Česk. Hyg.*, **7** (2–3), 84–94.

Protocol from the planning meeting on international collaborative twin studies (unpublished) (1973). Miami Beach, December 1973.

PUGH, T. F. and MACMAHON, B. (1960). *Epidemiologic findings in United States mental hospital data*. London: Churchill.

QUINTON, D. and RUTTER, M. (1976). Early hospital admissions and later disturbances of behavior: an attempted replication of Douglas' findings. *Develop. Med. Child Neurol.*, **18**, 447–59.

—— and —— (1980a). Parents with children in care: 1 Current circumstances and parenting skills (submitted for publication).

—— and —— (1980b). Parents with children in care: 2 Intergenerational continuities (submitted for publication).

——, ——, and ROWLANDS, O. (1976). An evaluation of an interview assessment of marriage. *Psychol. Med.*, **6**, 577–86.

RAEBILD, I. (1967). Unpublished data.

RAHE, R. H. (1969). Life crisis and health change. In *Psychiatric drug responses: advances in prediction* (ed. P. R. A. May and J. R. Wittenborn), pp. 92–125. Springield, Illinois: Thomas.

—— (1974). The pathway between subjects. Recent life changes and their near-future illness reports: representative results and methodological issues. In *Stressful life events* (ed. B. S. Dohrenwend and B. P. Dohrenwend), pp. 73–86. New York: Wiley.

RÄIHA, C. -E. (1964). Prematurity, perinatal mortality and maternal heart volume. *Guy's Hosp. Rep.*, **113**, 96–110.

—— (1968). Prevention of prematurity. *Advan. Pediat.*, **15**, 137–90.

—— and KAUPPINEN, M. (1963). An attempt to decrease perinatal mortality and the rate of premature birth. *Develop. Med. Child Neurol.*, **5**, 225–32.

RANK, T. (1962). Schulleistung und Persönlichkeit [Achievement at school and personality]. *Wissenschaftliche Jugendkunde*, vol. 4, Munich: J. A. Barth.

RAURAMO, L., GRONROOS, M., and KIVIKOSKI, A. (1961). A comparative study of the obstetrical history of pupils in school for backward children and elementary school pupils. *Acta Obstet. Gynecol. Scand.*, **40**, 321–9.

REICHARD, S., LIVSON, F., and PETERSEN, P. G. (1962). *Aging and personality*. New York: Wiley.

REID, D. D. (1960). *Epidemiological methods in the study of mental disorder*. (Public health papers no. 2). Geneva: World Health Organization.

REID, W. J. and SHYNE, A. W. (1969). *Brief and extended casework*. New York: Columbia University Press.

REISBY, N. (1967). Psychoses in children of schizophrenic mothers. *Acta Psychiat. Scand.*, **43**, 8–20.

RENIER, E. (1957). La privation de la présence au retour de l'école. *Enfance*, **4**, 491–504.

Report of WHO meeting of investigators (1966). The use of twins in epidemiological studies. *Acta Genet. Med. (Roma)*, **15**, 111–28.

RICH, A. R. (1944). *The pathogenesis of tuberculosis*. Springfield, Illinois: Charles C. Thomas.

RICHARDS, M., RICHARDSON, K., and SPEARS, D. (1972). Conclusions: intelligence and society. In *Race, culture and intelligence* (ed. K. Richardson and D. Spears), pp. 179–96. Harmondsworth, England: Penguin Books.

RICHARDS, M. P. M. (1978). Possible effects of early separation on later development of children: a review. In *Separation and special-care baby units* (ed. F. S. W. Zimblecombe, M. P. M. Richards and N. P. C. Robertson). Clinics in Developmental Medicine No. 68, pp. 12–32. London: Heinemann Medical.

RICHARDSON, K. (1977a). The writing productivity and syntactic maturity of eleven-year-olds in relation to their reading habits. *Reading*, **11**, 46–53.

—— (1977b). Reading attainment and family size: an anomaly. *Brit. J. educ. Psychol.*, **47** (1), 71–5.

——, CALNAN, M., ESSEN, J., and LAMBERT, L. (1976). The linguistic maturity of eleven year olds. *J. Child Lang.*, **3** (1), 99–115.

——, HUTCHISON, D., PECKHAM, C., and TIBBENHAM, A. (1977). Audiometric thresholds of a national sample of British sixteen-year-olds. *Develop. Medium*, December issue.

RICHARDSON, S. A., DOHRENWEND, B. S., and KLEIN, D. (1965). *Interviewing: its forms and functions*. New York: Basic Books.

—— (1975). Reactions to mental subnormality. In *The mentally retarded and society* (ed. M. J. Begab and S. A. Richardson). Baltimore: University Park Press.

—— (1978). Careers of mentally retarded young persons: services, jobs and interpersonal relations. *AJMD*, **82**(4), 349.

—— (in press). Family characteristics associated with mild mental retardation. In *Prevention of retarded development in psychosocially disadvantaged children* (ed. M. Begab and H. Garber).

——, KATZ, M., KOLLER, H., McLAREN, J., and RUBINSTEIN, B. (in press, a). Some characteristics of a population of mentally retarded young adults in a British city. *JMDR*.

——, KOLLER, H., KATZ, M., and McLAREN, J. (in press, b). Severity of intellectual and associated functional impairments of those placed in mental retardation services between ages 16 and 22. Implications for planning services. In *Proceedings of NICHD-UCLA conference on impact of specific setting on the development and behavior of retarded persons, September 1979* (ed. R. Edgerton, M. Begab and K. Kerman).

RICHMAN, N. (1977a). Is a behavioural check-list for pre-school children useful? In *Epidemiological approaches in child psychiatry* (ed. P. J. Graham). London: Academic Press.

—— (1977b). Short-term outcome of behavioural problems in three-year-old children. In *Epidemiological approaches in child psychiatry* (ed. P. J. Graham). London: Academic Press.

RIEGEL, K. F. and RIEGEL, R. M. (1960). A study on changes of attitudes and interests during later years of life. *Vita Humana*, **3**, 177–206.

—— and —— (1972). Development, drop and death. *Develop. Psychol.*, **6**, 306–19.

RIMMER, J., COLE, S., JACOBSEN, B., KETY, S. S., ROSENTHAL, D., SCHULSINGER, F., and WENDER, P. H. (1979). Personal and social characteristics differentiating between adoptive relatives of schizophrenics and non-schizophrenics: a preliminary report based on interviews. *Comprehensive Psychiatry*, **20**(2), 157–8.

RIVINUS, T. M., JAMISON, D. L., and GRAHAM, P. J. (1975). Childhood organic neurological disease presenting as psychiatric disorder. *Arch. Dis. Childh.*, **50**, 115–9.

ROBBINS, L. (1963). The accuracy of parental recall of aspects of child development and of child rearing practices. *J. abnorm. soc. Psychol.*, **66**, 261–70.

ROBERTSON, J. and ROBERTSON, J. (1971). Young children in brief separations: a fresh look. *Psychoanal. Study Child*, **26**, 264–315.

ROBINS, L. N. (1966). *Deviant children grown up*. Baltimore: Williams and Wilkins.

—— (1970). Follow-up studies investigating childhood disorders. In *Psychiatric epidemiology* (ed. E. H. Hare and J. K. Wing). London: Oxford University Press.

—— (1972a). Follow-up studies of behaviour disorders in children. In *Psychopathological disorders of childhood* (ed. H. C. Quay and J. S. Werry). New York: Wiley.

—— (1972b). An actuarial evaluation of the causes and consequences of deviant behavior in young black men. In *Life history research in psychopathology* (ed. M. Roff, L. N. Robins, and M. Pollack), vol. 2. Minneapolis: University of Minnesota Press.

—— (1973). Evaluation of psychiatric services for children in the United States. In *Roots of evaluation: the epidemiological basis for planning psychiatric services* (ed. J. K. Wing and H. Häfner). London: Oxford University Press.

—— (1977). Problems in follow-up studies. *Amer. J. Psychiat.*, **134**, 904–7.

—— (1978). Longitudinal methods in the study of normal and pathological development. In *Psychiatrie der Gegenwart, Band l, 'Grundlagen und Methoden der psychiatrie'* (ed. K. P. Kisker, J. -E. Meyer, C. Müller and E. Strömgren). Heidelberg: Springer-Verlag.

——, DAVIS, D. H., and WISH, E. (1977). Detecting predictors of rare events: demographic, family, and personal deviance as predictors of stages in the progression toward narcotic addiction. In *The origins and course of psychopathology* (ed. J. Strauss, H. M. Babigian and M. Roff). New York: Plenum.

—— and HILL, S. W. (1966). Assessing the contribution of family structure, class and peer groups to juvenile delinquency. *J. crim. Law Criminol. Pol. Sci.*, **57**, 325–34.

——, MURPHY, G. E., WOODRUFF, R. A., and KING, L. J. (1971). Adult psychiatric states of black school boys. *Arch. gen. Psychiat.*, **24**, 338–45.

——, RATCLIFF, K. S., and WEST, P. A. (1978). School achievement in two generations: a study of 88 urban black families. Paper presented at the Thistletown 1977 International Symposium, Toronto, Canada. In press.

——, WEST, P. A., and HERJANIC, P. L. (1975). Arrests and delinquency in two generations; a study of black urban families and their children. *J. Child Psychol. Psychiat.*, **16**, 125–40.

ROBINSON, J. O. (1963). A study of neuroticism and casual arterial blood pressure. *Brit. J. soc. clin. Psychol.*, **2**, 56–64.

—— and WOOD, M. M. (1968). Symptoms and personality in the diagnosis of physical illness. *Brit. J. prev. soc. Med.*, **22**(1), 23–6.

ROE, A. (1945). Children of alcoholic parentage raised in foster homes. *Alcoholism, science, and society*, pp. 115–27. Published by *Quarterly Journal of Studies on Alcohol*.

ROFF, M., SELLS, S. B., and GOLDEN, M. M. (1972). *Social adjustment and personality development in children*. Minneapolis: University of Minnesota Press.

RONGE, A. (1962). Die Umwelt der 'Nachkriegskinder' in Jahre 1955. In *Deutsche Nachkriegskinder* (ed. W. Hagen, H. Thomae, and A. Ronge), pp. 71–164. Munich: Barth.

ROSE, G. (1962). The diagnosis of ischaemic heart pain and internal claudication in field surveys. *Bull. W.H.O.*, **27**: 643.

—— and MARSHALL, T. F. (1974). *Counselling and school social work*. London: Wiley.

ROSE, H. K. and GLATT, M. M. (1961). A study of alcoholism as an occupational hazard of merchant seamen. *J. Ment. Sci.*, **107**(446), 18–30.

ROSENFELD, G. B. and BRADLEY, C. (1948). Childhood behaviour sequelae of asphyxia in infancy. *Pediat.*, **2**, 74–84.

ROSENTHAL, D. (1962). Familial concordance by sex with respect to schizophrenia. *Psychol. Bull.*, **59**, 401–21.

—— (ed.) (1963). *The Genain quadruplets*. New York: Basic Books.

—— (1970). *Genetic theory and abnormal behavior*. New York: McGraw-Hill.

—— (1974a). A program of research on heredity in schizophrenia. In *Genetics, environment and psychopathology* (ed. S. A. Mednick, F. Schulsinger, H. Higgins, and B. Bell). Amsterdam: North-Holland/American Elsevier.

—— (1974b). The concept of subschizophrenic disorders. In *Genetics, environment and psychopathology* (ed. S. A. Mednick, F. Schulsinger, H. Higgins and B. Bell). Amsterdam: North-Holland/American Elsevier.

—— (1974c). The genetics of schizophrenia. In *American handbook of psychiatry* (2nd edn.) (ed. S. Arieti), vol. 3, pp. 588–600. New York: Basic Books.

——WENDER, P. H., KETY, S. S., SCHULSINGER, F., WELNER, J., and ØSTERGAARD, L. (1968). Schizophrenics' offspring reared in adoptive homes. In *The transmission of schizophrenia* (ed. D. Rosenthal and S. S. Kety), pp. 377–91. Oxford: Pergamon.

——, ——, ——, ——, ——, and RIEDER, R. O. (1975). Parent–child relationships and psychopathological disorder in the child. *Arch. gen. Psychiat.*, **32**, 466–76.

——, ——, ——, WELNER, J. and SCHULSINGER, F. (1974). The adopted-away offspring of schizophrenics. In *Genetics, environment and psychopathology* (ed. S. A. Mednick, F. Schulsinger, H. Higgins, and B. Bell). Amsterdam: North-Holland/American Elsevier.

ROSS, E. (1973). Convulsive disorders in British children. *Proc. roy. Soc. Med.*, **66** (7), 703–4.

ROSVOLD, H. E., MIRSKY, A. F., SARASON, I., BRANSOME, E. D., and LLOYD, H. B. (1956). A continuous performance test of brain damage. *J. consult. Psychol.*, **20**, 343–50.

ROUMAN, J. (1956). School children's problems as related to parental factors *J. educ. Res.*, **50**, 105–12.

ROWBOTHAM, G. F., MacIVER, I. N., DICKSON, J., and BOUSFIELD, N. E. (1954). Analysis of 1400 cases of acute injury to the head. *Brit. Med. J.*, **1**, 726–30.

ROWNTREE, G. (1955). Early childhood in broken families. *Pop. Stud.*, **8**, 247.

ROZELLE, R. M. and CAMPBELL, D. T. (1969). More plausible rival hypotheses in the cross-lagged panel correlation technique. *Psychol. Bull.*, **71**, 74–80.

RUBIN, R. A., ROSENBLATT, C., and BARLOW, B. (1973). Psychological and educational sequelae of personality. *Pediat.*, **52**, 352–63.

RUDINGER, G. (1974) Eine

Querschnittuntersuchung im Altersbereich 20–90 Jahre. *J. Gerontol.*, **7**, 323–33.

—— (1976). Correlates of changes in cognitive functioning. In *Contributions to human development* (ed. H. Thomae), vol. 3, pp. 20–5. Basel: Karger.

RUPPEN, R., MUELLER, U., BAUMANN, U., and ANGST, J. (1973). Zur Prüfung der Aussagegenauigkeit bei einer Befragung uber Drogenkonsum. *Z. Praeventivmed*, **18**, 173–81.

RUSSELL, W. R. (1971). *The traumatic amnesias.* Oxford Neurological Monographs. London: Oxford University Press.

—— and SMITH, A. (1961). Post-traumatic amnesia in closed head injuries. *Arch. Neurol. (Chicago)*, **5**, 16–29.

RUTTER, M. (1965). Classification and categorization in child psychiatry. *J. Child psychol. Psychiat.*, **6**, 71–83.

—— (1966). *Children of sick parents: an environmental and psychiatric study.* Institute of Psychiatry Maudsley Monographs No. 16. London: Oxford University Press.

—— (1967). A children's behaviour questionnaire for completion by teachers: preliminary findings. *J. Child Psychol. Psychiat.*, **8**, 1–11.

—— (1969). Discussion of Lee Robins' paper: 'Follow-up studies of behavior disorders in children'. *WPA—RMPA Symposium of Psychiatric Epidemiology*, University of Aberdeen, July 1969.

—— (1970a). Autistic children: infancy to adulthood. *Sem. Psychiat.*, **2**, 435–50.

—— (1970b). Sex differences in children's responses to family stress. In *The child in his family* (ed E. J. Anthony and C. Koupernik). New York: Wiley.

—— (1970c). Follow-up studies investigating childhood disorders. Discussion. In *An international symposium on psychiatric epidemiology* (ed. E. H. Hare and J. K. Wing), pp. 69–86. London: Oxford University Press.

—— (1970d). Psychological development: predictions from infancy. *J. Child Psychol. Psychiat.*, **11**, 49–62.

—— (1971a). Parent–child separation: psychological effects on the children. *J. Child Psychol. Psychiat.*, **12**, 233–60.

—— (ed.) (1971b). *Infantile autism: concepts, characteristics and treatment.* Edinburgh: Churchill Livingstone.

—— (1972a). Relationships between child and adult psychiatric disorder. *Acta Psychiat. Scand.*, **48**, 3–21.

—— (1972b). *Maternal deprivation reassessed.* Harmondsworth: Penguin.

—— (1974). The development of infantile autism. *Psychol. Med.*, **4**, 147–63.

—— (1977a). Prospective studies to investigate behavioral change. In *The origins and course of psychopathology* (ed. J. S. Strauss, H. M. Babigian, and M. Roff). New York: Plenum.

—— (1977b). Brain damage syndromes in childhood: concepts and findings. *J. Child Psychol. Psychiat.*, **18**, 1–21.

—— (1977c). Surveys to answer questions. In *Epidemiological approaches in child psychiatry* (ed. P. J. Graham). London: Academic Press.

—— (1977d), Individual differences. In *Child psychiatry: modern approaches* (ed. M. Rutter and L. Hersov). Oxford: Blackwell Scientific.

—— (1978a). Language disorder and infantile autism. In *Autism: a reappraisal of concepts and treatment* (ed. M. Rutter and E. Schopler). New York: Plenum.

—— (1978b). Diagnosis and definition. In *Autism: a reappraisal of concepts and treatment* (ed. M. Rutter and E. Schopler). New York: Plenum.

—— (1978c). Diagnostic validity in child psychiatry. In *Adv. biol. Psychiat.*, **2**, 2–22. Basel: Karger.

—— (1978d). Family, area and school influences in the genesis of conduct disorders. In *Aggression and antisocial behaviour in childhood and adolescence* (ed. L. Hersov, M. Berger, and D. Shaffer). JCPP Monograph Series No. 1. Oxford: Pergamon.

—— (1978e). Early sources of security and competence. In *Human growth and development* (ed. J. S. Bruner and A. Garton). London: Oxford University Press.

—— (1979a). Protective factors in children's responses to stress and disadvantage. In *Primary prevention of psychopathology III: social competence in children* (ed. M. W. Kent and J. E. Rolf). Hanover, N. H.: University Press of New England.

—— (1979b). Autism: psychopathological mechanisms and therapeutic approaches. In *Cognitive growth and development—Essays in honor of Herbert G. Birch* (ed. M. Bortner). New York: Brunner/Mazel.

—— (1979c). *Changing youth in a changing society: patterns of adolescent development and disorder.* London: Nuffield Provincial Hospitals Trust. Cambridge, Mass.: Harvard University Press (1980).

—— and BARTAK, L. (1973). Special educational treatment of autistic children: a comparative study. II. Follow-up findings and implications for services. *J. Child Psychol. Psychiat.*, **14**, 241–70.

—— and BROWN, G. W. (1966). The reliability and validity of measures of family life and relationships in families containing a psychiatric patient. *Soc. Psychiat.*, **1**, 38–53.

——, CHADWICK, O., SHAFFER, D., and BROWN, G. (1980). A prospective study of children with head injuries. I. Design and methods. (Submitted for publication.)

—— and COX. A. (1977). *The assessment of diagnostic interviewing techniques in child psychiatry.* Final report to the Social Science Research Council, London.

——, ——, TUPLING, C., BERGER, M., and YULE, W. (1975a). Attainment and adjustment in two geographical areas. I. The prevalence of psychiatric disorder. *Brit. J. psychiat.*, **126**, 493–509.

—— and GRAHAM, P. (1968). The reliability and validity of the psychiatric assessment of the child: I. Interview with the child. *Brit. J. Psychiat.*, **114**, 563–79.

——, ——, CHADWICK, O. F. D., and YULE, W. (1976b). Adolescent turmoil: fact or fiction? *J. Child Psychol. Psychiat.*, **17**, 35–56.

——, ——, and YULE, W. (1970a). *A neuropsychiatric study in childhood.* Clinics in Developmental Medicine 35/36. London: Heinemann Medical/SIMP.

——, GREENFELD, D., and LOCKYER, L. (1967). A five to fifteen year follow-up study of infantile psychosis. II. Social and behavioural outcome. *Brit. J. Psychiat.*, **113**, 1183–99.

—— and LOCKYER, L. (1967). A five to fifteen year follow-up of infantile psychosis. I. Description of sample. *Brit. J. Psychiat.*, **113**, 1169–82.

—— and MADGE, N. (1976). *Cycles of disadvantage: a review of research.* London: Heinemann.

——, MAUGHAN, B., MORTIMORE, P., OUSTON, J., with SMITH, A. (1979) *Fifteen thousand hours: secondary schools and their effects on children.* London: Open Books. Cambridge, Mass.: Harvard University Press

—— and QUINTON, D. (1977). Psychiatric disorder: ecological factors and concepts of causation. In *Ecological factors in human development* (ed. H. McGurk). Amsterdam: North Holland.

——, TIZARD, J., and WHITMORE, K. (eds.) (1970b). *Education, health and behaviour.* London: Longmans.

——, ——, YULE, W., GRAHAM, P., and WHITMORE, K. (1976a). Research report: Isle of Wight studies, 1964–1974. *Psychol. Med.*, **6**, 313–32.

——, YULE, B., QUINTON, D., ROWLANDS, O., YULE, W., and BERGER, M. (1975b). Attainment and adjustment in two geographical areas. III. Some factors accounting for area differences. *Brit. J. Psychiat.*, **126**, 520–33.

—— and YULE, W. (1973). Specific reading retardation. In *The first review of special education* (ed. L. Mann and D. Sabatino). Philadelphia: Buttonwood Farms.

—— and —— (1975). The concept of specific reading retardation. *J. Child Psychol. Psychiat.*, **16**, 181–97.

——, BERGER, M., and HERSOV, L. (1977). The evaluation of a behavioural approach to the treatment of autistic children. Final Report to the Department of Health and Social Security, London.

——, and GRAHAM, P. (1973). Enuresis and behavioural deviance: some epidemiological considerations. In *Bladder control and enuresis* (ed. I. Kolvin, R. MacKeith, and S. R. Meadows). Clinics in Developmental Medicine Nos. 48/49. London: Heinemann/SIMP.

SAMEROFF, A. J. and CHANDLER, M. J. (1975). Reproductive risk and the continuum of caretaking casualty. In *Review of child development research* (ed. F. D. Horowitz) (vol. 4). London: University of Chicago Press.

SAMPHIER, M. L. (1975). A method of translating binary punched Hollerith cards to computer data files. *Int. J. Bio-med. Comput.*, **6**, 61–3.

SAND, E. A. (1966). Contribution à l'étude du développement de l'enfant. Aspects médico-sociaux et psychologiques. Thèse présentée en vue de l'obtention du grade légal d'Agrégé de l'Enseignement Supérieur. Université Libre de Bruxelles, Laboratoire de Médecine Sociale. Les Editions de l'Institut de Scoiologie de l'Université Libre de Bruxelles.

SARNA, S. (1977). Zygosity diagnosis in epidemiological twin studies by blood markers and by questionnaire. Thesis, University of Helsinki.

——, KAPRIO, J., SISTONEN, P., and KOSKENVUO, M. (1978). The diagnosis of twin zygosity by mailed questionnaire. *Human Heredity*, **28**, 241–54.

——, KOSKENVUO, M., KAPRIO, J., RANTASALO, I. (1976). *Data processing procedures of the*

Finnish Twin Register: compilation and mailing. Department of Public Health Science, University of Helsinki.

SASAKI, T. T. (1960). *Fruitland, New Mexico: a Navaho community in transition.* Ithaca, New York: Cornell University Press.

SAVIOZ, E. (1968). *Die Anfaenge der Geschwisterbeziehung.* Verhaltensbeobachtung in Zweikinderfamilien. Berne: Huber.

SAXEN, L. and RAPOLA, J. (1969). *Congenital defects.* New York: Holt, Rinehart and Winston.

SCHACHTER, F. F. and APGAR, V. (1959). Perinatal asphyxia and psychological signs of brain damage in childhood. *Pediat.,* 24, 1016–25.

SCHADENDORF, B. (1958). *Zur Entwicklung von aktiven Kindern im Grundschulalter.* Diploma Thesis, Univ. Erlangen.

—— (1960). Verlaufsformen hoher Anregbarkeitsvarianten. Diploma Thesis, Bonn.

—— (1964). Uneheliche Kinder. Untersuchungen zu ihrer Entwicklung und Situation in der Grundschule [Studies on the development of illegitimate children of elementary school age]. *Wissenschaftliche Jugendkunde,* vol. 7. Munich: J. A. Barth.

SCHAIE, K. W. (1965). A general model for the study of developmental problems. *Psychol. Bull.,* 64, 92–107.

—— and LABOUVIE-VIEF, G. (1974). Generation versus ontogenetic components of change in adult cognitive behaviour: a fourteen-year cross-sequential study. *Develop. Psychol.,* 10, 305–20.

SCHÄPPI-FREULER, S. (1976). *Zur Entwicklung fruehkindlicher Aengste.* (Dissertation, Zurich). Zurich: Juris Druck und Verlag.

SCHARFETTER, C. (1970). On the hereditary aspects of symbiotic psychoses—a contribution towards the understanding of the schizophrenia-like psychoses. *Psychiat. Clin.,* 3, 145–52.

—— (ed.) (1972). *AMP-System Manual* (2nd edn.). Berlin: Springer.

——, MOERBT, H., and WING, J. (1976). Diagnosis of functional psychoses. *Arch. Psychiat. Nervenheilk.,* 222, 47–60.

SCHMIDT, D. W. (1972). *Analysis of alcohol consumption data. The use of consumption data for research purposes,* pp. 57–66. Report on conference on epidemiology of drug dependence. London (WHO).

SCHMIDT, M. (1965). Somatische und psychische Faktoren der Reifentwicklung. *Wissenschaftliche Jugendkunde,* vol. 9. Munich: Barth.

SCHMIDT, W. and DE LINT, J. (1972). Causes of death of alcoholics. *Quart. J. Stud. Alc.,* 33, 171–85.

SCHMITZ-SCHERZER, R., THOMAE, H., ANGLEITNER, A., BIERHOFF, H. W., GROMBACH, H., RUDINGER, G., and STEFFENS K. H. (1974). *Altenhilfe 2. Berichte der landesregierung von NRW,* pp. 81–105. Düsseldorf: Ministerium für Arbeit und Gesundheit.

SCHOFIELD, W. and BALIAN, L. (1959). A comparative study of the personal histories of schizophrenics and non-psychiatric patients. *J. abnorm. soc. Psychol.,* 59, 216–25.

SCHOLZ, E. (1963). Dynamik des Wachstums [Dynamics of growth]. *Wissenschaftliche Jugendkunde.* Munich: Barth.

The school study—a code book (1975). *Project Metropolitan research report series,* no. 3.

SCHREINER, A. (1963). Auswirkungen mütterlicher Erwerbstätigkeit auf die Entwicklung von Grundschülern. [Effects of mother's work on the development of children]. *Arch. Gesam. Psychol.,* 115, 334–61.

SCHUHAM, A. I. (1967). The double-blind hypothesis a decade later. *Psychol. Bull.,* 68, 409–16.

SCHWAB, J. J., McGINNIS, N. H., and WARHEIT, G. J. (1973). Social change, culture change and mental health. In *Proceedings of the V World Congress of Psychiatry* (Excerpta Medica International Congress Series No. 274), pp. 703–9. New York: American Elsevier.

SCHWARZ, K. (1974). Voraussichtliche Entwicklung der Zahl älterer Menschen und ihrer Lebenserwartung. In *Schwerpunkte in der geriatrie* (ed. R. Schuber and A. Störmer), vol. 3, pp. 17–9. Werk Verlag.

SCHULSINGER, F. (1972). Psychopathy: heredity and environment. *Int. J. ment. Hlth,* 1, 190–206.

—— (1974). Psychopathy: heredity and environment. In *Genetics, environment and psychopathology* (ed. S. A. Mednick, F. Schulsinger, H. Higgins, and B. Bell). Amsterdam: North-Holland/American Elsevier.

—— (1977). *Nogle undersøgelser til belysning af sammenhaeng mellem arv og miljø i psykiatrien. Disputats.* Copenhagen: FADL's forlag. [In Danish].

—— and JACOBSEN, B. (1975). The heredity–environment issue in psychiatry. Perspectives from research at the Psykologisk Institut, Department of Psychiatry, Kommunehospitalet. *Acta Psychiat. Scand. Suppl.* 261, 44–58.

——, MEDNICK, S. A., VENABLES, P. H., RAMAN, A. C., and BELL, B. (1975). Early detection and prevention of mental illness: the Mauritius Project. *Neuropsychobiol.,* 1, 166–79.

SCHULSINGER, H. (1976). A ten year follow-up of children of schizophrenic mothers: clinical assessment. *Acta Psychiat. Scand.,* 53, 371–86.

SCOTT, E. M. and NISBET, J. D. (1954). Intelligence and family size in an adult sample. *Eugen. Rev.,* 46, 233–5.

SEARS, R. R., MACCOBY, E. E., and LEVIN, H. (1957). *Patterns of child rearing.* Evanston, Ill.: Row, Peterson.

SEGLOW, J., PRINGLE, M. L., and WEDGE, P. J. (1972). *Growing up adopted.* Slough: National Foundation for Educational Research.

SEIDEL, U., CHADWICK, O., and RUTTER, M. (1975). Psychological disorders in crippled children. A comparative study of children with and without brain damage. *Develop. Med. Child Neurol.,* 17, 563–73.

SELYE, H. (1956). *The stress of life.* New York: McGraw-Hill.

SEWELL, W. H. and MUSSEN, P. H. (1952). The effects of feeding, weaning, and scheduling procedures on childhood adjustments. *Child Develop.,* 23.

SHAFFER, D., CHADWICK, O., and RUTTER, M. (1975). Psychiatric outcome of localised head injury in children. In *Outcome of severe damage to the central nervous system* (ed. R. Porter and D. W. FitzSimons), pp.

191–213. Amsterdam: CIBA Foundation Symposium No. 34.

SHAPIRO, R. W. (1970) *A twin study of non-endogenous depression.* Copenhagen: Munksgaard.

SHEPHERD, M., COOPER, B., BROWN, A. C., and KALTON, G. W. (1966). *Psychiatric illness in general practice.* London: Oxford University Press.

——, OPPENHEIM, B., and MITCHELL, S. (1971). *Childhood behaviour and mental health.* London: University of London Press.

——, ——, and —— (1973). *Auffälliges Verhalten bei Kindern.* Göttingen: Vandenhoeck and Ruprecht.

SHEPS, M. C. (1958). Shall we count the living or the dead? *New Engl. J. Med.,* 259, 1210–14.

SHERIDAN, M. D. (1972). Reported incidence of hearing loss in children of seven years. *Develop. Med. Child Neurol.,* 14(3), 296–303.

—— (1973). Children of seven years with marked speech defects. *Brit. J. Disord. Commun.,* 8(1), 9–16.

—— and PECKHAM, C. (1975). Follow-up at eleven years of children who had marked speech defects at 7 years. *Child: Care, Hlth Develop.,* 1(3), 157–66.

—— and —— (1978). A follow-up to 16-years of school children who had marked speech defects at seven years. *Child:Care, Hlth Develop.,* 6, 3.

SHIELDS, J. and DUNCAN, J. (1964). *The state of crime in Scotland.* London: Tavistock.

——, HESTON, L. L., and GOTTESMAN, I. I. (1975). Schizophrenia and the schizoid: the problem for genetic analysis. In *Genetic research in psychiatry* (ed. R. R. Fieve, D. Rosenthal, and H. Brill), pp. 167–98. Baltimore: Johns Hopkins Press.

—— and SLATER, E. (1956). An investigation into the children of cousins. *Acta Genet. Statist. Med.,* 6, 60–79.

SHURE, M. B. and SPIVACK, G. (1978). Interpersonal problem-solving thinking and adjustment in the mother–child dyad. In *Primary prevention of psychopathology* (ed. M. W. Kent and J. E. Rolf), vol. 3. Hanover, N. H.: University Press of New England. In press.

SIDDLE, D. A. T. (1977). Electrodermal activity and psychopathy. In *Biosocial bases of criminal behavior* (ed. S. A. Mednick and K. O. Christiansen), pp. 199–212. New York: Gardner Press.

SIEGEL, S. (1956). *Nonparametric statistics.* New York: McGraw-Hill.

SIGURÐSSON, J. F. and ÓSKARSSON, Th. (1976). Brottfall nemanda úr Skólakerfinu með Tilliti til Félags-Uppeldis- og Sálfræðilegra Breyta [School-drop-out and its relationship to social, educational and psychological variables]. Unpublished B.A. thesis. Psychological Department, University of Iceland.

SILLANPÄÄ, M. (1973). Medico-social prognosis of children with epilepsy. Epidemiological study and analysis of 245 patients. *Acta Paediat. Scand.* (Suppl. 237).

SILVERMAN, J. (1964). Scanning-control mechanism and cognitive filtering in paranoid and nonparanoid schizophrenia. *J. consult. Psychol.,* 28, 385–93.

——, BERG, P. S., and KANTOR, R. (1966). Some perceptual correlates of institutionalization. *J. nerv. ment. Dis.*, **141**, 651–7.

SIMON, N. (1954), Spurious correlational analysis. *J. Amer. statist. Assoc.*

SINGER, H., GERARD, H. B., and REDFEARN, D. J. (1975). Achievement. In *School desegregation* (ed. H. B. Gerard and N. Miller). New York: Plenum Press.

SJÖBRING, H. (1973). Personality structure and development. A model and its application. *Acta Psychiat. Scand.* Suppl. 244.

SLATER, E. (1965). Diagnosis of hysteria. *Brit. med. J.*, **1**, 1395–9.

SLOTKIN, J. S. (1960). *From field to factory: new industrial employees.* Glencoe, Illinois: Free Press.

SMITH-MEYER, H., VALEN, H. A., FLEKKØY, K., FLØISTAD, I., HAASETH, K., and ASTRUP, C. (1976). Psychophysiological studies of a geographically defined area. *Activ. nervos superior*, **18**, 145–56.

SMULDERS, F. J. H. (1963). *Stutsman Intelligentietest voor kleuters. Nederlandse bewerking van Mental measurement of preschool children van R. Stutsman.* Nijmegen: Berkhout.

SNIJDERS, C. J. (1971). On the form of the human thoracolumbar spine and some aspects of its mechanical behaviour. Voorschoten: VAM.

SOBEL, D. E. (1961). Children of schizophrenic patients. Preliminary observations on early development. *Amer. J. Psychiat.*, **118**, 512–7.

ŠOBOVÁ, A. (1959). *Growth and development of children up to three years.* Materialy i prace antropologiczne. [In Polish]. Wroclaw: Polish Academy of Sciences.

Social Science Research Council (1975). *Longitudinal studies: report of an SSRC working party.* London: SSRC.

SOROKIN, P. A. (1957). *The crisis of our age: the social and cultural outlook.* New York: E. P. Dutton.

SOUTHGATE, V. (1962). *Southgate Group Reading Tests: manual of instructions.* London: University of London Press.

SPECK, O. (1956). *Kinder erwerbstätiger Mütter.* Stuttgart: Enke.

SPIETH, W. (1964). Cardiovascular health status, age, and psychological performance. *J. Gerontol.*, **19**.

SPIVACK, G., PLATT, J. J., and SHURE, M. B. (1976). *The problem solving approach to adjustment.* San Francisco: Jossey-Bass.

—— and SWIFT, M. (1972). *The Hahnemann High School Behavior Rating Scale (HHSB).* Philadelphia: Hahnemann Medical College and Hospital.

SPREEN, O. and GADDES, W. H. (1969). Developmental norms for 15 neuropsychological tests age 6 to 15. *Cortex*, **5**, 170–91.

SROLE, L., LANGNER, T. S., MICHAEL, S. T., OPLER, M. K., and RENNIE, T. A. C. (1962). *Mental health in the metropolis—The midtown Manhattan study,* Vol. 1. New York: McGraw Hill.

STANINCOVÁ, V. and DITTRICHOVÁ, J. (1964). [The development of infants with a low-birth weight up to the age of three years.] (In Czech.) Hálkova sb. 5, Praha SZdN.

STARFIELD, S. B. (1967). Functional bladder capacity in enuretic and non-enuretic children. *J. Paediat.*, **70**, 777–81.

STATTIN, H. (1979). Ungdomsbrottslighet och relativ prestationsutveckling i skolan : en longitudinell analys. (Juvenile delinquency and changes in relative achievement: a longitudinal perspective). Report from the Department of Psychology, University of Stockholm: Utbildningsförlaget. (English summary).

STECHLER, G. A. (1964). A longitudinal follow-up of neonatal apnea. *Child Develop.*, **35**, 333–48.

STEEGE, F. W. (1966). Untersuchungen zur motirischen Entwicklung 6–14 Jähriger Kinder. Phil. Diss., Bonn.

STEFANSSON, J. G. and HELGASON, T. (1969). First admissions to Kleppsspítalinn 1953–1957. Ten-year outcome survey. Presented at a meeting of the Reykjavík Medical Society.

——, MESSINA, J. A., and MEYEROWITZ, S. (1976). Hysterical neurosis, conversion type: clinical and epidemiological considerations. *Acta Psychiat. Scand.*, **53**, 119–38.

STEINDÓRSSON, B., JÓHANNSDÓTTIR, G., EINARSDÓTTIR, M., ERLINGSSON, O., and MAGNÚSSON, T. (1975). Afbrot Reykvískra unglinga [Juvenile delinquency in Reykjavík] Unpublished B.A. thesis. Department of Psychology, University of Iceland.

ŠTEMBERA, Z., ZEZULÁKOVÁ, J. and DITTRICHOVÁ, J. (1975). Comparison of some factors of risk pregnancy as to their influence on perinatal mortality and morbidity. *Čs. Gynek.*, **40**, 6, 401–6.

——, —— and ZNAMENÁČEK, K. (1972). [Evaluation of the importance of individual factors of risk pregnancy.] (In Czech.) *Čs. Gynek.*, **37**, 193.

STERN, C. (1973). *Principles of human genetics* (3rd edn). San Francisco: W. H. Freeman and Co.

STERN, S., MEDNICK, S. A., and SCHULSINGER, F. (1974). Social class, institutionalization and schizophrenia. In *Genetics, environment and psychopathology* (ed. S. A. Mednick, F. Schulsinger, J. Higgins, and B. Bell), pp. 283–91. Amsterdam: Elsevier-North Holland.

STEWART, A. L. (1977). The survival of low birth weight infants. *Brit. J. hosp. Med.*, **18**, 182–90.

STEWART, D. B. and BERNARD, R. M. (1954). A clinical classification of difficult labour and some examples of its use. *J. Obstet. Gynaecol. Brit. Emp.*, **61**, 318–28.

STONE, A. A. and ONQUÉ, G. C. (1959). *Longitudinal studies of child personality.* Cambridge, Mass.: Harvard University Press.

STONE, J. L. and NORRIS, A. H. (1966). Activities and attitudes of participants in the Baltimore longitudinal study. *J. Gerontol.*, **21**, 575–80.

STOTT, D. H. (1958). Some psychosomatic aspects of casualty in reproduction. *J. psychosom. Res.*, **3**, 42–55.

—— (1963). *The social adjustment of children: manual to the British Social Adjustment Guides* (2nd edn). London: University of London Press.

—— (1966). A general test of motor impairment for children. *Develop. Med. Child Neurol.*, **8**, 523–31.

STRAUSS, J. S., BABIGIAN, H. M., and ROFF, M. (eds.) (1977). *The origins and course of psychopathology.* New York: Plenum.

—— and CARPENTER, W. T. (1972). The prediction of outcome in schizophrenia. I. Characteristics of outcome. *Arch. Gen. Psychiat.*, **27**, 739–46.

—— and —— (1974a). Prediction of outcome: II. Relationships between predictor and outcome variables. *Arch. gen. Psychiat.*, **31**, 37–42.

—— and —— (1974b). The evaluation of outcome in schizophrenia. In *Life history studies in psychopathology* (ed. A. Thomas, M. Roff, and D. Ricks), vol. 3. Minneapolis: University of Minnesota Press.

STRAUSS, R. and WINTERBOTTOM, M. T. (1949). Drinking patterns of an occupational group: domestic servants. *Quart. J. Stud. Alc.*, **10**, 441–60.

STRICKMANN, R. (1957). *Untersuchungen zur Frage der Beziehungen von somatischer und psychischer Entwicklung.* Bonn: Bouvier.

STRÖMGREN, E. (1968). Contributions to psychiatric epidemiology and genetics. *Acta Jutland.*, **40**, 1–86.

STROOP, J. R. (1935). Studies of interference in serial verbal reactions. *J. Experiment. Psychol.*, **18**, 643–61.

STRUTT, G. F. and WATT, N. F. (1975). Primary prevention of adult psychological disorder through the school system. In *Proceedings of the Eighth Congress of the International Association for Psychiatry and Allied Professions* (ed. E. J. Anthony). Library of Congress, Washington D. C.

SUDNOW, D. (1965). Normal crimes—sociological features of the penal code. *Soc. Prob.*, **12**, 255–70.

SULLIVAN, C., GRANT, M. Q., and GRANT, J. D. (1957). The development of interpersonal maturity: applications to deliquency. *Psychiat.*, **20**, 373–85.

SUMMERS, T. (1970). Validity of alcoholics self-reported drinking history. *Quart. J. Stud. Alc.*, **31**, 972–4.

SUNDBY, H. S. and KREYBERG, P. C. (1968). *Prognosis in child psychiatry.* Baltimore: Williams and Wilkins.

SVALOSTOGA, K. (1959). *Prestige, class, and mobility.* Copenhagen: Gyldendal.

—— (1976). Analytic strategy in sequential research. *Project Metropolitan Research Report Series*, No. 6.

SWEETSER, F. L. (1968). Factorial ecology: Helsinki, 1960. *Demography*, **2**, 372–86.

TÄGERT, J. (1962). Entwicklungsverläufe bei antriebsstarken Kindern in der Anamnese. Dipl. Thesis, Bonn.

TAIT, C. D. and HODGES, E. F. (1962). *Delinquents, their families and the community.* Springfield, Ill.: Chas. C. Thomas.

TALLAND, G. A. (1965). *Deranged memory: a psychonomic study of the amnesia syndrome.* New York: Academic.

TANNER, J. M. (ed.) (1960). *Human growth.* London: Pergamon Press.

—— (1970). Physical growth. In *Carmichael's manual of child psychology* (ed. P. H. Mussen) (3rd edn.), pp. 77–155. New York: Wiley.

——, WHITEHOUSE, R. H., and TAKAISHI, M. (1966). Standards from birth to maturity for height, weight, height velocity, and weight velocity: British children 1965. *Arch. Dis. Childh.*, **41**, 454–71; 613–35.

——, ——, MARSHALL, W. A., HEALY, M. J. R., and GOLDSTEIN, H. (1975). *Assessment of skeletal maturity and prediction of adult height (TW2 method).* London: Academic Press.

TAVECCHIO, L. W. C., SPLINTER, P. G., KEMPER, H. C. G., RAS, J. G. A., SNEL, T., and

VERSCHUUR, R. (1976). Influence of physical education IV. Development and application of a physical education analysis system (PEIAS). *Proceedings of ICHPER*, Rotterdam, **18**, 375–82.

THIERY, M. (1969). Fetal and maternal lactate–pyruvate ratios. In *Fetal homeostasis* (ed. R. M. Wijnn), vol. 4, pp. 56–84. New York: Appleton-Century-Crofts.

THIESSEN, D. D. (1972). *Gene organization and behavior*. New York: Random House.

THOMAE, H. (1954). Der psychologische gesamteindruck. In *Deutsche nachkriegskinder* (ed. C. Coerper, W. Hagen, and H. Thomae), pp. 149–216. Stuttgart: Thieme.

—— (1957). Problems of character change. In *Perspectives in personality theory* (ed. H. P. David and H. V. Bracken), pp. 242–55. New York: Basic Books.

—— (1960a). Psychophysical relationships in personality development. In *Perspectives in personality research* (ed. H. P. David and I. C. Brengelmann), pp. 260–4. New York: Springer.

—— (1960b). Beziehungen zwischen Freizeitverhalten, sozialen Faktoren und Persönlichkeitsstruktur. *Psychol. Rundschau*, **11**, 151–9.

—— (1962). *Probleme der seelischen Reifung bei Jugendlichen in dieser Zeit*. Göthenburg: Vanderhoek.

—— (1963a). *Beobachtung und Beurteilung von Kindern und Jugendlichen* (Observation and assessment of children and juveniles). Basel: Karger.

—— (1963b). Persönlichkeitsmerkmale und soziale Merkmale von guten und schlechten Schülern. *Gawein Tidschr. Psychol.*, **12**, 60–75.

—— (1968a). *Das Individuum und seine Welt. Eine Persönlichkeitstheorie*. Göthenburg: Verlag für Psychologie.

—— (1968b). Psychische und soziale Aspekte des Alterns. *Z. Gerontol.*, **1**, 43–55.

—— (1969). Ansätze zu einer Theorie der Reifezeit. In *Vita Humana* (ed. H. Thomae). Frankfurt: M. Athenäum.

—— (1970). Theory of aging and cognitive theory of personality. *Human Develop.*, **13**, 1–16.

—— (1976). Patterns of 'successful' aging. In *Contributions to human development* (ed. H. Thomae), vol. 3, pp. 147–61. Basel: S. Karger.

THOMAS, A., CHESS, S., and BIRCH, H. (1968). *Temperament and behavior disorders in children*. New York: New York University Press.

THOMPSON, B., and AITKEN-SWAN, J. (1973). Pregnancy outcome and fertility control in Aberdeen. *Brit. J. prev. soc. Med.*, **27** (3), 137–45.

—— and ILLSLEY, R. (1969). Family growth in Aberdeen. *J. biosoc. Sci.*, **1**, 23–9.

THOMSON, A. M., CHUN, D., and BAIRD, D. (1963). Perinatal mortality in Hong Kong and in Aberdeen, Scotland. *J. Obstet. Gynaecol. Brit. Commonwlth*, **70**, 871–7.

THORN, I. (1968). *Cerebral symptoms in the newborn*. Copenhagen: Munksgård.

THORSTEINSSON, G. A. (1974). Inläggningar och vårdtider på det psykiatriska sjukhuset i Reykjavík, Kleppsspítalinn, 1951–1970. *Nord. Psykiat. Tidskr.*, **28**, 14–22.

THURSTON, J. R. and MUSSEN, P. H. (1951).

Infant feeding gratification and adult personality. *J. Personal.*, **19**, 449–58.

TIBBENHAM, A., ESSEN, J., and FOGELMAN, K. (1978a). Ability-grouping and school characteristics. *Brit. J. ed. Stud.*, **26**, 1.

——, PECKHAM, C. S., and GARDINER P. A. (1978b). Vision screening in children tested at 7, 11 and 16 years. *Brit. med. J.*, **1**, 1312–4.

TIZARD, B. (1977). *Adoption: a second chance*. London: Open Books.

—— and HODGES, J. (1978). The effect of early institutional rearing on the development of eight-year-old children. *J. Child Psychol. Psychiat.*, **19**, 98–118.

TOMASSON, H. (1938). Further investigation on manic-depressive psychosis. *Acta Psychiat. Scand.*, **13**, 519–23.

TOMKINS, G. M., GELEHRTER, T. D., GRANNER, D., MARTIN, D., JR., SAMUELS, H. H., and THOMPSON, E. B. (1969). Control of specific gene expression in higher organisms. *Science*, **166**, 1474–80.

TORREY, E. F., HERSH, S. P., and McCABE, K. D. (1975). Early childhood psychosis and bleeding during pregnancy: a prospective study of gravid women and their offspring. *J. Autism Child. Schizophren.*, **5**, 287–98.

TOUWEN, B. C. L., and PRECHTL, H. F. R. (1970). *The neurological examination of the child with minor nervous dysfunction*. Philadelphia: Lippincott.

—— (1971). A study on the development of some motor phenomena in infancy. *Develop. Med. Child Neurol.*, **13**, 435–6.

TRUAX, C. B. and CARKHUFF, R. R. (1967). *Towards effective counseling and psychotherapy: training and practice*. Chicago: Aldine.

TSUANG, M. T. and WINOKUR, G. (1977). A combined thirty-five year follow-up and family study of schizophrenia and primary affective disorders: sample selection, methodology of field follow-up and preliminary mortality rates. In *The origins and course of psychopathology* (ed. J. S. Strauss, H. M. Babigian, and M. Roff). New York: Plenum.

TUUTERI, L., DONNER, M., EKLUND, J., LEISTI, L., RINNE, A.-L., SANDSTRÖM, G., and YLPPÖ, L. (1967). Incidence of cerebral palsy in Finland. *Ann. Paediat. Fenn.*, **13**, 41–5.

UHR, R. (1965). Verlaufsformen der Entwicklung bei Jugendlichen [Forms of development in adolescents]. Phil Diss. Thesis, Bonn.

——, THOMAE, H., and BECKER J. (1969). Entwicklungsverläufe im Kindes- und Jugendalter. *Z. Entwicklungspsychol. pädagog. Psycholog.*, **1**, 151–64.

VAILLANT, G. E. (1964). An historical review of the remitting schizophrenias. *J. nerv. ment. Dis.*, **138**, 48–56.

VANDENBERG, S. G. (ed.) (1968). *Progress in human behavior genetics. Recent reports on genetic syndromes, twin studies and statistical advances*. New York: Johns Hopkins Press.

VAN LIESHOUT, C. F. M. (1965). Auffällige Kinder im psychologischen Gesamteindruck. Thesis voor Candidaatsexamen, University Nijmegen.

VAN'T HOF, M. A., PRAHL-ANDERSEN, B., and KOWALSKI, C. J. (1976). A model for the study of developmental processes in dental research. J. Dent. Res., **55**(3), 359–66.

——, VELING, S. H. J., and KOWALSKI, C. J. (1977). Data processing problems for multidisciplinary mixed-longitudinal studies with application to the Nijmegen Growth Study. *Meth. Inf. Med.*, **16**(4), 210–5.

VENABLES, P. H., MEDNICK, S. A., SCHULSINGER, F., RAMAN, A. C., BELL, B., DALAIS, J. C., and FLETCHER, R. P. (1978). Screening for risk of mental illness. In *The nature of schizophrenia* (ed. L. C. Wynne, R. L. Cromwell, and S. Matthysse). New York: Wiley.

VILLUMSEN, A. L. (1970) *Environmental factors in congenital malformations*. Copenhagen: F.A.D.L.

VLACH, V. and ZEZULÁKOVÁ, J. (1976). Method of examining infants from high risk pregnancies. In *High risk pregnancy and child* (ed. Z Štembera, K. Znamenáček and K. Poláček). Hage: Martinus Nijnhoff.

WADDINGTON, C. H. (1957). *The strategy of the genes*. London: Allen and Unwin.

WADSWORTH, M. E. J. (1976). Delinquency, pulse rates and early emotional deprivation. *Brit. J. Criminol.*, **16**, 245–56.

—— (1979a). Early life events and later behavioural outcomes in a British longitudinal study. In *Human functioning in longitudinal perspective* (ed. S. B. Sells, R. Crandall, M. Roff, J. S. Strauss, and W. Pollin). Baltimore: Williams and Wilkins.

—— (1979b). *Roots of delinquency: infancy, adolescence, and crime*. Oxford: Martin Robertson.

WALKER, A. and LEWIS, P. (1977). Career advice and employment experiences of a small group of handicapped school-leavers. *Careers Quart.*, **29**, 5–14.

WALKER, R. N. (1975). Standards for somatotyping children. *Ann. Human Biol.*, **1**, 149–58.

WALL, W. D. and WILLIAMS, H. L. (1970). *Longitudinal studies and the social sciences*. London: Heinemann Educational.

WALLACE, A. F. C. (1961). *Culture and personality*. New York: Random House.

WALLINGA, J. V. (1956). Severe alcoholism in career military personnel. *U. S. Armed Forces Med. J.*, **7**, 551–61.

WALSH, B., and WALSH, D. (1970). Mental illness in the Republic of Ireland—first admissions. *J. Irish med. Assoc.*, **63**, 365–70.

WALSH, D. (1968). Hospitalised psychiatric morbidity in the Republic of Ireland. *Brit. J. Psychiat.*, **114**, 11–14.

WARNER, R. and ROSETT, H. (1975). The effects of drinking on offspring. *J. Stud. Alc.*, **36**(11), 1395–420.

Warnock Committee (1978). Report of the Committee of Enquiry into the Education of Handicapped Children and Young People. *Special educational needs*. London: HMSO.

WASSERMAN, M. S. (1975). 'Personality system, social system and cultural system influences on juvenile delinquency: a Tokyo birth cohort analysis'. Rutgers University, Ph.D. Dissertation.

WATSON, J. D. and CRICK, F. H. C. (1953). Genetic implications of the structure of deoxyribonucleic acid. *Nature*, **171**, 964–7.

WATT, N. F. (1978). Patterns of childhood social development in adult schizophrenics. *Arch. gen. Psychiat.*, **35**, 160–5.

—— and LUBENSKY, A. W. (1976). Childhood

roots of schizophrenia. *J. consult. clin. Psychol.*, **44**, 363–75.

——, STOLOROW, R. D., LUBENSKY, A. W., and McCLELLAND, D. C. (1970). School adjustment and social behavior of children hospitalized for schizophrenia as adults. *Amer. J. Orthopsychiat.*, **40**, 637–57.

WECHSLER, D. (1944). *The measurement of adult intelligence.* Baltimore, Maryland: Williams and Wilkins.

WECHSLER, D. (1945). A standardized memory scale for clinical use. *J. Psychol.*, **19**, 87.

—— (1949). *Wechsler Intelligence Scale for Children (manual).* New York: The Psychological Corporation.

WEDGE, P. J. and PETZING, J. (1970). Housing for children. *Housing Rev.*, **19**(6). 165–6.

—— and PROSSER, H. (1973). *Born to fail?.* London: Arrow Books in association with National Children's Bureau.

WEINBERG, W. (1920). Methodologische Gesichtspunkte für die statistische Untersuchung der Vererbung bei Dementia praecox. *Z. Gesamte Neurol. Psychiatrieorig.*, **59**, 39–50.

WEINER, J. S. and LOURIE, J. A. (eds) (1969). *IBP Handbook No. 9 Human Biology, a guide to field methods.* Oxford: Blackwell.

WEINTRAUB, S., NEALE, J. M., and LIEBERT, D. E. (1975). Teacher ratings of children vulnerable to psychopathology. *Amer. J. Orthopsychiat.*, **45**(3), 838–45.

WENDER, P. H. (1971). *Minimal brain dysfunction in children.* New York: Wiley.

——, ROSENTHAL, D., KETY, S. S., SCHULSINGER, F., and WELNER, J. (1974). Cross fostering: a research strategy for clarifying the role of genetic and experiential factors in the etiology of schizophrenia. *Arch. gen. Psychiat.*, **30**, 121–8.

WEST, D. J. (1963). *The habitual prisoner.* London: Heinemann.

—— (1969). *Present conduct and future delinquency.* London: Heinemann.

—— and FARRINGTON, D. P. (1973). *Who becomes delinquent?* London: Heinemann.

—— and —— (1977). *The delinquent way of life.* London: Heinemann.

WHITTAM, H., SIMON, G. B., and MITTLER, P. J. (1966). The early development of psychotic children and their sibs. *Develop. Med. Child Neurol.*, **8**, 552.

WILKINS, R. H. (1974). *The hidden alcoholic in general practice.* London: Elek.

WILLERMAN, L. (1973). Social aspects of minimal brain dysfunction. *Ann. N.Y. Acad. Sci.*, **205**, 164–72.

WILLIAM, R. H. and WIRTHS, C. G. (1965). *Lives through the years.* New York: Wiley.

WILSON, G. B. (1940). *Alcohol and the nation.* London: Nicholson and Watson.

WILSON, R. S. (1977). Twins and siblings: comparisons of developmental trends during infancy. Program, Behavior Genetics Association, Louisville, KY. April 27–30, 1977. (Abstract).

WINDLE, W. F. (1969). Brain damage by asphyxia at birth. *Sci. Amer.*, **221**, 76–84.

WINER, B. J. (1962). *Statistical principles of experimental design.* New York: McGraw-Hill.

WING, J. K. (1976). A technique for studying psychiatric morbidity in inpatient and outpatient series and general population samples. *Psychol. Med.*, **6**, 665–71.

——, BIRLEY, J. L. T., COOPER, J. E., GRAHAM, P., and ISAACS, I. D.(1967). Reliability of a procedure for measuring and classifying 'present psychiatric state'. *Brit. J. Psychiat.*, **113**, 499–515.

——, COOPER, J. E., and SARTORIUS, N. (1974). *The description and classification of psychiatric symptomatology. An introduction manual for the PSE and Catego system.* London: Cambridge University Press.

—— and HAILEY, A. M. (1972). *Evaluating a community psychiatric service. The Camberwell Register, 1964–71.* London: Oxford University Press.

WINICK, M. (1976). *Malnutrition and brain development.* New York: Oxford University Press.

WISEMAN, S. (1967) The Manchester Survey. In *Central Advisory Council for Education, Children and their Primary Schools, 2*, pp. 347–400. London: H.M.S.O.

WOERNER, M., POLLACK, M., and KLEIN, D. (1973). Pregnancy and birth complications of schizophrenic patients: a comparison of schizophrenic and personality disorder patients with their siblings. *Acta Psychiat. Scand.*, **49**, 712–21.

WOLFF, H. G. (1950). *Life stress and bodily disease.* Association for Research in Nervous and Mental Diseases, Proceedings (vol. 19). Baltimore: Williams and Wilkins.

WOLFGANG, M. E. (1973). Crime in a birth cohort. *Proc. Amer. phil. Soc.*, **117**, 404–11.

WOLKIND, S., HALL, F., and PAWLBY, S. (1977). Individual differences in mothering behaviour: a combined epidemiological and observational approach. In *Epidemiological approaches in child psychiatry* (ed. P. J. Graham). London: Academic Press.

——, KRUK, S., and CHAVES, L. P. (1976). Childhood separation experiences and psychosocial status in primiparous women: preliminary findings. *Brit. J. Psychiat.*, **128**, 391–6.

WOOD, M. M. and ELWOOD, P. C. (1966). Symptoms of iron deficiency anaemia: a community survey. *Brit. J. prev. soc. Med.*, **20**(3), 117–21.

WOOTON, B. (1959). *Social science and social pathology.* London: Allen and Unwin.

World Health Organization (1951). WHO Technical Report series, No. 42. (Report on the first session of the Alcoholism Subcommittee).

World Health Organization (1973). *International pilot study of schizophrenia,* vol. 1. (WHO Offset Publications No. 2). Geneva.

WRIGHT, S. (1934). The results of crosses between inbred strains of guinea pigs, differing in number of digits. *Genetics*, **19**, 537–51.

WYNNE, L. C., SINGER, M., and TOOHEY, M. L. (1976). Communication of the adoptive parents of schizophrenics. In *Schizophrenia 75: psychotherapy, family studies, research* (ed. J. Jøorstad and E. Ugelstad), pp. 412–51. Oslo: Universitetsforlaget.

YARROW, M. R., CAMPBELL, J. R., and BURTON, R. V. (1970). Recollections of childhood: a study of retrospective methods. *Monogr. Soc. Res. Child Develop.*, **35**(5).

YOLLES, S. and KRAMER, M. (1969). Vital statistics. In *The schizophrenic syndrome* (ed. L. Bellak and L. Loeb). New York: Grune and Stratton.

YULE, W. (1967). Predicting reading ages on Neale's Analysis of Reading Ability. *Brit. J. educ. Psychol.*, **37**, 252–5.

—— (1973). Differential prognosis of reading backwardness and specific reading retardation. *Brit. J. educ. Psychol.*, **43**, 244–8.

—— and RIGLEY, L. (1969). A four-year follow-up of severely backward readers into adolescence. In *Reading: influences and progress* (ed. M. Clark and S. Maxwell). Edinburgh: United Kingdom Reading Association.

ZACHAU-CHRISTIANSEN, B. (1972) *Development during the first year of life.* Helsingør: Paul A. Andersen.

—— and Ross., E. M. (1975). *Babies: human development during the first year.* New York: Wiley.

ZAZZO, R. (1960). *Les jumeaux, le couple et la personne.* Tomes I & II. Paris: Presses Universitaires de France.

ZEITLIN, H. (1972). A study of patients who attended the children's department and later the adults' department of the same psychiatric hospital. M. Phil. Dissertation, University of London.

ZERSSEN, D. v. (1973). Selbstbeurteilungsskalen zur abschätzung des subjektiven befundes in psychopathologischen querschnitts- und längsschnittuntersuchungen. *Arch. Psychiat. Nervenheilk.*, **217**, 299–314.

——, KOELLER, D.-M., and REY, E.-R. (1969). Objektivierende Untersuchung zur prämorbiden Persönlichkeit endogen depressiver (Methodik und vorläufige Ergebnisse). In *Das Depressive Syndrom* (ed. H. Hippius and H. Selbach), pp. 183–205. Munich: Urban and Schwarzenberg.

——, ——, and —— (1970). Die prämorbide Persönlichkeit von endogen Depressiven. *Confin. Psychiat.*, **13**, 156–79.

Zetland Constabulary Chief Constable's (Annual) Report (1963–8). Lerwick, Shetland.

Zetland County Council (1973). *Interim county development plan.* County Development Office, March 1973.

ZETTERGREN, P. (1979). Utstötthet och isolering i ett flerårigt perspektiv. (Social rejection and isolation in a longitudinal perspective). Report from the Department of Psychology, University of Stockholm, No. 31.

—— (1980). Den sociala situationens betydelse för utstötta och isolerade barns utveckling. (The role of the social situation for the development of rejected and isolated children). Report from the Department of Psychology, University of Stockholm, No. 33.

ZEZULÁKOVÁ, J. (1974). *Infants of diabetic mothers—development and relationship to pre- and postnatal risk factors.* Fourth European Congress of Perinatal Medicine, Prague.

ZIGLER, E. and PHILLIPS, L. (1962). Social competence and the process-reactive distinction in psychopathology. *J. abnorm. soc. Psychol.*, **64**, 215–22.

ZNAMENÁČEK, K. and JIRSOVÁ, V. (1956). [Neurological examination of the newborn with CNS trauma.] (In Czech.) *Čs. Pediat.*, **11**, 830.

ZONNEVELD, R. J. van. (1954).

Gezondhiedsproblemen bij bejaarden [Health problems of the aged]; with English summary and tables. Assen: Royal Van Gorcum.

—— (1961). *The health of the aged* (in English). (An investigation into the health and a number of social and psychological factors concerning 3149 aged persons in The Netherlands, carried out by 374 general practitioners, under the direction of the Organization for Health Research TNO). Assen: Royal Van Gorcum.

Further references on the long-term mental health programme of the WHO regional office for Europe

COOPER, J. E. (1979). *Crisis admission units and emerging psychiatric services.* Copenhagen: WHO Regional Office for Europe. *(Public health in Europe).*

WORLD HEALTH ORGANIZATION (1973). *Report on a conference on comprehensive psychiatric services and the community* (EURO 5414 I). Copenhagen: WHO Regional Office for Europe.

—— (1973). *Report on a conference on the epidemiology of drug dependence* (EURO 5436 IV). Copenhagen: WHO Regional Office for Europe.

—— (1973). *Report on a working group on psychiatry and primary medical care* (EURO 5427 I). Copenhagen: WHO Regional Office for Europe.

—— (1974). *Report on a symposium on major issues in juvenile delinquency* (EURO 5430 III). Copenhagen: WHO Regional Office for Europe.

—— (1978). *Report on a conference on the care of the mentally retarded in the community* (EURO 5440 I). Copenhagen: WHO Regional Office for Europe.

—— (1976). *Report on a conference on suicide and attempted suicide in young people* (ICP/MNH 015 III). Copenhagen: WHO Regional Office for Europe.

—— (1977). *Report on a working group on forensic psychiatry* (ICP/MNH 028 I). Copenhagen: WHO Regional Office for Europe.

—— (1976). *Report on a symposium on planning and organizaton of services for alcoholism and drug dependence* (ICP/MNH 024 IV). Copenhagen: WHO Regional Office for Europe.

—— (1977). *Report on a working group on cost-benefit analysis in mental health services* (ICP/MNH 006 II). Copenhagen: WHO Regional Office for Europe.

—— (1978). *Report on a working group on constraints in mental health services development* (ICP/MNH 030 II). Copenhagen: WHO Regional Office for Europe.

—— (1978). *Report on a working group on the future of mental hospitals* (ICP/MNH 019 II). Copenhagen: WHO Regional Office for Europe.

Additional Project Readings

Chapter 23

BLACKMORE, J. (1974). The relationship between self-reported delinquency and official convictions among adolescent boys. *Brit. J. Criminol.*, **14**, 172–6.

FARRINGTON, D. P. (1972). Delinquency begins at home. *New Society*, **21**, 495–7.

—— (1973). Self-reports of deviant behavior: predictive and stable? *J. crim. Law Criminol.*, **64**, 99–110.

—— (1976). Statistical prediction methods in criminology. Paper given at NATO Advanced Study Institute, Cambridge.

—— (1977). Young adult delinquents are socially deviant. *Justice of the Peace*, **141**, 92–5.

—— (1978). The family backgrounds of aggressive youths. In *Aggressive and anti-social behaviour in childhood and adolescence*, (ed. L. Hersov, M. Berger and D. Shaffer). Oxford: Pergamon.

—— (1979). Environmental stress, delinquent behaviour, and convictions. In *Stress and anxiety*, vol. 6 (ed. I. G. Sarason and C. D. Spielberger). Washington: Hemisphere.

—— (1980). Truancy, delinquency, the home and the school. In *Out of school: modern perspectives in truancy and school refusal* (ed. I. Berg and L Hersov). Chichester: Wiley.

——, GUNDRY, G. and WEST, D. J. (1975). The familial transmission of criminality. *Med. Sci. Law*, **15**, 177–86.

——, OSBORN, S. G., and WEST, D. J. (1978). The persistence of labelling effects. *Brit. J. Criminol.*, **18**, 277–84.

—— and WEST, D. J. (1970). Research into early signs of violent attitudes and behavior: seven measures of aggressive attitude and behavior among adolescent boys. Paper given at 4th National Conference on Research and Teaching in Criminology, Cambridge.

—— and —— (1971). A comparison between early delinquents and young aggressives. *Brit. J. Criminol.*, **11**, 341–58.

GIBSON, H. B. (1963). A slang vocabulary test as an indicator of delinquent association. *Brit. J. soc. clin. Psychol.*, **2**, 50–5.

—— (1964). A lie scale for the Junior Maudsley Personality Inventory. *Brit. J. educ. Psychol.*, **34**, 120–4.

—— (1964). The Spiral Maze: a psychomotor test with implications for the study of delinquency. *Brit. J. Psychol.*, **55**, 219–25.

—— (1965). A new personality test for boys. *Brit. J. educ. Psychol.*, **35**, 244–8.

—— (1966). The validation of a technique for measuring delinquent association by means of vocabulary. *Brit. J. Soc. clin. Psychol.*, **5**, 190–5.

—— (1967). Self-reported delinquency among schoolboys, and their attitudes to the police. *Brit. J. soc. clin. Psychol.*, **6**, 168–73.

—— (1967). Teachers' ratings of schoolboys' behavior related to patterns of scores on the New Junior Maudsley Inventory. *Brit. J. educ. Psychol.*, **37**, 347–55.

—— (1968). Self-reported delinquency: preliminary results of an on-going study. Paper given at 3rd National Conference on Research and Teaching in Criminology, Cambridge.

—— (1968). The measurement of parental attitudes and their relation to boys' behavior. *Brit. J. educ. Psychol.*, **38**, 233–9.

—— (1969). The Tapping Test: a novel form with implications for personality research. *J. clin. Psychol.*, **25**, 403–5.

—— (1969). The Gibson Spiral Maze Test: retest data in relation to behavioral disturbance, personality and physical measures. *Brit. J. Psychol.*, **60**, 523–8.

—— (1969). Early delinquency in relation to brokem homes. *J. Child Psychol. Psychiat.*, **10**, 195–204.

—— (1969). The significance of 'lie responses' in the prediction of early delinquency. *Brit. J. educ. Psychol.*, **39**, 284–90.

—— (1971). The factorial structure of juvenile delinquency: a study of self-reported acts. *Brit. J. soc. clin. Psychol.*, **10**, 1–9.

—— and HANSON, R. (1969). Peer ratings as predictors of school behavior and delinquency. *Brit. J. soc. clin. Psychol.*, **8**, 313–22.

——, ——, and WEST, D. J. (1967). A questionnaire measure of neuroticism using a shortened scale derived from the Cornell Medical Index. *Brit. J. soc. clin. Psychol.*, **6**, 129–36.

——, MORRISON, S., and WEST, D. J. (1970). The confession of known offences in response to a self-reported delinquency schedule. *Brit. J. Criminol.*, **10**, 277–80.

—— and WEST, D. J. (1964). Family patterns and juvenile delinquency. Paper given at 1st National Conference on Research and Teaching in Criminology, Cambridge.

—— and —— (1968). Some concomitants of early delinquency. Paper given at 3rd National Conference on Research and Teaching in Criminology, Cambridge.

—— and —— (1970). Social and intellectual handicaps as precursors of early delinquency. *Brit. J. Criminol.*, **10**, 21–32.

KNIGHT, B. J., OSBORN, S. G., and WEST, D. J. (1977). Early marriage and criminal tendency in males. *Brit. J. Criminol.*, **17**, 348–60.

—— and WEST, D. J. (1975). Temporary and continuing delinquency. *Brit. J. Criminol.*, **15**, 43–50.

—— and —— (1977). Criminality and welfare dependency in two generations. *Medicine, Science and the Law*, **17**, 64–7.

OSBORN, S. G. (1980). Moving home, leaving London and delinquent trends. *Brit. J. Criminol.*, **20**, 54–61.

—— and WEST, D. J. (1978). The effectiveness of various predictors of criminal careers. *J. Adol..*, **1**, 101–17.

—— and —— (1979). Conviction records of fathers and sons compared. *Brit. J. Criminol.*, **19** 120–33.

—— and —— (1979). Marriage and delinquency: a postscript. *Brit. J. Criminol.*, **19**, 254–6.

WEST, D. J. (1973). Are delinquents different? *New Society*, **26**, 456–8.

Chapter 26

BENGTSSON, C., BLOHMÉ, G., HALLBERG, L., HÄLLSTRÖM, T., ISAKSSON, B., KORSAN-BENGTSEN, K., RYBO, G., TIBBLIN, E., TIBBLIN, G., and WESTERBERG, H. (1973). The study of women in Gothenburg 1968–1969. A population study. *Acta med. scand.*, **193**, 311.

——, HALLBERG, L., HÄLLSTRÖM, T., HULTBORN, A., ISAKSSON,B., LENNARTSSON, J., LINDQUIST, O., LINDSTEDT, S., NOPPA, H., REDVALL, L., and SAMUELSSON, S. (1978). The population study of women in Göteborg 1974–1975. The second phase of a longitudinal study. General design, purpose and sampling results. *Scand. J. soc. Med.*, **6**, 49.

——, HÄLLSTRÖM, T., and TIBBLIN, G. (1973). Social factors, stress experience, and personality traits in women with ischaemic heart disease, compared to a population sample of women. *Acta med. scand.*, Suppl. 549, 82.

HÄLLSTRÖM, T. (1970). Depressions among women in Gothenburg. *Acta psychiat. scand.*, Suppl. 217, 25.

—— (1973). *Mental disorder and sexuality in the climacteric. A study in psychiatric epidemiology.* Göteborg: Scandinavian University books, Esselte Studium.

—— (1975). Mental disorder in women in Gothenburg. In *Tromsø seminar in medicine 1975 on social, somatic and psychiatric studies of geographically defined populations* (ed. C. Astrup), p. 217.

—— (1977). Sexuality in the climacteric. *Clin. Obstet. Gynaec.*, **4**, 227.

—— (1977). Life-weariness, suicidal thoughts and suicidal attempts among women in Gothenburg. *Acta psychiat. scand.*, **56**, 15.

—— (1979). Sexuality of women in middle age: the Göteborg study. *J. biosoc. Sci.*, Suppl. 6, 165.

Chapter 28

ZONNEVELD., R. J. van (in press). Les etudes epidemiologiques sur l'etat desante et les besoins sanitaires des personnes agees.

—— and BEEK, A. (1976). Examination of blood and circulatory tract in old age. Some data from a longitudinal study in the Netherlands. *Giorn. di Geront. (Italy)*, **24**, 718–23.

—— and —— (1977). Some biological values in transversal and longitudinal studies of old people. In *Proceedings of the Vth European symposium on basic research in gerontology (Weimar, DDR)*. Erlangen DDR: Verlag Straube.

Chapter 30

BINDER, J., SIEBER, M., and ANGST, J. (1979). Verzerrungen bei postalischen Befragungen: das Problem der Nichtantworter. *Zeitschr. exp. ang. Psychol.*, **26**(1), 53–71.

SIEBER, M. F. (1979). Social background, attitudes and personality in a three-year follow-up study of alcohol consumers. *Drug Alc. Dependence*, **4**, 407–17.

—— (1979). Zur Zuverlässigkeit von Eigenangaben bei einer Fragebogenuntersuchung. *Zeitschr. exp. ang. Psychol.*, **26**(1), 157–67.

—— (1979). Zur Erhöhung der Rücksendequote bei einer postalischen Befragung. *Zeitschr. exp. ang. Psychol.*, **26**(2), 334–40.

—— and ANGST, J. (1977). Zur Epidemiologie des Drogen-, Zigaretten- und Alkoholkonsums bei jungen Männern. *Schweiz. med. Wschr.*, **107**, 1912–20.

—— and —— (1979). Risikofaktoren für starkes Zigarettenrauchen bei jungen Männern. Eine Längsschnittuntersuchung. *Schweiz. med. Wschr.*, **109**, 115–22.

Chapter 34

ESSEN-MÖLLER, E. (1980). 25-jährige Verläufe einer ganzen Bevölkerungsgruppe ('Lundbyproject'). Symposium in Hamburg, June 9–10, 1978: *Psychiatrische Verlaufsforschung, Methoden und Ergebnisse*. Bern: Verlag Hans Huber, pp. 58–61.

—— Intrafamilial correlations in Sjöbring's dimensions of personality. *Acta psychiat. scand.*, in press.

——, HAGNELL, O. and ÖJESJÖ, L. Psychiatric morbidity through 25 years in a socially healthy population individually defined at the outset. *Acta psychiat. scand.*, in press.

HAGNELL, O. and RORSMAN, B. (1978). Suicide and endogenous depression with somatic symptoms in the Lundby Study. *Neuropsychobiology*, **4**, 180–7.

—— and —— (1978). Maskerad depression – en svar och viktig psykiatrisk diagnos i somatisk sjukvard. *Lakartidningen*, **75**, 779–80.

—— and —— (1979). Suicide in the Lundby study: a comparative investigation of clinical aspects. *Neuropsychobiology*, **5**, 61–73.

—— and ——. Suicide in the Lundby study: a controlled prospective investigation of stressful life events. Accepted for publication in *Neuropsychobiology*.

ÖJESJÖ, L. Prevalence of known and hidden alcoholism in the revisited Lundby population. *Soc. Psychiat.*, in press.

—— (1980). Alcoholism and labor, a comparison between occupation, class and employment. Paper presented at the 26th International Institute on the Prevention and Treatment of Alcoholism, ICAA, Cardiff, Wales, June 9–14, 1980.

—— (1980). What happened to the Lundby alcoholics? A prospective 15 year follow-up study of 96 Swedish men from a general population cohort. Paper presented at the 26th International Institute on the Prevention and Treatment of Alcoholism, ICAA, Cardiff, Wales, 9–14 June 1980.

——, HAGNELL, O., and LANKE, J. On the incidence of alcoholism among men by age and class. The Lundby study. In preparation.

Chapter 35

DE BORGGRAEF-RAUTS, F., EMERY-HAUZEUR, C., and SAND, E. A. (1976). Etude longitudinale du développement intellectuel de la naissance à 18 ans. (In press).

—— and SAND, E. A. (1971). Constance et inconstance du développement intellectuel. *Enfance*, **1–2**.

——, ——, SMETS, P. and ROBAYE, E. (1975). Evaluation des attitudes parentales selon le P.A.R.I. de Schaefer et Bell. *Enfance*, **1**.

EMERY-HAUZEUR, C. and SAND, E. A. (1974). Naissances désirées et non désirées. Etude descriptive. Association avec diverses variables sociales et biologiques. *Population Famille*, **31**(1), 1–26.

—— and WACHHOLDER, A. (1974). Les études longitudinales du développement de l'être humain. *Bull. Musée d'anthropol. Préhist. Monaco*, **19**, 125–45.

SAND, E. A. (1972). Symptômes de comportements d'enfants belges observés par leur mère. Stabilité de 3 à 9 ans. *Revue Neuropsychiat. infant.*, **20**, (3–4), 239–51.

—— (1972). Symptômes de comportement d'enfants belges observés par leur mère. Association entre symptômes (3 à 9 ans). *Revue Neuropsychiat. infant.*, **20**(3–4), 253–365.

—— (1972). Développement psycho-social de l'enfant normal. In *Pediatrie sociale* (ed. R. Mande, N. P. Masse, and M. Manciaux) 114–52. Paris: Flammarion.

—— (1978). Specialized mental health services for children and adolescents in France, Belgium and Frenchspeaking Switzerland. *Int. J. ment. Hlth*, **7**,(1–2), 75–89.

—— (1978). Uber Längsschnittstudien zur kindlichen Entwicklung. *Der Kinderarzt*, **7–9**(26), 895–7.

—— (1978). Effet de la structure familiale sur le développement psychologique de l'enfant. Santé et planification familiale. Recueil de textes publiés sous l'égide de Bureau Régional pour l'Europe de l'Organisation Mondiale de la Santé et du Centre International de l'Enfance. Paris, pp. 46–53.

—— (1979). Exposé d'introduction au travaux du Groupe de Réfexion: D'une pseudo-évidence à une formulation des problèmes. 'Facteurs psycho-sociaux et santé des enfants et des adolescents. In *Facteurs psycho-sociaux et santé* (ed. E. A. Sand and F. Baro). pp. 32–9, 119–22. Bruxelles: l'Université Libre de Bruxelles.

—— (1980). Faut-il favoriser la socialisation précoce du jeune enfant? *Cahiers Médicaux*, **5**, 861–2.

—— and EMERY-HAUZEUR, C. (1973). Prévalence de l'allaitemept maternel en Belgique. *Arch. françaises Pédiat.*, **30**, 363–80.

—— and —— (1973). Etude des comportements agressifs chez l'enfant entre trois et neuf ans. *Enfance*, **1–2**, 1–21.

—— and —— (1975). L'échec scolaire précoce. Variables associées – Prédictions. Collection *Recherche en education* (éd. Ministère de l'Education Nationale et dela Culture française). Bruxelles: Direction Générale de l'Organisation des Etudes.

—— and —— (1974). Quelques problèmes psycho-sociaux de la puberté et de l'adolescence chez la fille. *Compte-Rendu de la XIIème réunion des Equipes chargées des Etudes de la Croissance et du Développement*

de *l'Enfant normal*. Paris: Centre International de l'Enfance.

——, HAUZEUR, C. and DEBORGGRAEF-RAUTS, F. (1978). Etude des aspects psycho-sociaux du développement de l'enfant, de la naissance à 18 ans. Rapport sur l'analyse longitudinale des données du Centre d'Etude de la Croissance. Rapport présenté au Fonds de la Recherche Scientifique Médicale, Bruxelles.

WACHHOLDER, A. (1974). Etude de la puberté chez les filles. Association de paramètres somatiques et sociaux. *Compte-Rendu de la XIIème Réunion des Equipes chargées des Etudes de la croissance et du développement de l'enfant normal*. Paris: Centre International de l'Enfance.

—— and BEGHIN, D. (1974). La taille et le poids des écoliers et écolières du Cap Bon – Tunisie. Premières données. *Arch. l'Inst. Pasteur Tuni*, **51**, 201–10.

—— and —— (1975). La taille et le poids des écoliers et écolières du Cap Bon – Tunisie. *Bull. Soc. Belge Méd. trop.*, **55**(4), 341–58.

——, COLIN, F. C., and CANTRAINE, F. (1972). Etude de la croissance de la taille, du poid du périmètre céphalique et de la longueur du troisième métacarpien selon la méthode longitudinale mixte, des enfants de 1 mois à 10 ans, suivis au Centre d'Etude de la Croissance de Bruxelles. *Compte-Rendu de la XIème Réunion des Equipes chargées des études de la croissance et du développement de l'enfant, Londres*. Paris. Centre International de l'Enfance.

—— and GRAFFAR, M. (1973). *Courbes de croissance – en percentiles des mesures biométriques (poids, taille, périmètre céphalique) des enfants belges de 0 à 15 ans, garçons et filles*. Centre d'Etude de la Croissance de Bruxelles.

Chapter 38

KAPRIO, J., KOSKENVUO, M., and SARNA, S. (1977). The Finnish twin registry: a study of coronary heart disease in twins. *Cardiovasc. Dis. Epidemiol. Newsletter II*, 43 (abstract).

——, —— and —— (1978). The coronary heart disease study of the Finnish twin registry. *Cardiovasc. Dis. Epidemiol. Newsletter*, 25 (abstract).

—— and TEPPO, L. (1978). Basal cell carcinoma in identical twins. *Brit. med. J.*, **436**. (Letter to the editor.)

SARNA, S. (in press). Probabilities of concordance of twins with respect to genetic markers. *Acta Genet. Med. Gemellol.*

—— and KAPRIO, J. (in press). Dependency of concordance probability on gene frequencies in genetic systems for the diagnosis of twin zygosity. *Acta Genet. Med. Gemellol.*

—— and —— (in press). Optimization procedures in twin zygosity diagnosis by genetic markers. *Acta Genet. Med. Gemellol.*

—— and —— (1980). Use of multiple logistic analysis in twin zygosity diagnosis. *Human Heredity*, **30**, 71–80.

—— and —— (in press). Applicability of Selvin's Efficiency Measure in twin zygosity diagnosis by genetic systems. *Acta Genet. Med. Gemellol.*, **28**. (Letter to the editor.)

——, KOSKENVUO, M., KAPRIO, J., and RANTASALO, I. (1976). The data processing procedures of the Finnish twin register: compilation and mailing. Helsinki:

Publications of the Department of Public Health Science, M19.

SISTONEN, P. and ENHOLM, C. (in press). On the heritability of serum high density lipoprotein in twins. *Amer. J. hum. Genet.*

——, JOHNSSON, V., KOSKENVUO, M., and AHO, K. (In press). Serum IgE levels and allergy in twins. *Human Heredity.*

TEPPO, L., KAPRIO, J., KOSKENVUO, M., and PUKKALA, E. (1978). Risk of cancer among twins: record linkage between the Finnish twin registry and the Finnish cancer registry. Paper presented at the Symposium on Genetic Factors in Neoplastic Diseases of Man, 21 June 1978, Iceland.

Chapter 39

BRANDRUP, F., HAUGE, M., HENNINGSEN, K., and ERIKSEN, B. (1978). Psoriasis in an unselected series of twins. *Arch. Dermatol.*, **114**, 874–8.

FISCHER, M. (1971). Psychoses in the offspring of schizophrenic monozygotic twins and their normal co-twins. *Brit. J. Psychol.*, **118**, 43–52.

—— (1973). *Genetic and environmental factors in schizophrenia* Copenhagen: Munksgård.

HARVALD, B. and HAUGE, M. (1956). A catamnestic investigation of Danish twins. *Dan. med. Bull..*, **3**, 150–8.

—— and —— (1958). A catamnestic investigation of a Danish twin series. *Acta Genet.*, **8**, 287–94.

—— and —— (1963). Selection in diabetes in modern society. *Acta med. scand.*, **173**, 459–65.

—— and —— (1963). Heredity of cancer elucidated by a study of unselected twins. *J. Amer. med. Ass.*, **186**, 749–53.

—— and —— (1965). Hereditary factors elucidated by twin studies. In *Genetics and the epidemiology of chronic diseases* (ed. J. V. Neel, M. Shaw, and W. J. Schull) Washington: U.S. Department of Health, Education and Welfare.

—— and —— (1970). Coronary occlusion in twins. *Acta Genet. Med. Gemellol.*, **19**, 248–51.

—— and —— (1976). Diabetes in twins. *Nordic Council Arct. med. Res. Rep.*, **15**, 13–5.

HAUGE, M. and HARVALD, B. (1961). Malignant growths in twins. *Acta genet.*, **11**, 372–8.

——, —— and DEGNBOL, B. (1964). Hereditary factors in longevity. In *Age with a future* (ed. P. F. Hansen). Copenhagen: Munksgård.

JUEL-NIELSEN, N. and VIDEBECH, T. (1970). A twin study of suicide. *Acta Genet. Med. Gemellol.*, **19**, 307–11.

MØLLER, M., HORSMAN, A., HARVALD, B., HAUGE, M., HENNINGSEN, K. and NORDIN, B. E. C. (1978). Metacarpal morphometry in elderly twins. *Calcif. Tiss. Res.*, **25**, 197–201.

RAASCHOU-NIELSEN, E. (1960). Smoking habits in twins. *Dan. med. Bull.*, **7**, 82–8.

Chapter 67

LUTHI, R. and VUILLE, J.-C. (In press). Präventives Elterntraining. *Der Kinderarzt*, **11**.

VUILLE, J.-C. (1979). Prophylaktische Familienhilfe. In *Krise der Kleinfamilie?* (ed. M. Perrez). Bern: H. Huber.

Author Index

Subject Index